Developing Practical Adult Nursing Skills

Developing Practical Adult Nursing Skills

Third Edition

Edited by

Lesley Baillie RGN, ONC, BA(Hons), RNT, MSc(Nurs), PhD
Principal Lecturer (Clinical Skills Development)
London South Bank University
London, UK

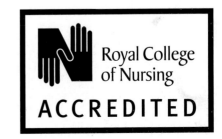

Royal College of Nursing
ACCREDITED

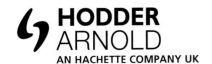

HODDER
ARNOLD
AN HACHETTE COMPANY UK

First published in Great Britain in 2001 by Arnold
Second edition 2005
This third edition published in 2009 by
Hodder Arnold, an imprint of Hodder Education, an Hachette UK Company
338 Euston Road, London NW1 3BH

http://www.hoddereducation.com

Hachette UK's policy is to use papers that are natural, renewable and recyclable products and
made from wood grown in sustainable forests. The logging and manufacturing processes are expected to
conform to the environmental regulations of the country of origin.

Whilst the advice and information in this book are believed to be true and accurate at the date of
going to press, neither the author[s] nor the publisher can accept any legal responsibility or liability
for any errors or omissions that may be made. In particular (but without limiting the generality of the
preceding disclaimer) every effort has been made to check drug dosages; however it is still possible that
errors have been missed. Furthermore, dosage schedules are constantly being revised and new side-effects
recognized. For these reasons the reader is strongly urged to consult the drug companies' printed
instructions before administering any of the drugs recommended in this book.

British Library Cataloguing in Publication Data
A catalogue record for this book is available from the British Library

Library of Congress Cataloging-in-Publication Data
A catalog record for this book is available from the Library of Congress

ISBN   978 0 340 974 209

2 3 4 5 6 7 8 9 10

Commissioning Editor:	Naomi Wilkinson
Project Editors:	Clare Patterson and Joanna Silman
Production Controller:	Rachel Manguel
Cover Designer:	Laura De Grasse

Typeset in 10/14 Minion Regular by MPS Limited, A Macmillan Company. (www.macmillansolutions.com)
Printed and bound in India

What do you think about this book? Or any other Hodder Arnold title?
Please visit our website: www.hoddereducation.com

CONTENTS

This book has a companion website available at: http://www.hodderplus.co.uk/adultnursingskills
To access the interactive MCQs, PowerPoint slides and image bank included on the website, please register on the website using the following access details:

Serial number : 543wgv682ks

Contributors

Janine Ashton RGN, MSc
Tissue Viability Sister, Buckinghamshire Hosptials NHS Trust

Lesley Baillie RGN, BA(Hons), RNT, MSc(Nurs), PhD
Principal lecturer in Clinical Skills Development, London South Bank University

Dee Burrows PhD, BSc(Hons), RGN, RNT
Consultant Nurse and Director, Pain Consultants Limited

Veronica Corben RGN, BSc(Hons), RCN TPGDE, Diploma Cancer Nursing, MSc(Nurs)
Assistant Director of Nursing, Chelsea and Westminster Hospital NHS Trust

Patricia Folan RGN, BSc, Diploma Tropical Disease Nursing, MSc
Infection Control Matron, The Whittington Hospital NHS Trust, London

Rachel Leaver RN, MSc, BSc(Hons), PGCE
Lecturer/Practitioner, London South Bank University and University College London Hospital

Sue Maddex RGN, BSc(Hons), RNT, PGDip, MSc
Senior Lecturer, London South Bank University

Lesley Marsh RGN, BSc(Hons)
Interim Deputy Director of Nursing, Whipps Cross University Hospital NHS Trust

Nicola Neale RGN, RNT, MA(Ed) PGDip, Diploma in Nurse Education, Diploma in Nursing
Senior Lecturer, Buckinghamshire New University

Glynis Collis Pellatt RN, Dip N(Lond), BA(Hons), Diploma in Nurse Education, MA, PhD
Senior Lecturer, University of Bedfordshire

Jenni Randall RN, BSc(Hons), PGDip(Education)
Head of Nursing-Education, Whipps Cross University Hosptial NHS Trust

Joanne Sale RMN, RN, MSc, BSc
Senior Lecturer, University of Bedfordshire

Tracey Valler-Jones RSCN, RN, MEd, PGCE, BSc
Academic Lead for Skills and Practice, University of Worcester

Preface to the third edition

This book, fully updated and expanded from the 2nd edition, aims to assist readers to develop the practical skills necessary to care for adults with physical health needs in varied health care settings. Practical nursing skills, carried out with competence and compassion, are highly valued by patients/clients and their families: these skills promote health, recovery and comfort, making an essential contribution to positive healthcare experiences. The Nursing and Midwifery Council (2007) recently highlighted the importance of fundamental skills by explicitly identifying them in their Essential Skills Clusters for pre-registration nursing students. This 3rd edition covers all of the NMC's essential skills as well as other skills which are important in nursing practice. In some environments nurses are more likely to supervise or support others than directly carry out these practical skills. To supervise others in providing quality fundamental care requires a sound knowledge and understanding of these skills, and a commitment to their value.

The book's first chapter explains the caring context for skills, emphasising the importance of the underpinning knowledge and attitudes of the caregiver, as well as the practical components of skills. This chapter also provides guidance to help students maximise learning from their practical experiences. Dignity in care is explored and subsequent chapters address how to promote the dignity of patients and clients when undertaking specific skills in practice. Each chapter starts with practice scenarios related to adults who have physical health conditions, mental health conditions and learning disabilities. The importance of promoting the physical health of people with mental health needs or learning disabilities is increasingly emphasised (Department of Health 2006, 2007). Therefore nurses working in mental health and learning disability settings need sound practical skills, as nurses working primarily with adults with physical health needs do. In this book, skills are discussed with application to the patient/client scenarios, emphasising problem-solving skills and a person-centred, caring approach. The book is interactive, evidence-based and promotes theory-practice links and reflective practice.

While this 3rd edition is particularly applicable to pre-registration nursing students following the adult, mental health and learning disability branches, it is also relevant to care assistants who are studying for qualifications in care, students on a range of assistant practitioner (foundation degree) healthcare-related programmes, and to all those involved in the teaching of practical skills, including university and college lecturers, and practitioners.

Nurses care for people in a wide range of settings in different circumstances so no single term is appropriate to use in every situation. In this book, the terms 'person' and 'people' are often used but in some contexts the terms 'patient', 'client', 'individual' or 'service user' are referred to in relation to people nurses are caring for.

I hope that this book will be really helpful to students who are learning skills for nursing adults and I wish all those using the book a successful and rewarding career.

Lesley Baillie
January 2009

REFERENCES

Department of Health 2006. *Best Practice Competencies and capabilities for pre-registration mental health nurses in England: the Chief Nursing Officer's review of mental health nursing.* London: DH.

Department of Health 2007. *Good Practice in Learning Disability Nursing.* London: DH.

Nursing and Midwifery Council 2007. *Introduction of Essential Skills clusters for pre-registration Nursing programmes.* NMC Circular, July 2007

Acknowledgements

The editor and contributors would like to thank the following people for their help in preparing the manuscript.

Alan Baillie
RN(Mental Health), BA(Hons), MSc, PGDipE
Senior lecturer (Mental health branch leader)
Buckinghamshire New University
(Reviewed and gave guidance on mental health content)

Jessica Baillie
RN, BN(Hons)
Staff Nurse, University Hospital of Wales, Cardiff
Formerly student nurse, Cardiff University
(Reviewed all chapters from student perspective and critically read the website material)

Pauline Pepperell
RN (Learning disability)
Community Learning Disability Nurse, Cancer Awareness Team Leader Nurse
(Reviewed all chapters for learning disability content)

Heartfelt thanks also to:
- Friends, family and colleagues for their invaluable support and encouragement during the 3rd edition's preparation
- Alan, Emily and Jessica Baillie who lived with the 3rd edition and helped in so many ways
- Ebenezer Osowo of London South Bank University for his assistance with images
- The staff at Hodder publishers for their support and encouragement throughout the 3rd edition's development

Practical Nursing Skills: A Caring Approach

Lesley Baillie

This book aims to assist readers to develop a caring approach to a range of practical skills that can be applied with adults in different healthcare settings. Practical nursing skills comprise not only the 'hands-on' (psychomotor) element, but require evidence-based knowledge, effective interpersonal skills, an ethical approach, creative and reflective thinking, and an appropriate professional attitude. These elements are considered throughout the text.

To become a registered nurse requires more than an ability to carry out practical skills. However, all student nurses need to develop the ability to perform a range of practical skills safely (Nursing and Midwifery Council [NMC] 2004; NMC 2007a). Healthcare support workers and assistant practitioners also need to acquire practical skills. This book specifically addresses this element of nursing; there are many other texts that cover other subjects underpinning nursing practice (see later in this chapter: 'Recommended reading').

This chapter discusses the nature of practical skills in nursing, how these skills can be learned, and how this book can help you to develop your nursing skills. This chapter emphasises developing and valuing these practical skills as holistic, caring skills, which give you the opportunity to develop the therapeutic use of self.

This chapter includes:
- What are practical nursing skills?
- Practical skills included in this book and the use of practice scenarios
- Practical skills: affective, cognitive and motor dimensions
- A caring approach to practical nursing skills
- Cultural competence and practical nursing skills
- Patient/client dignity and practical nursing skills
- How can you develop your practical nursing skills?

WHAT ARE PRACTICAL NURSING SKILLS?

Nurses need to master a range of skills, including practical, communication and management skills. These are often integrated within the nursing role, because carrying out practical nursing skills effectively also requires skills in, for example, communication and teamwork. Bjork (1999a) defines practical nursing skills as 'hands-on actions that promote the patients' physical comfort, hygiene and safe medical treatment [which are] ... commonly referred to as procedures or psychomotor skills'. Although this definition implies a purely physical perspective, practical skills undoubtedly enhance social and psychological comfort and well-being too, oral hygiene being a good example. Bradshaw (1994) notes that physical, social, psychological and spiritual care is actually an integrated whole and cannot be separated. Thus while a practical nursing skill may appear to be a physical procedure, its effect is not only physical.

Romyn (1999) argues that deciding what constitutes a practical nursing skill is problematic, as many skills that nurses carry out are not solely their domain; for example, doctors give injections too. This book takes the stance that practical nursing skills are those involving 'hands-on' care by nurses with patients/clients, although some of these skills are also performed by other professionals. Healthcare support workers and assistant practitioners carry out many of these skills and so this book is relevant for these staff too. There is a vast range of practical skills that nurses use which they must adapt in different situations with varied groups of people.

The range of practical skills used in nursing

Traditionally there was a hierarchy of skills within nursing, with experienced nurses undertaking more technical, medical skills (for example, administering medicines) and junior staff carrying out what was sometimes referred to as 'basic nursing care'; that is, assisting people with activities of daily living such as hygiene and elimination. McMahon (1998) described this system as biomedical and task-focused rather than being client-focused, with a nurse delivering all of an individual person's care.

The term 'basic' has often been used in a derisory manner, implying that these skills are not as important as more technical ones. Indeed student nurses have been found to view learning technical skills as more important than other aspects of care (Randle 2001). The notion of delivering individualised care for clients, operationalised through the nursing process (assessing, planning, implementing and evaluating care), and based on the framework of a nursing (rather than medical) model, has become widely accepted within nursing. However, with registered nurses' roles expanding, often taking on skills previously carried out by doctors, and healthcare support workers increasingly carrying out skills that were formerly the domain of registered nurses, it is probably unrealistic to deny that a skills hierarchy exists.

In Rogers et al.'s (2000) survey, a respondent commented: 'The nurses were very nice and worked very hard, but I think they have become technicians rather than providing what we used to consider "nursing care".' Randle (2001) commented that engaging with the biomedical model of practice led to deteriorating nurse–patient relationships, her research portraying 'a picture of students actively engaging with technology whilst at the same time disengaging from the emotional care of patients' (p. 162). However, in Alliex and Irurita's (2004) Australian study, nurses described making additional efforts to meet patients' humanistic needs in the presence of technology, which they referred to as 'maximising'. Maximising consisted of:

- maintaining presence: offering help, popping in, giving time;
- minimising the impact of technology: social interaction, using humour appropriately, understating and manipulating technology; and
- individualising interactions: considering patients' likes, doing little things, portraying a caring demeanour and being kind and cheerful.

Thus use of technology need not diminish a caring approach. This book emphasises that practical skills can be person-centred and delivered within the context of a caring philosophy, with value attached to fundamental as well as technical care. Helping an older person regain the ability to wash and dress after a stroke, or assisting a person with confusion to maintain continence, can be more complex than technical, medically focused skills, such as recording an electrocardiogram.

Over the past decade there have been increasing concerns about fundamental care being neglected in healthcare settings. In 1997, the *Observer* newspaper launched a media campaign 'Dignity on the Ward', due to concerns about the poor quality of care delivered to older people. The campaign triggered an independent inquiry, commissioned by the Department of Health (DH), into the care of older people in hospital (Health Advisory Service 2000 1998). These research findings led to the launching of *The Essence of Care: Patient-focused benchmarking for health care practitioners* (DH 2001a), which laid out benchmarking standards for fundamental care for people of all ages, which have continued to be developed and updated. Box 1.1 presents the areas of care now included in 'The Essence of Care'. Where relevant, these standards of best practice are referred to in this book. Reviews of mental healthcare have highlighted the need for skilled physical care too (DH 2006a). The other UK governments have also published care standards, accessible

---

Box 1.1 *The Essence of Care: Patient-focused benchmarks for clinical governance* **(NHS Modernisation Agency 2003)**

- Continence and bladder and bowel care
- Personal and oral hygiene
- Food and nutrition
- Pressure ulcers
- Privacy and dignity
- Record keeping
- Safety of clients/patients with mental health needs in acute mental health and general hospital settings
- Principles of self-care
- Communication

Additional benchmarks
- 'Promoting health' (DH 2006b)
- 'Care environment' (DH 2007a)

on their websites. The NMC's (2007a) 'Essential Skills Clusters' emphasise that nurses must acquire a range of skills including fundamental, caring skills as well as technical skills (see next section).

PRACTICAL SKILLS INCLUDED IN THIS BOOK AND THE USE OF PRACTICE SCENARIOS

This book includes a range of practical skills that student nurses need to develop during their pre-registration programme. Many are addressed in courses for healthcare support workers too. Within the UK, student nurses must achieve proficiencies within four domains of practice (professional and ethical practice, care delivery, care management, and personal and professional development) to enter the register (NMC 2004). The proficiencies include practical skills, but the NMC has now published specific guidance about skills to be developed during pre-registration nursing programmes in the 'Essential Skills Clusters' (NMC 2007a). The Essential Skills Clusters, and the chapters in this book focusing on these care aspects, are:

- 'Care, communication and compassion' (Chapters 1, 2, 8, 9, 10 and 12);
- 'Organisational aspects of care' (Chapters 4, 6 and 11);
- 'Infection control' (Chapters 3 and 7);
- 'Nutrition and Fluid balance' (Chapter 10);
- 'Medicines management' (Chapter 5).

To meet a patient's comfort needs requires integration of a range of skills (for example, hygiene care and pain management). The final chapter examines pain management and how comfort can be promoted, drawing on skills explored in earlier chapters. Interprofessional team working is essential for holistic patient care and is discussed throughout the book.

For general first aid procedures you are advised to consult the most current *First Aid Manual*, at the time of writing, the eighth revised edition (British Red Cross *et al.* 2006). This can be bought at any bookseller's and is very detailed and fully illustrated. The St John Ambulance website covers most first aid procedures (see www.sja.org.uk/ sja/first-aid-advice.aspx). All healthcare staff should be able to assess a collapsed person and administer basic life support (BLS). These procedures are updated regularly by the Resuscitation Council (UK) and outlined in detail on their website (www.resus.org.uk). Therefore these procedures, though referred to where appropriate, are not reproduced in detail here. The Resuscitation Council's (UK) very informative website includes other interesting sections as well as guidelines; for example, information about legal aspects of resuscitation and 'Do not attempt resuscitation' policies. You must undergo supervised BLS practice in the skills laboratory with a trained instructor, and it is mandatory for all healthcare staff to attend these sessions annually. Chapter 6 covers some principles underpinning moving and handling skills. However, these skills are frequently updated and you must attend the training sessions provided for you, both as a student and as a registered nurse, so you can practise and update your skills under supervision.

Each chapter begins with scenarios of adults in physical healthcare, learning disability and mental healthcare settings, and the chapter links the content back to these patients/clients, thus encouraging theory–practice links. The book aims to include a selection of scenarios, from a variety of settings, but it is not intended that all possible situations are represented. All scenarios have been developed from experience with similar people with health needs. Any identifying details have been changed or omitted, and pseudonyms were allocated at random.

PRACTICAL SKILLS: AFFECTIVE, COGNITIVE AND MOTOR DIMENSIONS

ACTIVITY

Almost everyone has had an injection at some stage and you may have had recent immunisations before starting to study nursing. You probably took it for granted that the skill would be performed competently. What are the different elements of carrying out this skill?

You probably considered technical aspects such as drawing up the correct drug accurately using sterile equipment; but may also have identified the need for underlying knowledge of the drug's actions and potential side-effects, and that the nurse should use a calm and friendly approach to relax you and relieve anxiety. This example illustrates that effective practical nursing skills require a skilled motor performance (the 'doing' element), a sound knowledge (based on best evidence), and an appropriate attitude towards patients/clients. Bjork (1999a) reviewed the concept of nursing practical skills and concluded that they were for many years commonly considered to make up the art of nursing but that more recently the technical, motor element has been emphasised.

Oermann (1990) suggested that the motor (doing) element of a practical (psychomotor) skill is often emphasised to the exclusion of the cognitive and affective component. She highlighted the importance of the cognitive base (the scientific principles underlying the performance of the skill) and the affective domain, which reflects the nurse's values and concern for the person while the skill is being performed. To provide high-quality care, nurses must be competent to apply theory and skill in each clinical situation, which includes knowledge, and mastery in each of the psychomotor, cognitive and affective domains (Fitzpatrick *et al.* 1992). These three aspects are now discussed.

The affective domain

A practical skill's affective domain includes the nurse's attitude and approach to the person as well as the ethical dimension. Bush and Barr's (1997) study of critical care nurses' experiences of caring identified the affective process as including sensitivity, empathy, concern and interest. One participant was quoted saying: 'instead of just saying, "I'm taking your blood pressure, your temperature", you really care about what the patient is going through – how they must feel – you kind of put yourself in their position, and how you'd want to be taken care of yourself instead of just a mechanical (action)'. Bjork (1999a) argued that caring intentions are necessary in practical nursing actions because 'they can transform the acts of handling and

> ### Box 1.2 Illustrative example of the significance of the nurse's approach to a patient while assisting with showering
>
> About 5 days after I had had major abdominal surgery, after which I had been seriously ill, a nurse got me up for the first time and took me in a wheelchair to the bathroom for a shower. I was weak, afraid of being naked in front of her, and I felt uncomfortable about my wound being on show. She helped me off with my clothes and helped me have a shower, during which she sensitively used humour to make me relaxed. She washed my body and hair, and at intervals put her hand gently on my shoulder in a comforting way. At one point she knelt down and gently put her hands either side of my large wound and said 'It looks beautiful – it's going to heal up really well. You'll be back in a bikini within a month.' (I was!) I got this tremendous sense of relief that even though I had this massive scar I would still be me again. She had encouraged me to accept my scar. By the end of the whole episode of care I felt wonderfully clean from top to toe, relaxed, and had begun to recover a sense of self. The fear had just disappeared.

helping into tolerable or even meaningful experiences for the patient'. She suggested that nurses can demonstrate respect for and interest in patients while carrying out skills, conveying the message that 'it is not just a body that is being handled'. While carrying out practical skills, such as bathing, nurses can foster confidence and develop trusting relationships with patients.

Bjork (1999a) also suggested being aware of the meaning of the practical skill for the individual and how it fits into the person's overall experience. For example, a wound dressing may exemplify the change in body image following invasive surgery, and bathing someone may highlight their loss of independence due to physical or mental health problems. Box 1.2 details the positive experience of Dee Burrows (one of Chapter 12's authors) of being assisted with a shower postoperatively. Her story illustrates the significance of the nurse's approach while carrying out her care, and its impact on her recovery. Each time you carry out a practical skill with a patient/client, you convey a message about your state of being (Paterson and Zderad 1988); for example, are you anxious, in a hurry, distracted or uninterested? Chapter 2 considers the nurse's approach to patients and clients during practical nursing skills application.

Valuing people

Mencap (a UK charity campaigning for equal rights for children and adults with a learning disability) (2004; 2007) identified that people with learning disabilities face unequal healthcare and have worse treatment than those without disabilities. Therefore, all nurses should be familiar with the document *Valuing People: A new strategy for learning disability for the 21st century* (DH 2001b). *Valuing People* stressed that people with learning disabilities are people first and there should be a focus on what they can do rather than what they cannot. All people with learning disabilities should have a health facilitator (who may be a keyworker, a nurse or another health or social care professional) appointed to ensure they get the healthcare they need, and a Health Action Plan. An individual's Health Action Plan includes details of health interventions, oral health and dental care, fitness and mobility, continence, vision, hearing, nutrition, emotional needs, medication, and records of screening. Any nurses carrying out practical skills with people with learning disabilities, or supporting their carers in doing so, should do so with an appropriate attitude and with reference to their Health Action Plan.

Valuing People Now: From progress to transformation (DH 2007b) reviewed progress made and set out the priorities for service provision for people with learning disabilities from 2008 to 2011. The role of learning disability nurses in acting as an expert resource to other professionals was emphasised. The DH acknowledged that, while progress had been made in some aspects, progress in other areas like good-quality healthcare had been disappointing. Most people with learning disabilities have poorer health and die younger than the rest of the population, yet their access to the National Health Service is often poor, and personalisation, dignity and safety are undermined (DH 2007b). Nurses caring for adults in all settings, including mental health, acute and primary care services will care for people with learning disabilities so everyone has a responsibility to demonstrate commitment to improving health experiences for this client group.

In *Good Practice in Learning Disability Nursing*, the DH (2007c) emphasised that learning disability nurses are essential for making the 'Valuing People' vision happen and they can help people with learning disabilities to stay healthy as long as possible. The document sets out benchmarks with recommendations for learning disability nurses. Other UK countries have published documents regarding services for people with learning disabilities (Department of Health and Social Security 2005; Scottish Executive 2000; Learning Disability Advisory Group 2001). The Royal College of Nursing (2006) provided helpful guidance for nurses about meeting the health needs of people with learning disabilities.

The cognitive domain

The cognitive domain reflects the 'thinking' element behind the skill, including the application of research to practice and problem-solving; it is what makes nurses 'knowledgeable doers'. Being able to adapt a skill in the practice setting requires a sound underlying knowledge of why it is being performed and the rationale for each stage. For example, understanding the principles behind oxygen therapy administration enables nurses to choose an administration method that is safe and acceptable to people in specific healthcare situations. All healthcare professionals should apply best evidence to their practice as there is increasing emphasis on 'evidence-based care'. In many situations, evidence is derived from research, but it may also be based on experience, and through reflection on practice. Benner (1984) identified that practice is always more complex and presents many more realities than theory ever can, and she highlighted the value of theory derived from practice (see later section: 'Learning from experience and reflection').

Nurses are accountable for their actions and so they must be able to explain the knowledge base underpinning their practice. Benner (1984) explored how expert nurses develop knowledge from their practice, learning to recognise, for example, subtle changes in people's conditions. Not all nursing skills have a firm evidence base on which to implement practice, but in many areas such research-based knowledge is obtainable. Within this book, authors have searched for up-to-date evidence on which to base practical skills and systematic reviews and they refer to evidence-based guidelines where available. Health service users should be able to assume that practical skills carried out by nurses are based on sound, current evidence, rather than on out-of-date, ritual or unsubstantiated knowledge.

Increasingly NHS Trusts and other healthcare organisations have their own clinical guidelines, based on best evidence, to assist nurses and other healthcare professionals to implement evidence-based practice. You should always work with your employer's guidelines if available. Also, the National Patient Safety Agency regularly produces guidelines and alerts relating to safe practice. If you are searching for evidence, an excellent source of information is the National Library for Health, which includes access to resources for evidence-based practice, such as Bandolier, the Cochrane Library, National Institute for Health and Clinical Excellence (NICE), Protocols and Care Pathways, search databases, the *British National Formulary,* and the NHS Centre for Reviews and Dissemination. The standards in the National Service Frameworks, and other government guidelines, are based on best evidence too. See 'Useful websites' at the end of this chapter for all these sources.

The motor domain

Mastering the motor dimension of a skill is important for an effective outcome as lack of a skilled motor performance jeopardises both safety and comfort. Knowing how to do a practical skill can be termed 'know-how' type of knowledge – practical expertise and skill that is really acquired through practice and experience (Manley 1997). Nursing skills are performed in a changing clinical environment, with people who respond and react in different ways. Therefore, nurses need to adapt skills accordingly so practical nursing skills can never be wholly automatic in nature.

A CARING APPROACH TO PRACTICAL NURSING SKILLS

When asked your reasons for wanting to be a nurse you might well have responded that you wanted to care for people. Many nursing theorists have recognised that caring and nursing are interrelated. Watson (1979) stated that 'the practice of caring is central to nursing' (p. 9). Benner and Wrubel (1989) asserted that the 'nature of the caring relationship is central to most nursing interventions' (p. 5). They identify that the same act done in a non-caring way, as opposed to a caring way, has very different consequences, so that 'nursing can never be reduced to mere technique' (p. 4). Roach (2002) identified caring both as a natural attribute of being human and as the core of nursing. Bjork (1999b) presents a model of practical skill performance, which includes aspects such as sequence and fluency, but also includes caring comportment, explained as being how the nurse creates a respectful, accepting and encouraging atmosphere, which includes concern for the whole person.

The experience of non-caring versus caring

Arman and Rehnsfelt's (2007) study led them to conclude that 'the essence of uncaring was that patients were not seen as whole human beings and their existential suffering was not noticed by caregivers' (p. 373). Box 1.3 provides an example of unkindness to a patient who was clearly vulnerable and the staff member, instead of being understanding, was impatient and harsh. Halldorsdottir's (1991) study identified the detrimental effects of skills being implemented without a caring context. Her in-depth interviews highlighted the vulnerability of patients who found uncaring encounters with nurses were discouraging and distressing. Patients described being initially puzzled and disbelieving, followed by feelings of anger and resentment, and then despair and helplessness. She found that dependent people being uncared for developed feelings of a sense of loss, and of being betrayed by those counted on for caring. Non-caring nurses were described as being 'cold human beings, like computers'. Halldorsdottir described this feeling as 'dehumanisation', with the person feeling that they have no value as a person and are 'an object': 'I was ... a piece of dust on the floor'. The uncaring nurse, Halldorsdottir found, did carry out the routine tasks but was perceived as not 'caring about the patient as a person'. In Thorsteinsson's (2002) study, participants reported that poor-quality nursing care made them feel angry and stressed. One person said: 'It made me mad – I did not feel that I deserved it. When you are in my position you are unable to defend yourself – it was an unpleasant feeling.'

Therefore, to measure a person's blood pressure in a technically competent manner would not, in itself, be perceived as caring. In Thorsteinsson's study, nurses perceived as giving high-quality care were described as 'joyful, warm, tender, smiling, positive, polite and understanding'. All these attributes relate to the nurse's approach; clinical competence was also expected but did not lead to an experience of high-quality care unless accompanied by these other aspects. Kralik *et al.*'s (1997) research identified that patients saw nurses as being either engaged or detached in their care. Nurses who were engaged with their care were friendly and warm, behaved as if nothing was too much trouble, and had a gentle touch. Care by detached nurses was viewed negatively by patients. They felt that they were treated as if they were a number or an object, the nurses were sharp/cold in their approach to their care, and were rough with their physical care. In Cortis's (2000)

Box 1.3 An uncaring approach (from Baillie 2007, p. 155)

An older, frail man had been admitted to a surgical ward in the night. He was confused and had a hearing impairment (his hearing aid lay on his bedside locker). The nurse (or healthcare assistant) approached him to find out what he wanted for breakfast but was impatient and clearly irritated by his inability to answer coherently. Two other patients observed the interaction and found it quite upsetting. Mr A said of the situation: '*This poor chap opposite me who was clearly quite deaf and obviously very confused – didn't know where he was – and she was shouting at him – she was a bully. She shouldn't be in that job.*'

study, a patient commented: 'Some nurses do not want to listen, and they do not want to talk to you. They come and go and [do] not say anything' (p. 113).

Woodward's (1997) analysis of the literature on professional caring identified two dimensions of caring: *instrumental* caring (the technique comprising skills and knowledge) and *expressive* caring (the emotional element which includes respect for the individual). She suggested that it is expressive caring which transforms nursing actions into caring. Halldorsdottir (1991) identifies a 'life-sustaining mode of being with a patient' which includes 'compassionate competence, genuine concern for the patient as a person, undivided attention when the nurse is with the patient, and cheerfulness'. This approach is described as 'professional caring'. Research participants felt relief when they felt cared for and they believed that their diminished anxiety gave them time to concentrate on getting better.

The above review highlights the importance of a caring approach from patients' perspectives. Roach (2002) made a study of caring in relation to nursing and developed a framework: 'the 6Cs'. These are compassion, competence, confidence, conscience, commitment and comportment. She explained that her theory developed over time in response to the question: What is a nurse doing when she or he is caring? The 6Cs are a broad framework 'suggesting categories of human behaviour within which professional caring is to be understood' (2002, p. 66).

Roach's 6Cs: a framework for caring

Compassion

Roach defined compassion as 'a way of living born out of an awareness of one's relationship to all living creatures. It engenders a response of participation in the experience of another; a sensitivity to the pain and brokenness of the other and a quality of presence that allows one to share with and make room for the other' (p. 50). Compassion is 'a simple unpretentious presence to each other, a gift that we seem to have lost even as we have developed sophisticated techniques in our efforts to acquire it' (p. 51). Roach argued that compassion is needed more than ever to humanise the ever-increasing cold and impersonal technology used within healthcare. Box 1.4 illustrates this with a nurse's act of compassion that occurred in the highly technical environment of the intensive therapy unit.

Competence

To ensure safe and effective care, practical skills must be carried out competently. The NMC (2008a) specify that nurses must provide a high standard of practice, displaying up-to-date knowledge and skills for safe and effective practice. Roach defined competence as having the 'knowledge, judgement, skills, energy, experience and motivation required to respond adequately to the demands of one's professional responsibilities' (p. 54). Roach goes on to state that 'while competence without compassion can be brutal and inhumane, compassion without competence may be no more than a meaningless, if not harmful, intrusion into the life of a person or persons needing help' (p. 54).

Wallis's (1998) in-depth study of patients' experiences of being cared for in a coronary care unit found that patients viewed competence as essential in a caring

> ### Box 1.4 Compassion: an illustrative example from an intensive therapy unit
>
> James was in the final stages of heart and lung failure and his nurse, about to go home after a 12-hour shift and knowing that she would not see him again, asked him if there was anything she could get him before she left. He replied 'Oh, a port and brandy please!' Phone calls around the hospital were unsuccessful in locating any and the nurse went off shift. She returned half an hour later with a small glass of port and brandy brought from home. As James was unable to swallow she dipped sponge mouth sticks into the drink and put them in his mouth for him to suck. James grinned and said it was 'wonderful'. This act of compassion brought tenderness to this patient's final hours and made an immeasurable difference to his relatives' feelings about his death.

nurse: 'You have got to have a competent nurse to start with.' It seemed that technical competence was reassuring to patients, and that this competence then allowed the nurse to 'transcend' the technology and become close to patients.

Confidence

Roach defined confidence as 'the quality that fosters trusting relationships' (p. 56). She discussed the importance of not deceiving clients, stating that 'Caring confidence fosters trust without dependency, communicates truth without violence and creates a relationship of respect without paternalism or without engendering a response borne out of fear or powerlessness' (p. 58). For example, a person may have fallen, sustaining a hip fracture, and is regaining mobility and independence. The person may lack confidence and be afraid of falling again, but the nurse's approach enables a trusting relationship to be built. The nurse can help the person to work towards realistic goals in mobilisation, giving praise for achievements, and helping them to believe in their abilities.

Conscience

Conscience is, according to Roach, a 'state of moral awareness' (p. 60) which nurses can portray through their approach when undertaking practical skills. Roach considers that conscience grows out of experience, 'out of a process of valuing self and others' (p. 61). Nurses can demonstrate whether they value people and respect their rights to dignified and humane care and should speak out if they feel that care is compromised in any way.

Commitment

Roach defined commitment as 'a complex affective response characterised by a convergence between one's desires and one's obligations, and by a deliberate choice to act in accordance with them' (p. 62). The implication is a sense of duty, ensuring that nurses will endeavour to carry out necessary care in a timely way, regardless of barriers and constraints.

Henderson *et al.* (2007) found that nurses needed to respond to patients' needs in a timely manner to be perceived as caring. Patients were dissatisfied when nurses apparently forgot patients and their needs. In Box 1.4 the nurse's action exemplified compassion but also demonstrated commitment to James, by bringing the drink from home despite just finishing a 12-hour shift.

Comportment

In relation to this aspect of caring, Roach asked the question: 'Are dress and language of caregivers consistent with the belief that the patient-client is of incalculable worth, and that the caregiver him/herself is a person of intrinsic worth and dignity?' (p. 65). She proposed that how nurses present themselves represents their beliefs about the worth of those they are caring for. She argued that 'caring is reflected in bearing, demeanour, dress and language' (p. 65), and that 'we usually dress and use language consistent with our attitude towards the person or the occasion' (p. 64). Thus we would not usually wear casual clothes to a funeral. Duffy *et al.* (2007) found that patients perceived nurses who were poised and cheerful as caring, a finding they viewed as consistent with Roach's comportment factor.

Roach's 6Cs act as a useful framework when considering how practical skills can be carried out in a caring manner.

Therapeutic nursing

The term 'therapeutic nursing' can be defined as nursing that 'deliberately leads to beneficial outcomes for the patient' (McMahon 1998, p. 7). At first glance it might seem obvious that this is what nursing seeks to attain. However, in the DH's (2006c) 'Dignity in Care' survey, one relative wrote: 'When my father went into hospital, I saw food and drinks for people who were unable to eat and drink unaided being left on trolleys. I always went in at meal times to make sure my father got something to eat.' Unfortunate examples such as these illustrate that nursing does not always have a therapeutic effect on individuals. McMahon (1998) even argues that some patients get better *despite* their nursing care, not because of it.

Ersser (1998) identified three core categories which he found reflected views about nurses' therapeutic actions:

* presentation of the nurse, such as non-verbal communication and greeting the patient;
* relating to patients as when developing rapport;
* specific actions of the nurse, which are largely instrumental or procedural, for example, dressing a wound.

When carrying out any practical nursing skill you need to consider how your actions can be therapeutic. For example, what will turn the taking of someone to the toilet into a therapeutic action, as opposed to simply assisting with elimination? Reflecting on your practice can help you to identify how you could provide a more positive outcome for patients and clients (see later section: 'Learning from experience and reflection').

CULTURAL COMPETENCE AND PRACTICAL NURSING SKILLS

Britain is a multicultural society and practical nursing skills must be carried out with sensitivity and in a culturally appropriate manner for each individual and family. The American nurse and anthropologist, Madeleine Leininger, studied transcultural caring over many years, and identified how acts of caring such as comforting and physical care, and the meaning attached to them, can vary between cultures (Leininger 1981). Leininger suggested that culture and caring cannot be separated within nursing actions and decision-making; Reynolds and Leininger (1993) provide an overview of Leininger's theory. Papadopoulos (2006a) presents the Papadopoulos–Tilki–Taylor model for transcultural nursing and health, consisting of four linked elements: cultural awareness, cultural knowledge, cultural sensitivity and cultural competence.

- **Cultural awareness** includes examining and questioning one's personal value-base and beliefs. Chapter 2 of this book will help you to develop self-awareness.
- **Cultural knowledge** may be drawn from sources such as sociology, anthropology and research, and from experience of people. Where appropriate to specific practical skills, cultural variations (particularly related to religious beliefs) are considered in this book. However, there are often individual and regional variations so it is important to avoid stereotyping and making ethnocentric judgements; these are barriers to cultural sensitivity. In Cioffi's (2005) Australian study, the nurses used experiences of caring for culturally diverse patients to develop their knowledge; sources were bilingual health workers and colleagues, patients, their families and support persons. Some nurses used stereotypical views of the patient's cultural group to give care but others used the individual patient's perspective: 'You actually have to ask the person. You can't assume they're going to be the traditional Chinese or Arabic lady' (Cioffi 2005).
- **Cultural sensitivity** can be achieved by nurses working with people as partners, offering choices in care. In Cioffi's study, one nurse said that when caring for culturally diverse patients: 'If I am not sure, I just say to the patient "What is the right thing for me to do?", "Can I do this" or "Would you mind if I do this?".' Another nurse said: 'It's just finding out what they believe and what they don't believe in and then you can work it out from there with them and individualise their care.' Communication skills, respect and empathy are all very important for cultural sensitivity (see Chapter 2).
- **Cultural competence** requires the application of cultural awareness, knowledge and sensitivity to achieve effective healthcare which addresses people's cultural beliefs, behaviour and needs. The culturally competent nurse also challenges prejudice, discrimination and inequality. Leishman (2006) highlighted the importance of mental health nurses developing cultural competence in an increasingly culturally diverse UK society.

In Cortis's (2000) UK study, Pakistani adults provided some examples of good healthcare experiences where staff were sensitive to their rights for privacy, provided for their need to pray, and offered opportunities to maintain cultural practices in the hospital environment. However, nurses were generally perceived as seriously lacking cultural knowledge about this community; they lacked awareness of appropriate support systems, hygiene practices, the significance of Halal food, and practices associated with caring and spiritual needs. One participant said: 'Nurses are not particularly interested to find out about our way of life. I feel that it is [the] nurses' duty to get to know some things about our customs or at least learn from us. This will be a great help to nurses as well, but they do not ask us anything either' (Cortis 2000, p. 114). This comment indicated the willingness of the participant to share cultural knowledge but their perception that nurses were not interested in learning.

ACTIVITY

Reflect on your own cultural competence at this stage. Jot down a few notes about your personal values and beliefs, your cultural knowledge, and your skills which will aid you to demonstrate cultural sensitivity.

Papadopoulos' (2006b) textbook *Transcultural Health and Social Care: Development of culturally competent practitioners* provides a comprehensive guide to this important dimension of practice and is recommended further reading. In this book we address cultural aspects of communication in Chapter 2.

PATIENT/CLIENT DIGNITY AND PRACTICAL NURSING SKILLS

It is essential that nurses promote people's dignity while carrying out practical nursing skills. Respecting patients/clients' dignity is a requirement from the Human Rights Act (Great Britain 1998), and the NMC's (2008a) Code of Professional Conduct asserts this requirement of registered nurses:

> Make the care of people your first concern, treating them as individuals and respecting their dignity.

Dignity can be difficult to define, however, and people may have different interpretations of its meaning.

ACTIVITY

Spend a few minutes writing down what you see as being 'dignity'. Now ask someone else for their view and compare with your own.

How similar were your views? Did you find it difficult to put 'dignity' into words? The Social Care Institute for Excellence (SCIE) (2006) stated that:

> While dignity may be difficult to define, what is clear is that people know when they have not been treated with dignity and respect.

The SCIE suggested that dignity comprises many overlapping aspects such as respect, privacy, autonomy and self-worth. A definition developed from patients' views is:

> Patient dignity is feeling valued and comfortable psychologically with one's physical presentation and behaviour, level of control over the situation, and the behaviour of other people in the environment.

(Baillie 2007, p. 247)

How does this compare with your views?

Research studies in various settings have confirmed that dignity is important to patients (Chochinov *et al.* 2002; Matiti 2002; Joffe *et al.* 2003), and health policy documents increasingly emphasise dignified care. Whether people are treated with dignity in healthcare affects perceptions of their whole experience. In November 2006, the DH launched a 'Dignity in Care' campaign, aimed across health and social care (see www.dh.gov.uk/dignityincare). The campaign initially focused mainly on dignity for older people, but in 2007 it was extended to mental health services to focus on tackling stigma, inpatient services (the therapeutic environment, safety and privacy, extending rights to advocacy) and older people's mental health. The key point is that all patients/clients in all settings, and their relatives, should be treated with dignity. The campaign has a 'Dignity Challenge' which is a ten-point plan, available on pocket-size cards (see Box 1.5). Other UK health departments have emphasised dignity in care in policy documents too.

ACTIVITY

Look at the Dignity Challenge in Box 1.5. From your healthcare experiences to date, as either a patient, relative or professional, which of the ten challenges do you feel are usually achieved? Are there any that you feel are rarely achieved? If so, reflect on what barriers might stop these being achieved in healthcare.

While government health policies have often focused on dignity of older people, studies have indicated that adults of all ages are concerned about their dignity and can be vulnerable to a loss of dignity in healthcare (Matiti 2002; Baillie 2007). The Royal College of Nursing (RCN) launched a Dignity campaign in 2008 and published a survey of nurses' experiences of providing dignified care for patients

---

Box 1.5 The Dignity Challenge (DH 2006d). Reproduced with permission from the Department of Health. www.dh.gov.uk/dignityincare

High-quality services that respect people's dignity should:
- show zero tolerance towards all forms of abuse;
- treat people with the same respect as you would want for yourself and your family;
- treat each person as an individual;
- ensure people are able to maintain maximum levels of independence, choice and control;
- support people in expressing their needs
- respect people's rights to privacy;
- ensure people can complain without fear of retribution;
- work with patients' families and their partners in their care;
- help people to maintain confidence and self-esteem;
- alleviate people's loneliness and isolation.

and clients across the age range in diverse settings (RCN 2008). The report highlighted these key areas which impact on dignity:

- **Place**: the physical environment and organisational culture
- **People**: the attitudes and behaviour of nurses and others
- **Processes**: care activities and how they are carried out.

In the survey, nurses identified many care activities during which patients were vulnerable to a loss of dignity, but they described in detail the actions they took to prevent dignity being lost, which related to privacy, communication and physical actions (see Table 1.1). When carrying out skills with people in practice, you need to ensure that your behaviour promotes their dignity. Chapter 2 focuses in detail on your communication, and how this can portray care and compassion. Other chapters highlight dignity in relation to specific skills.

Table 1.1: How nurses protect dignity during care activities. Reproduced with permission from RCN (2008, p. 36).

Privacy	Communication	Physical care actions
Physical environment	Interactions that make patients feel comfortable	Preparation
• Side rooms	• Sensitivity	• Procedure
• Quiet/private room/area	• Empathy	• Environment
• Bathroom/toilet use	• Developing relationships	• Timeliness
• Curtains/screens/blinds	• Non-verbal communication	• Equipment
• Curtain clips/pegs/signs	• Conversation	Staff management
• Managing smells	• Reassurance	Promoting independence
• Auditory privacy	• Professionalism	Physical comfort
Staff behaviour	• Family involvement	
• Discretion	Interactions that make patients feel in control	
• Respect for personal space	• Explanations and information giving	
• Prevent/manage interruptions	• Choices and negotiation	
• Sensitivity to culture/religion	• Gaining consent	
Managing people in the environment	Interactions that make patients feel valued	
• Staff: number present, gender	• Giving time	
• Other patients	• Concern for patients as individuals	
• Family	• Courteousness	
• Ward visitors/public		
Bodily privacy		
• Covering body		
• Minimising time exposed		
• Privacy during undressing		
• Clothing		

In Baillie's (2007) research, one man's description of the nurse who promoted his dignity was that she:

> . . . is sensitive, explains what she's going to do before she does it, she's cheerful, she has a sense of humour, she appears interested in me as an individual, she has a caring approach, appears to enjoy her work – doesn't appear as though it's a chore *(p. 205)*.

Baillie found that in situations where dignity was threatened, staff behaviour could prevent dignity being lost. One man said that the student nurse who inserted his suppositories (a procedure that he felt could have threatened his dignity) 'did it nicely' so he did not lose his dignity. A woman in her fifties with terminal cancer identified that she could have lost her dignity in the bathroom but her 'bath had been handled well' as she had been given choices which promoted her dignity.

The SCIE produced a series of practice guides on Dignity in Care, focusing on 'respect', 'autonomy' and 'privacy' (see www.scie.org.uk/publications/practiceguides). These include many examples of where dignity has been promoted in a wide range of care settings. The RCN's learning zone (which you can access if an RCN member) has an excellent on-line learning package about dignity.

HOW CAN YOU DEVELOP YOUR PRACTICAL NURSING SKILLS?

To make the most of opportunities to learn practical skills, it is helpful to think about how skills are learned.

ACTIVITY

Reflect back on a practical skill which you have learned, for example learning to drive. How did you learn this skill?

You may recall that you built up the skill in step-by-step stages, learning each sub-skill one at a time. You could probably focus only on the skill, and found that it was difficult to do anything else (e.g. have a conversation) at the same time. Benner (1984) identified that when learning any new skill, the performance is initially 'halting and rigid' (p. 37) and that one must pay careful attention to the explicit rules relating to the skill.

As a student you are not expected to be an expert in your practical skills! Benner's research adapted a skill acquisition model by Dreyfus and Dreyfus to describe different levels of performance in nurses. She conducted paired interviews with beginners and experienced nurses as well as using participant observation to study nurses with various levels of experience. The five stages of performance identified are outlined below.

Stages of skill performance

- **Stage 1 – Novice.** Novice nurses have no experience on which to draw (this applies not only to new students but also to experienced nurses moving to an unfamiliar area of practice). Benner describes the novice as being 'rule-governed' in behaviour. By this she means that the novice needs explicit guidelines about what to do and in which sequence. However, these guidelines need to be adapted to the actual situation, and novice nurses need help and guidance to do this.
- **Stage 2 – Advanced beginner.** At this stage nurses can use previous experience and apply it in practice but continue to need adequate support, particularly with aspects that are situational, such as prioritising. They have difficulty seeing a situation as a whole and focus on the specific skill to be carried out, regardless of additional situational factors.
- **Stage 3 – Competent.** Competent nurses are able to carry out conscious and deliberate planning, and prioritise and manage their work. However they lack the flexibility and speed of proficient nurses.
- **Stage 4 – Proficient.** Proficient nurses perceive situations holistically, recognise important and less important elements, and make decisions quickly. Benner found proficiency in nurses who have worked in an area for some time.
- **Stage 5 – Expert.** Expert nurses have a deep understanding and an intuitive grasp of situations, gained from substantial experience in the practice setting. You may observe this level in some practitioners with whom you work. In her book, Benner gives many examples of expert nurses' care for clients. Such nurses may be excellent and inspirational role models but it is important not to feel inadequate or overawed by such expertise.

Developing the affective, cognitive and motor dimensions of a skill

Knight (1998) provides a detailed review of theories about learning psychomotor skills.

The affective dimension

Woodward's (1997) analysis indicates that developing the affective dimension of a skill requires practice and perseverance, just as will the motor element. Roach (1992) suggested that, while nursing students may start their course with rudimentary expressive caring skills, these sometimes go unrecognised and unvalued and may be eroded rather than developed further. This book includes activities throughout which focus on the affective dimension, asking you to think about, for example, how a patient might be feeling in a particular situation. Chapter 2 concentrates on the affective dimension of practical skills, and will help you to understand the concept of self-awareness and how your values might affect how you carry out your care.

The cognitive dimension

Learning the cognitive elements of skills involves you acquiring and understanding the underpinning knowledge and rationale. Throughout this book the evidence base for practical skills is discussed, but there are also activities encouraging you to draw on other sources of knowledge, such as reflecting on your experience. These activities will help you to develop an enquiring and problem-solving approach to your nursing practice.

The motor dimension

Learning the motor dimension of a psychomotor skill requires practice – the opportunity to try out and repeat performance. It is only with practice that movement becomes refined and a smooth coordinated performance can develop. The amount of practice needed varies according to motivation to learn the skill, previous related skills learning, familiarity with equipment, level of anxiety, the physical resources and the learner's coordination (Oermann 1990). More complex skills need more practice. Motivation affects mastery as many skills are initially difficult, but highly motivated students will persevere. If you have had previous experience of a related skill, some of the skill's component parts will be familiar, so then your practice can focus on parts of the skill not already learned. Familiarity with equipment also eases the learning of a new skill.

There are key points a facilitator can do to help when you are learning a new skill (see Box 1.6).

You yourself can be active about promoting these conditions. For example, the best time to ask a nurse to supervise you drawing up an injection for the first time is not in the middle of an emergency situation, as the stress and anxiety in the environment are unlikely to be conducive to learning. Thus when asking to be supervised carrying out a skill, pick the right moment! Be open about your prior knowledge, saying explicitly that you have, for example, practised injection technique in the skills laboratory, have observed injection administration in practice, and now feel ready to be supervised preparing and administering an injection.

De Tornyay and Thompson (1987) highlighted that learners need to handle equipment as this diffuses anxiety; therefore always take opportunities to become familiar with equipment that you are likely to use. This book will help by explaining what type of equipment is used for the skills discussed and includes illustrations

---

Box 1.6 How a facilitator can help a student learn a practical skill (adapted from Quinn and Hughes 2007)

- Provide an atmosphere conducive to learning.
- Carry out a skills analysis.
- Determine the procedure sequence.
- Assess the student's prior knowledge.
- Demonstrate the skill at normal speed.
- Teach the procedure sequence.
- Teach the skill by either whole learning or part learning.
- Allocate sufficient time to practise.
- Provide feedback on performance.
- Prompt student to self-evaluate.
- Encourage transfer of skills.

of equipment. There is also advice about where you can access equipment with which to become familiar. De Tornyay and Thompson suggested that adult learners can be self-conscious when trying out new skills. You need to be supervised when practising a new skill, but you may wish to ensure that there won't be too big an audience if you feel that you will be self-conscious! A warm and accepting learning environment helps to reduce excess anxiety that might adversely affect your performance. Although supervisors should avoid the temptation to 'take over', they will need to do so if safety is compromised. Learning practical skills requires the opportunity to practise and gain feedback (Quinn and Hughes 2007) to reinforce correct behaviour and eliminate error.

The importance of obtaining feedback

Gaining feedback when you are developing skills is important for your learning. From whom can you gain feedback? Obviously staff supervising you can give you feedback. It is best if the comments are as specific as possible rather than a general comment such as 'very good', or 'you need to be quicker'. It will help your supervisor if you identify any aspects in particular that you want feedback about. For example, you might state that when performing the skill last time, the supervisor said that you needed to give a clearer explanation to the client, and ask that they give you feedback on this aspect in particular. Patients and clients can also give you feedback. They may make spontaneous comments, such as that they feel 'much more comfortable now', but you can also seek feedback specifically, by asking how they feel at different stages. If you are approachable in the way you seek feedback, people are more likely to give honest responses. Your observation of patients/clients while you are carrying out practical skills will also give you feedback; for example, you can observe for facial expressions that might indicate fear or discomfort.

The sources of feedback outlined so far will provide *extrinsic* feedback. Combined with *intrinsic* feedback, this should give you a balanced view of your performance. Intrinsic feedback involves you reflecting on your performance, and asking yourself what were the strengths and weaknesses and how you could improve your performance next time.

Learning from experience and reflection

You need to become skilled at learning from experience so that you can benefit fully from your practice experience. To develop competency, practice is necessary, but is it inevitable that experience leads to learning and improved performance? Bjork's (1999b) study followed the progress of four newly qualified nurses' practical skill development and focused on the skill of mobilising a patient postoperatively. In fact the nurses' skills performance did not necessarily improve over time. Some aspects in some nurses improved while other aspects deteriorated. Bjork's findings led her to question why nurses with 8–14 months' experience 'do not give the patient sufficient physical support during ambulation, or that basic attention to the patient's clothing and comfort is missing?' She also found that nurses became quicker and seemingly more efficient, but learned to cut corners in a way that was apparently acceptable. Andrews *et al.* (1998) suggest that continued repetition of skills may lead to merely habitual behaviour, rather than conscious analysis of actions.

Bjork (1999b) theorised a number of possible reasons why these nurses' performance did not necessarily improve with experience. She questioned whether their knowledge base was adequate, suggesting that some skills are inadequately described in nursing textbooks. She identified, therefore, that nurses cannot use in practice knowledge that they do not have, but equally, they may not use in practice the knowledge that they do have. However, she also identified lack of reflection on experience as a possible cause. She suggested that nurses are often intent on long-term outcomes and that opportunity to reflect and learn from practice is delayed or embedded in a broader context. The results of our actions in everyday life are often clear and direct, therefore making an obvious connection between our action and its result. For example, if you leave a cake in the oven too long it will burn, so you might take more care next time. The result of nurses' failure to wash their hands after dealing with patients is unlikely to be immediately obvious.

Dewey, an educational theorist, argued that we do not 'learn by doing' but by 'doing and realizing what came of what we did' (Dewey 1929, p. 367). Dewey's theories were developed further by Kolb and Fry (1975), and then more fully by Kolb (1984). The theory of how we learn from experience is often referred to as 'experiential learning', and is portrayed as a cycle. The process starts at the point of a concrete experience or event, after which observations and reflections occur, followed by abstract conceptualisation, where new ideas are developed, linked to other knowledge and experience, and then the new knowledge arising from the experience is tested out in a new situation. This new experience then starts the experiential learning cycle once again.

Reflection enables you to consider what you did and why, and provides opportunities to develop knowledge from experience and link theory and practice. Johns (2004) defined reflection as:

> ... being mindful of self, either within or after experience, as if a window through which the practitioner can view and focus self within the context of a particular experience, in order to confront, understand and move toward resolving contradiction between one's vision and actual practice. *(p. 3)*

Thus reflection can assist practitioners to become aware of conflicts between aims of care and the reality of practice, and these insights can enable nurses to become more effective. Johns (2004, p. 2) identified 'reflection-on-experience', which occurs after the event with insights gained informing future practice. Knowledge gained from reflection on practice has been termed 'practical knowledge' (Schon 1987) and reflection can enable the uncovering of knowledge embedded in practice (Lawler 1991). Johns also identified other layers of reflection, including 'reflection-in-action', where the person pauses during a situation to make sense of it and then proceeds more effectively, and 'mindful practice' – being aware of self during 'an unfolding moment with the intention of realising desirable practice' (p. 2). See Johns (2004) for an in-depth exploration of how you can become a reflective practitioner.

To think over or mull over an event is commonplace, but without an analytical and purposeful approach it may not lead to new ways of thinking or behaving (Andrews *et al.* 1998). To help you to develop your reflective skills you could write reflective accounts which may be included in your portfolio, recording significant events which you experience in your nursing practice. This activity can assist you to develop evaluative and decision-making skills, and help you to link theory and practice (Howard 2004). Remember: you must not identify patients or clients (either by name or by using other identifying material) in your reflective writing, to maintain confidentiality. You may take part in reflective activities within the classroom setting where you will be encouraged to reflect on specific incidents from practice. You may be recommended to use a reflective model, which can help you to be more structured and systematic about your reflection.

Skills laboratories and simulation

As students need opportunities to rehearse skills in a safe environment, most universities have simulation facilities: skills laboratories or centres where you can practise skills. In simulation, students learn in a realistic clinical environment where they practise a range of skills without the risk of harming patients and then apply these skills in the clinical setting (Wilford and Doyle 2006). Simulation is increasingly commonplace in healthcare education (Bradley 2003; Feingold *et al.* 2003), and the NMC (2007b) has endorsed the benefits of simulation in nurse education. Learning in the skills laboratory can help to reduce anxiety about clinical placement experience and develop confidence. Skills laboratories also provide a more controlled environment for familiarisation with skills than do practice settings.

Skills laboratories vary in complexity and resources but usually contain clinical equipment for practising technical procedures. Some skills, such as blood pressure measurement, can be practised safely on your peers and there will be simulation models for practising other skills. Some skills laboratories organise volunteer 'patients' for students' practice. Universities have different systems for learning in skills laboratories, which you should become familiar with. There may be compulsory sessions, optional workshops, and formal or informal sessions. Activities within the chapters of this book often suggest that you access equipment to practise with if possible. You will need to find out about your local policies/procedures for use of equipment in the skills laboratory and there may be a code of behaviour for users to ensure safety. Your placement provider or employing organisation may also have simulation facilities for skills learning.

Some skills laboratories include video equipment so that students can analyse their performance afterwards (Knight and Mowforth 1998). Watching the video objectively and identifying your strengths and areas for improvement will help you to enhance your skills performance. Increasingly students' skills are tested in the classroom, through a process termed 'objective structured clinical examination' (OSCE). OSCEs require students to carry out practical skills with simulated patients or manikins, in response to a given scenario, and their performance is assessed against pre-set criteria (Nicol and Freeth 1998).

Learning in the practice setting

Skills laboratory practice does not replace skills practice within clinical placements; practising skills with patients/clients in the healthcare environment is essential to develop competence. It is important, however, not to see clients as just people to be practised on, thereby objectifying them. Roach (1992) suggested that, instead, students should see themselves as being 'in a helping therapeutic relationship with clients who freely collaborate in the educational enterprise' (p. 120). Practical skills development and practice should therefore take place within the context of the relationship between you and the client, as part of their holistic care. Obviously you should take every opportunity to develop new skills, but not within a task-orientated framework that is dehumanising and objectifies people. Learning practical skills should thus occur within the total care required for each individual.

When starting a new clinical placement you may well feel anxious or even fearful, but be reassured that you are not alone in these feelings. Starting a new placement has been likened to starting a new job! Each practice setting has its own culture and you need to familiarise yourself with the environment, staff and routines (Nolan 1998). Until you 'settle in' and start to feel part of the team, effective learning can be difficult. Some practice settings send you information prior to your placement to help you feel welcome and reduce anxiety, and often a pre-placement visit is encouraged. Alternatively this information may be available to you on the intranet; do make sure you access it and make good use of this facility.

In *Standards to Support Learning and Assessment in Practice,* the NMC (2008b) detail how students' effective learning and assessment in practice can be facilitated. When students enter a new practice setting they can sometimes feel overwhelmed by the range of learning opportunities. Placement areas often identify what specific learning opportunities are available and these will include learning practical skills.

In any practice setting you will have an assigned mentor, whose remit includes supporting you in:

- identifying your learning needs
- addressing these learning needs through enabling you to practise, and giving feedback
- assessing your performance.

The NMC (2008b) identifies the mentor's role in detail. Your role should be an active one throughout this learning process.

Identifying your learning needs

When identifying your learning needs you should take into account:

- the learning outcomes for your stage of the course;
- your prior learning, from previous practice placements, and any relevant experience prior to entering nurse education

- any learning needs that were identified during your previous practice placements
- the specific learning opportunities identified by this placement.

Your mentor will discuss these learning needs with you, and can advise of the learning opportunities in the practice area that can assist you, but you must be honest about your strengths and areas needing improvement. Your learning needs are likely to include practical skills but will address other needs too.

Addressing your learning needs

The earlier section 'Learning from experience and reflection' gives you insight into how you can most benefit from your clinical experience. You need to be active in seeking out your learning opportunities. Being aware of how practical skills are learned will help you to make the best use of opportunities available, ensuring that you observe a skill first, and ask for supervised practice until you feel confident to practise the skill independently. While some skills need minimal practice, others are much more complex and need repeated practice. You should not attempt a skill unsupervised unless you are confident of your ability. You will be given feedback during practice placements to guide your learning. As discussed before, the practical skills you develop should be considered within the holistic care of patients, and not as isolated tasks which you have learned to perform.

You can be more proactive about learning in the practice setting if you are aware of different learning methods. There is much you can learn from observing others in the practice setting, but you need to distinguish between 'good' professional role models and 'poor' ones. In some practice settings there may be formal teaching sessions organised. This might be particularly appropriate when there are several students in a placement area, and where workload is predictable so a specific time can be set aside for teaching sessions. Formal teaching sessions enable you to prepare, by pre-reading for example. Informal teaching occurs more spontaneously 'on the spot'. Such sessions can be particularly meaningful as they are likely to be linked with the clinical practice occurring at that time. Sometimes a critical incident can be used as a basis for reflection in the practice setting. This might be a situation that has occurred which was difficult or challenging, such as where a relative has complained about lack of care by staff. Critical incident analysis can aid reflection and learning from such a situation.

Here is an example of how you might employ different learning methods in the practice setting. When taking part in medicine administration, you can actively observe a qualified nurse, either asking questions at the time (if appropriate) or making a note of questions for later or of specific medicines you want to find out about. The nurse you are with might ask you questions to check your understanding and encourage you to think about what is happening. You may be able to take part in practical elements such as dispensing of tablets or preparing a nebuliser. If a difficult situation occurs, for example a patient declines his tablets, you could use this incident to reflect afterwards and develop knowledge from this experience. You could consider, for example, whether a different approach to the patient would have made any difference, or whether an adequate explanation about the tablets was given. You could also follow up later by looking up information about medicines that you encountered and were not familiar with.

RECOMMENDED READING

As stated earlier, the remit of this book is to help you to develop a foundation in practical nursing skills. For guidance about reading material for other aspects you should refer to the recommended reading list for your course.

Many practical nursing skills require an underlying biological knowledge base. For example, when taking and recording blood pressure it is necessary to understand what blood pressure is and how it is maintained. A foundation in biology is not, however, within the scope of this book and you should gain your biological knowledge from the biology texts available, many of which are aimed specifically at student nurses.

When working through each chapter of this book it is sensible to have an understanding of the related biology, so each chapter includes biology questions. Use your recommended text to check your biological knowledge by finding out the answers to the questions posed. Studying the relevant biology and then working through the chapter can help to make the biology more comprehensible and memorable, as you can see its immediate relevance and applicability to nursing practice.

Your recommended reading list is likely to include ethics, sociology and psychology texts, all of which also provide underpinning knowledge for nursing skills, assisting you to care for people holistically.

CHAPTER SUMMARY

All nurses must be competent in a range of practical nursing skills. This book addresses skills that are generally applicable to nurses working with adults in a range of settings and all the Essential Skills Clusters (NMC 2007a) are included.

Practical nursing skills should be carried out therapeutically and within the context of caring. They include motor, affective and cognitive dimensions, and to become competent requires all three aspects to be developed.

In today's multicultural society, nurses need to develop cultural competence which was also introduced in this chapter. Nurses applying skills with people in any healthcare setting must ensure that they promote their dignity while carrying out care.

To develop competence requires practice and experience, which should include gaining feedback and reflection, thus maximising learning from experience. Through classroom preparation in a skills laboratory or equivalent setting, students can develop familiarity with equipment and the sequential steps of a skill, and the cognitive and affective domains can also be introduced. Carrying out practical skills in the dynamic and variable environment of the clinical setting is affected by many factors. Repeated practice in the clinical setting is needed to become competent and confident in practical skills, and students need to be proactive in seeking out opportunities for learning.

REFERENCES

Alliex, S. and Irurita, V.F. 2004. Caring in a technological environment: how is this possible? *Contemporary Nurse* **17**(1–2), 32–43.

Andrews, M., Gidman, J. and Humphreys, A. 1998. Reflection: does it enhance professional nursing practice? *British Journal of Nursing* **7**, 413–17.

Arman, M. and Rehnsfeldt, A. 2007. The 'Little Extra' that alleviates suffering. *Nursing Ethics* **14**, 372–86.

Baillie, L. 2007. *A Case Study of Patient Dignity in an Acute Hospital Setting*. Unpublished thesis. London South Bank University.

Benner, P. 1984. *From Novice to Expert*. Boston: Addison-Wesley.

Benner, P. and Wrubel, J. 1989. *The Primacy of Caring*. Boston: Addison-Wesley.

Bjork, I.T. 1999a. What constitutes a nursing practical skill? *Western Journal of Nursing Research* **21**, 51–70.

Bjork, I.T. 1999b. Practical skill development in new nurses. *Nursing Inquiry* **6**, 34–47.

Bradley, P., 2003. Simulation in clinical learning. *Medication Education* **37** (Suppl 1), 1–5.

Bradshaw, A. 1994. *Lighting the Lamp: The spiritual dimension of nursing care*. Harrow: Scutari Press.

British Red Cross, St Andrew's Ambulance Association and St John Ambulance 2006. *First Aid Manual*, 8th revised edn. London: Dorling Kindersley.

Bush, H.A. and Barr, W.J. 1997. Critical care nurses' lived experiences of caring. *Heart and Lung* **26**, 387–98.

Chochinov, H.M., Hack, T., McClement, S., Kristjanson, L. and Harlos, M. 2002. Dignity in the terminally ill: a developing empirical model. *Social Science and Medicine* **54**, 433–43.

Cioffi, J. 2005. Nurses' experiences of caring for culturally diverse patients in an acute care setting. *Contemporary Nurse* **20**(1), 78–96.

Cortis, J.D. 2000. Perceptions and experiences with nursing care: a study of Pakistani (Urdu) Communities in the United Kingdom. *Journal of Transcultural Nursing* **11**, 111–18.

Department of Health (DH) 2001a. *The Essence of Care: Patient-focused benchmarking for health care practitioners*. London.

— 2001b. *Valuing People: A new strategy for learning disability for the 21st century*. London.

— 2006a. *Best Practice Competencies and Capabilities for Pre-registration Mental Health Nurses in England: The Chief Nursing Officer's review of mental health nursing*. London.

— 2006b. *Essence of Care: Benchmarks for promoting health*. London.

— 2006c. *Dignity in Care Public Survey*. Available from www.dh.gov.uk/dignityincare. Accessed 22 November 2006.

— 2006d. *About the Dignity in Care Campaign*. Available from www.dh.gov.uk. Accessed 22 August 2006.

— 2007a. *Essence of Care: Benchmarks for the Care Environment*. London.

— 2007b. *Valuing People Now: From progress to transformation*. London.

— 2007c. *Good Practice in Learning Disability Nursing*. London.

Department of Health and Social Security (DHSS) 2005. *Equal Lives: Review of policy and services for people with a learning disability in Northern Ireland*. Belfast.

de Tornyay, R. and Thompson, M.A. 1987. *Strategies for Teaching Nursing*, third edn. New York: Delmar Publishing.

Dewey, J. 1929. *Experience and Nature*. New York: Grove Press.

Duffy, J.R., Hoskins, L. and Seifert, R.F. 2007. Dimensions of caring: psychometric evaluation of the caring assessment tool. *Advances in Nursing Science* **30**(3), 235–45.

Ersser, S. 1998. The presentation of the nurse: a neglected dimension of therapeutic nurse–patient interaction? In McMahon, R. and Pearson, A. (eds) *Nursing as Therapy,* 2nd edn. Cheltenham: Stanley Thornes, 36–63.

Feingold, C.E., Calaluce, M. and Kallen, M.A. 2003. Computerized patient model and simulated clinical experiences: evaluation with baccalaureate nursing students. *Journal of Nursing Education* **43**(4), 156–63.

Fitzpatrick, J.M., While, A.E. and Roberts, J.D. 1992. The role of the nurse in high-quality patient care: a review of the literature. *Journal of Advanced Nursing* **17,** 1210–19.

Great Britain 1998. *Human Rights Act* c. 42. London: HMSO.

Halldorsdottir, S. 1991. Five basic modes of being with another. In Gaut, D.A. and Leininger, M.M. (eds) *Caring: The compassionate healer.* New York: National League for Nursing Press, 37–49.

Health Advisory Service 2000. 1998. *'Not because they are Old': An independent inquiry into the care of older people on acute wards in general hospitals.* London: Health Advisory Service 2000.

Henderson, A., van Eps, M.A., Pearson, K. *et al.* 2007. 'Caring for' behaviours that indicate to patients that nurses 'care about' them. *Journal of Advanced Nursing* **60**(2), 146–53.

Howard, A. 2004. Learning and teaching in practice. In Hinchliff, S. (ed.) *The Practitioner as Teacher,* 3rd edn. Edinburgh: Baillière Tindall, 61–105.

Joffe, S., Manocchia, M., Weeks, J.C. and Cleary, P.D. 2003. What do patients value in their hospital care? An empirical perspective on autonomy centred bioethics. *Journal of Medical Ethics* **29**(2), 103–8.

Johns, C. 2004. *Becoming a Reflective Practitioner,* 2nd edn. Oxford: Blackwell.

Knight, C. 1998. Evaluating a skills centre: the acquisition of psychomotor skills in nursing – a review of the literature. *Nurse Education Today* **18,** 441–7.

Knight, C.M. and Mowforth, G.M. 1998. Skills centre: why we did it, how we did it. *Nurse Education Today* **18,** 389–93.

Kolb, D.A. 1984. *Experiential Learning: Experience as the source of learning and development.* London: Prentice Hall International.

Kolb, D.A. and Fry, R. 1975. Towards an applied theory of experiential learning. In Cooper, C.L. (ed.) *Theories of Group Processes.* London: John Wiley, 33–57.

Kralik, D., Koch, T. and Wotton, K. 1997. Engagement and detachment: understanding patients' experiences with nursing. *Journal of Advanced Nursing* **26,** 399–407.

Lawler, J. 1991. *Behind the Screens: Nursing somology and the problem of the body.* London: Churchill Livingstone.

Learning Disability Advisory Group 2001. *Fulfilling the promises: Report of the learning disability advisory group.* Cardiff: National Assembly for Wales.

Leishman, J.L. 2006. Culturally sensitive mental health care: a module for 21st century education and practice. *International Journal of Psychiatric Nursing Research* **11**(3), 1310–21.

Leininger, M. 1981. Transcultural nursing: its progress and its future. *Nursing and Health Care* **2,** 365–71.

Manley, K. 1997. Knowledge for nursing practice. In Perry, A. and Jolley, M. (eds) *Nursing: A knowledge base for practice,* 2nd edn. London: Arnold, 301–33.

Matiti, M.R. 2002. *Patient Dignity in Nursing: A phenomenological study.* Unpublished thesis, University of Huddersfield School of Education and Professional Development.

McMahon, R. 1998. Therapeutic nursing: theory, issues and practice. In McMahon, R. and Pearson, A. (eds) *Nursing as Therapy,* 2nd edn. Cheltenham: Stanley Thornes, 1–20.

Mencap 2004. *Treat Me Right! Better healthcare for people with a learning disability.* London: Mencap.

Mencap 2007. *Death by Indifference: Following up the Treat Me Right! report.* London: Mencap.

NHS Modernisation Agency 2003. *Essence of Care: Patient-focused benchmarks for clinical governance.* London: NHS Modernisation Agency.

Nicol, M. and Freeth, D. 1998. Assessment of clinical skills: a new approach to an old problem. *Nurse Education Today* **18,** 601–9.

Nolan, C.A. 1998. Learning on clinical placement: the experience of six Australian student nurses. *Nurse Education Today* **18,** 622–9.

Nursing and Midwifery Council (NMC) 2004. *Standards of Proficiency for Pre-registration Nursing Education.* London.

— 2007a. *Introduction of Essential Skills Clusters for Pre-registration Nursing Programmes.* NMC Circular 07/2007.

— 2007b. *Supporting Direct Care through Simulated Practice Learning in the Pre-registration Nursing Programme.* NMC Circular 36/2007.

— 2008a. *The Code: Standards of conduct, performance and ethics for nurses and midwives.* London.

— 2008b. *Standards to Support Learning and Assessment in Practice,* 2nd edn. London.

Oermann, M.H. 1990. Psychomotor skill development. *Journal of Continuing Education in Nursing* **21,** 202–4.

Papadopoulos, I. 2006a. The Papadopoulos, Tilki and Taylor model of developing cultural competence. In Papadopoulos, I. (ed.) *Transcultural Health and Social Care: Development of culturally competent practitioners.* Edinburgh: Churchill Livingstone, 7–24.

Papadopoulos, I. (ed.) 2006b. *Transcultural Health and Social Care: Development of culturally competent practitioners.* Edinburgh: Churchill Livingstone.

Paterson, J. and Zderad, L. 1988. *Humanistic Nursing.* New York: League for Nursing.

Quinn, F. and Hughes, S.J. 2007. *Quinn's Principles and Practice of Nurse Education,* 5th edn. Cheltenham: Nelson–Thornes.

Randle, J. 2001. Past caring? The influence of technology. *Nurse Education Today* **1,** 157–65.

Reynolds, C.L. and Leininger, M. 1993. *Madeleine Leininger: Cultural care diversity and universality theory.* Newbury Park: Sage.

Roach, M.S. 1992. *The Human Act of Caring: A blueprint for the health professions,* revised edn. Ottawa: Canadian Hospital Association Press.

Roach, M.S. 2002. *Caring, the Human Mode of Being: A blueprint for the health professions,* 2nd revised edn. Ottawa: Canadian Hospital Association Press.

Rogers, A., Karlsen, S. and Addington-Hall, J. 2000. 'All the services were excellent. It is when the human element comes in that things go wrong': dissatisfaction with hospital care in the last year of life. *Journal of Advanced Nursing* **31,** 768–74.

Romyn, D.M. 1999. Commentary. *Western Journal of Nursing Research* **21,** 64–70.

Royal College of Nursing 2006. *Meeting the Health Needs of People with Learning Disabilities: Guidance for nursing staff.* London.

— 2008. *Defending Dignity: Challenges and opportunities for nurses.* London.

Schon, D. 1987. *Educating the Reflective Practitioner.* San Fransisco: Jossey-Bass.

Scottish Executive 2000. *The Same as You: A review of services for people with learning disability.* Edinburgh: Scottish Executive.

Scottish Government 2006. *Delivering Care, Enabling Health: Harnessing the nursing, midwifery and allied health professions' contribution to implementing delivering for health in Scotland.* Edinburgh: Scottish Government. Available from www.scotland.gov.uk/Publications/2006/10/23103937/4. Accessed 28 May 2008.

Social Care Institute for Excellence (SCIE) 2006. *Practice Guide 09: Dignity in care.* Available from www.scie.org.uk/publications/practiceguides/practiceguide09. Accessed 28 May 2008.

Thorsteinsson, L. 2002. The quality of nursing care as perceived by individuals with chronic illnesses: the magic touch of nursing. *Journal of Advanced Nursing* **11,** 32–40.

Wallis, M.C. 1998. Responding to suffering: the experience of professional nurse caring in the coronary care unit. *International Journal for Human Caring* **2,** 35–44.

Watson, J. 1979. *Nursing: The philosophy and science of caring.* Boston: Little Brown.

Wilford, A., Doyle, T.J., 2006. Integrating simulation training into the nursing curriculum. *British Journal of Nursing* **15**(11), 604–7.

Woodward, V.M. 1997. Professional caring: a contradiction in terms? *Journal of Advanced Nursing* **26,** 999–1004.

USEFUL WEBSITES

- Department of Health: www.dh.gov.uk
- Welsh Assembly Government: wales.gov.uk/topics/health
- Dignity in Care: www.dh.gov.uk/dignityincare
- Scottish Government: www.scotland.gov.uk/Topics/Health
- Department of Health, Social Security and Public Safety (Northern Ireland): www.dhsspsni.gov.uk
- National Library for Health: www.library.nhs.uk
- National Institute for Health and Clinical Excellence: www.nice.org.uk
- Nursing and Midwifery Council: www.nmc-uk.org
- National Patient Safety Agency: www.npsa.nhs.uk
- Resuscitation Council (UK): www.resus.org.uk
- University of York: NHS Centre for Reviews and Dissemination: www.york.ac.uk/inst/crd
- St John Ambulance first aid advice: www.sja.org.uk/sja/first-aid-advice.aspx
- Social Care Institute for Excellence (SCIE): www.scie.org.uk

The Nurse's Approach and Communication: Foundations for Compassionate Care

Nicola M. Neale and Joanne Sale

When we communicate with others they are inevitably influenced by our behaviour and our responses. Therefore our actions and those of others do not happen in isolation; they are a reflection of the internal and external environment of all involved in the interaction.

As we suggest above, any interaction is a two-way process and therefore nurses must be aware that their approach to clients/patients in any setting affects the outcome. This book focuses on practical nursing skills and in this chapter we explore nurse–client interactions while carrying out skills. The chapter addresses the 'Care, compassion and communication' theme in the Nursing and Midwifery Council's (NMC) (2007) Essential Skills Clusters (ESC), which outline expectations of student and newly qualified nurses.

> This chapter includes:
> - Understanding what influences the nurse's approach to care
> - The communication process
> - Developing and maintaining therapeutic relationships
> - Communication in challenging situations

PRACTICE SCENARIOS

The following scenarios, taken from later chapters, will be referred to in the text. *Definitions of medical terms in these scenarios can be found in the chapters in which they appear.*

Chapter 3 – Preventing cross-infection

Mrs Winifred Lewis, aged 87, was widowed many years ago and lives in wardened accommodation. She has a history of rheumatoid arthritis and type 2 diabetes, and recently fell and fractured her hip. This was operated on in hospital but the wound developed an infection, which grew MRSA. She was discharged home, under the care of the district nursing team and intermediate care, but her wound deteriorated and the surrounding skin showed signs of infection. Mrs Lewis appeared unwell and dehydrated, so her GP requested readmission. She is now being isolated in the side room of a surgical ward, and an intravenous infusion and intravenous antibiotics have been commenced. She has a commode in the room and can transfer with help.

Chapter 4 – Fundamental vital signs measurement

Natalie Turney is 21 years old. She has been admitted as a voluntary patient to an acute mental health ward with severe depression. After going home for a day she returns, appearing unsteady on her feet and she has a strong smell of alcohol. Her speech is very slurred and she is quite uncommunicative. When the staff ask her if she has taken any tablets she mentions some 'little yellow pills' and paracetamol. However, she won't give details about the quantity or when she took them.

Chapter 5 – Administration of medicines

Mercy Makumbe is 72 years old. She has recently had a below-knee amputation of her leg, has a long history of cardiovascular disease, and has now been transferred to her local community hospital, where she is currently receiving subcutaneous heparin, as well as oral morphine solution for pain. For years she has taken diuretics and other medication for her cardiac problems and she is concerned about having to take regular strong pain-relieving medicines too. She has had a known penicillin allergy for some time. Mercy has also been prescribed fucidin cream for a small infected area behind one ear. A recent urinalysis showed blood in her urine.

Chapter 8 – Meeting hygiene needs

William Newton, who likes to be called 'Bill', is a retired accountant aged 73. He is terminally ill with a history of oesophageal cancer and metastases in his lungs. He is cared for by his wife at home with the support of community nurses and the Macmillan nurse. He is taking regular oral morphine for pain control. He has a very low haemoglobin and has been admitted for a blood transfusion. He is weak and breathless and his general condition is poor. He has a body mass index (BMI) of 16. Bill can swallow only very small amounts of liquidised food and drink. He has some of his own teeth but also a partial denture which he likes to wear although it is now ill-fitting. His tongue appears coated and his mouth is dry.

Chapter 10 – Nutrition and fluid balance

Miss Alice West is 84 years old and has been transferred from a medical ward to a rehabilitation unit following a stroke which has caused right-sided weakness. The medical ward staff who transferred her handed over that although she initially had swallowing problems she has since been assessed as being able to swallow. However, her appetite is very poor and she often eats only a few small mouthfuls, refusing any more. The staff have been keeping a food chart and a fluid chart which confirm her poor intake. She has dentures but they appear loose. Her niece is concerned that she is 'looking thin' and seems depressed. Miss West is often uncommunicative but on occasions expresses herself clearly. She is also registered partially sighted. Her weight on admission was 58 kg and is now 53 kg. Her height is 1.64 metres.

Chapter 12 – Managing pain and promoting comfort

Maria is a 58-year-old woman with a moderate learning disability living in a group home. She was diagnosed with breast cancer eight years ago and underwent surgery and chemotherapy. However, the cancer has returned and she now has bony metastases in her left hip, making it painful to mobilise. She also has metastases in her ovaries, lungs and liver. The community learning disability nurse is her health facilitator and is coordinating her care plan. He is working with Maria and other professionals to understand her illness and treatment plan and gain Maria's consent. He and the occupational therapist are supporting Maria, with input from her family, friends and carers, to develop Maria's 'lifebook', which celebrates her life's experiences and includes many photos and Maria's wishes and aspirations. The nurse is also working with the staff team, Maria's family (she has three siblings, two of whom live locally with their families), the district nurse, physiotherapist and the palliative care team to establish an individual pain assessment scale and effective pain management. Maria mobilises with difficulty and is currently taking non-opiate analgesics.

Chapter 12 – Managing pain and promoting comfort

Violet Davies, aged 76, has advanced Alzheimer's disease. She has been admitted to a care home, as her husband is physically and emotionally exhausted and unable to cope. He has refused help in the past as he has been determined to look after his wife, but he has now agreed to her admission. Violet is physically well but she is also known to have osteoarthritis in her right hip. She looks permanently worried and agitated and keeps repeating the same phrase over and over again. Mr Davies looks shaky and tearful.

UNDERSTANDING WHAT INFLUENCES THE NURSE'S APPROACH TO CARE

LEARNING OUTCOMES

By the end of this section you will be able to:
1 understand the terms 'self-concept' and 'self-awareness' and apply them in a reflective manner within a caring context;
2 outline how personality may be important in nurse–client relationships;
3 discuss attitudes, values and beliefs and their impact in the care environment;
4 understand the terms 'stereotyping' and 'labelling' and their significance to the care environment.

Learning outcome 1: Understand the terms 'self-concept' and 'self-awareness' and apply them in a reflective manner within a caring context

Self-awareness can be defined as 'focussing on self as well as, recognising, knowing, and accepting of self' (Rungapadiachy 2007, p. 4). An awareness of self is essential to inform supportive therapeutic relationships. Rungapadiachy sees self-awareness as a skill that nurses need to develop, comprising three components: *cognitive* (how we think and form an understanding), *affective* (our feelings and emotions) and *behavioural* (the outward expression – verbal or non-verbal). There is a dynamic

	You know	You don't know
Others know	Public area	Blind area
Others don't know	Hidden area	Unknown area

Figure 2.1: Johari window (Luft and Ingram 1955).

relationship between these components. So, for example, you need to be aware of what you think about a client who has an alcohol problem and how this may affect your feelings and behaviour towards them.

One way of developing self-awareness is to use a model such as the Johari window (see Fig. 2.1), which was developed to help individuals to identify aspects of self. This model suggests that self-disclosure and receiving feedback – i.e. telling others about yourself and seeking feedback from them – helps increase your awareness of self. This occurs because the public area increases in relation to the other three areas as your understanding of your own strengths and weaknesses grows.

ACTIVITY

How might being self-aware be important for you when carrying out practical skills?

You may have considered several aspects. For example, if you have had an argument at home you may understand why you feel impatient with a person who appears to lack motivation to assist with hygiene needs. Acknowledging your emotional state will help you to understand your feelings and the subsequent effect on your caregiving. This increased awareness may highlight a need to adapt your behaviour.

Healthcare professionals should develop understanding of how and why they behave in certain circumstances because, as Jack and Smith (2007) suggest, having an increased self-awareness helps us to relate to others. Therefore the crucial point about self-awareness is its impact on our communication with others, and how it can help us to recognise the effects of our behaviour.

ACTIVITY

Reflect upon a recent situation where your behaviour might have had an impact. Recall your thoughts, feelings and emotions related to this incident and whether these affected your actions, choice of words or your relationship with others.

For example, you may have considered:

- If you were angry at the time, did you shout?
- Did you say things that you regretted? Did you 'storm off'?
- If you were sad, did you cry? Were you too emotional to speak?
- Were you able to listen effectively?

Now consider how your behaviour might have influenced the situation, either positively or negatively. If you raised your voice did the other person also raise their voice? Or did they become aggressive or cry? It is helpful for nurses to reflect upon their own behaviour and how it affects others' responses.

In Chapter 1, reflection was identified as being a conscious activity that usually involves a change in behaviour. Reflection, therefore, should help to increase awareness of how psychological, sociological, physical and contextual factors affect relationships with others. A lack of self-awareness can lead to serious problems in nurse–client relationships. Eckroth-Bucher (2001, p. 33) suggests that 'understanding another begins with understanding yourself'.

Self-concept can be defined as the information and beliefs that individuals have about their own nature, qualities and behaviour (Rogers 1961). However, Gross and Kinnison (2007, p. 295) suggest that it is a 'hypothetical construct' that each of us develops about ourselves: this is dynamic, never complete and helps us to understand not only who we are but how we fit into society. Schaffer (2004) suggests that self-concept is always affected by how other people evaluate us.

ACTIVITY

Describe yourself, including your strengths and weaknesses. Spend 5 minutes writing down the aspects of yourself that you would like a stranger to know. Then ask one of your friends to describe you and compare:
- Does their view match yours?
- Were there things that you did not know about yourself?
- What do any differences tell you about yourself? (the authors accept no responsibility for the break-up of friendships!).

It is generally accepted that there are three components to self-concept (Gross and Kinnison 2007): self-image, self-esteem and the ideal self. Look back to the strengths and weaknesses that you identified in the previous activity. How might the above three components be relevant?

Self-image

Self-image is the way in which we would describe ourselves. Kuhn and McPartland (1954) (cited by Gross and Kinnison 2007) suggest that this can be found by asking a person to answer the question 'Who am I?' 20 times. The answer might include social roles, physical characteristics (or body image), and personality traits (see Fig. 2.2). Looking back at your strengths and weaknesses, did your list include any of these three areas?

You may have thought about social roles. Did you consider the different roles you have in your life: student, friend, nurse? Did you consider your lifestyle and how this affects choices you make, your religious/spiritual beliefs, and how your sexuality affects your sense of who you are? You may have considered your personality: do you see yourself as an outgoing person or a shy person? Personality is discussed later. You may have included physical characteristics; how you view your body is referred to as 'body image'.

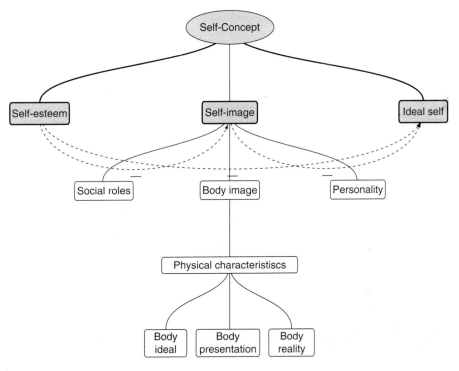

Figure 2.2: Pictorial representation of how self-concept links to other aspects of self.

Body image is the individual's interpretation of their bodily self which includes physical characteristics such as being tall, short, fat, thin, brown-eyed, blond-haired. Price (1990) identifies three aspects of body image:

- **Body ideal** is how we would like to look. Sometimes this is guided by society's views and is a dynamic process. An *Observer* (2003) survey found that Kylie Minogue was considered to have the most attractive body shape for a woman and David Beckham for a man. The ideal woman emerged as being short, slim, with long hair and tanned skin. Neither author unfortunately conforms to this ideal!

- **Body presentation** is how we present ourselves, for example our clothes, hair style, how we sit and walk. Social expectations may influence this; you would probably choose different clothes to wear to a party than for a job interview. The NMC (2007) identified that nurses should behave in a way that promotes a professional image and highlights the individual's responsibility for their behaviour. Consider the effect of a nurse having dirty nails; it is unlikely to demonstrate a 'professional' manner and might affect the client's/relatives' confidence in the nurse.

- **Body reality** is the way we are, which may be very far from our body ideal, which might be thinner, taller, stronger and/or weaker than we really are.

Self-esteem

Self-esteem is the extent to which we value and approve of ourselves and relates to how much we like ourselves. Childhood and adolescence are especially important periods in self-esteem development. This evaluation of ourselves can be general or specific (Gross and Kinnison 2007). For example, we might like ourselves generally but might not like a particular aspect, like the size of our nose, or our short temper. Society values certain characteristics more than others, which can affect self-esteem. Factors affecting self-esteem might include physical disfigurement or disability, particularly if it is visible by others, for example an adolescent with acne. Stigma, related to illness, may also be a factor: consider someone with an illness labelled as schizophrenia and how this might affect their self-esteem and how the illness affects how they value themselves.

The ideal self

The ideal self is the person we would like to be. This is not just about physical characteristics but also considers wider issues such as personality and relationships. We might want to change some aspects of ourselves, or we might wish we were a different person altogether, perhaps kinder or more intelligent.

ACTIVITY

Consider the scenarios at the beginning of this chapter. How might each person's perceptions of their self- image be influenced by what they are experiencing?

Mrs Lewis's sudden deterioration following her fractured hip and the related infection may have a negative effect upon her self-perception and her judgement of her ability to cope. Mercy's recent below-knee amputation could affect her self-perception due to the sudden alteration in body image. As this is a visible disfigurement, Mercy could experience psychosocial difficulties (Rumsey *et al.* 2004.) Maria may have difficulty understanding what is happening to her. Her diagnosis, her increasing lack of mobility and pain could affect her body image and self-esteem. Mrs Davies's advanced Alzheimer's disease might affect her sense of self from physical, psychological and social perspectives. Physical changes in her brain might have changed her perception. At some point in her illness she might have been aware of her loss of intellectual functioning. She might have observed other people's reactions change towards her. Now she may lack understanding of her surroundings and the people around her. Other examples include loss of hair due to treatment (e.g. Maria following chemotherapy), loss or gain of weight due to illness (e.g. Bill has a low BMI) and loss of function (e.g. Miss West, following her stroke).

The concept of self is complex and all of the above aspects are interrelated and dynamic. They are influenced by individual, family and societal experiences and expectations throughout the life-span. Self-esteem and self-image are connected: if your self-image is positive then you will probably have good self-esteem, and vice versa. Rogers (1961) suggests that the greater the gap between our self-image and our ideal self, the lower our self-esteem.

Many people in different care settings have changes to their self-concept due to their illness experiences. The nurse's approach while carrying out practical skills can negatively or positively affect patients' self-image or self-esteem.

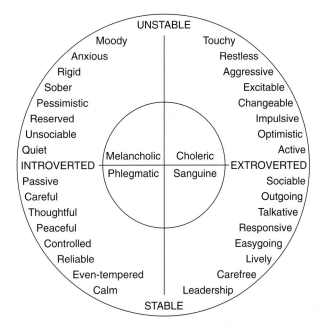

Figure 2.3: Dimensions of personality (Eysenck 1965). Reprinted with permission from *Personality Investigations Publications and Services*.

Learning outcome 2. Outline how personality may be important in nurse–client relationships

Personality is part of what makes people unique, but which at the same time allows people to be compared with each other. Personality is seen in psychological theories as being either a relatively stable component of the self, or as varying depending on an individual's situation. Eysenck (1965) proposed one approach to explaining personality, identifying two principal dimensions:

• introversion–extroversion
• neuroticism–stability.

Each individual lies within one of the four quadrants (see Fig. 2.3).

ACTIVITY

Where do you think you would lie in this diagram? What about a family member or a friend? Why would it be important to consider personality in healthcare settings?

An introverted nurse may find communicating with clients or colleagues in groups more stressful than an extrovert nurse would. However on a one-to-one basis there may be little difference. The client's personality can affect interactions. The behaviour that you observe may give small, but important, insights into a person's personality. For example, Natalie may be quiet and uncommunicative. What conclusions would you draw from this? You might decide that Natalie is introverted and shy, or that she is thoughtful and polite. You might be concerned about her psychological well-being. These views would indicate something about her personality *from your viewpoint,* but how accurate is this without a formalised approach to assessment? Nichols (2003) suggests that psychological care, of which communication is a key area, is often haphazard and rarely structured. Therefore, clients' psychological needs are often unmet – which can affect recovery, their compliance (concordance) with interventions and their response to illness.

Shaw (1999) proposes that understanding personality is important because personality appears to affect individuals' coping styles and psychological well-being. For example, whether Mercy was extrovert or an introvert, stable or unstable (see Fig. 2.3) would affect how she adapted to her new situation. Mr Davies may find changes in his wife's personality (one of the effects of Alzheimer's disease) hard to cope with. Gosling (1995), cited by Gross and Kinnison (2007), suggests that an understanding of personality can help nurses to understand patients and their illnesses, and how best to deliver individualised patient-centred care.

Learning outcome 3: Discuss attitudes, values and beliefs and their impact in the care environment

First some definitions (Gross and Kinnison 2007):

- **Value** – the person's sense of desirability, worth or utility of obtaining some outcome.
- **Belief** – an opinion held about something: the information, knowledge or thoughts about a particular thing.

Our values and beliefs underpin our attitudes and affect how we behave with others. Attitudes have been described as feelings that give order and shape to our lives but defining attitudes is difficult. For example, what is your opinion about smokers receiving healthcare? You may value life but believe in the right to freedom of choice; therefore your attitude might be ambivalent.

Similarly to self-awareness (discussed earlier), Rosenberg and Hoveland (1960, cited in Gross and Kinnison 2007) suggested that there are three components to attitudes:

- **Affective** – how we feel about a person, object or situation
- **Cognitive** – our thoughts and perceptions about the person, object or situation
- **Behavioural** – how we act toward the person, object or situation.

ACTIVITY

Consider the scenario concerning Mrs Davies. Would you feel any differently about her if you found out that her dementia was related to alcohol abuse in the past? Be as honest with yourself as possible.

You might feel less keen to care for Mrs Davies because you believe her condition to be her own fault, or you might even openly criticise her behaviour. Morrison and Burnard (1997) suggest that caregivers constantly make decisions about whether or not people deserve care, citing Rajecki (1982), who suggests that attitudes play a crucial part in influencing caring behaviours. However, the NMC (2008a) states that nurses should treat clients as individuals and respect their dignity, be kind and considerate and not discriminate in any way.

ACTIVITY

Are there other illnesses where health professionals may decide that the individual or their lifestyle is responsible for the health problem?

Some examples are:
- a person who is HIV-positive as a result of unsafe sex (in contrast to someone infected due to a contaminated blood transfusion);
- a person who has deliberately taken an overdose (in contrast to someone who has mistakenly taken an overdose);
- a cocaine addict who is experiencing hallucinations (in contrast to someone who is experiencing hallucinations either because of their treatment or due to an infection).

The examples above are linked to diagnosis. However, in reality there are many subtle, social factors that influence our judgements in client-centred relationships (Johnson and Webb 1995). It is therefore important to be aware that values, beliefs and attitudes are central to how we behave, and to examine whether these affect the quality of our communication, how we care, and our compassion for individuals and their circumstances.

Learning outcome 4: Understand the terms 'stereotyping' and 'labelling' and their significance to the care environment.

Stereotyping is the assigning of attributes to an individual based on their membership of a particular group (Walker *et al.* 2007). Geiger (2001) suggests that if patients from an ethnic minority are stereotyped by healthcare professionals this may lead to worse treatment. **Labelling** is a form of stereotyping where we categorise people by, for example, aspects such as their behaviour or their age.

ACTIVITY

When next in the practice setting, listen carefully to how nurses and other healthcare professionals speak about clients and their families. Are value judgements being made, and if so do these affect caring relationships? If so, how?

What did you notice about the words used to describe clients and their behaviour? Examples that we have heard include: 'difficult', 'attention-seeking', 'lovely', 'a pain in the neck', 'demanding' and 'bless him'. You might also have observed body language that reflects attitude: sighing, raising eyes to the ceiling, shrugging shoulders.

ACTIVITY

You are to admit a new patient. You are told his name is Albert Higginbottom and given limited other information: he is 67, lives in a hostel, fell while under the influence of alcohol, is reluctant to be admitted, and has a fractured right femur. Describe how you might imagine Albert to be; e.g. his personality and his physical characteristics.

You may have decided that Albert is elderly, scruffy, has an alcohol problem, has no supporting relatives and is uncooperative. You would thus already be forming judgements about the patient which might affect how you approach him. On the other hand, you might have decided to keep a completely open mind! The NMC's (2007) ESC for 'Care, Communication and Compassion' includes the need to be non-judgemental, stating that nurses must deliver care that is warm, sensitive and compassionate and free from discrimination and harassment.

As previously discussed, the judgements we make of others may affect the care that we give. Sometimes we make these judgements as a result of personal bias, thus failing to see the individual as a unique human being leading to prejudice in the care provided. The word *prejudice* means 'to pre-judge' and it is a constant challenge in our interpersonal relationships to remain as non-judgemental as possible.

There are two manifestations of prejudice – direct and indirect (Pettigrew and Meertens 1995). Direct or open prejudice is blatant and obvious; for example, a patient refusing to be looked after by a nurse who is black. Indirect or closed prejudice is more subtle; for example, a nurse who does not approve of a patient who has acquired HIV through their choice of lifestyle might provide the minimum acceptable level of care and not talk to them or make eye contact.

ACTIVITY	Consider the practice scenarios. How might both direct and indirect prejudice manifest itself?

Miss West might be seen as an older woman who would not understand the implications of possible treatment choices, leading to exclusion from the decision-making process. If Maria is judged as a result of her learning disability, staff may not explain what they are doing, assuming that she won't understand. Mrs Davies may be avoided by staff if she is agitated, as they might consider her 'difficult' resulting in her physical needs not being met.

We make attempts at ordering the world around us in an effort to understand what is happening, but this can lead to erroneous perceptions that can affect care delivery. Our communication with our patients/clients can reflect our underlying prejudices.

At one time, labelling of patients was considered fairly fixed in nature, so that once labelled, this would remain with the patient/client (Stockwell 1972). However, Johnson and Webb (1995) found that labels were more flexible and transient, changing with time and experience. When approaching patient care, you should be aware of whether your behaviour is affected by any labels or stereotypical views.

Hannigan (1999) suggests that negative representations and attitudes about mental illness are prevalent in the media and community. These negative representations are often associated with violence and are sensationalised, reducing the quality of life of people living within the community. Individuals who have a mental illness or learning disability are vulnerable to disadvantage and exclusion (Cabinet Office 2007), which has led to social inclusion being a key government agenda item. Nurses in any sector may care for people with learning disabilities or a history of mental health problems; if nurses hold stereotypical or prejudiced views this could affect their approach to care and their interactions. These points relate to the NMC's (2007) ESC for 'Care, Compassion and Communication', which identified that nurses must act professionally, ensuring that personal judgements, prejudices, values, attitudes and beliefs do not compromise care provision.

Summary

- An understanding of self-concept and related aspects informs and enhances nurse–client relationships.
- Developing self-awareness improves nurses' approach to patients/clients.
- Personality and attitudes are influential in affecting nurse–client relationships.
- Awareness of attitudes, prejudices and labelling – and responding to these appropriately – helps to reduce negative effects.

THE COMMUNICATION PROCESS

LEARNING OUTCOMES

By the end of this section you will be able to:
1 identify appropriate verbal and non-verbal communication skills;
2 identify barriers to communication;
3 discuss elements of effective written communication;
4 outline elements of appropriate telephone communication;
5 recognise the importance of effective communication between members of the multidisciplinary team.

Learning outcome 1: Identify appropriate verbal and non-verbal communication skills

In everyday life we constantly communicate, either verbally, or through the written word, or by our gestures or body language. Thompson (2003) suggests that communication involves not only transmitting information from one individual to another but that it is also important in relationships.

ACTIVITY

Write down as many different ways that you can think of to send a message.

You may have thought of speaking to someone either face to face individually or in a group. You may have considered the telephone, writing a note, sending a text message or an e-mail, or participating in an on-line forum. Did you think of sign language too? In 2003, the UK government recognised British Sign Language as a language in its own right (British Deaf Association 2008).

There are two aspects of interpersonal communication: *verbal* and *non-verbal*.

ACTIVITY

List under the headings 'Verbal' and 'Non-verbal' as many aspects of communication you can think of.

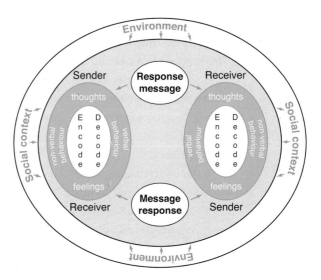

Figure 2.4: A framework for communication.

The verbal aspects you may have listed include tone of voice, pitch (or loudness), use of silence and pauses. These verbal components express our emotions and communicate information about our interpersonal attitudes. Sometimes clients' speed of speech indicates their emotional state – someone who is depressed may speak in a slow, flat, monotone voice. Mrs Davies, who is increasingly agitated, keeps repeating the same phrase over and over again and her speech may become faster and louder. Sometimes the way we use communication alters the meaning of the words used. For example, consider the different ways 'What do you want?' can be said. Non-verbal aspects include proximity, posture, body movements, touch, eye contact, facial expression and gesture. Both verbal and non-verbal behaviour are culturally determined (Arnold and Bloggs 1999) – which is further discussed in learning outcome 2.

Several authors have developed models or frameworks of the communication process, to portray the complexity of interpersonal interactions. Some suggest that communication is something that people do to one another, rather than a process where there is continual receiving, responding and interacting (Rungapadiachy 2007) Many frameworks now incorporate wider aspects in relation to communication. The framework in Fig. 2.4 has been developed from reviewing a number of previous models published in the literature: steps in the communication process (Porritt 1984, adapted from Berlo 1960), a conceptual model of message transmission and reception (Minardi and Riley 1997), a skill model of interpersonal communication (Hargie *et al.* 1994).

The framework in Fig. 2.4 illustrates that the social context and environment encompass and influence all areas of the interaction process. It also shows that, at any given moment, the sender of a message is also the receiver of messages. Our thoughts, feelings and behaviour (verbal and non-verbal) influence our interpretation and therefore our response to the message and its perceived meaning. *Encoding* entails turning our thoughts and feelings into a recognisable message which is in many cases reflected in our responses. *Decoding* is about how we interpret a message we have received, to make sense of it. Therefore we are continually receiving and sending messages in this dynamic process of interaction. We discuss some of these issues further in this chapter.

There are many different definitions of listening emphasising the aural (hearing), oral (spoken) and environmental aspects. However Stein-Parbury (2005) underlines the importance of recognising listening as an active process that requires concentration and effort to enable appropriate skills development.

ACTIVITY

Reflect on a recent occasion when you were speaking to a friend, a colleague or a client. What can you recall about:
* verbal ways that you showed that you were listening?
* body positions: your's and their's?
* eye contact and facial expressions?
* other non-verbal communication?

What can you remember about the content?

How we select, perceive and retain messages is influenced by our values and beliefs and our cultural upbringing. How are these aspects relevant to your reflections in the above activity? Was it easier to remember what you discussed with your friend rather than a colleague? This exercise may demonstrate how important attention and memory are within the listening process.

Egan (1990) uses the acronym SOLER to help us to remember how to use our body position when listening:

* **Sit** squarely in relation to the client.
* Maintain an **Open** position.
* **Lean** slightly towards the client.
* Maintain reasonable **Eye** contact.
* **Relax**.

Did you identify these aspects of body language? You may also have reflected on use of space, silence, touch and gestures, such as nodding in agreement or using facial expression to show interest or understanding. You or others may have used verbal signals to indicate that you were listening – for example, 'umm', 'aah', 'uh-huh', 'oh' or 'I see'. Sometimes when we are supposed to be actively listening, we can slip into automatic pilot and are not really fully responsive to the message. Stein-Parbury (2005) suggests that there are many barriers to effective listening, both external and internal, such as our own thoughts, value judgements and feelings.

When we are with clients it may be particularly useful to develop the skill of reflecting. Stein-Parbury explains that reflecting demonstrates that we have heard and understood both the emotional and factual content of the speaker's message. This, she suggests, is not always accurately interrupted, often requiring validation and further clarification from the client. Therefore we must also be alert to any non-verbal messages. For example, Natalie may say that she is 'OK', but you determine from her non-verbal cues that she is anxious.

To recognise incongruence between the verbal and non-verbal message, sensitive observational skills and an empathetic approach are required. Empathy can be described as 'a form of emotional knowing or the experience of another person's feelings' (Rungapadiachy 2007, p. 20). Being empathetic requires the appropriate use of skills mentioned earlier – touch, eye contact and use of voice. Vocal features may encompass not only the words we use but, just as importantly, the tone and manner perhaps through using a calm and soothing voice. Wiseman (2007) suggests that self-aware nurses are more likely to be empathetic. They may be more likely to be effective listeners too (Rungapadiachy 2007). Another skill that can show empathy is 'paraphrasing', whereby an individual's words are rephrased without losing the original meaning. Stein-Parbury (2005) proposes that paraphrasing is a fundamental component of expressing empathy.

The Code (Nursing and Midwifery Council 2008a, p. 1) states that the nurse must 'provide a high standard of care at all times'. This incorporates care that shows sensitivity and compassion towards individuals. The NMC (2007) confirmed the importance of nurses acquiring effective communication skills, including verbal and non-verbal aspects and identifying possible barriers.

Learning outcome 2: Identify barriers to communication

ACTIVITY

Identify factors that may act as barriers to your communication and relationships with clients.

The NMC (2007) identified that nurses should be able to recognise and overcome barriers affecting the development of therapeutic relationships. Barriers can be physical, psychological or social, although the distinction between these is not always clear-cut.

- **Physical barriers** could include visual, auditory or speech impairment, pain or how the surrounding environment is organised (a desk between two participants, one person sitting while the other is standing, or background noise).
- **Psychological barriers** may relate to personality (e.g. if someone is very shy), attitudes, beliefs and labelling (either the caregiver's or the client's), the emotional state of either party (e.g. anxiety), and cognition or thought processes, which may affect language and/or understanding. For example Maria, who has a learning disability, might understand what is said to her, but she may be unable to express herself verbally. Mrs Lewis, who is in isolation, may perceive a lack of attention from nursing staff and express feelings of loneliness (Newton *et al.* 2001). It is important that she understands the reason why she is in isolation; Myatt and Langley (2003) suggest that such explanations are often overlooked.
- **Social barriers** may include social status, culture, religious and spiritual beliefs. Social status may affect how we interact with others due to our place in the hierarchy or the context of the relationship. Is there a difference in how you would communicate with a doctor or a healthcare assistant?

The influence of an individual's culture and their religious and spiritual beliefs are important factors that are often overlooked in nurse–client interactions. The NMC (2007) requires that nurses be culturally competent (see Chapter 1 for an explanation of cultural competence). Leininger (1985, cited in Allen and Crouch 2007, p. 450) described 'culture' as the 'learned, shared and transmitted values and beliefs, norms and lifestyle practices of a particular group that guide thinking, decisions and actions in patterned fashions'. Vydelingum's (2000) study, which included Hindu, Sikh and Muslim clients, highlighted how communication difficulties led to patients feeling isolated due to language barriers. For example, nurses did not provide sufficient information in relation to diagnosis or medication. Furthermore, Gerrish (2001) found that 'patients who spoke little English were disadvantaged' (p. 571). Perceptions about causation of illness are also important because they affect cultural and religious experiences and responses and expectations during communication. For example, beliefs about possession by spirits have been demonstrated in some cultures. In Malaysia, 53 per cent of those diagnosed with a mental health problem attributed them to supernatural agents such as witchcraft (Razali *et al.* 1996).

There are differences in the use of eye contact, gesture, proximity and touch that may affect communication. For example, looking directly into the other person's eyes can be considered disrespectful or a sign of honesty, depending on the culture.

The unspoken conventions that accompany language in different cultures, such as politeness, degrees of directness, pace and the use of silence, can also cause misunderstandings. Fuller (2003) suggests ways to facilitate communication with individuals from different ethnic groups – for example, keeping an even tone, maintaining consistent speed of delivery and avoiding shouting.

Communication can be aided by using pictures, photos and mime and these strategies may help to ascertain understanding. Translators and interpreters may be necessary, but where possible professional interpreters should be used rather than untrained personnel or family members. Dein (2006) suggests that using informal interpreters may inadvertently alter the meaning of the message in translation leading to inadequate information or a lack of understanding. Family members may be reluctant to discuss sensitive and personal subjects with their relatives, particularly if communication is influenced by cultural taboos, for instance about bodily functions.

ACTIVITY

Looking at the section above, think about a recent clinical experience and list some of the factors that may have affected your ability to deliver culturally sensitive care.

You may have included whether individuals' food preferences were addressed (e.g. Halal meat or vegetarian), provisions were made for practising religious beliefs, or the number of visitors was limited making it difficult for extended families to visit.

The above points all highlight the importance of recognising a range of influences within the communication experience, how these aspects might affect nurse–client relationships and potential barriers.

Learning outcome 3: Discuss elements of effective written communication

Written communication is an important but often neglected area in nursing and is increasingly emphasised in relation to documentation and record-keeping. The NMC (2008b, p. 7) states that 'record-keeping is an integral part of nursing and midwifery practice. It is a tool of professional practice and one that should help the care process.' Good record-keeping helps to protect patients' welfare by promoting high standards of continuity and clinical care. It also ensures effective and accurate communication and dissemination of information between healthcare team members.

The NMC (2008b, p. 8) outlines crucial factors for effective record-keeping. Some of these are listed below with application to the scenarios. Patient and client records should:

- *be factual, consistent and accurate.* Mrs Davies' behaviour should be documented in an unbiased and non-judgemental way.
- *be written as soon as possible after the event has occurred, providing current information on the care and condition of the patient or client.* When Bill, who is terminally ill, is at home, he will be cared for by various community and specialist nurses. Therefore his care must be documented immediately and in sufficient detail.
- *be written clearly and in such a manner that the text cannot be erased.* Pencil and correcting solutions should not be used, and any errors should have a single line drawn through them and should be dated, timed and signed.
- *not include abbreviations, jargon, meaningless phrases, irrelevant speculation and offensive subjective statements.* Carry out the activity below and see how confusing and potentially dangerous using abbreviations can be.

ACTIVITY   What do the following abbreviations mean: CF, CPA, PID, TPR, BP, OE, RXT, ABC, ETA, DTA, DNA, ABS, DOA, GCS? All these can be found in healthcare settings. Discuss them with a friend or colleague.

How many of these did you know without further investigation? Were there any that could have more than one meaning? One example is that PID can mean either 'prolapsed intervertebral disc' or 'pelvic inflammatory disease'. Other examples are that BP could mean 'blood pressure' or 'bedpan', and DOA might mean 'dead on arrival' or 'date of admission'. You might think DNA is to do only with genetics but it is often used to abbreviate the phrase 'did not attend (an appointment)'. The context of the clinical environment may influence your interpretation of an abbreviation. Generally, although abbreviations are part of everyday life there are few that are acceptable in healthcare practice, especially in written records.

When completing nursing records, nurses must have a comprehensive awareness of all the pertinent issues contained in the NMC (2008b) guidelines as these are professional standards for practice.

The internet now plays a vital role in healthcare communications. Nurses should be aware of issues relating to the use of email. Redfern-Jones (2006) advises:

- Keep it concise.
- Do not include confidential information.

- Check your spelling and grammar.
- Avoid abbreviations and acronyms.
- Reply quickly.

More formal written communication or a telephone conversation is more appropriate for some issues.

Learning outcome 4: Outline elements of appropriate telephone communication

ACTIVITY

Reflect on the last time you telephoned someone to make an appointment or clarify something. Did you know who you were speaking to? Did they give you the information you wanted? How did it feel if your needs were met or not met; for example, you ended up being directed to a message box or a queue?

Increasingly telephones are an important mode of communication within healthcare settings (RCN 2006). However, there is little guidance about using them appropriately. Organisations provide their own corporate guidance about how telephones must be answered, telephone usage etc.; ensure you are aware of local policy.

- **Answering the telephone.** It is important that you clearly state where you are answering the telephone and who you are.
- **Maintaining confidentiality.** It is essential that confidentiality be ensured. You need to know who you are talking to at the other end of the phone. If someone asks about a client by name, you must ensure that the client is happy for information to be passed on. If possible, and the client has access to a telephone, they should be encouraged to make contact independently.
- **Acknowledging your level of competence.** For example, if you were asked to take down a message or a set of laboratory results and you did not understand what you were being told, you should explain to the caller that you need to get someone else to take the details.
- **Documenting and disseminating the information.** Make sure that messages are documented accurately and clearly and promptly passed on to the relevant individuals. This includes passing messages to patients; knowing that others are thinking of them is good for their sense of belonging and self-esteem.

Telephone consultations are becoming more common for nurses to engage in, and the RCN (2006) provides helpful specific guidelines for communicating with clients with long-term conditions.

Learning outcome 5: Recognise the importance of effective communication between members of the multidisciplinary team

Effective communication within the multidisciplinary team is important in all areas of nursing, both in hospital and community settings, and is essential for effective care management. Gibbons (2008) suggests that communication with colleagues is one of the most important areas for ensuring that we are working in the patients' best interests – it is vital that health professionals coordinate and share verbal and written information so that communication with patients about their care is clear and relevant. If you look back at the scenarios at the start of this chapter, you can see that nurses would need to communicate with a wide range of health care professionals. Later chapters will explore the multidisciplinary teamwork necessary for the effective care of these patients.

ACTIVITY	Look at Mercy Makumbe's scenario. Identify members of the multidisciplinary team between whom communication would be necessary as her care continues to prepare her for discharge. What form of communication would be used?

You might have identified that effective communication must occur between Mercy, her family, nurses (ward-based, community and specialist, e.g. pain specialist nurse), medical staff (hospital and community), the pharmacist, physiotherapist, occupational therapist, and prosthetist. Other staff might be involved too, depending on her assessed needs (e.g. dietician, chaplain, social worker, voluntary organisations). Communication will be verbal (including telephone) and written (including documentation, email, fax). The key principles relating to effective communication discussed in this chapter also apply to communication within the multidisciplinary team.

In relation to skills, nurses must ensure that information is recorded accurately and communicated unambiguously and concisely to other team members. For example, communicating with medical staff about changes to observations that may require medication adjustment or communicating with the physiotherapist to ensure analgesics are given if needed before exercise. Sometimes communication between team members occurs in urgent situations, for example a cardiac arrest situation.

Summary

- Communication can be both verbal and non-verbal.
- Identifying barriers to communication and having an awareness of how these might be overcome is important.
- Effective written communication skills are an essential component of nursing practice.
- Telephone communication is an important method of sharing information and must be conducted in a professional manner.
- Effective communication within the multidisciplinary team is essential for patients'/clients' well-being and safety.

DEVELOPING AND MAINTAINING THERAPEUTIC RELATIONSHIPS

LEARNING OUTCOMES

By the end of this section you will be able to:

1 understand important aspects of initiating successful interactions;
2 identify how to give clear explanations;
3 discuss how a range of questioning styles can be used appropriately;
4 summarise key features of gaining informed consent;
5 outline elements of appropriate professional behaviour.

Learning outcome 1: Understand important aspects of initiating successful interactions

Stein-Parbury (2005) suggests that the initial phase of a nurse–patient relationship is full of uncertainty and there is a need to reduce this. Therefore gaining trust is essential and can be achieved through learning about each other. For nurses, this should be within the boundaries of the professional role (NMC 2008a).

ACTIVITY

Imagine you are meeting the people from the scenarios at the beginning of the chapter. Write down how you think you would introduce yourself to each of them.

You might introduce yourself by giving your first name: for example, 'Hello, I'm Jane' or 'I'm Jane Smith', or perhaps 'Hello I'm student nurse Smith'. If you offer your first name you may make it difficult for clients not to give you their's. Some people prefer to be called by their formal titles, for example Miss West. Usually if the person wants you to call them by their first name, they will give you permission sometime in the relationship. Using a formal title is a sign of respect while first names imply intimacy or familiarity. Think back to the first time you met the practitioner in charge of a recent placement – how did you address them? It is likely that you adopted a formal approach until told otherwise.

Here again, cultural aspects should be considered. For example it would be disrespectful for a nurse to call a Sikh man by his first name or to ask him for his 'Christian' name. As highlighted earlier, cultural norms determine all aspects of the communication process, including the verbal and non-verbal.

ACTIVITY

Imagine that you have been asked to measure Natalie's blood pressure. You are meeting her for the first time. How would you establish rapport?

Opening introductions often involve some small talk. You might, for example, see that Natalie is wearing a scarf of a local football team. You could comment: 'I see you are wearing City's colours, how do you think they're doing this season?' Any introductory conversation should focus on putting the client at ease, thus enabling assessment to be more accurate. Trust can be achieved only if the client experiences the nurse as consistent in approach, be it in attitude, behaviour or communication. Therefore, how we initiate interactions is important for developing therapeutic relationships.

Learning outcome 2: Identify how to give clear explanations

Clear explanations are effective if they help people remember what has been said, so for example, the correct medication will be taken and for the correct period of time. Some relevant principles might include:

- identifying the client's understanding;
- using language that the client is able to understand;
- checking the client's understanding throughout;
- giving important information first and repeating it at the conclusion of the interaction;
- giving specific rather than general or vague advice;
- stressing the importance of certain information and repeating it where necessary (Ley 1997, cited by Walker *et al.* 2007, p. 78).

ACTIVITY

Consider the principles highlighted above. How might you explain to any of the clients in the scenarios what practical skill you are about to carry out?

You might have thought about how you would ensure Maria understands you when assessing her pain. You should use clear, short questions, and communication methods could include interpreting non-verbal cues, using pictures and signing. The nurse should work closely with Maria and her carers to explain things in an understandable manner. The Department of Health's *Valuing People Now* (DH 2007) emphasises that people with learning disabilities should be able to access healthcare as easily as any other member of the public, and this includes communication matters. The onus is on staff to adapt and use different approaches to meet individuals' needs. When discussing Bill's pain management you should check and re-check that he understands what you are saying, as his deteriorating condition may lead to confusion and an inability to concentrate. Having completed an explanation you should check that patients understand the information accurately (Nichols 2003).

An important part of giving explanations are the *words* that we use. Nurses should understand the power of language; Crawford (1999) argues that language shapes relationships. Thompson (2002) suggests language can reinforce social and cultural divisions, emphasising that it is not just the words we use but the way that we use them. When nurses explain to Mrs Lewis the reason for her being isolated, it would be easy to take a dominant stance, making it difficult for her to assert herself; for example, 'Don't be silly, you know you can't leave the room.' The way that nurses talk to clients can be beneficial and supportive or it can be detrimental by being patronising or debilitating. Imagine that Bill needed to wear an incontinence pad and the nurse said 'Let's put your nappy on.' How do you think he would feel?

How would you feel if someone spoke to your father or grandfather in this way? Crawford (1999, p. 49) emphasises the unacceptability of 'secondary baby talk' and the harmful effects it may have on nurse–client relationships.

Stein-Parbury (2005) suggests that acknowledging the client's experience encourages further interaction. Explanations should be high quality and adjusted to meet the individual's needs – who should receive comprehensive information about all aspects of their care.

Learning outcome 3: Discuss how a range of questioning styles can be used appropriately

There are many different types of questions that may be used.

| ACTIVITY | Make a list of some different types of questions and give an example for each. |

You may have identified the following types of questions:
- **Closed questions** (e.g. 'Would you like a cup of tea?', 'Have you got pain?'). These can gain factual information but they do not allow further exploration. They frequently require a yes/no answer and are helpful for gaining information from patients who can only respond briefly (e.g. in acute breathlessness). Often closed questions are used in initial patient assessments and lead to the second major type of question.
- **Open questions** (e.g. 'What symptoms have you experienced in the last week?', 'How would you describe your pain?'). These allow a fuller response, enabling people to reply in their own manner. Sometimes open questions precipitate a long and not necessarily relevant response and a closed question can refocus the conversation. Thus both closed and open questions are valuable when interviewing.
- **Probing questions** (e.g. 'You say that the pain is worse in the mornings. Tell me when else it is particularly bad?'). Probes or prompts can assist people to talk about their thoughts and feelings and express their concerns.
- **Leading questions** (e.g. 'You don't look as if you are in pain. Are you?'). These are best avoided as they can pressure people to respond in a particular way. However, nurses are often unaware of using them.
- **Affective questions.** These specifically address clients' emotions and indicate concern. For example, if Natalie is quiet and uncommunicative she could be asked how she feels about being in hospital. We need to have established a good rapport before asking this kind of question and should ensure that we can give time for responses. We should also know our own limitations in terms of helping responses.

Learning outcome 4: Summarise key features of gaining informed consent

Nurses must ensure that they gain consent before any care or treatment is given (NMC 2008a). Patients have a legal and ethical right to determine what happens to them within healthcare settings, so consent is needed before any action is taken with patients – for example, administering an injection or helping with personal hygiene. Seeking consent is also common courtesy between health professionals and patients (DH 2001a). Informed consent is an ongoing agreement by a person to receive treatment, undergo procedures or participate in research, after risks, benefits and alternatives have been adequately explained to them. The RCN (2005) advised that for informed consent to be valid, the patient must:

- be competent to make the particular decision;
- have received sufficient information to make the decision;
- not be acting under duress.

For example, if Miss West were to be asked if she consents to having a brain scan, then to be considered informed consent she needs to understand what the scan is and why the investigation is being suggested. She would also need to understand what would happen when she goes for the scan and the implications of not having the scan for her care.

People have different information needs and where possible these should be discussed as early as possible. Some clients would choose to have the minimum amount of information and prefer others to make the choices. Other clients will want to be involved throughout any decision-making process. Getting this correct minimises undue anxiety and distress.

Clients who for whatever reason are not considered sufficiently competent to consent or refuse treatment and have been treated under common law are said to have fallen into 'The Bournewood gap' (DH 2005). People may lack competence if they have:

- a learning disability;
- a severe mental illness such as dementia;
- a head/brain injury or disease.

Recent acts of Parliament, the Mental Capacity Act (MCA) (Great Britain 2005) and the Mental Health Act (Great Britain 2007) have strengthened protection for those who lack the mental capacity to consent to the care or treatment they need. The Mental Capacity Act 2005 Code of Practice (Department for Constitutional Affairs [DCA] 2007) provides a detailed guide to practical implementation of the Mental Capacity Act, including methods of communication, and is recommended further reading. One of the statutory principles of the MCA is that it is important to take all practical and appropriate steps to enable people to make decisions for themselves before deciding that an individual lacks capacity to make a particular decision (DCA 2007). A person's capacity (or lack of capacity) refers specifically to their capacity to make a particular decision at the time it needs to be made, and individual circumstances and needs must be taken into account. For example someone with a learning disability, such as Maria, may need a different approach, to a person with dementia, such as Mrs Davis.

The DCA's Code of Practice (2007, pp. 29–30) suggests the following good practice in relation to helping someone to make a decision for themselves:

Providing relevant information:

- Does the person have all the relevant information they need to make a particular decision?
- If they have a choice, have they been given information on all the alternatives?

Communicating in an appropriate way

- Could the information be explained or presented in a way that is easier for the person to understand (for example, by using simple language or visual aids)?
- Have different methods of communication been explored if required, including non-verbal communication?
- Could anyone else help with communication (for example, a family member, support worker, interpreter, speech and language therapist or advocate)?

Making the person feel at ease

- Are there particular times of day when the person's understanding is better?
- Are there particular locations where they may feel more at ease?
- Could the decision be put off to see whether the person can make the decision at a later time when circumstances are right for them?

Supporting the person

- Can anyone else help or support the person to make choices or express a view?

Care home staff should apply the above suggestions in the care of Mrs Davies, enabling her to make her own decisions wherever possible, for example, use of pictures may help her to make choices and Mr Davies may be able to help her to express her views. If decisions are made on her behalf they must be in her 'best interests' and the 'least restrictive interventions' should be employed (Great Britain 2005). These would need to be discussed within the multidisciplinary team and involve her husband too.

Learning outcome 5: Outline elements of appropriate professional behaviour

The Code (NMC 2008a) assumes that nurses are in positions of trust, and to justify this nurses must act with integrity to uphold the profession's reputation. They further highlight two areas of particular concern:

- *The receipt of gifts/money.* This specifically relates to anything that could be considered an attempt to receive preferential treatment or care.
- *The need to establish and maintain clear sexual boundaries with clients, their families and carers.* Thus any over-familiarity or intimacy is absolutely inappropriate and cannot be sanctioned under any circumstances.

Other relevant aspects to maintaining appropriate professional boundaries within therapeutic relationships include:

- being over-friendly;
- inappropriate self-disclosure;
- doing too much for a client at the expense of others;
- taking advantage of a client for one's own needs or gain;
- taking too much interest in the client beyond the confines of the supportive relationship.

Most clients and patients are vulnerable to some extent, including those with short episodes of illness and temporary dependence or individuals with severe and ongoing physical, emotional or cognitive impairments. For example, suppose you are the only person Natalie seems to communicate with: therefore when she asks for your mobile number you may be tempted to give her this. However this would be an inappropriate response which compromises the professional relationship, potentially making her more dependent in the relationship.

Summary

- Establishing initial rapport is an important stage in developing trusting nurse–patient/client relationships.
- Clear explanations are essential to ensure understanding.
- There are different types of question that should be used appropriately for effective interactions.
- Informed consent must be gained. Where clients lack the mental capacity for consent, care must be conducted in their best interests.
- It is vital to behave in an appropriate professional manner at all times, in accordance with the NMC's (2008a) Code.

COMMUNICATION IN CHALLENGING SITUATIONS

LEARNING OUTCOMES

By the end of this section you will be able to:
1 consider how anxiety is experienced and managed;
2 discuss how depression is recognised and managed;
3 identify how to recognise and manage anger;
4 consider ways of communicating with people who are confused;
5 discuss how to communicate with people who are receiving unwelcome news;
6 consider communication in relation to sensitive issues such as sexuality.

Learning outcome 1: Consider how anxiety is experienced and managed

Anxiety is one of our basic emotions and can range from mild to very severe, serving as a warning and helping us to cope with threatening situations. However, if anxiety is excessive and left untreated it may be detrimental and interfere with a person's normal day-to-day life and interactions. It can cause suffering and disability and can be costly at both an individual and societal level. The National Institute for Health and Clinical Excellence (NICE) (2007) asserts that anxiety disorders are common across all care settings.

If you think about the scenarios, Mrs Lewis may be anxious because she is in isolation or she may be a naturally anxious person. She may be lonely and have more time to worry about what is happening to her (Myatt and Langley 2003).

ACTIVITY

- What are the cues that may lead you to think a person is anxious?
- What aspects of Mercy's situation may give rise to anxiety?

In answer to the first question you might have considered facial expression, restlessness, wringing hands and profuse sweating, which are some indicators that an individual is anxious due to a feeling of impending doom. The resulting fear (which can be intense) may also cause some or all of the following: dryness of the mouth, racing heart, butterflies in the stomach, shortness of breath and having to go to the toilet repeatedly, irregular heart beats (palpitations), cognitive impairment including poor concentration, impatience, irritability, painful or missed periods, and difficulty in falling or staying asleep (NHS Direct 2008).

Anxiety about illness and implications for the future are often linked to fearfulness and/or uncertainty. Mercy could have fears for the future and uncertainty about her situation causing anxiety; for example, how she will cope at home following her amputation. She may also fear being harmed; for example, her belief that taking a combination of strong medication for pain and her cardiac problems may be detrimental to her health. Other factors that may cause healthcare recipients anxiety include:

- awaiting and fear of a life-threatening or life-changing diagnosis;
- fear of operative procedures or treatments and their effects;
- fear of pain and how successfully it will be managed;
- fear of the unknown environment, leading to feelings of vulnerability and insecurity;
- a perceived loss of control.

Any or all of the above may be relevant to individuals, so we should make no assumptions about what may be causing their anxiety. Careful assessment (including observation and information gathering) and the development of trusting relationships can enable nurses to accurately identify causes of anxiety.

Anxiety management techniques include:

- explanation of the process of anxiety and the symptoms experienced;
- breathing control;
- relaxation therapy;
- challenging of cognition (thoughts);
- assertiveness training.

These techniques are mainly longer-term strategies, used by healthcare professionals with enhanced skills. Nichols (2003) suggests that effective communication and information-giving skills can reduce anxiety, fear and uncertainty, enabling clients to work in partnership and follow treatment in a more relaxed manner, while positively contributing to recovery.

Learning outcome 2: Discuss how depression is recognised and managed

Depression is a common mental disorder characterised by sadness, loss of interest in activities, and decreased energy. It is differentiated from normal mood changes by the extent of its severity, the symptoms and the duration of the disorder. It is estimated that 5–10 per cent of the population at any given time are suffering from identifiable depression and need psychiatric treatment or psychosocial intervention.

This can mean as many as 2.85 million people in the United Kingdom (World Health Organization 2008).

A depressed mood is common when a patient has a life-threatening illness and is often a stage of adjustment. Depression is difficult to diagnose and can be unrecognised in acute hospital care settings. It is estimated that 50 per cent of people who are terminally ill can suffer from some degree of depression (Davis 2007). It is important to differentiate between someone who is sad, perhaps due to receiving unwelcome news about their prognosis, and someone who is in need of clinical support for depression. Nurses need to be able to assess patients accurately in order to recognise these differences and ensure appropriate referral for those in need of specialist support (Gamlin 2002). Nurses have an important role in identifying depression and their communication skills can help the effective assessment and screening of vulnerable clients. Assessment can highlight those at risk – for example, those who have a past history of brain pathology, those who have not maintained good relationships with healthcare professionals in the past or clients who have poor social support.

NICE (2004) guidelines for managing depression, which are recommended further reading, detail the assessment of depression and recommend a stepped care approach. These guidelines assist nurses and other healthcare professionals to identify patients at risk of depression, thus differentiating between those who are feeling low, sad or depressed as opposed to those who have depression as a clinical condition.

Depression has various physical and psychological symptoms but may not be identified in the clinical setting for various reasons, including the knowledge and attitudes of healthcare staff or resource and time issues. Clients may also not complain of depression, or depression may manifest itself in other symptoms – for example pain that is difficult to control. Nurses have a vital role in recognising the physical and psychological changes that may indicate a client is in need of support.

ACTIVITY

What might indicate to you that a client is depressed? List signs that you are aware of. Then access Mind's website (www.mind.org.uk) and read their client information about signs of depression. Have you seen any assessment tools used in practice to help assess depression?

As detailed on Mind's website, there are many signs and symptoms of depression. People who are depressed may also be anxious and it is not always clear whether the anxiety leads to the depression or whether depression causes the anxiety. Various assessment tools are used in healthcare settings to assess depression and anxiety – for example, the Hospital Anxiety and Depression Scale (Zigmund and Snaith 1983) and the Beck Depression Inventory (Beck *et al.* 1961) – so you may have seen these or similar tools.

Barraclough (1999) suggests that the guiding principles in caring for someone who is depressed are to:

- Give information.
- Encourage the patient to participate in care decisions.

- Allow expression of emotional distress.
- Ensure continuity of care.

This learning outcome has highlighted the importance of recognising 'normal' responses to adverse events/life-threatening illnesses, as opposed to responses which indicate a client needs further psychological assessment and support.

Learning outcome 3: Identify how to recognise and manage anger

Anger is a natural response to feeling attacked, injured or violated. It is part of being human; it is energy seeking expression (Mind 2006). Nurses are sometimes confronted with people who are displaying strong emotions such as anger and aggression. It is important to employ good interpersonal skills at these times to minimise the psychological impact of the emotions.

ACTIVITY

How would you recognise that a client was becoming angry? Divide your answers into verbal and non-verbal indications.

Examples of verbal indications include a raised voice, fast speech or using obscenities. Non-verbal indications include changes in body language: the person may display exaggerated movements, clenched fists, pace back and forth, throw or kick objects. There may be changes in facial expression; for example, frowning, and eye contact may be negligible or it might be extended – glaring. These are just some indications that an individual is becoming angry.

A nurse who has recognised these signs should act to disperse the anger.
- Listening actively to what the person has to say, thus showing a non-judgemental stance. However, eye contact that is held for too long may be seen as threatening (Williams 1996).
- Acknowledge the anger. This demonstrates empathy with what the person is feeling (Williams 1996).
- Encourage the person to identify the cause of the anger, through use of skilful questioning.
- Where possible, empower the person to resolve any causes.

Thus the aim is peaceful resolution of the situation. However, confronting anger with anger – through direct confrontation, defensiveness or questioning of the person's feelings – will probably lead to an escalation in anger, maybe to aggression. You may find it useful to reflect upon situations where you have encountered anger and try to identify possible causes.

Learning outcome 4: Consider ways of communicating with people who are confused

Confusion is defined as not being aware of or oriented to time, place or self (Tabers Cyclopedic Medical Dictionary 2005).

| ACTIVITY | On arrival at the care home, Mrs Davies appears confused. Identify the possible causes of this. |

Confusion may be a relatively permanent feature of Mrs Davies's condition, related to dementia. However, we must avoid making assumptions as her confusion may be due to physical factors such as malnutrition, dehydration, constipation or an acute infection. She may also be disorientated by being taken away from the familiar environment of her home. This would be compounded if she had a visual or hearing impairment.

| ACTIVITY | You think that Mrs Davies needs to use the toilet as she is becoming more agitated. Suggest strategies you could use to help her in this confused state. |

Strategies to consider include:
- orientation to time and place;
- use of appropriate and understandable language;
- a calm, clear voice;
- a calm manner, for example avoiding sudden or exaggerated movements;
- use of active listening skills.

Sometimes, despite all attempts to help a patient, their confusion makes it difficult for them to make their needs known and for nurses to identify appropriate interventions. In these situations the patient's safety and best interests are paramount, with reference to the Mental Capacity Act (Great Britain 2005) a consideration. The Code (NMC 2008a, p. 4) highlights the nurse's responsibility to ensure that 'people who lack capacity remain at the centre of decision-making and are fully safeguarded'. Dignity and privacy should be observed in line with benchmarks for best practice (DH 2001b).

Learning outcome 5: Discuss how to communicate with people who are receiving unwelcome news

Breaking unwelcome or 'bad' news is often medical staff's role but increasingly specialist nurses and other healthcare professionals are involved. Nurses should understand how to facilitate the situation to minimise distress for patients and relatives. It is often at times of intimate contact (e.g. bed-bathing) that patients ask searching questions. Buckman (1984, cited in Buckman 2005, p. 138) defines bad news as 'any news that adversely and seriously affects an individual's view of his or her future'. Therefore nurses should recognise the physical and emotional consequences for both patients and families. Brixey (2006) suggests that the badness of the news is the gap between the client's expectations and the medical reality.

Giving bad news is often cited as the most difficult part of the healthcare professional's role and can engender feelings of guilt, distress and fear for one's own mortality. Healthcare staff may sometimes avoid telling the whole truth either because they fear the reactions of patients and relatives or they fear acknowledging their own feelings. Although it can be distressing for patients and relatives to receive bad news, it is rarely acceptable to withhold the truth from them. Society holds the belief that truth is a fundamental and valued principle and is essential for establishing effective relationships. Furthermore, patients need correct information for making informed choices in decision-making (Ryan and McQuillan 2006).

Patients generally want to be told the truth, and the Code (NMC 2008a) states that nurses must be open and honest. Collis (2006) outlines arguments relating to deception in healthcare and stresses the importance of respecting patient autonomy. This involves acknowledging aspects such as individual preference and establishing an environment of trust that enables clients to feel accepted, respected and involved in their care (Kruijer *et al.* 2001; Collis 2006). A supportive environment helps patients to disclose their concerns, enabling nurses to adapt information according to individuals' emotional needs. Price (2004) emphasises the importance of conducting interviews in a sensitive and structured way to elicit information about clients' beliefs, attitudes and values.

Buckman's (2005) SPIKES strategy centres on addressing and recognising the emotional aspects of the patient experience:

- **Setting** – ensuring privacy, adequate time, set up of room, removing the chance of interruptions, listening mode.
- **Perception** – how the person views the seriousness of their situation and the language and vocabulary they use to describe it.
- **Invitation** – finding out how much the patient would like to know about their situation.
- **Knowledge** – giving a warning that you are going to give bad news, using similar language to the patient, avoiding technical jargon.
- **Empathy** – listening for and identifying emotions and their source and acknowledging these.
- **Strategy and summary** – checking understanding, summarising and allowing time for questions and clarification.

Although SPIKES is directed primarily towards medical staff, it provides valuable insights for nurses dealing with patients at this sensitive time. Both Barraclough (1999) and Buckman (2005) suggest that if breaking bad news is perceived to have been handled insensitively it can have adverse long-term consequences for the patient and family in adjusting to the illness.

Barraclough (1999) proposes that the choice of words, facial expression and tone of voice are dependent on individual situations and outlines possible guidelines when giving patients potentially unwelcome news (see Table 2.1). Rancour (2000) suggests that talking with patients and their families does not mean that hope need be removed.

Learning outcome 6: Consider communication in relation to sensitive issues such as sexuality

There are various sensitive issues that nurses may need to discuss with patients and clients; sexuality is one such area. Sexuality plays an important part in the development of self-concept and who we are as human beings. The way individuals perceive themselves sexually affects self-image, body-image and self-esteem (Volman

Table 2.1: Giving unwelcome news: some do's and don'ts (Barraclough 1999)

Do:	Don't:
Allow time and ensure privacy	Assume
Respect confidences	Give false reassurance
Allow patient time to talk	Try to predict what will happen
Listen	Give too much information at one time
Be sensitive to non-verbal cues	Fill silences
Permit silence and difficult topics	Make judgements or criticise
Take account of individual need for information at an appropriate level	Give direct advice
Allow for hope	

and Landeen 2007). Indeed the nurse's own sexuality may have an impact on their assessment of situations and behaviour. It is important that nurses are aware of the various ways individuals may identify in relation to their sexuality, for example gay, lesbian, transgender or bisexual. Explorations of how illness affects an individual's sexuality is often neglected due to nurses' own inhibitions about discussing intimate issues and other institutional and client-related factors (Magnan *et al.* 2006).

Gregory (2000) outlines the difference between sexuality (concepts of identity) and sexual functioning (bodily function). Major illness such as cancer, stroke and arthritis can affect sexuality either because of the effects of the illness itself or due to hospitalisation, treatments or medication.

ACTIVITY   Reflect upon situations where clients' sexuality needed to be considered.

Did you think of:
- how the client identifies in relation to their sexuality?
- following mastectomy or other surgery that alters body image?
- where appearance has altered due to medication (e.g. chemotherapy may cause a loss of hair and steroid therapy may cause weight gain)?
- effects of long-term medication use (e.g. some medications used for hypertension and mental illnesses can cause impotence/sexual dysfunction)?
- people with long-term urinary catheters?
- people who are paralysed or following a stroke?
- patients who have had genital or reproductive surgery?

Assessment can help to discover the physical, psychological and relational aspects of an individual's sexual needs, but a sensitive and skilled approach is vital. Gregory (2000) outlines the importance of a structured approach, suggesting that the benefits of including sexuality in patient assessment include:
- helping patients to understand their situation/condition and possible effects on their sexual functioning;
- helping to relieve fear and anxiety;
- helping towards an understanding of treatment options.

Gregory (2000) suggests that managing sexual problems is primarily about giving information and allowing patients to respond to options in care and treatment. Davis (2006) highlights research that suggests that patients often do not voice concerns about their sexuality as they prefer nurses to raise the subject. However, Krebs and Marrs (2006) suggest that the nurses' own beliefs may hinder their exploration and communication with clients about sexuality. Nurses might be unsure about when to raise the topic and be concerned that patients themselves might feel uncomfortable. However, it is important that nurses are able to discuss sensitive issues; as we have seen, illness often affects sexuality.

Summary

- This section highlighted and raised awareness of communication with people who are angry, depressed, confused or who have sensitive issues to address.
- Breaking bad news is one of the most difficult aspects of a healthcare professional's role and demands sensitive, compassionate care.
- Excellent interpersonal communication skills are particularly needed in challenging situations.
- Key aspects of communication in challenging situations are:
  - Be prepared to listen and hear what clients are saying.
  - Give clients permission to raise their concerns.
  - Ask questions sensitively.
  - Give timely information.
  - Respond and refer appropriately.

CHAPTER SUMMARY

Understanding influences such as self-awareness, personality, attitudes and stereotyping are important aspects in the provision of sensitive, compassionate communication – and therefore of care. Communication takes many forms and has verbal and non-verbal components. Nurses need to use a range of interpersonal skills effectively. In relation to practical nursing skills, initiating interactions, listening, non-verbal communication, questioning and giving explanations are all of particular importance. There are many situations where communication is challenging which requires nurses to be skilled and empathetic.

In conclusion, this chapter aimed to provide insights into the importance of nurse–client relationships. It included a discussion about the impact of self within this relationship, and how this affects communication and thus the care of people. The scenarios highlighted how communication principles are applied in a variety of care settings with different clients and within multidisciplinary teams. In the following chapters, where specific practical nursing skills are focused on, effective communication is paramount throughout. As suggested by Niven and Robinson (1994), one of the most crucial features of communicating with others is that we understand ourselves as well as those with whom we are communicating.

REFERENCES

Allen, S. and Crouch, A. 2007. Cultural and spiritual health assessment. In: Amugi-Crouch A. and Meurier C. (eds) *Vital Notes for Nurses: Health assessment* Oxford: Blackwell, Chapter 10.

Arnold, E. and Bloggs, K. 1999. *Interpersonal Relationships: Professional communication skills for nurses*, 3rd edn. London: Saunders.

Barraclough, J. 1999. *Cancer and Emotion: A practical guide to psycho-oncology.* Chichester: Wiley.

Beck, A.T., Ward, C.H., Mendelssohn, M.J. and Erbaugh, J. 1961. An inventory for measuring depression. *Archives of General Psychiatry* **4,** 561–71.

British Deaf Association 2008. *About British Sign Language* (BSL). London: BDA. Available from http://bda.org.uk/British_Sign_Language-i-14.html. Accessed 21 June 2008.

Brixey, L. 2006. The difficult task of delivering bad news. *Dermatology Nursing* **16**(4), 347–56.

Buckman, R.A. 2005. Breaking Bad News: the S-P-I-K-E-S strategy. *Community Oncology* **2,** 138–42.

Cabinet Office Social Exclusion Task Force. 2007. *Prioritising the Most Disadvantaged Adults.* Available from www.cabinetoffice.gov.uk/social_exclusion_task_force/psa.aspx. Accessed 21 June 2008.

Collis, S.P. 2006. The importance of truth-telling in health care. *Nursing Standard* **20**(17), 41–5.

Crawford, P. 1999. Nursing language: uses and abuses. *Nursing Times* **95**(6), 48–9.

Davis, C. 2007. Depression and cancer. *Cancer Nursing Practice* **6**(9), 10–11.

Davis, T.B. 2006. Using the extended PLISSIT model to address sexual healthcare needs. *Nursing Standard* **21**(11), 35–40.

Dein, S. 2006. *Culture and Cancer Care: Anthropological insights in oncology.* Maidenhead: Open University Press.

Department for Constitutional Affairs. 2007. *Mental Capacity Act 2005 Code of Practice.* The Stationery Office. Available from www.dca.gov.uk/legal-policy/mental-capacity/mca-cp.pdf.

Department of Health (DH) 2001a. *Good Practice in Consent Implementation Guide.* London.

— 2001b. *The Essence of Care: Patient-focused benchmarking for health care practitioners.* London.

— 2005. *'Bournewood' Consultation: The approach to be taken in response to the judgment of the European Court of Human Rights in the Bournewood case.* London.

— 2007. *Valuing People Now: From progress to transformation.* London: DH

Eckroth-Bucher, M. 2001. The philosophical basis and practice of self-awareness in psychiatric nursing. *Journal of Psychosocial Nursing and Mental Health Services* **39**(2), 32–9.

Egan, G. 1990. *The Skilled Helper: A systematic approach to effective helping*, 4th edn. California: Brooks/Cole.

Eysenck, H.J. 1965. *Fact and Fiction in Psychology.* Harmondsworth: Penguin Books.

Fuller, J. 2003. Effective cross-cultural communication. In Kai, J. (ed.) *Ethnicity, Health and Primary Care: A practical guide.* Oxford: Oxford University Press.

Gamlin, R. 2002. Diagnosing and dealing with depression. *International Journal of Palliative Nursing* **8**(3), 153.

Geiger, H. 2001. Racial stereotyping and medicine: the need for cultural competence. *Canadian Medical Association Journal* **164**(12), 1699–70.

Gerrish, K. 2001. The nature and effect of communication difficulties arising from interactions between district nurses and South Asian patients and their carers. *Journal of Advanced Nursing* **33,** 566–74.

Gibbons, P. 2008. Ethical dimensions of care. In Hinchliff, S., Norman, S. and Schoeber, J. (eds) *Nursing Practice and Health Care*, 5th edn. London: Hodder Arnold, Chapter 9.

Great Britain 2005. *Mental Capacity Act.*

— 2007. *Mental Health Act.*

Gregory P. 2000. Patient assessment and care planning: sexuality. *Nursing Standard* **15**(9), 38–41.

Gross, R. and Kinnison, N. 2007. *Psychology for Nurse and Allied Health Professionals.* London: Hodder Arnold.

Hannigan, B. 1999. Mental health care in the community: an analysis of contemporary public attitudes towards, and public representations of, mental illness. *Journal of Mental Health* **8,** 43–40.

Hargie, O., Saunders, C. and Dickson, D. 1994. *Social Skills in Interpersonal Communication,* 3rd edn. London: Routledge.

Jack, K. and Smith, A. 2007 Promoting self-awareness in nurses to improve nursing practice. *Nursing Standard* **21**(32), 47–52.

Johnson, M. and Webb, C. 1995. Rediscovering unpopular patients: concept of social judgement. *Journal of Advanced Nursing* **21,** 466–75.

Krebbs, L. and Marrs, J.A. 2006. What should I say? Talking with patients about sexuality issues. *Clinical Journal of Oncology Nursing* **10**(3), 313–15.

Kruijer, I.P.M., Kerstra, A., Bensing, J.M. and van de Wiel, H.B.M. 2001. Communication skills of nurses during interactions with simulated cancer patients. *Journal of Advanced Nursing* **34**(6), 772–9.

Luft, J. and Ingram H. 1955. *The Johari Window: A graphic model of interpersonal relations.* Los Angeles: University of Los Angeles Press.

Magnan, M.A., Reynolds, K.E. and Galvin, E.A. 2006. Barriers to addressing patient sexuality in nursing practice. *Dermatology Nursing* **18**(5), 448–54.

Minardi, H.A. and Ritey, M.J. 1997. *Communication in Health Care: A skills based approach.* Oxford: Butterworth Heinemann.

Mind 2006. *How to deal with anger.* Available from www.mind.org.uk/Information/Booklets/ How+to/How+to+deal+with+anger.htm. Accessed 21 June 2008.

Morrison, P. and Burnard, P. 1997. *Caring and Communicating: The interpersonal relationship in nursing,* 2nd edn. Basingstoke: Macmillan.

Myatt, R. and Langley, S. 2003. Changes in infection control practice to reduce MRSA infection. *British Journal of Nursing* **12**(11), 675–81.

National Institute for Health and Clinical Excellence (NICE) 2004. *Depression: Management of depression in primary and secondary care.* London.

— 2007. *Quick Reference Guide. Anxiety: Management of anxiety (panic disorder, with or without agoraphobia, and generalised anxiety disorder) in adults in primary, secondary and community care.* London.

Newton, J., Constable, D. and Senior, V. 2001. Patients' perceptions of methicillin-resistant *Staphlococcus aureus* and source isolation: a qualitative analysis of source isolated patients. *Journal of Hospital Infections* **48**(4), 275–80.

NHS Direct 2008. *Anxiety Symptoms.* Available from www.nhsdirect.nhs.uk/articles/article. aspx?articleId=28&sectionId=10. Accessed 21 June 2008.

Nichols, K. 2003. *Psychological Care for Ill and Injured People: A clinical guide.* Maidenhead: Open University Press.

Niven, N. and Robinson, J. 1994. *The Psychology of Nursing Care.* London: Macmillan.

Nursing and Midwifery Council (NMC) 2007. *Essential Skills Clusters for Pre-registration Nursing Programmes.* Annexe 2 to NMC Circular 07/2007.

— 2008a. *The Code: Standards of conduct, performance and ethics for nurses and midwives.* London.

— 2008b. *Guidelines for Records and Record-Keeping.* London.

Observer 2003. The poll: body uncovered, 26 October, 14–23.

Pettigrew, T. and Meertens, R. 1995. Subtle and blatant prejudice in Western Europe. *European Journal of Social Psychology* **25,** 55–75.

Porritt, L. 1984. *Communication: Choices for Nurses.* London: Churchill Livingston.

Price, B. 1990. *Body Image: Nursing concepts and care.* London: Prentice-Hall.

Price B. 2004. Conducting sensitive patient interviews. *Nursing Standard* **18**(38), 45–52.

Rancour P. 2000. Those tough conversations. *American Journal of Nursing* **100**(4), 24–6.

Razali, S.M., Kahn, U.A. and Hasanah, C.I. 1996. Belief in super-natural causes of mental health illness among Malay patients: impact on treatment. *Acta Psychiatrica Scandanavica* **94**(4), 229–33.

Redfern-Jones, J. 2006. Sending the right message. *Nursing Standard* **20**(41), 72.

Rogers, C.R. 1961. *On Becoming a Person.* Boston: Houghton Mifflin.

Royal College of Nursing (RCN) 2005. *Informed Consent in Health and Social Care Research: RCN guidance for nurses.* London.

— 2006. *Telephone Advice Lines for People with Long-term Conditions: Guidance for nurse practitioners.* London.

Rungapadiachy, D.M. 2007. *Self Awareness in Health Care.* Hampshire: Palgrave Macmillan.

Rumsey, N., Clarke, A., White, P. *et al.* 2004. Altered body image: appearance-related concerns of people with visible disfigurement. *Journal of Advanced Nursing* **48**(5), 443–53.

Ryan, K. and McQuillan, R. 2006. Ethical decision-making. In: Read, S. (ed.) *Palliative Care for People with Learning Disabilities.* London: MA Healthcare Ltd, Chapter 6.

Schaffer, H.R. 2004. *Introducing Child Psychology.* Oxford: Blackwell.

Shaw, C. 1999. A framework for study of coping, illness behaviour and outcomes. *Journal of Advanced Nursing* **29,** 1246–55.

Stein-Parbury, J. 2005. *Patient and Person: Developing interpersonal skills in nursing*, 3rd edn. London: Churchill Livingstone.

Stockwell, F. 1972. *The Unpopular Patient.* London: Royal College of Nursing.

Taber's Cyclopedic Medical Dictionary 2005. Available from www.tabers.com/tabersonline/ub? Accessed 21 June 2008.

Thompson, N. 2002. *People Skills,* 2nd edn. Hampshire: Palgrave Macmillan.

Thompson, N. 2003. *Communication and Language: A handbook of theory and practice.* Hampshire: Palgrave Macmillan.

Volman, L. and Landeen, J. 2007. Uncovering the sexual self in people with schizophrenia. *Journal of Psychiatric and Mental Health Nursing* **14,** 411–17.

Vydelingum, V. 2000. South Asian patients' lived experience of acute care in an English hospital. *Journal of Advanced Nursing* **32,** 100–7.

Walker, J., Payne, S., Smith, P. and Jarrett, N. 2007. *Psychology for Nurses and the Caring Professions.* Maidenhead: Open University Press.

Williams, D. 1996. *Communication Skills in Practice: A practical guide for health professionals.* London: Jessica Kingsley.

Wiseman, T. 2007. Toward a holistic conceptualization of empathy for nursing practice. *Advances in Nursing Science* **30**(3), E61–72.

World Health Organization 2008. *Depression.* Available from www.who.int/topics/depression/en/. Accessed 21 June 2008.

Zigmund, A.S. and Snaith, R.P. 1983. The hospital anxiety and depression scale. *Acta Psychiatrica Scandinavica* **67**(6), 361–70.

CHAPTER 3

Preventing Cross-infection

Patricia Folan and Lesley Baillie

Preventing cross-infection is an essential activity for all nurses in their everyday practice. Nurses have an ethical and legal duty to protect patients against infection (Cochrane 2000; Department of Health [DH] 2006a) but within hospital and residential situations, where many nurses work, the risk of cross-infection is high. In any healthcare setting, unless adequate care is taken, nurses can unwittingly transmit microorganisms from one person to another. The media regularly report concerns about lack of cleanliness and associated infection rates in hospitals and other healthcare settings.

Hospital-acquired infection, sometimes referred to as 'nosocomial infection', is a serious problem, causing as many as 5000 patients' deaths each year in the UK (Pratt *et al.* 2001). With the increasing emphasis on community care, including GPs' surgeries and care homes carrying out invasive procedures, and earlier patient discharges from hospitals, hospital-acquired infection often first becomes evident in the community. The term 'healthcare-associated' infection (HCAI) is therefore used more often now, defined as: 'Infection acquired as a result of the delivery of healthcare either in an acute (hospital) or non-acute setting' (Pratt *et al.* 2007, S62). The Nursing and Midwifery Council (2007) specified infection-control Essential Skills Clusters for student nurses, all of which are incorporated in this chapter.

This chapter includes:
- Principles for preventing healthcare-associated infection: an introduction
- Hospital environmental hygiene and multi-use equipment
- Hand hygiene
- Use of personal protective equipment including gloves, aprons and gowns
- Aseptic technique
- Specimen collection
- Isolation procedures
- Sharps disposal
- Healthcare waste disposal and linen management

Recommended biology reading

These questions will help you to focus on the biology underpinning the skills required to prevent cross-infection. Use your recommended textbook to find out:
- What are microorganisms? Where are they found? Are all microorganisms harmful?

- Identify some of the beneficial roles of microorganisms.
- How do microorganisms enter the body?
- How are microorganisms classified?
- What are the structure and properties of bacteria, viruses, prions, fungi, yeasts and protozoa?
- How do bacteria grow and multiply?
- What factors influence the proliferation of microorganisms?
- What is meant by the terms 'commensal', 'pathogen' and 'normal flora'?
- Distinguish between endogenous and exogenous sources of infection.
- What mechanisms does the body employ to defend itself from infection? Think about non-specific defences, e.g. secretions, reflexes, barriers etc., as well as specific mechanisms. Review the structure of the skin.
- How does the body fight infections?
- What are the clinical signs of infection? What role does histamine play?
- Which cells are involved in the specific immune response? Where are they found?
- What is the difference between humoral and cell-mediated immunity?
- What are antibodies? How do they help protect us from infection?
- How do we achieve an immunological memory?
- What factors can affect an individual's immune system?

PRACTICE SCENARIOS

As discussed above, prevention of cross-infection is part of the nurse's role in all practice settings. The following scenarios will be referred to throughout the text, when discussing the practical skills covered in this chapter.

Adult

Mrs Winifred Lewis, aged 87, was widowed many years ago and lives in wardened accommodation. She has a history of rheumatoid arthritis and type 2 diabetes, and recently fell and fractured her hip. This was operated on in hospital but the wound developed an infection, which grew MRSA. She was discharged home, under the care of the district nursing team and intermediate care, but her wound deteriorated and the surrounding skin showed signs of infection. Mrs Lewis appeared unwell and dehydrated, so her GP requested readmission. She is now being isolated in the side room of a surgical ward, and an intravenous infusion and intravenous antibiotics have been commenced. She has a commode in the room and can transfer with help.

Learning disability

James Smith is a 59-year-old man with a learning disability who lives alone in a farm cottage and works on the adjacent farm. Following an accident, James has an open wound on his lower left leg that shows signs of infection. There is a large amount of exudate, which has an offensive odour. The district nurse has been visiting the farm to carry out dressings and a wound swab has been taken. James is

---

Rheumatoid arthritis
An inflammatory disease often affecting a number of joints (initially smaller ones), causing pain, swelling, stiffness and deformity. It is often accompanied by systemic ill-health.

Type 2 diabetes
Type 2 diabetes develops when the body makes insufficient insulin, or when the insulin that is produced does not work effectively (known as insulin resistance). See www.diabetes.org.uk.

Infection
The successful invasion, establishment and growth of microorganisms within the tissues of the host.

MRSA
A strain of *Staphylococcus aureus* which is highly resistant to many commonly used antibiotics.

Health Action Plan
A personal plan developed for each individual who has a learning disability, detailing their health interventions, medication, oral health, nutrition, etc. (DH 2001).

keen to carry on with his usual work on the farm. The district nurse is liasing with the community nurse for learning disabilities to help to teach James how to care for his leg in between dressings. This information is now included in James's Health Action Plan. As the district nurse runs a clinic at the local GP's surgery, James is being encouraged to attend this for dressings instead of receiving visits at his home.

Mental health

Stacey is 28 years old and has been addicted to opiates for six years. She is living with her parents who are very supportive. Recently Stacey began a community-based detoxification programme with support from her local drug and alcohol team. During detoxification, Stacey experienced severe withdrawal symptoms, including very high blood pressure and vomiting. As a result she was admitted as an emergency to the acute mental health admission unit. She arrived feeling very unwell, and soon after arrival vomited over her bed. She was prescribed intramuscular metoclopramide (an antiemetic) to stop her vomiting. Stacey is known to have hepatitis B.

PRINCIPLES FOR PREVENTING HEALTHCARE-ASSOCIATED INFECTION: AN INTRODUCTION

Colonise
The establishment of pathogenic microorganisms at a specific body site with little or no host response. This can lead to a large number of microorganisms, forming a reservoir for infection and cross-infection.

Many microorganisms exist but not all cause infection in individuals. Those that cause disease are called **pathogens**. When pathogens are acquired from another person, or from the environment, they are described as **exogenous**. The transmission of pathogens, between people and across environments, is termed **cross-infection**. When microorganisms colonise one site on the host and enter another site on the same person causing further infection, this is called self-infection or **endogenous** infection.

In the third national prevalence survey (DH 2007a), the prevalence of HCAI in England was 8.2 per cent, compared with 7.6 per cent for the UK and Ireland collectively (excluding Scotland). The most common types of infections were gastrointestinal system infections (22 per cent), urinary tract infections (19.7 per cent), pneumonia (13.9 per cent) and surgical site infections (13.8 per cent).

LEARNING OUTCOMES

On completion of this section you will be able to:
1 discuss key policies influencing infection control practices;
2 identify the composition and role of infection control teams;
3 understand the chain of infection including the routes by which microorganisms are spread.

Learning outcome 1: Discuss key policies influencing infection control practices.

Concern about HCAI has led to many government publications, providing recommendations for infection control. *Clean, Safe Care: reducing infections and saving lives* (DH 2008) provides an overview of initiatives in England. Key publications are mentioned below.

- *Saving Lives: Reducing infection, delivering clean and safe care* (revised edition, DH 2007b). This provides evidence-based 'high impact interventions' (HIIs) or 'care bundles' for key clinical procedures which can increase the risk of infection if not performed appropriately. The HIIs highlight the critical elements of particular procedures, the key actions required, and a means of demonstrating reliability using compliance measurement. The HIIs aim to minimise unwarranted variation in practice by identifying where compliance needs to be increased and measuring how often all elements are performed for a given procedure. The tool enables results to be quickly fed back to staff, actions can be agreed and implemented and progress can be tracked.
- *The Health Act: Code of Practice for the Prevention and Control of Health Care-associated Infections* (DH 2006a). This aims to assist National Health Service providers to plan and implement how they can control HCAIs. It led to a legal requirement for acute hospitals and other care providers to prevent infection. Failure to observe the Code may result in an 'improvement notice' or 'special measures'.
- *National Evidence-based Guidelines for Preventing Healthcare-associated Infections in NHS England* (Pratt *et al.* 2007). In these updated DH-commissioned evidence-based infection control guidelines (referred to as EPIC2), the authors noted that standard infection control precautions need to be applied by all healthcare practitioners to the care of all patients. It is planned that revised guidelines will be published in 2011.

The other UK countries' administrations also provide guidance and policy on infection control: for Scotland see www.hps.scot.nhs.uk; for Wales see www.wales. nhs.uk; and for Northern Ireland see www.dhsspsni.gov.uk.

Standard infection control precautions relevant to all areas of practice are:

- hospital environmental hygiene;
- hand hygiene;
- the use of personal protective equipment;
- isolation of patients;
- the use and disposal of waste and sharps.

In this chapter you will encounter each of these precautions and focus on the skills that are associated with them. These precautions are consistent with – and build on – the 'universal precautions' that were established in the 1980s in response to the growing problems of blood-borne infections. In the 1990s, the terminology changed to 'standard precautions'. Universal/standard precautions recognised a few simple practices that could be used to care for all patients to minimise the risk of cross-infection to patients and staff alike. The National Institute for Health and Clinical Excellence (NICE) (2003) produced guidelines for preventing HCAIs in primary and community care. These apply the standard precautions of hand hygiene, use of personal protective equipment and sharps disposal to various aspects of community-based care.

Standard precautions combine the major features of universal precautions and Body Substance Isolation (BSI) and are based on the principle that all blood, body fluids, secretions, excretions except sweat, non-intact skin and mucous membranes may contain transmissible infectious agents. Standard precautions include infection prevention practices that apply to all patients, regardless of suspected or confirmed infection status, in any setting in which healthcare is delivered.

Learning outcome 2: Identify the composition and role of infection control teams

As you read above, there are many national infection control policies. These are implemented at local level by an **infection control team (ICT).**

ACTIVITY

When next in the practice setting, find out who the members of the local infection control team are and where they are located. Also, find out where your local infection control policy is kept and familiarise yourself with its content.

The ICT generally comprises an infection control nurse (ICN) and an infection control doctor. Their roles include planning, implementing and monitoring the infection prevention and control programme. They are available to offer advice on all matters relating to infection control. They also provide education to healthcare personnel and develop local policy. An infection control committee from a variety of hospital departments provides advice and support for the ICT.

Many community healthcare trusts also employ ICNs who work closely with the consultant for communicable disease control. The consultant is responsible for monitoring and controlling the spread of infection in the community, as well as other environmental hazards (Wilson 2006). Many hospitals also use infection control link nurses (or 'champions') to improve awareness of infection control in clinical areas. They receive basic training and help provide education, training, audit and surveillance in clinical areas. There should also be close liaison between the occupational health department and the ICT to ensure the health and safety of patients and staff alike (Wilson 2006).

Learning outcome 3: Understand the chain of infection including the routes by which microorganisms are spread

The 'chain of infection' can help you to understand how to prevent spread of infection (see Fig. 3.1). Prevention of cross-infection is about breaking the chain of infection. Each link in the chain will now be discussed.

Infectious agent

An infectious agent is a microorganism with the ability to cause disease. This includes bacteria (most common in hospitals), viruses (more common in the community) and fungi (e.g. Candida, which causes 'thrush'). To identify the specific infectious agent, specimens are collected and sent to the laboratory for microscopy,

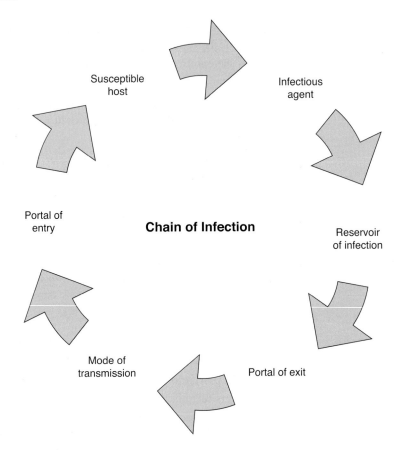

Figure 3.1: Chain of infection.

culture and sensitivity ('M,C&S'). For example, if a urinary tract infection (UTI) is suspected, a specimen of urine will be sent to the laboratory. A later section in this chapter focuses on the collection of a specimen.

Two microorganisms that have caused particular concern in healthcare settings and are regularly covered in the media are MRSA and *Clostridium difficile*.

MRSA

Mrs Lewis is an example of a person who is infected with MRSA. This is a strain of *Staphylococcus aureus* that has become resistant to the antibiotic methicillin – hence the name 'methicillin-resistant *Staph. aureus*'. Strains of MRSA are usually resistant to all penicillins and all cephalosporins. They may also be resistant to other first-line antibiotics. *Staph. aureus* commonly colonises normal skin, particularly warmer parts such as the axillae, groins, perineum and nose. *Staph. aureus* and MRSA are usually carried 'silently'. Healthy people do not usually develop an infection though they can become colonised (Wilson 2006). Serious staphylococcal infection usually occurs in people who are vulnerable because of underlying illness or medical interventions. Mrs Lewis, as a frail older person with diabetes and rheumatoid arthritis, fits into this category.

MRSA can cause a range of superficial infections of the skin as well as hospital-acquired wound infections, as with Mrs Lewis. In the third national prevalence survey, 1.28 per cent of patients had an MRSA infection, and MRSA was the causative organism in 15.5 per cent of all HCAIs (DH 2007a). *Staph. aureus* can also cause boils and abscesses and serious systemic infections, such as septicaemica and pneumonia (Wilson 2006). Unfortunately, the few drugs currently available that have reliable activity against MRSA are very expensive and difficult to administer. They necessitate blood levels being monitored since they are highly toxic.

MRSA is most likely to be spread on the hands of staff as transient organisms. If staff have certain skin conditions, such as eczema or dermatitis, or have cuts on their skin, they are at increased risk of harbouring the organism and can spread it to other staff and patients. The organism can also be carried on skin scales from an infected patient or member of staff and may contaminate uniforms or clothing, especially if the clothing is damp.

Clostridium difficile

Clostridium difficile-associated disease (CDAD) is transmitted through chlostridial spores, which can survive long periods in the environment and are shed in large numbers by infected patients (DH 2007c). *C. difficile* is usually controlled by the gut's normal flora, but when these are killed off by antibiotics *C. difficile* is able to multiply, produce toxins and cause diarrhoea.

In the third national prevalence survey, 1.98 per cent of patients surveyed had CDAD. Patients most at risk are older people and those who have recently taken antibiotics (DH 2007c), so Mrs Lewis fits into this category and could be at risk. CDAD causes mild or severe diarrhoea, and outbreaks have led to clusters of patient deaths, which you may remember being reported in the media.

Reservoir of infection

A reservoir of infection is a place within which microorganisms grow and reproduce and can include people (healthcare workers, patients), the environment, equipment and water. Mrs Lewis's and James's wounds provide reservoirs for infection.

Portal of exit

A portal of exit provides a way for microorganisms to leave the reservoir and includes excretions (e.g. faeces from the bowel) or droplets (via the mouth or nose by sneezing or coughing). If Stacey cut herself, this would provide a means for the hepatitis B microorganism to leave her body.

Mode of transmission

Microorganisms can spread through a number of routes.

ACTIVITY

Read Table 3.1, which presents the routes by which pathogenic microorganisms can be transmitted or spread between people. Then reread the practice scenarios. Can you work out which transmission route would feature mostly strongly for these patients?

Table 3.1: Routes of transmission (adapted from Parker 1999).

Route	Explanation	Examples
Direct or indirect contact	Transfer from body surface to body surface *directly* between an infected or colonised person and a susceptible host, or *indirectly* via an intermediate object	*Direct:* Patient to patient (e.g. through touch), or staff to patient when carrying out patient care activities such as moving and handling. *Indirect:* Patient touched by a nurse's unwashed hands or gloves that have not been changed after contact with a patient who is infected/colonised
Inanimate objects and equipment (fomites)	Susceptible host infected by an object that is contaminated with microorganisms	Beds, curtains, toys, bedpans, tables, keyboards can all be contaminated and spread infection, sometimes via hands of staff acting as transmitters
Droplet	Microorganisms transmitted through the air within droplets, mainly saliva	Coughing, sneezing, talking and singing can transmit, as well as during procedures (e.g. bronchoscopy or suctioning)
Air-borne	Microorganisms carried in droplet nuclei (small particle residue), or by dust particles consisting of dead skin scales, clothing fibres, etc.	Carried by air currents in the environment and breathed in by a susceptible host, or settle on horizontal surfaces. Some bacteria form spores and survive for months in such conditions
Ingestion	Ingested into the body with food or water, causing gastrointestinal infections and excreted in faeces. Known as the faecal–oral route	Food may be contaminated when hands that have been in contact with faeces transfer the organisms to food
Vector	Transmission via insects or rodents	Cockroaches, rats, mice and ants cause contamination of food; mosquitoes spread malaria and yellow fever; ticks spread Lyme disease and typhus

It is likely that direct or indirect contact via hands of carers is the principal cause of spread. For Mrs Lewis, infection can be spread via the air-borne route, but direct and indirect contact transmission is likely. Stacey has hepatitis B and this is transmitted via blood and serum-derived fluids such as vaginal secretions, so direct and indirect contact with these fluids is a major source of transmission. Hands could spread infection from James's leg wound, especially since there is a large amount of exudate.

Whilst all routes of transmission are important, this short activity points out that the most common route of spread is via hands. The DH (2003) reports that healthcare workers are a major route through which patients become infected and that high levels of compliance with hand hygiene protocols are essential. Attention to hand hygiene has the potential to break the chain of infection.

Portal of entry

This is the opening allowing microorganisms to enter the body.

ACTIVITY   Identify Mrs Lewis's portals of entry.

Mrs Lewis's wound (already infected) is one portal of entry, but her intravenous site is another. While we have many defences to prevent microorganisms entering the body, patients/clients often have increased routes for entry because of invasive procedures (e.g. urinary catheters, intravenous cannulae and chest drains) and wounds. Intravenous infusions provide a route for bacteria and other microorganisms to enter the body directly (DH 2007d). The Department of Health (DH) (2003) reported that 80 per cent of urinary tract infections can be traced back to urinary catheters and 60 per cent of blood-borne infections are linked to medical devices, such as intravenous cannulae and urinary catheters.

Susceptible host

Most patients/clients are vulnerable to infection because of their immunity, age, underlying disease and medical interventions.

ACTIVITY   Discuss with a colleague the people in the scenarios and the factors that make them susceptible to cross-infection.

Individuals vary widely in their ability to resist infection. Patients are especially vulnerable to infection if they have underlying disease. Mrs Lewis's chronic diseases of rheumatoid arthritis and diabetes and Stacey's hepatitis B will render them more susceptible. Mrs Lewis's impaired defence mechanisms could have led to her infection being more severe than in healthy people. Serious diseases, such as cancer, and associated treatments (e.g. powerful drugs, including steroids and chemotherapy), affect the immune system too. Local factors, such as a poor blood supply to a wound, increase the likelihood of infection developing, and people who have diabetes, like Mrs Lewis, can have impaired circulation. Age (especially very young or very old), and previous exposure to infection and vaccinations, all affect levels of risk (Wilson 2006). Mrs Lewis, as an older adult, is therefore more vulnerable to infection.

The presence of a wound, as in the cases of Mrs Lewis and James, increases susceptibility to infection as the skin, which is an important bodily defence, is breached. Other reasons for susceptibility to infection include poor nutrition, which could apply to any of the people in the scenarios. You should look out for underlying susceptibilities when you are in clinical practice.

Summary

- HCAI is a major concern to governments. Infection control policies are regularly produced for implementation at local level by ICTs.

● It is important to keep up to date with policy developments and to be familiar with local policy.
● An understanding of the chain of infection can assist in understanding the rationale behind infection control measures.

HOSPITAL ENVIRONMENTAL HYGIENE AND MULTI-USE EQUIPMENT

Pratt *et al.* (2007) highlight that microorganisms including MRSA have been found in the hospital environment and can be harboured by dust. While cleaning cannot eradicate microorganisms from the environment, hospital environments must be 'visibly clean, free from dust and soilage and acceptable to patients, their visitors and staff' (Pratt *et al.* 2007, S3). Ward surfaces (floor, furniture, equipment or walls) that are physically clean and dry are unlikely to provide a substantial infection risk (Ayliffe *et al.* 2000).

LEARNING OUTCOMES

On completion of this section you will be able to:
1 discuss issues relating to healthcare environments and their cleanliness;
2 identify how and when multi-use equipment should be cleaned.

Learning outcome 1: Discuss issues relating to healthcare environments and their cleanliness

The Department of Health (DH) (2006a, p. 5) states that healthcare providers have a duty to 'provide and maintain a clean and appropriate environment for healthcare'.

ACTIVITY

What is the environment, in relation to healthcare? List all the items you can think of.

You probably thought of the floor, furniture like beds and bedside lockers, and toilets. Did you identify curtains/screens, light switches, doors and door handles too? Health Protection Scotland (HPS) (2008a) provides guidelines for standard infection control precautions relating to the environment. They highlight that stores must not be placed on the floor, that furniture should be easily cleaned and with smooth surfaces, and that damaged items should be removed as they can harbour microorganisms. They also recommend a clutter-free environment which is easier to keep clean.

ACTIVITY

Whose responsibility is it to ensure healthcare environments are clean? How should you deal with body fluid spillages, e.g. blood, vomit or urine?

You probably identified the key role that domestic staff have in ensuring that healthcare environments are kept clean. HPS (2008a) recommends that routine cleaning should generally occur daily or twice-daily depending on the risk assessment for the area but must also be carried out if it is visibly soiled/dusty and immediately following any body fluid spillages. General-purpose detergent and hot water should be used and the mechanical action of cleaning is particularly valuable (HPS 2008a). Pratt *et al.* (2007, S3) advise that all healthcare staff should be aware of 'their individual responsibility for maintaining a safe care environment for patients and staff'. Clinical staff should be observant and proactive to ensure environments are kept clean, particularly when unexpected events occur, such as body fluids being spilt. Pratt *et al.* (2007) advise that hypochlorite and detergent should be used where microorganisms are surviving for long periods in the environment and may be contributing to spread of infection.

Following Mrs Lewis's discharge from the sideroom it will be the nursing staff's responsibility to request that the room and any multi-use equipment be thoroughly cleaned and dry before other patients are in contact with it. Disposable equipment must be disposed of as infective waste.

HPS (2008b) identified that blood and body fluid spillages pose cross-infection risks so they must be dealt with immediately and appropriately. HPS provided detailed guidelines for dealing with different body fluids. For any body fluid spillages, staff must perform hand hygiene before and after, wear personal protective equipment, use paper towels for initial fluid absorption, followed by use of recommended cleaning solutions and disposal of the used items appropriately (see later sections). Local infection control policies must be followed when dealing with spillages; practice differs according to type of body fluid. HPS (2008b) identified actions for three groups of body fluid spillage:

* *Blood, body fluids including cerebrospinal, peritoneal, pleural, pericardial, synovial, amniotic, semen, vaginal secretions, breast milk and any other body fluids containing blood* (except urine). Apply an approved disinfectant (e.g. sodium hypochlorite, at 10 000 ppm), used as per manufacturer's instructions as this inactivates blood-borne viruses. Then wash area with detergent and water, rinse and dry.
* *Faeces, vomit, sputum and pus.* Wash the area with detergent and water, rinse and dry. If these fluids contain blood, treat as for blood; but if organic material is present (e.g. faeces), wash with detergent first before applying disinfectant.
* *Urine.* Wash with water and detergent, rinse and dry. If it contains blood an approved disinfectant (e.g. sodium hypochlorite, at 1000 ppm) is used first.

Learning outcome 2: Identify how and when multi-use equipment should be cleaned.

HPS (2008c) advises that single-use equipment should be used where available and appropriate. However, many items are multi-use, for example, infusion pumps, drip stands and stethoscopes. Pratt *et al.* (2007) recommend that shared equipment in clinical settings must be decontaminated after use appropriately. Decontamination aims to ensure reusable items are safe to use by other patients; equipment should be decontaminated according to manufacturers' instructions and includes cleaning, **disinfection** and **sterilisation** (DH 2006a). Wilcox *et al.* (2003) found that over half of commodes were contaminated by *C. difficile*.

Disinfection
A process to reduce the number of viable microorganisms but it may not inactivate some microbial agents (e.g. spores).

Sterilisation
A process which renders an item free from microorganisms including spores.

While patients coming into contact with multi-use equipment generally have intact skin and therefore infection may not be introduced by contaminated equipment, nevertheless equipment may transmit microorganisms between patients which could result in infection (Pratt *et al.* 2007).

Consider each of the patients in the scenarios. What multi-use equipment will be used in their care? How and when might you clean this equipment?

When James's wound was dressed at home, there should have been no multi-use equipment used in his care. At the doctor's surgery, the dressing trolley used will be multi-use. Dressing trolleys are unlikely to become contaminated during the dressing procedure, but they should be cleaned before and after use (see 'Aseptic technique').

Stacey's blood pressure monitoring equipment will be multi-use. However, in some settings patients are allocated their own blood pressure cuff to use until their discharge. Other equipment used is disposable (injection equipment) or washable (bed-linen). Her bed and bedside locker should be cleaned following her discharge and kept socially clean while in her use.

As Mrs Lewis has MRSA and is isolated, any non-disposable equipment (e.g. commode, blood pressure monitoring equipment) should be designated for her use only. Following discharge, the equipment must be cleaned effectively before use by other patients.

Pratt *et al.* (2007) advise that detergent and water is adequate for cleaning equipment, but that in outbreaks of infection, detergent and hypochlorite are recommended.

Summary

- All healthcare workers have a duty to ensure that healthcare environments are clean.
- Multi-use equipment must be effectively cleaned between patients.

HAND HYGIENE

Adequate hand hygiene is the single most important practice in reducing the spread of infection during care delivery (HPS 2008d). Pratt *et al.* (2007) identified standard principles for hand hygiene and these are referred to throughout this chapter, with application to practice and this chapter's scenarios.

The term 'hand decontamination', used throughout these principles, is defined as 'the process for the physical removal of blood, body fluids, and transient microorganisms from the hands – that is, handwashing and/or the destruction of microorganisms – hand asepsis' (NICE 2003, p. 46). Handwashing is the key skill used for hand hygiene. Hand decontamination can also be achieved, in some circumstances, by using an alcohol-based handrub containing isopropyl alcohol (70%).

By the end of this section you will be able to:

1 state the purpose and importance of hand decontamination for the care and safety of both patients and nurses;

2 assess when hand decontamination is needed;

3 carry out hand hygiene effectively;

4 understand the factors that influence effective handwashing practice.

Learning outcome 1: State the purpose and importance of hand decontamination for the care and safety of both patients and nurses

Hungarian obstetrician Ignaz Semmelweis (1815–65) succeeded in reducing the death rate of his patients from around 1 in 8 to 1 in 79 by persuading his colleagues and medical students to wash their hands in a solution of chlorinated lime. Since then it has become widely recognised that the hands of those employed in healthcare settings are an important route for the transmission of infection (Pratt *et al.* 2007). People requiring healthcare are often more vulnerable to infection for a variety of reasons, meaning that infection control measures, like hand hygiene, are central to their care.

Microorganisms are important in an ecological balance on earth; some live in humans and other animals and are needed to maintain health. However, as some microorganisms cause disease, how individuals interact with the environment is important. James's work environment may not have been conducive to keeping his wound free from infection, especially if it was not adequately covered. As you will read in Chapter 7, 'Principles of wound care', traumatic wounds are nearly always contaminated so infection poses a high risk in these situations.

Like everyone in the general population, James requires a basic knowledge of hygiene and infection control, including handwashing to reduce his susceptibility to infection. Now that he has an infected wound, the community nurse for learning disabilities should check that he has the cognitive and physical dexterity to care for his wound in between dressing changes and to carry out handwashing. The nurse could demonstrate effective handwashing to James and ensure he can carry this out. She could provide photos of the different stages in handwashing as an *aide-memoire*. Handwashing can help to reduce the risk of infection being transferred to other sites in his body or prevent re-infection. James's Health Action Plan should include this information and the other care associated with his leg, documenting the role of the different professionals involved in his care.

For some people with learning disabilities, a structured behavioural programme may be necessary to teach effective handwashing. The nurse would assess the individual's comprehension level and adapt the programme for the individual. Sometimes a backward chaining technique is used, which involves teaching the final stage of the skill first, and then working consecutively backwards. Encouragement and reinforcement by nurses are very important. Carr and Wilson (1987) cover in detail the techniques for teaching self-help skills such as handwashing.

Bacteria on hands

In a series of classic studies, Price (1938) discovered two populations of bacteria present on hands: *resident* organisms and *transient* organisms. Resident microorganisms, sometimes called **normal flora,** lie deep in the stratum corneum of the skin and are difficult to remove, and are therefore less likely to be implicated in cross-infection. Transient microorganisms are acquired from the environment and are carried temporarily on the hands. These organisms may be transferred between nurse and client, resulting in cross-infection as the nurse moves from one person to another, or handles different sites on the same person. The aim of hand hygiene is to remove transient bacteria to below the level likely to cause infection.

ACTIVITY	Consider how you might pick up transient microorganisms on your hands during everyday nursing practice.

Some examples are:
1. following the care of a person who has been incontinent;
2. when emptying urine bags and bedpans;
3. when handling the bed-linen of a person who has an infection or has been incontinent;
4. when bed-bathing and handling wash bowls;
5. when touching fomites, such as computer keyboards, patients' notes, lockers or beds;
6. during bed-making;
7. when taking a patient's pulse or temperature.

Ayliffe *et al.* (2001) state that studies in their laboratories, using finger impressions, indicate that significant contamination can follow activities 1, 2, 3 and 4 and less so 5, 6 and 7. However, it is important to note that you can pick up microorganisms in any of these ways that involve direct or indirect contact with patients/clients. Wilson *et al.* (2006) found that over a third of keyboards tested in their study were contaminated with MRSA, regardless of the position of the keyboard. Hand hygiene rarely accompanied keyboard contact. Transferring bacteria from your hands to a patient can lead to them acquiring colonisation or infection. Effective hand hygiene can reduce the incidence of HCAIs in all settings.

Learning outcome 2: Assess when hand decontamination is needed

ACTIVITY	With a colleague, make a list of the times when you think it is important to decontaminate your hands in the practice setting.

The standard principle you should adhere to is that you should decontaminate your hands immediately 'before each and every episode of direct patient contact/ care and after any activity or contact that potentially results in hands becoming contaminated' (Pratt *et al.* 2007, S3). Some examples you might have thought of are:

- before aseptic procedures;
- before and after handling invasive devices;
- before and after handling food;
- after removing gloves;
- when hands become visibly soiled;
- after using the toilet;
- when leaving the clinical area.

Pathogens are likely to be acquired on the hands in greatest numbers when handling moist, heavily contaminated substances, such as body fluids. Hand decontamination must be carried out at this time.

ACTIVITY

For each of the practice scenarios, identify care activities when nurses would decontaminate their hands.

You could have thought of many situations for Mrs Lewis; for example, before and after any direct contact such as assisting with personal hygiene, before and after using gloves (see later discussion), when dealing with a used commode, and when carrying out her wound dressing. With James, nurses should decontaminate their hands before and after redressing his wound. With Stacey, hand decontamination would be necessary before and after dealing with her vomit and soiled bed-linen and before and after giving her intramuscular injection.

The nurses caring for Stacey know that she has hepatitis B, but in many other situations this information is not known. Therefore, following the principles of hand decontamination and the other principles discussed in this chapter (personal protective equipment, use and disposal of sharps) for each and every patient will protect you and other patients from the unwitting transmission of dangerous pathogens such as hepatitis B. The DH (2007e) also recommends that all appropriate healthcare staff should be up to date with immunisations for hepatitis B, tuberculosis (TB), measles, mumps and rubella, influenza and chickenpox.

Learning outcome 3: Carry out hand hygiene effectively

Most people learn about washing their hands at an early stage in their lives as part of personal health and hygiene. However, because of the susceptibility of people in healthcare settings, professionals must take particular care to decontaminate hands carefully and thoroughly.

Hand-cleaning preparations

Pratt *et al.* (2007) reviewed hand-cleaning preparations. They concluded that, generally, washing hands effectively with soap and water removes transient microorganisms and renders hands socially clean, which is sufficient for most care activities. They found that soap containing an antiseptic reduces transient and resident microorganisms and

> **Box 3.1   Steps for an effective handwashing technique (Pratt** *et al.* **2007)**
>
> At the start of each shift, remove all wrist and hand jewellery and cover all cuts/abrasions with waterproof dressings.
>
> Preparation
> - Wet hands under running water before applying liquid soap or an antimicrobial preparation.
>
> Washing
> - The handwash solution must come into contact with all the surfaces of the hands.
> - The hands must be rubbed together vigorously for a minimum of 10–15 seconds.
> - Particular attention must be paid to the tips of the fingers, the thumbs and the areas between the fingers.
>
> Drying
> - Hands should be rinsed thoroughly prior to patting dry with good-quality paper towels.

that some antiseptics have a residual effect, which is useful when carrying out surgery or other invasive procedures. Alcohol-based handrub, too, reduces both transient and resident flora but it should not be used when hands are visibly soiled or contaminated with blood or body fluids, and it is not effective against *C. difficile*. Alcohol handrubs are advantageous in situations where handwashing facilities are absent or poor, such as in some community settings. They also reduce the need to leave patients during procedures, like wound dressings, to carry out handwashing.

Effective handwashing technique involves three processes: preparation, washing and rinsing, and drying. Pratt *et al.*'s recommendations for these are summarised in Box 3.1. These processes are now discussed.

Preparation for handwashing

ACTIVITY   What do you think you would need to do to prepare for handwashing?

First ensure you have the necessary equipment at the sink area – liquid soap and paper hand-towels. Based on best evidence, the DH (2007f) identified good practice for uniform/dress of healthcare professionals and recommended that the following should *not* be worn: false nails (they can harbour microorganisms), watches and jewellery such as rings (excluding plain wedding rings) and bracelets, and neckties (they are rarely laundered and have been found to be heavily colonised). Staff should keep nails short, free of nail varnish and clean. Preparation also includes covering cuts and abrasions with a waterproof dressing. This prevents the risk of acquiring infections such as hepatitis B and C and human immunodeficiency virus (HIV)

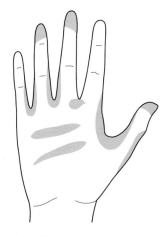

Figure 3.2: Areas commonly missed with poor handwashing. Reproduced with permission from Ayliffe *et al.* (2001).

and may also prevent infection from bacteria and fungi. Preparation before handwashing requires that you wet your hands under tepid running water before applying liquid soap or an antimicrobial cleaning agent.

Washing and rinsing

ACTIVITY

> Find out if you can access pink-dye handwashing solution. This may be available in the skills laboratory or via the infection control nurse. Wash your hands with this solution in your usual fashion and then take note of those areas that you have not covered with the dye. Alternatively you may have access to 'germ powder' and a light-box. Follow the instructions to assess your handwashing technique.

Figure 3.2 shows a diagram of the areas most commonly missed (Ayliffe *et al.* 2001). How does this compare with your handwashing result?

Pratt *et al.* (2007) stressed that all surfaces of the hands must be included during handwashing. Figure 3.3 is an example of a technique that can help you to cover all surfaces of your hands during hand decontamination. You should finish by washing your wrists.

ACTIVITY

> Re-wash your hands using the principles in Box 3.1 and the technique in Fig. 3.3 as a guide. If available, use pink dye or 'germ powder' for this activity so you can note any improvement: did you manage to cover all areas of your hands this time? Ensure you time your handwashing with a watch and adhere to the recommended minimum of 10–15 seconds.

The amount of time you wash your hands for is important, as the mechanical action helps to remove bacteria. As you can see, Pratt *et al.*'s guidelines suggest you spend a minimum of 10–15 seconds; when timing this in the last activity did this

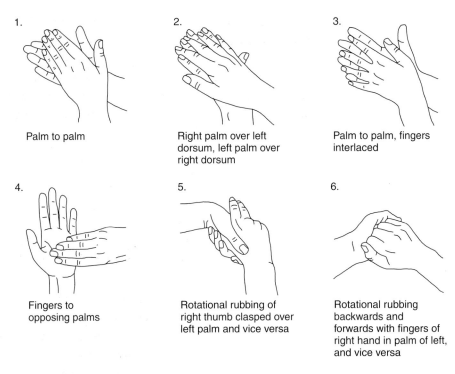

Figure 3.3: An example of handwashing technique to cover all skin surfaces. From Ayliffe, G.A., Babb, J.R. and Quoraishi, A.H. 1978. A test for 'hygienic' hand disinfection. *Journal of Clinical Pathology* 31, 923. Reproduced with permission from the BMJ Publishing group.

feel longer than usual? Hands should be rinsed thoroughly prior to patting dry with good-quality paper towels (Pratt *et al.* 2007). When disposing of paper towels, using foot-operated pedal bins reduces the risk of re-contaminating hands after washing.

Alcohol-based handrubs

The Hand Hygiene Liaison Group (2001) highlighted the benefits of alcohol-based handrubs. They are quick to use and effective. Seventy per cent alcohol decontaminates hands more effectively than soap and water for a wide range of microorganisms, including *Staph. aureus*, *Pseudomonas aeruginosa*, *Klebsiella* and *Rotavirus*. As previously mentioned, alcohol-based handrub can be used only when hands are visibly clean, and it does not kill *C. difficile* spores. It is also preferable that hands are washed with soap and water following glove removal (Pratt *et al.* 2007).

ACTIVITY   Are the principles for performing handwashing and drying that you have read about any different when using an alcohol-based handrub? If so, how?

The principles are similar. The preparatory measures for handwashing discussed also apply to decontamination of hands with alcohol-based handrubs. Pratt *et al.* (2007) advise that the handrub solution must come into contact with all surfaces of the hands, with the hands rubbed together vigorously, giving particular attention to the tips of the fingers, the thumbs and the areas between the fingers, until the solution has evaporated and the hands are dry. After several consecutive uses of alcohol-based handrub the hands should be washed with soap and water.

Learning outcome 4: Understand the factors that influence effective handwashing practice

According to the DH (2003), it is widely believed that failure to wash hands is due to laziness or carelessness; however, there are a number of other barriers to good hand hygiene. In a large hospital-wide survey, Pittet *et al.* (1999) identified predictors of non-compliance with hand hygiene during routine patient care. In 2834 observed opportunities for hand hygiene, average compliance was 48 per cent, being highest among nurses. Non-compliance was higher in intensive therapy units rather than medical wards, during procedures with a high risk for bacterial contamination, and when intensity of patient care was high. The results indicated organisational factors must be considered and that hand hygiene could improve if focused on certain wards, groups of staff and patient interventions.

The importance of staff champions or role models in hand hygiene improvement is critical to improving compliance. Each member of staff can exert a very powerful influence on fellow staff. Adequate preparation for involving patients in hand hygiene improvement is important. The need for commitment from all levels of the organisation is necessary to support this aspect of improving compliance.

ACTIVITY	What factors can you think of that might influence effective handwashing? In particular, think about when you would need to wash your hands either in the community or in a hospital setting. Referring to the scenarios will help you.

By referring to the scenarios you will probably have identified how frequently nurses need to wash their hands. Frequent handwashing can cause damage to skin, especially if antiseptic solutions are used, or if hands are not dried properly. Cracked skin may harbour more bacteria and increase the risk of cross-infection. Therefore you should apply an emollient handcream regularly to protect skin from the drying effects of regular hand decontamination; and if a particular soap or antimicrobial handwash or alcohol-based product causes skin irritation, then occupational health advice must be sought (Pratt *et al.* 2007).

You may have thought of other reasons that could deter nurses from washing their hands. Did your reasons include the following?

- Inadequate and inconveniently placed handwashing facilities. Lack of time may deter handwashing when facilities are some distance away. Water may be too hot and no mixer taps present (Dancer 2002). Taps and dispensers should be elbow-operated, and good facilities should exist for dispensing and disposing of paper towels.
- Lack of education concerning the importance of handwashing.
- Lack of emphasis on handwashing by peers and managers.
- The use of gloves, incorrectly seen as obviating the need for handwashing. Flores and Pevalin (2007) found that hand hygiene compliance was significantly worse after inappropriate glove usage.

You may be aware of campaigns to improve hand hygiene. The National Patient Safety Agency's (NPSA) 'cleanyourhands' campaign aims to 'minimise the risk to patient safety of low compliance with hand hygiene by NHS staff through a national strategy of improvement' – see www.npsa.nhs.uk/cleanyourhands for details. You may have seen campaign posters in care settings. For HPS's hand hygiene campaign, see www.washyourhandsofthem.com

---

Summary

- Effective hand hygiene is an essential tool in the prevention of cross-infection.
- There are various decontamination agents and techniques and nurses need to be aware of which are appropriate in different situations. For example, alcohol-based handrubs are an acceptable alternative to handwashing when hands are not visibly soiled.
- Handwashing must be performed thoroughly, paying attention to preparation, washing and rinsing, and drying, and for an adequate length of time.
- Hands must be patted dry carefully with paper towels.
- There are a number of barriers to effective handwashing but these must be overcome to prevent cross-infection.
- An Infection Control Champion in each clinical area can assist in improving compliance.
- Commitment from all levels of the organisation is needed to support aspects of improving compliance with hand hygiene.

USE OF PERSONAL PROTECTIVE EQUIPMENT, INCLUDING GLOVES, APRONS AND GOWNS

Pratt *et al.* (2007, p. S20) advise that selection of protective equipment (aprons, gowns, gloves, eye protection and face masks) should be based on an assessment of:

> the risk of transmission of microorganisms to the patient or to the carer and the risk of contamination of healthcare practitioners' clothing and skin by patients' blood, body fluid, secretions or excretions.

This section focuses on glove and apron usage as they are commonly used for protection. Masks and visors must be worn when there is a risk of blood, body fluids, secretions and excretions splashing into the face and eyes. Respiratory protective equipment (a particulate filtrate mask) must be fitted when caring for patients with some air-borne respiratory infections.

LEARNING OUTCOMES

On completion of this section you will be able to:
1 identify the procedures for which gloves, sterile or non-sterile, are recommended and key factors in their usage;
2 discuss when plastic aprons and gowns should be worn, stating the rationale.

Pratt *et al.* (2007, S20) point out that gloves are worn for two main reasons:

- to protect hands from contamination with organic matter and microorganisms;
- to reduce the risks of transmission of microorganisms to both patients and staff.

They go on to advise that gloves should not be worn unnecessarily as prolonged and indiscriminate use can lead to adverse reactions and skin sensitivity. Therefore risk assessment should be carried out considering who is at risk and whether sterile or non-sterile gloves are needed, the potential for exposure to blood, body fluids, secretions and excretions, and the likelihood of contact with non-intact skin or mucous membranes. In the next activities you consider situations where sterile gloves are needed, situations where non-sterile gloves are sufficient, and situations where no gloves are needed.

Situations where sterile gloves are used

ACTIVITY

> Referring to each scenario at the beginning of the chapter, write down those clinical procedures and situations for which you think sterile gloves should be worn.

For Mrs Lewis and James, an aseptic technique (see later section) using sterile gloves will be necessary when re-dressing their wounds to reduce the risk of cross-infection. For Stacey, sterile gloves are not necessary from the information given in the scenarios.

From the above activity you can conclude that sterile gloves are used most frequently for invasive procedures and for direct contact with non-intact skin. Another example of a procedure where sterile gloves are necessary is urinary catheterisation (more information in Chapter 9).

When applying sterile gloves you must avoid contaminating the outer surface of the glove. Using the inner surface of the folded cuff, push your hand into the glove. If you line up your thumb with the thumb of the glove you will find the glove goes on more easily. The second glove is easier to put on as you can use your other, gloved, hand to help but it must not touch ungloved areas.

Situations where non-sterile gloves are satisfactory

ACTIVITY

> Look again at the practice scenarios and list those clinical procedures and situations when nurses and other staff should use non-sterile gloves.

As Mrs Lewis has MRSA, gloves should be used by all staff entering her room (Coia *et al.* 2006). Gloves must always be worn when there is potential contact with faeces, urine or any other body fluid (Pratt *et al.* 2007), so non-sterile gloves must be worn when dealing with her commode. Additionally the domestic cleaner should be instructed to wear gloves (and apron) when cleaning the room and to dispose of them before leaving.

For James, probably no gloves are required. However, when the district nurse removes James's soiled dressing, any outer layers (such as a cotton bandage keeping the dressing in place) might be removed using non-sterile gloves, with sterile gloves preserved for the aseptic dressing procedure itself.

Considering Stacey, contact with vomit (a body fluid) necessitates the use of non-sterile gloves. Whether gloves would be worn for other procedures with Stacey depends on individual risk assessment and local policy. Non-sterile gloves are advised for drawing up and administering injections (due to the small risk of bleeding occurring) (NPSA 2007). Wearing gloves also protects from potential harm to nurses during preparation of specific drugs, such as antibiotics and cytotoxic materials.

Key factors in using gloves

All gloves can perforate and should therefore be checked for defects. Keeping fingernails short helps to avoid perforations. Pratt *et al.*'s (2007) standard principles include the following points.

- Gloves are single-use items and must be put on immediately before an episode of care and discarded after each care activity for which they were worn. This is to prevent the transmission of microorganisms to other sites in that individual or other patients. However, Flores and Pevalin (2007) observed nurses wearing the same pair of gloves for more than one task, for example, making a bed and then manipulating an intravenous line.
- Hands should be decontaminated after removing gloves, preferably with soap and water.
- All gloves should be disposed of appropriately (see later section).

Situations where gloves are not necessary

ACTIVITY

With reference to the scenarios, make a list of the procedures and situations for which gloves are usually unnecessary. Think particularly of all the individuals who may come into contact with the patient/client and try to decide if they need to wear gloves.

The risk to Mrs Lewis's visitors is minimal as most do not have contact with body fluids and they do not therefore need to wear gloves. Nevertheless, they should be instructed to wash their hands before leaving the room. If Mrs Lewis visits another department (e.g. X-ray), whether their staff require gloves depends on their level of contact with her. As porters transferring Mrs Lewis are unlikely to be in contact with her or infectious material directly, gloves are not needed.

Concerning James, gloves are needed only when changing wound dressings. For any other aspects of his care they are not required. Similarly, for most of Stacey's care – for example, checking her blood pressure, administering oral medication and giving psychological support – gloves are not required.

Flores and Pevalin (2007) identified considerable over-use of gloves, observing them being worn for collecting equipment, answering the telephone, talking to patients, writing notes and measuring vital signs.

ACTIVITY	When next in the clinical area, take note of the different types of gloves available to practitioners.

All gloves must meet the European Standard (Pratt *et al.* 2007). Types of disposable gloves include natural rubber latex (NRL), vinyl and nitrile. Pratt *et al.* make the following points about these:

- NRL is the material of choice due to the degree of protection offered and level of dexterity.
- Some staff and patients have sensitivities to latex, so non-latex alternatives must be available and allergies must be documented.
- Nitrile gloves offer good protection but can also cause sensitivities.
- Polythene gloves should not be used due to their permeability and tendency to damage.
- Powdered gloves should not be used.

Learning outcome 2: Discuss when plastic aprons and gowns should be worn, stating the rationale

ACTIVITY	Make a list of those occasions when you have seen plastic aprons worn by nurses in practice settings and when you have seen gowns worn.

You may be able to relate your experiences to Pratt *et al.*'s (2007, S21–2) advice about apron and gown usage:

- *Disposable plastic aprons* must be worn when close contact with the patient, materials or equipment are expected, **or** when there is a risk that clothing may become contaminated with pathogenic microorganisms or blood, body fluids, secretions and excretions (with the exception of perspiration).
- *Full-body gowns* are worn if there is a risk of extensive splashing of blood, body fluids, secretions and excretions (with the exception of perspiration) on to the skin of the healthcare practitioner (e.g. during childbirth).

As with gloves, aprons and gowns must be worn as single-use items for one care activity and then disposed of.

In community settings, such as small staffed residences, there is an emphasis on social aspects of care and normalisation, so the use of plastic aprons is likely to be greatly reduced. However, when dealing with body fluids, they are still advisable.

In some care settings, different coloured aprons are used for different care activities. Check your local policy about this.

Normalisation
Normalisation is a concept that has seen much development over the past 30 years. Currently it is viewed as a system that seeks to value positively devalued individuals and groups; see, for example, Emerson (1992) and Swann (1997).

Summary
- Selection of appropriate personal protective equipment should be based on risk assessment.
- Gloves and aprons are single-use items and should be disposed of appropriately, followed by hand decontamination.

ASEPTIC TECHNIQUE

Aseptic technique (also referred to as 'aseptic non-touch technique' or ANTT) is used to prevent cross-infection during procedures where body defences are breached by preventing microbial contamination of body tissues during the procedure. An important component of aseptic technique is to use a sterile field and sterile equipment and to ensure that equipment that must remain sterile is not contaminated. This is achieved by using a non-touch technique (handling equipment in such a way that the important sterile parts are not touched), and by using sterile gloves in some situations. Effective hand hygiene is a fundamental aspect of aseptic technique.

LEARNING OUTCOMES

By the end of this section you will be able to:
1 assess when aseptic technique is required;
2 prepare the patient and the appropriate equipment for aseptic technique, with special reference to wound dressings;
3 outline how aseptic technique is performed and its underpinning rationale, with special reference to wound dressings.

Learning outcome 1: Assess when aseptic technique is required

ACTIVITY

For the following list, identify whether it is true or false that an aseptic technique is required:
1 giving food to patients
2 removal of sutures or clips
3 inserting a urinary catheter
4 taking a patient's temperature
5 assisting with oral hygiene
6 wound dressings.

You should have identified that the answers for 2, 3 and 6 are true, as these are procedures that could introduce infection. For the three remaining procedures, 1, 4 and 5, hand hygiene is required but not aseptic technique. For oral hygiene, non-sterile gloves may be used (more information in Chapter 8).

Generally, aseptic technique should be used following surgery when skin integrity has been interrupted, following trauma to skin tissue, such as experienced by James, and during invasive procedures such as catheterisation. Mrs Lewis would require aseptic technique during her wound care, and her intravenous cannula would have been inserted using an aseptic technique. Any other invasive techniques that may be performed as part of her investigations and treatment would require an aseptic technique. A clean, rather than aseptic, technique is sufficient in some wound care situations, such as with 'chronic' wounds (Gilmour 2000). See Chapter 7, 'Principles of wound care', for further discussion.

Learning outcomes 2 and 3 now explain the use of aseptic technique, as applied to wound dressings, as this is one of the most common reasons for using aseptic technique.

Learning outcome 2: Prepare the patient and the appropriate equipment for aseptic technique, with special reference to wound dressings

ACTIVITY

To maintain asepsis, can you identify what might be the single most important action you can perform prior to performing aseptic technique?

The answer is hand hygiene. Take this opportunity to revisit the section concerned with hand hygiene. Aseptic technique is a prime example of when effective hand hygiene is of utmost importance.

Because hands are not sterile, forceps were traditionally used during wound dressing. However, forceps are awkward to use and do not prevent the transfer of bacteria from wound to hands (Thomlinson 1987). Also, when a patient moves suddenly forceps can be dangerous. Sterile disposable gloves are used for most wound dressings now. Good gloving technique is required to prevent contamination of gloves (see previous section).

ACTIVITY

Discuss with a colleague how you would prepare James to have his wound dressed.

You would need to explain the procedure to James and gain his consent and cooperation. The accident that caused James's wound, followed by ongoing wound dressings, could cause him anxiety, so nurses should be understanding and patient. The community nurse for learning disabilities could help prepare James for his dressings and will be familiar with how to communicate with him effectively. Pictures and photos may be useful to aid understanding. Dressings should be changed when exudate is visible on the surface, as the dressing will no longer act as an impermeable barrier preventing bacteria from the outside reaching the open wound. If a wound is infected, then the moist exudate on the surface of the dressing will contaminate any surfaces it comes into contact with.

ACTIVITY

How might you prepare the environment before carrying out a wound dressing, either in the community as for James, or in a hospital setting, as for Mrs Lewis?

In the community, good lighting and James's comfort and privacy are key factors to consider. James has been having his dressing changed at his home near the farm and community nurses are used to adapting within the home environment. When James attends the local surgery for his dressings, there should be a clean treatment room and good handwashing equipment. In hospital, privacy should be maintained. Mrs Lewis is in a sideroom, but for other patients privacy will be provided by screening or a designated treatment room may be available which should ideally be mechanically ventilated (Ayliffe *et al.* 2000). In open wards, Ayliffe *et al.* (2000) recommend that cleaning activities should be minimised in the immediate vicinity while wound dressings are performed.

The dressing trolley or other surface should be clean and dry. Alcohol-based wipes are commonly used for decontamination, follow local policy.

ACTIVITY

Next you should consider what equipment is required. Drawing on experience in practice, make a list of the equipment you think will be needed for carrying out a wound dressing. Then compare your list with that in Box 3.2.

Dressing packs vary in content but typically include medium-size sterile gloves, gauze swabs, a disposal bag, a paper towel and a container in which fluid can be poured. Commercially manufactured packs often state the content on the wrapper. If there is no waste bag included, you will need to take one. If your hands are small or large you will need separately wrapped sterile gloves in your size. You should check the dressing pack for integrity; if the pack is damaged or torn it should be discarded as the contents can no longer be guaranteed sterile. You should also check that the pack has been sterilised and that the expiry date has not elapsed. For some wound dressings, additional instruments are needed. If these are from the Central Sterile Supplies Department, a receptacle for these used instruments will be needed so they can be returned.

Box 3.2 Equipment for carrying out a wound dressing

- A dressing trolley or surface that can be used for the equipment
- A sterile dressing pack
- Sterile cleansing solution (if cleansing required) and alcohol swab to clean its outer packaging
- Wound dressing appropriate for wound, based on assessment, as per patient's care plan (see Chapter 7), and any additional equipment needed to apply this dressing
- Hypoallergenic tape (if tape is needed)
- Sterile scissors (if needed for the dressing)
- Clean disposable apron
- Alcohol-based handrub

A sterile solution such as normal saline can be used to clean and irrigate the wound, if indicated, and is available in sachets and aerosol cans. A syringe can be used for irrigation and would need adding to the equipment list. Aerosol cans of saline must not be contaminated. It may be preferable for each patient to have their own can, and certainly if the wound is known to be infected or contaminated (Williams 1996). When the district nurse was carrying out James's dressing at home, a can of saline could have been kept in his cottage. Chapter 7, 'Principles of wound care', discusses when and how wound cleansing should take place.

As both James and Mrs Lewis have heavily exuding wounds due to their infections, cleansing will be necessary. The choice of wound dressing depends on many factors (see Chapter 7). The wound care for each patient, including type of dressing, frequency of dressing change and cleansing agent, should all be in the care plan. If tape is to be used, it should be hypoallergenic, in good condition and clean. Sterile scissors should be taken if the dressing will need cutting.

Learning outcome 3: Outline how aseptic technique is performed and its underpinning rationale, with special reference to wound dressings

Before starting aseptic technique, try to ensure you will not be disturbed by telephones etc. Box 3.3 outlines a set of guidelines which you could use to change a wound dressing. These guidelines are intended for use when alone. If you have a second nurse available then this person can, after decontaminating hands, open the pack, be available to observe and support the patient throughout the procedure and open additional items on to the sterile field when required. Before starting aseptic technique, tell the patient that you will minimise talk during the procedure to avoid contamination. This is because, during speech, you could spread microorganisms from your oral mucosa.

The guidelines in Box 3.3 can be adapted as long as the underlying principles are maintained, and you should follow local policy for aseptic technique. The important principles of aseptic technique when applied to wound dressings are that the open wound should not come into contact with any item that is not sterile, and that any items that have been in contact with the wound should be discarded safely or decontaminated (Wilson 2006). This same principle applies to any other procedure using aseptic technique. For example, during catheterisation (see Chapter 9) the sterile catheter, which will be inserted into the sterile urinary tract, must not be contaminated by anything that is non-sterile. Stacey's injection must also be carried out using aseptic technique. The needle will be piercing the skin (the protective barrier) and entering the sterile muscle. Therefore, the needle, syringe and drug must be sterile and should be prepared and administered using a non-touch technique (see Chapter 5), but non-sterile gloves can be worn as these will not touch sterile parts of the equipment.

ACTIVITY

If you have access to a skills laboratory and equipment, collect the equipment listed in Box 3.2 and, following the instructions in Box 3.3, practise carrying out a wound dressing on a colleague. Take particular care to ensure that you do not contaminate the sterile gloves or your sterile field.

> **Box 3.3   Guidelines for aseptic technique, applied to a wound dressing**
>
> *Note*: throughout the procedure continually observe patient's condition and take into account their comfort and privacy.
> * Check patient's notes regarding wound management plan.
> * Explain the procedure, gain consent and cooperation.
> * Wash hands and put on plastic apron.
> * Prepare the environment. Clean the trolley surfaces.
> * Collect equipment and place on bottom of trolley.
> * Position the patient and adjust clothing to expose required area.
> * Loosen the dressing covering the wound (wear non-sterile gloves if necessary).
> * Decontaminate hands.
> * Open the outer packaging of the pack and slip the inner package onto the trolley top.
> * Open the dressing pack using corners only. The sterile field should lie flat on the trolley. Avoid touching sterile inner surfaces and content.
> * Use the sterile disposal bag over one hand to arrange the equipment. Then remove the used dressing with your hand inside the bag, invert the bag and attach it to the side of the trolley, between you and the patient.
> * Open any additional equipment onto the sterile field.
> * Pour solution (if using) into container, avoiding splashing.
> * Decontaminate hands and put on sterile gloves.
> * Place sterile towel near wound.
> * Irrigate/cleanse the wound, if required.
> * Apply new dressing according to manufacturer's instructions.
> * Make patient comfortable.
> * Dispose of all equipment safely. Remove and dispose of apron and gloves.
> * Clean the trolley and wash hands.
> * Document the care, reporting any significant findings or effects on the patient.

Summary

● There are many situations where aseptic technique is necessary to prevent cross-infection during invasive procedures.

● Effective aseptic technique requires good hand hygiene, sterile equipment and ensuring sterile items are not contaminated by using a non-touch technique.

● Understanding the underlying principles of aseptic technique enables guidelines to be adapted safely to each individual situation.

SPECIMEN COLLECTION

Laboratory tests can assist with diagnosing an infection, and successful laboratory diagnosis depends on effective collection of a specimen. This requires appropriate and timely collection of specimens, the correct technique and equipment, along with rapid and safe transport (Meers *et al.* 1995). The sooner a specimen arrives at a laboratory, the greater the chance of organisms surviving and being identified. In general, the larger the quantity of material sent for laboratory examination, the greater the chance of isolating causative organisms. Specimens can be contaminated by poor technique giving rise to confusing or misleading results. Ideally samples should be collected before the beginning of treatments with, for example, antibiotics or antiseptics, or the laboratory should be informed of which are being used. Both antiseptics and antibiotics affect the outcome of laboratory results.

LEARNING OUTCOMES

By the end of this section you will be able to:
1 identify the general principles relating to the collection of any specimen;
2 understand the principles of MRSA screening;
3 show awareness of the general principles underpinning the collection of wound swabs and pus.

Note: For urine and stool specimen collection, refer to Chapter 9. For sputum specimen collection, refer to Chapter 11.

Learning outcome 1: Identify the general principles relating to the collection of any specimen

General principles of collecting any specimen include:
- explaining the procedure to the person, and gaining consent;
- maintaining privacy while the procedure takes place;
- ensuring that hands are washed before and after the procedure;
- wearing non-sterile gloves if handling of body fluids is likely;
- ensuring that tissue and fluid is collected from the suspected site of infection;
- preserving any microorganisms collected in the relevant medium/container and preventing it becoming contaminated by other organisms;
- placing the specimen in an appropriate and correctly labelled container and ensuring the request form is filled out correctly.

The microbiology laboratory may be the provider of the correct specimen container. **Do not** label the container until after the specimen is collected, to prevent contamination of the label, and mistakes.

If specimens cannot be sent to a laboratory immediately they should be stored in a dedicated specimen refrigerator at 4°C. Blood cultures, however, go in an incubator at 37°C. Cotton-wool swab sticks are used to take specimens from mucous membranes. The specimen stick is then inserted into a tube of soft agar, which preserves any microorganisms for up to 24 hours. Bottles for transporting viruses are usually acquired from the laboratory and need prompt transport to the laboratory as soon as possible after the swab is taken.

Without full information it is impossible to examine a specimen adequately or to report it accurately. Also, if specimens are not correctly labelled the laboratory cannot process the specimen and a further specimen will have to be obtained, thus delaying treatment.

Make a list of the information that you think would be essential to document and accompany the specimen. Why is full and correct information important?

You may have identified the following:
- patient's name and location (e.g. address, ward);
- hospital number and patient's date of birth;
- consultant's/GP's name;
- date and time specimen collected;
- clinical details of relevance to the specimen, for example signs of infection;
- date of onset of the illness;
- any antibiotic therapy being taken by the patient – failure to provide this information could lead to a false report (Donovan 1998);
- type of specimen and site;
- name and telephone/bleep number of the doctor/nurse requesting the investigation – it may be necessary to telephone the result before the report is despatched.

The specimen must be correctly labelled to ensure that it can be identified and matched with its corresponding request form so results of the tests are related to the correct patient. Specimens are potentially hazardous to staff who could be exposed to people's body fluids. Wilson (2006) advises that the person collecting the specimen must ensure the specimen container is sealed securely and is leakproof, that all body fluid traces have been removed from the container's outside, that the specimen container is not over-filled, that biohazard labels are attached to the container and form if appropriate, and that the container is sealed in a plastic bag.

Learning outcome 2: Understand the principles of MRSA screening

There has been variability across the NHS regarding which patients to screen for MRSA, how to screen them, and when (DH 2007g). Coia *et al*.'s (2006) guidelines for the control and prevention of MRSA recommend an active approach to MRSA screening linked to isolation and cohorting facilities (see next section).

In practice, how have you seen decisions made about who to screen for MRSA? Should Mrs Lewis have been screened when she was first admitted to hospital after fracturing her hip?

The Department of Health (DH) (2007g) suggests that there is good evidence to support the following patients being screened for MRSA.
- *Preoperative patients in surgical specialities where MRSA infection is particularly serious* (elective orthopaedics, cardiothoracic, neurosurgery). This is to prevent

patients becoming infected by their own MRSA while also preventing transmission to other vulnerable patients. These patients should be screened before admission so that, if necessary, they can first be decolonised.

- *Emergency orthopaedic and trauma admissions.* Many of these are older people from care homes or in regular contact with healthcare personnel, so the risk of them being colonised with MRSA is increased. Mrs Lewis fits into this category and should have been screened on admission. It is possible that her wound infection was endogenous – she could have been colonised with MRSA on admission, which then led to her wound infection.
- *Critical care.* Intensive treatment unit and high-dependency unit patients have the highest risk of MRSA transmission and bacteraemia. They should be screened on admission to critical care and on a weekly basis. Decolonisation should be instigated for patients found to be positive, but the DH (2007g) suggests that there is a case for decolonisation being started before results are available and then discontinued if the patient's result is negative.
- *Renal medicine.* Patients on dialysis have a very high risk of bacteraemia due to MRSA and should therefore be screened on admission and at regular intervals.

The DH (2007g) suggests that other groups of patients screened should be determined according to local risk assessments and practicality, but might include:

- all patients previously known to be positive for MRSA;
- all elective surgical patients at pre-admission clinics;
- oncology/chemotherapy patients (as they have a high risk of MRSA bacteraemia due to immunosuppression and vascular access for treatment);
- patients admitted from high-risk settings, including those with frequent contact with healthcare settings or who are care-home residents (around 20 per cent of care-home residents are colonised with MRSA);
- all emergency admissions – some trusts consider it simpler and more reliable if screening is conducted on all patients admitted through A&E or on to medical reception units.

The DH contends that the most logical approach is the universal screening of all people admitted to hospital, which should commence by 2011.

ACTIVITY

Have you observed or been involved in MRSA screening in the practice setting? If so, what sites were swabbed and how was this performed?

The DH (2007g) advises that the essential site to swab is the nose as it is the most common site for MRSA and most patients positive at other sites also have positive nose swabs. Secondary sites are the axilla and perineum/groin and skin lesions should be swabbed too. Coia *et al.* (2006) also advise catheter sites, catheter urine, tracheostomies, sputum if the patient has a productive cough, and possibly also throat swabs.

You should act according to local policy when collecting specimens, but the following procedures have been recommended for swabs. A transport (culture) medium is required and swabs taken from drier areas, like the nose and skin, should first be moistened by dipping them into sterile saline or the culture medium.

Obtaining a nose swab
- The patient should sit facing a strong light source with the head tilted back.
- The moistened swab is rubbed several times firmly around the anterior nares of each nostril (Ayliffe *et al.* 2001).

Obtaining a throat swab
- A tongue depressor and a good light source are needed. This procedure is unpleasant and may cause the patient to gag.
- The swab, taken quickly but gently, should be rubbed over the pharyngeal wall and/or the tonsillar fossa. Saliva contamination should be avoided (Ayliffe *et al.* 2001).

Patients who are MRSA positive should be isolated if possible or cohort-nursed with other MRSA-positive patients, and a decolonisation programme will commence (covered in the next section, 'Isolation procedures').

Learning outcome 3: Show awareness of the general principles underpinning the collection of wound swabs and pus

Collection of a wound swab is indicated when signs of infection (e.g. purulent discharge, swelling, redness, pain, pyrexia and delayed healing) are present. As you read in the scenarios, James had a wound swab taken from his clinically infected wound. The Health Protection Agency (HPA) (2006a) advises that collecting samples of pus or exudate, if present, is preferable to swabbing wounds. Pus can be withdrawn using a syringe and sent to the laboratory in a universal container (Ayliffe *et al.* 2001). If only minute amounts of pus are present, it can be collected on a swab which is put into transport medium (HPA 2006a). There is little point swabbing dry areas (HPA 2006a). Miller (1998) highlights that many wounds are colonised rather than infected, and that microorganisms grown from the swab may not in fact be the causation of the infection. Wilson (2006) agrees and states that wound infection should be recognised by clinical signs of infection rather than just isolation of bacteria from a swab.

Wound swabs or pus should be obtained at the beginning of the dressing procedure, after the dressing has been removed, and dressing material traces should be first cleansed away using saline. Donovan (1998) reviewed the literature on how best to take a wound swab and her recommendations can be found in Box 3.4. The swab should be taken from the infected site, avoiding surrounding skin and mucous membranes, and then placed in transport medium. The site of the wound must be stated on the request form so that the appropriate media can be set up. Different areas of the body have different natural flora, which can be pathogenic elsewhere (Donovan 1998). One swab only should be taken from a wound on any one occasion.

> ### Box 3.4 Wound swabbing technique (references cited by Donovan 1998)
>
> - Irrigate the wound with a gentle stream of normal saline at body temperature (Lawrence 1997), to remove surface contamination.
> - Moisten the wound swab with normal saline (Rudensky *et al.* 1992) or transport medium (Wound Care Society 1993).
> - Move the swab across the whole wound surface, by using a zigzag movement across the wound while rotating the swab between the fingers (Cooper and Lawrence 1996).
> - Sample the whole surface area (Gilchrist 1996) or 1 cm^2 if the surface is large (Levine *et al.* 1976).
> - Place the swab straight into the transport medium. Label and package it appropriately.

Summary

- Specimens can be important diagnostic aids and should be collected carefully, using recommended techniques.
- It is essential to prevent cross-infection and contamination of the specimen.
- Specimens should be labelled accurately, and full accompanying information supplied.
- MRSA screening should be carried out for patients as recommended.
- Clinical signs of a wound infection should be looked for. Collection of pus is preferable to wound swabs.

ISOLATION PROCEDURES

Isolation procedures are used to prevent the spread of infection from an infected or colonised person to others in healthcare settings. This type of isolation procedure is termed 'source isolation'. 'Protective isolation' is used to protect people who are highly susceptible to infections from others in healthcare settings. In both types of isolation, standard precautions, including hand hygiene, personal protective equipment and waste disposal, are central. The DH (2007h) recommends that single rooms are always preferable for isolating infected patients but that cohort nursing for a group of patients with the same organism (e.g. MRSA) is an alternative if single-room capacity is exceeded. For cohort nursing they advise these key points:

- Patient movements for non-clinical reasons should be minimal.
- There should be designated staff for these patients.
- If there is no designated ward, use a bay within a ward – but bays should have doors that can be closed, thus physically separating them from other patients.
- In critical care, cohorting may need to occur in a specific area of the unit.

LEARNING OUTCOMES

By the end of this section you will be able to:

1 identify when source isolation is necessary and key principles of care;
2 discuss when protective isolation is necessary and what it entails;
3 consider the importance of communication and be aware of whom to inform
   when isolation is required.

*Learning outcome 1: Identify when source isolation is necessary and key
principles of care*

ACTIVITY

Mrs Lewis is being nursed in isolation as she has MRSA. Why is this necessary?
What infection control measures would underpin her care?

When patients, like Mrs Lewis, are identified as MRSA positive, either because
they have an MRSA infection or were identified through screening as being an
asymptomatic carrier by screening, they should be isolated to reduce the risk of
transmission to other patients. However, the DH (2007g) recommends that when a
patient is identified as an MRSA carrier a decolonisation regimen should commence,
irrespective of the availability of isolation facilities. Decolonisation comprises an
antibacterial shampoo and body wash daily, and application of an antibacterial nasal
cream thrice daily for 5 days (DH 2007g). The aim is to prevent an endogenous
MRSA infection and transmission of MRSA to other patients. After each shampoo
and hairwash, new bed-linen, towels and clothing must be provided (Coia *et al.* 2006).

You probably identified that infection control measures underpinning Mrs Lewis's
care include hand hygiene, personal protective equipment and correct waste disposal –
and all these are important. Coia *et al.* (2006) advise that a standard approach to
isolation should be taken using sound infection control principles rather than specific
precautions for patients with MRSA. The DH (2007h) identified these key points for
any patient being isolated; all are relevant to Mrs Lewis:

- Regardless of glove usage, there should be high standards of hand decontamination,
  with hand hygiene before and after each direct patient contact.
- All staff and visitors assisting with patient care or in contact with their immediate
  environment should wear aprons.
- Disposable gloves should be worn when in contact with bodily fluids or
  contaminated items. In addition, Coia *et al.* (2006) advise gloves should be worn
  by any staff entering the isolation room of a patient with MRSA.
- Fans should not be used.
- Notes and charts should be kept outside the room/bay/area.
- Where possible, equipment should be single use. Multi-use equipment must be
  decontaminated as per manufacturer's instructions.
- Linen should be treated as infectious.
- All waste should be disposed of as hazardous waste.

- Cleaning procedures should be rigorously applied with enhanced and terminal cleaning procedures.
- Transfer and movement of patients should be minimised and only take place for clinical reasons. The receiving area must be informed. Hand hygiene and personal protective equipment should be used when transferring. Equipment used for transferring (e.g. a trolley) should be decontaminated.

Any other special precautions used depend on the type of infection and its specific route of transmission. Check back to Table 3.1 if you need to recap on these. Patients with air-borne infections (e.g. chickenpox, pulmonary tuberculosis) should, as a minimum, be nursed in a well-ventilated side-room with the door closed, but ideally a negative-pressure ventilated isolation room would be used (Wilson 2006). In most cases, when a single room is necessary for isolation, the door should be kept shut; but the ICT can advise concerning individual cases; for example, when a patient is confused and their safety could be jeopardised by closing the door. Patients, such as Stacey, with blood-borne infections (unless bleeding) can often be managed in the open ward using standard infection control precautions. This includes the safe management of sharps and the routine use of protective clothing where contact with body fluids or blood is likely.

ACTIVITY

To prevent spread of infection to other people, what precautions should be taken if someone develops diarrhoea and vomiting? Consider both small community-based units and hospital situations.

For a community setting you might have identified the following:
- Good personal hygiene is required, particularly handwashing before eating and after using the toilet.
- Normal crockery and cutlery are usually sufficient. Bacteria are easily removed by washing in hot water and detergent. However, cleaning of crockery and cutlery is best done at high temperatures in a dishwasher.
- If dishes are washed by hand, then clean hot water should be used with detergent. The items should be rinsed and left to drain, rather than being dried with a cloth, as these are easily contaminated. Dishcloths should be disposable.
- If possible, the person should be allocated a toilet for their sole use.
- If there is a suspected outbreak of gastrointestinal illness – defined as when two or more clients or staff are affected by unexplained diarrhoea or vomiting – then further action may be needed, particularly if there are other vulnerable people within the residence. In small staffed units, the other residents' GPs and the ICT need to be informed. Stool specimens should be obtained from those affected even if they no longer have symptoms.

If gastroenteritis occurs in an institutional setting, such as a hospital, affected patients must be transferred to single rooms where at all possible. Standard isolation procedures should then be put in place (as previously discussed) and the infection control department informed.

C. difficile-associated disease

In the care bundle to prevent the spread of *C. difficile*-associated disease (CDAD), the DH (2007c) identifies the following elements:

- Prescribing of antibiotics should be prudent.
- Hands should be washed with soap and water after each contact with a patient with CDAD. Alcohol-based handrub is not effective for these patients.
- Gloves and aprons should be worn when handling bodily fluids and when caring for patients with CDAD.
- Environmental decontamination involves enhanced cleaning for areas with CDAD patients, using chlorine-based disinfectants or other sporicidal products.
- There should be a deep clean and decontamination of rooms following discharge of CDAD patients.
- Patients with CDAD should be isolated in single rooms if possible, but cohort care can be applied if they are unavailable.

Learning outcome 2: Discuss when protective isolation is necessary and what it entails

Isolation is used also for patients who are extremely vulnerable to infectious diseases because their immune system is compromised. 'Protective isolation' is used to protect patients from infection risks from themselves and others rather than to protect others from any risk that they pose.

ACTIVITY

What conditions might lead to patients being severely immunocompromised? What precautions would be necessary?

Examples include patients with prolonged neutropenia as a result of chemotherapy for leukaemia, lymphoma and bone marrow transplant (Gould and Brooker 2000). Patients in protective isolation should not be cared for by staff with infections or who are looking after people with infections on the same shift (Wilson 2006). Protective isolation requires single rooms, thorough handwashing, and use of aprons and gloves.

Management of these patients includes consideration of the food they eat. Most food contains microorganisms and these are not usually harmful in small numbers. Wilson (2006) advises that food for immunocompromised patients must be served without delay and must not be reheated. Eggs must be cooked thoroughly and fresh fruit should be washed and peeled. These patients should avoid soft cheeses, undercooked meat and fish, patés and freshly made salad. Wilson (2006) advises that fresh tapwater and pasteurised milk are acceptable. Bottled water is not recommended due to variable storage and manufacturing conditions.

Invasive procedures are a major threat to immunosuppressed patients and strict protocols must be followed when these are used (Gould and Brooker 2000). Finally, visitors should have no obvious signs of infection and must decontaminate their hands prior to visiting the patient.

Learning outcome 3: Consider the importance of communication and be aware of who to inform when isolation is required

List the key people who should be informed when a decision is made to isolate a patient. Try to link your answer to Mrs Lewis's case.

You may have identified the following: Mrs Lewis herself, her family and friends, domestic staff, the ICT, and possibly other departments (e.g. Radiography). Further details about these will now be discussed.

Explanations to patients and relatives

Infections cause emotional as well as physical distress. There is some evidence that some patients do not understand the reasons for isolation and need to receive explanations about this in order to support treatment (Myatt and Langley 2003). The DH (2007h) advises that staff should provide affected patients and visitors with explanations of their infection, isolation procedures and treatment. Patient information leaflets are available for certain infections, such as chickenpox and MRSA, and these can back up verbal explanations and should be available in different languages. Providing information to patients about being isolated has been found to reduce the negative psychological effects (Gammon 1999).

Some clinical areas ask that visitors enter isolation rooms only after obtaining permission and instruction from the nurse in charge. While children and susceptible visitors should be advised of the risks of visiting, for most infections the risks are minimal, as the visitors do not have contact with body fluids (Wilson 2006). They should be advised to wash their hands before leaving the room.

Explanations to domestic staff

The domestic supervisor should be informed of any patients who are being isolated. A dedicated mop, bucket and disposable cleaning cloths should be provided for the room. The domestic will need to wear apron and gloves when cleaning and these must be disposed of before leaving the room.

Most microorganisms are not able to survive on clean, dry surfaces for long (Wilson 2006), so the environment need not be a major factor in the transmission of infections. The normal standard of cleaning should be maintained and domestic staff should be reassured that the risks to their own health are minimal if protective clothing is worn and careful handwashing takes place. This is very important as otherwise the standard of cleaning may suffer (Wilson 2006).

There is some evidence that increasing domestic cleaning time with emphasis on removal of dust by vacuum cleaning and allocation of responsibility for the routine cleaning of medical equipment can help to terminate prolonged outbreaks of MRSA (Rampling *et al.* 2001).

Infection control team

The clinical area will often have a list of communicable infections which indicates if isolation is necessary and highlights which material from the patient is potentially infectious. If in doubt, the ICT can offer advice. The ICT must be contacted if a patient has MRSA, or has been infected, colonised or transferred from a ward with MRSA cases in the recent past (usually defined as six months). Those patients isolated because of other infectious diseases should also be notified to the ICT. Certain infectious diseases are notifiable to local authorities, usually by the doctor making the diagnosis (Wilson 2006).

Nationally, there are organisations who advise on control of infectious diseases: the HPA (www.hpa.org.uk), and in Scotland, HPS (www.hps.scot.nhs.uk).

Visits to departments

Staff in other departments and areas that the patient may need to visit should be informed so that any special arrangements can be made. If possible, investigations should be carried out immediately so that patients do not wait in communal areas in contact with other patients (Coia *et al.* 2006). This would be relevant to Mrs Lewis if she requires a hip X-ray. Porters need not wear protective clothing, but should be advised to wash their hands on completion of the journey (Wilson 2006). Any transporting staff with skin abrasions should wear gloves and the trolley or chair should be cleaned with detergent and hot water, or in accordance with local policy. Linen use should comply with local guidelines.

Managing the psychological effects of isolation

ACTIVITY

• How might Mrs Lewis feel, being isolated in a side-room?
• What might nurses do to reduce the effects of isolation?

Gammon (1999) states that source isolation can be an extremely frightening and anxiety-provoking experience for both patients and relatives. He goes on to suggest that the psychological effects of source isolation are not well understood and that more research is needed. He describes how patients may feel confined, imprisoned and shut in. Moreover, depression, irregular sleep patterns, and even hallucinations, disorientation and regression are described. A small qualitative study by Oldham (1998) cites patients saying 'There are times when I am completely forgotten' and 'I feel very shut out at the moment.'

Nurses should be sensitive to the psychological implications of being labelled infectious and of being isolated. Patients who are isolated may receive less attention and contact from nurses as they are not in immediate view, and because nurses must put on gloves and apron before entering, quick casual contact is reduced. It is important for nurses to try to reduce patients' fears and problems of isolation and ensure that they approach people in an understanding manner (see also Chapter 2).

Summary

- While standard precautions are sufficient to prevent cross-infection in many circumstances, in some situations additional measures are necessary in the form of source isolation.
- Source isolation requires correct use of hand hygiene, gloves, aprons and waste disposal, and usually a single room for the person who is identified as a source of infection – with, if possible, equipment for their sole use.
- For patients who are severely immunocompromised, protective isolation may be required.
- When isolation is necessary, good communication with patients, relatives and staff is essential.
- Nurses should be aware of the psychological impact of isolation and provide support and information.

SHARPS DISPOSAL

Safe disposal of sharps, such as needles, blood glucose lancets, intravenous cannulae and catheter stylets, is important to maintain a safe environment and prevent cross-infection. The HPA (2006b) reported that occupational exposures to needlestick injuries increased by 49 per cent between 2002 and 2005, and that almost half of all exposures occur in nurses. Needle protection devices are in use in some areas which could reduce the number of needlestick injuries, but Pratt *et al.* (2007) concluded that further evaluation of these is needed.

LEARNING OUTCOMES

By the end of this section you will be able to:
1 understand the need and reasons for the safe disposal of sharps;
2 explain the principles for the safe use and disposal of sharps;
3 identify the actions required following needlestick injury.

Learning outcome 1: Understand the need and reasons for the safe disposal of sharps

ACTIVITY

Identify with a colleague two possible reasons for the importance of disposing of sharps safely.

The main reason for disposing of sharps safely is the physical prevention of cross-infection through needlestick injuries. Pratt *et al.* (2007) report that the average risk of transmission of blood-borne pathogens following a single percutaneous exposure, without post-exposure prophylaxis or prior vaccination (if available), has been estimated as:

- hepatitis B virus 33.3 per cent (1 in 3)
- hepatitis C virus 3.3 per cent (1 in 30)
- HIV 0.31 per cent (1 in 319).

The staff who are caring for Stacey know that she has hepatitis B. Therefore if they sustain a needlestick injury from her used injection needle they will be at risk of acquiring hepatitis B, if they are not immune. However, this information is not always available. Patients themselves may not know that they are carrying a blood-borne disease. Therefore sharps disposal should be carried out in the same way for all patients. In the first instance, it is the injured healthcare professional who is at risk of contamination from a patient source. However, the professional may then pass the infection back to other patients if the correct procedures are not followed.

A second important reason for ensuring the safe disposal of sharps is the professional responsibility of nurses to protect patients and colleagues from risk (NMC 2008). The distress that almost invariably occurs following sharps injuries is concerned with individuals' understandable fear of the blood-to-blood transmission of bacteria and viruses.

ACTIVITY   Discuss with a colleague how you would feel if you sustained a needlestick injury where the patient source was suspected of having a blood-borne infection.

You might have identified fear, anxiety and panic among your emotions. It is clearly much better to prevent needlestick injuries.

Learning outcome 2: Explain the principles for the safe use and disposal of sharps

ACTIVITY   Make a list of the key safety factors you think you should take into account when using and disposing of sharps.

There are many factors to take into account. Pratt *et al.* (2007) includes these standard principles:
* Sharps must not be passed directly from hand to hand, and handling should be kept to a minimum.
* Needles must not be bent, recapped, dissembled or broken after use.
* Used sharps must be discarded into the sharps container (conforming to UN3291 and BS7320 standards) at the point of use.
* The sharps container must not be filled above the mark indicating that it is full.
* Containers should be placed out of reach of children at a height that enables safe disposal by staff, and they should be secured to prevent spillage.

Other important points

Sharps boxes placed more than 1.2 m (4 ft) above the ground are associated with increased risk of sharps injuries (Weltman *et al.* 1995), so ensure they are positioned appropriately. Preferably take a sharps bin to the patient. Always place sharps carefully into the container and never drop or throw them from a distance. Never put fingers into the sharps container, nor kick or shake the container in order to make more room. Do not attempt to clean the sharps container, particularly around the lip. The responsibility for the disposal of sharps lies with the individual who has been using them.

The DH (2006b) explains that, due to waste disposal legislation, sharps bins should have different coloured lids according to the sharps used:

- purple lid for sharps used for cytotoxic drugs;
- yellow lid for sharps containing non-cytotoxic drugs (e.g. syringe with residual medicine);
- orange lid for sharps not containing drugs and not used for cytotoxics (e.g. sharps used for venepuncture).

It is advised that sharps should not be discharged of medicines just so that an orange-topped bin can be used. In the community (and some other settings) it may be more practical to use only yellow-topped sharps boxes to avoid having to segregate sharps. Self-medicating community patients (e.g. people with diabetes) should be provided with a sharps bin and taught to seal and label it and return it to the surgery or pharmacy for disposal when it is three-quarters full. Policies for hospital community trusts, and care homes may vary, and you should ensure that you are familiar with the relevant policies for the areas that you study and work in.

ACTIVITY	What should you do when a sharps box is full (i.e. reached the 'full' mark on the box)?

Containers should be sealed according to the manufacturer's instructions, which are often found on the outside of the box. If you observe that a sharps box is full, be proactive about sealing it. Do not leave someone else to deal with an overfilled sharps bin as this is very hazardous. Sealed containers should be left at identified collection points in the manner prescribed by the local policy, and labelled with date and source. It is usual for portering staff to remove the boxes and take them to a central point for transporting. The correct sealing and disposal of sharps bins is essential to protect the many people who could be injured otherwise, including porters, transport staff and waste disposal staff.

Learning outcome 3: Identify the actions required following needlestick injury

ACTIVITY	With a colleague, discuss what you think should be done following a needlestick injury.

All healthcare employers are required to develop mechanisms for dealing with sharps injuries. These include identifying the employee's responsibility to report the injury and their subsequent entitlement to be provided with counselling and testing services. However, before this stage is reached, emergency action should be taken. Now check your ideas with Table 3.2.

Table 3.2: Action after a needlestick injury.

	Note that you should consult and follow your local policy throughout. It is the responsibility of the member of staff involved and their manager to see that all procedures are carried out.
Emergency action	• Encourage bleeding at the site by squeezing. • Wash wound with soap and water. • For splashes to eyes, mouth or into broken skin, rinse thoroughly with plenty of running water. • Call for assistance. • Cover wound with waterproof dressing.
Reporting	• Inform your manger immediately. • Complete accident/incident form. • Identify patient source if possible. • Report to the occupational health department immediately, or if closed attend the emergency department for further advice.
Follow up	• Make use of counselling if required. • Attend for testing if indicated. • Follow medical advice.

The policies outlined above are also used if blood or body fluid is splashed into the eyes or mouth, or on to broken skin.

ACTIVITY

When you are next in the practice setting, seek out and read the local clinical policy on the action to be taken following a sharps injury.

Summary

- Sharps pose a potential hazard to nurses, other staff and the public.
- All nurses must follow national and local policy and handle and dispose of sharps safely in order to prevent the risk of needlestick injury to themselves and colleagues.
- All healthcare organisations have agreed procedures to follow in the event of a needlestick injury and these should be adhered to carefully.

HEALTHCARE WASTE DISPOSAL AND LINEN MANAGEMENT

The DH (2006b) points out that, historically, 'clinical waste' was the term used, in accordance with the Controlled Waste Regulations (Statutory Instrument 1992), to refer to waste that was either infectious or medicinal. In recent years both UK and European legislation have led to changes in how waste is classified and disposed of. The DH (2006b) provides a detailed background to how legislation has changed waste disposal procedures in healthcare and recommends new methods for identifying and classifying infectious and medicinal waste, a revised colour-coded waste segregation and packaging system, the use of European Waste Catalogue (EWC) codes, and an offensive/hygiene waste stream to describe waste that is non-infectious (human hygiene waste). There is a statutory duty of care which applies to all those involved in the waste management chain; this includes nurses.

The EWC is produced by the European Commission in accordance with the European Waste Framework Directive (75/442/EEC) to provide common terminology for describing waste throughout Europe. The EWC is implemented in England, Wales and Northern Ireland by the Hazardous Waste Regulations (Statutory instrument 2005a) through the List of Wastes Regulations, and in Scotland by the Special Waste Amendment (Scotland) Regulations (Statutory instrument 2004). HPS (2008e) outlined safe disposal of healthcare waste in Scotland.

The Health and Safety Executive (2006) advised that key changes in waste disposal practice are as follows.

- The new term 'healthcare waste' is introduced, defined as waste from maternity care, diagnosis, treatment or prevention of disease in humans or animals. Healthcare waste includes infectious waste, laboratory cultures, anatomical waste, sharps waste, medicinal waste, laboratory chemicals, and offensive/hygiene waste from wards or other healthcare areas.
- Infectious waste is defined as waste that contains viable microorganisms or their toxins, which are known or reliably believed to cause disease in humans or living organisms.
- Medicinal waste and a methodology for its classification are defined.
- The new term 'offensive/hygiene' waste is introduced, defined as non-infectious non-hazardous waste which does not require specialist treatment or disposal, but which may cause offence to those coming into contact with it.

LEARNING OUTCOMES

By the end of this section you will be able to:
1 define different types of waste arising from healthcare and identify how they are dealt with;
2 identify the colours used for different waste streams and apply this in practice;
3 discuss how used linen should be dealt with.

Learning outcome 1: Define different types of waste arising from healthcare and identify how they are dealt with

Table 3.3 summarises the waste streams now used. In England and Wales, it is a legal requirement of the Hazardous Waste Regulations to segregate infectious waste (waste that is subject to special requirements) from other wastes. This duty is not specified in the Hazardous Waste Regulations in Northern Ireland (Statutory instrument 2005b) nor in the Special Waste Regulations in Scotland, but source segregation of infectious waste is considered best practice (DH 2006b).

Hazardous waste may be *infectious* or *medicinal*.

ACTIVITY

Identify waste from Mrs Lewis and James that you think is infectious waste.

Table 3.3: Waste streams (adapted from DH 2006b)

Waste type	Definition	Examples
Hazardous waste	Waste classified as hazardous by the Hazardous Waste Regulations and the List of Wastes Regulations In Scotland, the term 'special waste' is used instead of 'hazardous waste' May be infectious or medicinal	*Infectious:* Used dressing materials from infected wounds *Medicinal:* Expired liquid medicines and tablets
Offensive/hygiene waste	May cause offence due to recognisable healthcare waste items or body fluids Does not possess any hazardous properties, does not need disinfection, or any other treatment, to reduce microorganisms present	Incontinence and other waste produced from human hygiene, sanitary waste, nappies, medical items and equipment which do not pose a risk of infection (e.g. old plaster casts)
Domestic waste	Same as, or similar to, household waste and which is suitable for disposal to landfill	Newspapers, flowers

Infectious waste is waste that poses a known or potential risk of infection, regardless of the level of infection posed, so even minor infections are included within the definition of infectious (DH 2006b). You might have identified Mrs Lewis's and James's old wound dressings as examples of infectious waste. The DH (2006b) advised that whether healthcare waste is infectious must be assessed by healthcare staff. In the community, domestic waste – which includes items like minor first aid and self-care items (e.g. nappies, sanitary products and plasters) which do not need healthcare practitioner input – is assumed to be non-infectious unless a healthcare practitioner indicates otherwise.

The DH (2006b) explained that, in healthcare premises, infectious waste is healthcare waste from patients with diseases caused by a microorganism or its toxin, where the causal pathogen or toxin is present in the waste. Examples are:

- waste from wound infections and other HCAIs;
- hygiene products from patients with UTIs;
- waste from patients with diarrhoea and vomiting caused by infectious agents or toxins (e.g. noroviruses, *C. difficile*);
- blood-contaminated dressings from a patient with HIV, hepatitis B, rubella, measles, mumps, influenza or other infection that may be present in the blood;
- respiratory materials from patients with pulmonary tuberculosis, influenza, respiratory syncytial virus (RSV) or other respiratory infections;
- contaminated waste from provision of general healthcare to patients with known or suspected underlying or secondary microbial diseases and healthcare waste that may cause infection to any people coming into contact with it.

ACTIVITY   What do you think medicinal waste might be?

You might have considered boxes of tablets that are out of date, medicine bottles not fully used, ampoules and syringes with drug residue. The DH (2006b) identifies three groups of medicinal waste:

- cytotoxic and cytostatic;
- pharmaceutically active but not cytotoxic and cytostatic;
- not pharmaceutically active and possessing no hazardous properties (e.g. saline and glucose).

Only cytotoxic and cytostatic medicines are classified as a hazardous waste, although other medicines often possess hazardous properties and therefore require appropriate treatment and disposal.

Learning outcome 2: Identify the colours used for different waste streams and apply this in practice

The DH (2006b) advises that staff segregating waste should be provided with clear instructions on the segregation process and should be provided with appropriate training, and colour-coded waste receptacles should be supplied for each waste stream. The options for waste management are recycling, landfill, treatment or incineration and the colour coding relates to these.

ACTIVITY	What colour receptacles have you seen used in practice for waste disposal?

The colours you are likely to have seen will depend on the type of healthcare settings you have worked in and the type of waste produced and how it should be disposed of. Here are the colours now recommended for different types of waste (DH 2006b):

- **Yellow** *is for waste requiring incineration.* This includes anatomical waste (e.g. placenta), diagnostic specimens, reagent or test vials, and kits containing chemicals. Examples include anatomical waste from theatres (e.g. if bone was removed from Mrs Lewis during her hip surgery).
- **Orange** *is for waste which may be treated at a licensed facility.* This includes infectious and potentially infectious waste (as discussed previously).
- **Purple** *is for cytotoxic and cytostatic waste,* which requires incineration.
- **Yellow with black stripe** *is for deep landfill disposal.* This includes offensive/hygiene waste which is not infectious or hazardous (as discussed previously).
- **Black or clear bag** *is for landfill/recycling.* Domestic – general refuse, flowers, confectionery.

Note: Colour-coding for sharps bins was discussed in the previous section.

ACTIVITY	If waste is not dealt with safely spillage can occur, causing harm to anyone in contact with it. How can you avoid this occurring?

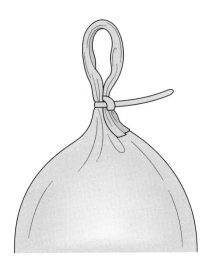

Figure 3.4: Swan-neck technique for sealing waste bags.

Receptacles (bags or rigid containers) must be no more than three-quarters full when they are sealed. The 'swan-neck' method is recommended for sealing bags (see Figure 3.4). The bags/containers must be labelled or tagged with their origin so they can be traced back to source. Waste bags must be provided as near to usage as possible.

Healthcare workers who generate waste in the community have a duty of care to ensure the waste is managed correctly.

ACTIVITY   How should the waste from James's infected wound dressing have been dealt with by the district nurse at his cottage?

As this was infected material, it should have been put into an orange waste disposal bag, labelled appropriately and arrangements for collection made (e.g. a contractor or local authority). The waste should be stored safely (i.e. where children, pets and pests etc. do not have access).

The DH (2006b) recommended using the European Wound Management Association's (2005) criteria when assessing if wounds are infected. A high risk for wound infection is identified as: the presence of erythema, pus/abscess, an offensive smell, increase in wound pain, and the patient being treated with antibiotics for wound infection. See Chapter 7 for further details about wound infection recognition.

While small amounts of non-infectious healthcare waste (e.g. non-infectious dressings, disposable instruments, stoma bags, catheter bags, incontinence pads) can be mixed with household refuse, large amounts of non-infected dressings and medicinal dressings must go into the offensive/hygiene waste stream. If any healthcare waste is assessed as infected (e.g. incontinence pad from a patient with a UTI), it must by put into an orange bag. Healthcare packaging should be put in a plastic bag before putting it in the black bag.

The DH (2006b) advised that the healthcare waste from community patients with MRSA is not necessarily infectious – the likelihood must be assessed. Therefore, the wound dressing waste from a patient known to have an MRSA wound infection should be disposed of in an orange bag, but the incontinence pads from the same patient may not be if they are not likely to have a UTI.

Learning outcome 3: Discuss how used linen should be dealt with

Used linen requires careful handling, bagging and disposal as it can become contaminated with microorganisms from patients' body fluids or the infections they have. The laundry process decontaminates linen through the mechanical process of washing, the detergent used and the temperature of the water. The process must include sufficient time for all parts of the load to be washed at an adequate temperature. Any microorganisms that remain after washing can be destroyed by tumble drying and ironing (Wilson 2006).

ACTIVITY

Can you name three different types of linen bag and the category of linen that should be placed in each? Why are the different categories needed? Which colour would be used for Mrs Lewis' used sheets and which colour for Stacey's vomit-covered bed-linen?

The categories are needed to protect laundry staff from cross-infection. Additionally the categories protect other staff and patients by ensuring that linen is adequately decontaminated during the laundering process. There are three main types of linen bag. The first is white linen or clear plastic and is used for used, soiled and foul linen. This is appropriate for Stacey's bed-linen. This should be washed at 65ºC for 10 minutes or 71ºC for 3 minutes for thermal disinfection. Duvets should withstand washing at 71ºC and comply with DH standards of retardancy (Wilson 2006). For infected linen a water-soluble bag with a red outer bag is required. This is used for infectious diseases or at other times as advised by the ICT and would be used for Mrs Lewis's bed-linen. The laundry staff do not open and sort the linen in the inner bag and the linen is washed and thermally disinfected as for used linen. A third type of bag with an orange stripe is used for fabric likely to be damaged by thermal disinfection, for example wool. These items are washed at 40ºC and hypochlorite added to the penultimate wash.

Summary

- Nurses and other healthcare workers have a duty of care to ensure that they dispose of waste appropriately to prevent hazards to themselves, colleagues, patients and the public.

- It is important to differentiate between different categories of waste, assessing whether it is hazardous (infectious or medicinal), offensive/hygiene waste or household.
- Used linen must be disposed of correctly according to whether it is infectious or soiled only.

CHAPTER SUMMARY

This chapter has highlighted the problem of healthcare-associated infection and covered important practices for preventing cross-infection. Infection control polices and principles underpinning cross-infection were introduced. Standard principles and precautions for preventing cross-infection were outlined and each chapter section has focused on the practical skills involved and how they can be applied in different situations. Having worked your way through this chapter you should now be aware of the fundamental principles that underpin the prevention of cross-infection. The principles are relevant to all other practical nursing skills, and this chapter will, therefore, be referred to within many other chapters in this book.

The Code of Professional Conduct (NMC 2008) demands that nurses protect and support the health of individual patients and clients and the health of the wider community whilst at the same time being personally accountable for their practice. Therefore there is a professional as well as moral imperative to aid the prevention of cross-infection. This is of fundamental importance to the health, safety and well-being of patients, nurses and other healthcare practitioners alike.

ACKNOWLEDGEMENT

This chapter has been revised and updated. The authors acknowledge the work of Vickie Arrowsmith on this chapter in the previous two editions of this book.

REFERENCES

Ayliffe, G.A.F., Graise, A.P., Geddes, A.M. and Mitchell, K. 2000. *Control of Hospital Infection: A practical handbook.* London: Arnold.

Ayliffe, G.A.J., Babb, J.R. and Taylor, L.J. 2001. *Hospital-acquired Infection: Principles and prevention,* 3rd edn. London: Arnold.

Carr, J. and Wilson, B. 1987. Self-help skills: washing, dressing and feeding. In Yule, W. and Carr, J. (eds) *Behaviour Modification for People with Mental Handicaps.* London: Croom Helm, 143–60.

Cochrane, J. 2000. Moral precepts of hand washing in a community healthcare setting. *Journal of Community Nursing* **14,** 19–20.

Coia, J.E., Duckworth, G.J., Edwards, D.I. *et al.* 2006. Guidelines for the control and prevention of meticillin-resistant *Staphylococcus aureus* (MRSA) in healthcare facilities *Journal of Hospital Infection* **63S**: S1–44.

Dancer, S.J. 2002. Handwashing hazard? *Journal of Hospital Infection* **52,** 76.

Department of Health (DH) 2001. *Valuing People: A new strategy for learning disability for the 21st century.* London.

— 2003. *Winning Ways: Working together to reduce healthcare associated infection in England.* London.

— 2006a. *The Health Act 2006. Code of Practice for the Prevention and Control of Healthcare-associated Infections.* London.

— 2006b. *Environment and Sustainability. Health Technical Memorandum 07-01: Safe management of healthcare waste.* London.

— 2007a. *The Third Prevalence Survey of Healthcare Associated Infections in Acute Hospitals in England – 2006 Report.* London.

— 2007b. *Saving Lives: Reducing infection, delivering clean and safe care,* revised edn. London.

— 2007c. *High Impact Intervention No. 7: Care bundle to reduce the risk from* Clostridium difficile. London.

— 2007d. *High Impact Intervention No. 2: Peripheral intravenous cannula care bundle.* London.

— 2007e. *Immunization against Infectious Disease.* London.

— 2007f. *Uniforms and Workwear: An evidence base for developing local policy.* London.

— 2007g. *Screening for Methicillin-resistant* Staphylococcus aureus *(MRSA) Colonisation. A Strategy for NHS Trusts: Summary of best practice.* London.

— 2007h. *Isolating Patients with Healthcare-associated Infection: Summary of best practice.* London.

— 2008. *Clean, Safe Care: Reducing infections and saving lives.* London.

Donovan, S. 1998. Wound infection and swabbing. *Professional Nurse* **13,** 757–9.

Emerson, E. 1992. What is normalisation? In Brown, H. and Smith, H. (eds) *Normalisation: A reader for the nineties.* London: Routledge, 1–15.

European Wound Management Association. 2005. *Position Paper: Identifying criteria for wound infection.* London: Medical Education Partnership. Available from www.ewma.org/pdf/fall05/pos_doc_eng.pdf.

Flores, A. and Pevalin, D.J. 2007. Glove use and compliance with hand hygiene. *Nursing Times* **103**(38), 46–8.

Gammon, J. 1999. Isolated instance. *Nursing Times* **95**(2), 57–60.

Gilmour, D. 2000. Is aseptic technique always necessary? *Journal of Community Nursing* **14**(4).

Gould, D. and Brooker, C. 2000. *Applied Microbiology for Nurses.* London: Macmillan.

Hand Hygiene Liaison Group 2001. Hand hygiene. *British Medical Journal* **323,** 411–12.

Health Protection Agency (HPA) 2006a. *Investigation of Skin, Superficial and Non-surgical Wound Swabs.* National Standard Method BSOP, 11, Issue 4. Available from www.hpa-standardmethods.org.uk/pdf_sops.asp. Accessed 1 June 2008.

— 2006b. *Eye of the Needle: UK surveillance of significant occupational exposure to BBVs in health care workers.* London.

Health Protection Scotland (HPS) 2008a. *Control of the Environment: Policy and procedure* (an element of standard infection control precautions). Available from http://hps.scot.nhs.uk.

— 2008b. *Management of Blood and Other Body Fluid Spillages: Policy and procedure* (an element of standard infection control precautions). Available from http://hps.scot.nhs.uk.

— 2008c. *Management of Care Equipment: Policy and procedure* (an element of standard infection control precautions). Available from http://hps.scot.nhs.uk.

— 2008d. *Hand Hygiene: Policy and procedure* (an element of standard infection control precautions). Available from http://hps.scot.nhs.uk.

— 2008e. *Safe Disposal of Waste: Policy and procedure* (an element of standard infection control precautions). Available from http://hps.scot.nhs.uk.

Health and Safety Executive 2006. *Management of Healthcare Waste.* London: HSE.

Meers, P., Sedgwick, J. and Worsley, M. 1995. *The Microbiology and Epidemiology of Infection for Health Science Students.* London: Chapman & Hall.

Miller, M. 1998. How do I diagnose and treat wound infection? *British Journal of Nursing* **7,** 335–8.

Myatt, R. and Langley, S. 2003. Changes in infection control practice to reduce MRSA infection. *British Journal of Nursing* **12,** 675–81.

National Institute for Health and Clinical Excellence (NICE) 2003. *Infection Control: Prevention of healthcare-associated infection in primary and community care.* London: NICE. Available from www.nice.org.uk. Accessed 29 May 2008.

National Patient Safety Agency 2007. *Promoting Safer Use of Injectable Medicines: NPSA template standard operating procedure for use of injectable medicines.* London: NPSA. Available from www.npsa.nhs.uk/health/alerts. Accessed 1 June 2008.

Nursing and Midwifery Council (NMC) 2007. *Essential Skills Clusters for Pre-registration Nursing Programmes.* Annexe 2 to NMC Circular 07/2007.

— 2008. *The Code: Standards of conduct, performance and ethics for nurses and midwives.* London.

Oldham, T. 1998. Isolated cases. *Nursing Times* **94**(11), 67–9.

Parker, L.J. 1999. Current recommendations for isolation practices in nursing. *British Journal of Nursing* **8,** 881–7.

Pittet, D., Mourouga, P., Perneger, T.V. *et al.* 1999. Compliance with handwashing in a teaching hospital. *Annals of Internal Medicine* **130**(2), 126–30.

Pratt, R.J., Pellowe, C. Loveday, H.P. *et al.* 2001. The epic project: developing national evidence-based guidelines for preventing healthcare associated infections. Phase 1: Guidelines for preventing hospital-acquired infections. *Journal of Hospital Infection.* **47** Suppl, S1–82.

Pratt, R.J., Pellowe, C., Wilson, J.A. *et al.* 2007. National evidence-based guidelines for preventing healthcare-associated infections in NHS, England. *Journal of Hospital Infection* **65S,** S1–64.

Price, P.B. 1938. The classification of transient and resident microbes. *Journal of Infectious Disease* **63,** 301–8.

Rampling, A., Wiseman, S., Davis, L. *et al.* 2001. Evidence that hospital hygiene is important in the control of methicillin-resistant *Staphylococcus aureus. Journal of Hospital Infection* **49,** 109–6.

Statutory Instrument 1992. *No. 588: The Controlled Waste Regulations* Available from www.opsi.gov.uk/si/si1992/Uksi_19920588_en_1.htm.

— 2004. *No. SSI 112: Special Waste Amendment (Scotland) Regulations.* Available from www.opsi.gov.uk/legislation/scotland/ssi2004/20040112.htm.

— 2005a. *No. 894: The Hazardous Waste (England and Wales Regulations.* Available from www.opsi.gov.uk/si/si2005/20050894.htm.

— 2005b. *No. SR 300: The Hazardous Waste Regulations (Northern Ireland).* Available from www.opsi.gov.uk/sr/sr2005/20050300.htm.

Swann, C. 1997. Development of services. In Gates, B. (ed.) *Learning Disabilities,* 3rd edn. London: Churchill Livingstone, 39–54.

Thomlinson, D. 1987. To clean or not to clean? Cleaning discharging surgical wounds. *Nursing Times* **83**(9), 71, 73, 75.

Weltman, A.C., Short, L.J., Mendelson, M.H. *et al.* 1995. Disposal-related sharps injuries at a New York city teaching hospital. *Infection Control and Hospital Epidemiology* **16,** 268–74.

Wilcox, M.H., Fawley, W.N., Wigglesworth, N. *et al.* 2003. Comparison of the effect of detergent versus hypochlorite on environmental contamination and incidence of *Clostridium difficile* infection. *Journal of Hospital Infection* **54,**109–114.

Williams, C. 1996. Irriclens: a sterile wound cleanser in an aerosol can. *British Journal of Nursing* **5,** 1008–10.

Wilson, J. 2006. *Infection Control in Clinical Practice,* 3rd edn. London: Baillière Tindall.

Wilson, A., Hayman, S. and Folan, P. *et al.* 2006. Computer keyboards and the spread of MRSA. *Journal of Hospital Infection* **62**(3), 390–2.

Measuring Vital Signs

Sue Maddex

Nurses spend millions of hours each year monitoring vital signs (Salvage 2000). These observations contribute to overall nursing assessments of patients, establish a baseline for future comparison, and help to identify abnormalities. All student nurses should learn to measure and record vital signs accurately (Nursing and Midwifery Council 2007). This chapter aims to prepare nurses to undertake these measurements skilfully, based on best evidence, and to begin to interpret findings.

When carrying out nursing observations, effective non-verbal and verbal communication skills are essential (covered in Chapter 2). It is important to promote patients'/clients' confidence in your ability to perform these techniques accurately. Uncertainty of your skills may produce fear and anxiety in people, thus altering their vital signs measurements. Documenting and reporting observations is also crucial to ensure that abnormalities or potential problems are identified and addressed.

This chapter includes:
- Measuring and recording temperature
- Measuring and recording the pulse
- Measuring and recording respirations
- Measuring and recording blood pressure
- Measuring oxygen saturation by pulse oximetry
- Neurological assessment

Vital signs monitoring forms part of many hospitals' early-warning 'track and trigger' systems which alert staff to patients' potential deterioration (see Chapter 11). Pain assessment is also a vital sign (see Chapter 12).

Recommended biology reading:

The following questions will help you to focus on biology underpinning this chapter's skills. Use your recommended textbook to find out:
- What is homeostasis, and why is it important?

Temperature control
- Which body systems are involved in thermoregulation?
- How is heat generated within the body?
- How is heat lost from the body?

- What effect does temperature have on cellular function?
- What happens if the body starts to get too hot or too cold?
- Why do we appear flushed when too warm?

Cardiovascular system
- What are the components of the cardiovascular system?
- Which vessels usually carry oxygenated blood?
- Why does blood travel in one direction?
- Name the four chambers of the heart, the great vessels and valves. Draw a diagram of the heart and label these structures. Indicate the direction in which oxygenated and deoxygenated blood flows through the heart.
- What are the layers of the heart wall and what types of tissue are they composed of?
- How does the heart contract in such a coordinated way? Explore the route taken by impulses through the myocardium.
- Myocardial tissue needs its own blood supply. Where are the coronary vessels located and what would result from their blockage?
- Compare the structures of arteries, capillaries and veins. Which vessels permit gaseous exchange and why? Which vessels contain valves?
- When tissues are damaged, an inflammatory process is initiated to repair the damage. What are the clinical signs of inflammation? What role does histamine play in inflammation? Why is inflammation of brain tissue potentially life-threatening?
- What role does blood play in maintaining cellular homeostasis?
- What are the components of blood and what specific roles do they play?
- Where are blood cells produced?
- What is haemostasis, and why is it important?
- What is blood pressure and how is it maintained?

Respiratory system
- What are the components of the respiratory system (e.g. airways, respiratory muscles, control mechanisms) and what are their functions?
- How do these functions contribute towards maintaining homeostasis?
- Where does gaseous exchange occur? Which gases are being exchanged?
- Why does this exchange occur? What may affect this exchange?
- How does inspiration occur? What is the stimulus for us to breathe?
- What are the proportions of gases in atmospheric, alveolar and expired air?
- What factors are required for adequate tissue oxygenation to occur? Consider the role blood plays in this.

PRACTICE SCENARIOS

Observation and recording of a person's vital signs are carried out for many reasons. The following scenarios are used to assist you to relate your learning of these skills to patients/clients you might encounter in practice settings.

Adult

Mrs Anne Parkinson is a 56-year-old woman who has been taken to the A&E unit by ambulance following a head injury after falling from her bicycle. She cannot remember the accident but was apparently unresponsive for 2–3 minutes afterwards. She is alert but appears disorientated. Her husband is present.

Learning disability

> **Down's syndrome**
> This congenital condition is caused by an extra chromosome, often leading to a characteristic physical appearance and a low intelligence quotient (IQ). Other physical effects (e.g. heart disease) are often associated with it. There is an increased risk of dementia at a younger age.

Ken O'Reilly is a 49-year-old man with **Down's syndrome** and a moderate learning disability. He has some verbal communication difficulties. He lives in a small group home with a live-in staff team. Ken is known to the Community Learning Disability Nurse (CLDN) as he is prone to chronic chest infections. He has oxygen therapy and a nebuliser at home, which the staff team have been trained to support him with. The nurse, while carrying out routine **Health Facilitator's** training with the staff team, is informed that Ken is unwell and is asked for advice. The nurse records Ken's vital signs and advises the staff to arrange for the GP to visit to carry out further health assessment.

Mental health

> **Health facilitator**
> A member of the community learning disabilities team (often a nurse) who supports a person with learning disabilities to access the healthcare they need. See *Valuing People* (DH 2001).

Natalie Turney is 21 years old. She has been admitted as a voluntary patient to an acute mental health ward with severe depression. After going home for a day she returns, appearing unsteady on her feet and she has a strong smell of alcohol. Her speech is very slurred and she is quite uncommunicative. When the staff ask her if she has taken any tablets she mentions some 'little yellow pills' and paracetamol. However, she won't give details about the quantity or when she took them.

EQUIPMENT REQUIRED FOR THIS CHAPTER

Before working through this chapter, find out what vital signs recording equipment is available within the skills laboratory or your practice area. Look for:
* thermometers: may be tympanic, electronic probes, chemical disposable;
* sphygmomanometers: electronic and/or manual equipment;
* pulse oximeter for recording oxygen saturations.

You also need a watch with a second hand, a pen torch and observation charts for temperature, pulse, respiration, pulse oximetry, blood pressure and neurological assessment. You may wish to work through the sections with a colleague so that you can practise this chapter's skills.

MEASURING AND RECORDING TEMPERATURE

Nurses frequently measure temperature to assess whether body temperature is within the normal range. A person's body temperature is measured by a thermometer in degrees Celsius (°C). Body temperature results from a balance between heat production within the body and heat loss from the body (Marieb 2006). In a healthy individual the normal core body temperature (the temperature of the organs within the cranial, thoracic and abdominal cavities) is maintained within a range of 35–37.5°C (Montague *et al.* 2005).This process is called **thermoregulation** and is controlled by the hypothalamus, which acts as a thermostat (Tortora and Grabowski 2003). There may be times when this process is ineffective for various reasons. Body temperature which is higher than 37.5°C is termed **pyrexia** and a body temperature lower than 35°C is termed **hypothermia** (Montague *et al.* 2005).

LEARNING OUTCOMES

By the end of this section you will be able to:
1 explain the rationale for monitoring temperature;
2 identify the sites and equipment used for measuring temperature;
3 accurately measure a person's temperature.

Learning outcome 1 : Explain the rationale for monitoring temperature

Temperature readings can be used to help identify disease or dysfunction.

ACTIVITY What factors might influence a person's body temperature?

You may have identified the following factors:

- **Age.** Older people often have a lower body temperature as metabolic rate falls after the age of 50 years (Childs 2006).
- **Environment.** Heat loss is influenced by environmental temperature and humidity. The body's ability to thermoregulate cannot accommodate extremes of heat and cold for long periods. Hence hypothermia may result from prolonged exposure to cold, and heat exhaustion from a very hot environment. If thermoregulation is impaired, people become susceptible to overheating or cooling. Older people are less able to respond metabolically to falling body temperature and may have decreased perception of cold (Tortora and Grabowski 2003), increasing hypothermia risk. People with impaired cognitive function, confusion or perceptual disturbance may be unable to recognise and respond appropriately to environmental temperature changes, for example, going out inadequately dressed in cold weather.
- **Level of physical activity.** Muscular activity produces heat energy that contributes to maintaining body temperature; changes to muscle activity are an important part of thermoregulation (Marieb 2006). Intense muscular contraction, such as shivering, produces a large amount of heat (Brooker 1998) and is a physiological response to cold, an attempt by the body to raise its temperature. Strenuous exercise may lead to a higher core body temperature for several hours afterwards due to heat production by muscles (Childs 2006). People with diminished mobility, due to conditions such as cerebral palsy or arthritis, may be susceptible to cold and unable to respond behaviourally by, for example, adding extra clothing, without assistance.

- **Metabolic rate.** The body's metabolic processes are a source of heat production. People with an excessive metabolic rate, for example those with an overactive thyroid gland, may have a higher than normal body temperature (Edwards 1997). Underactivity of the thyroid gland results in a condition termed 'myxoedema' and a low metabolic rate. Low metabolic rates may cause low body temperatures.
- **Time of day.** Body temperature normally falls during sleep, so tends to be lowest at night and rises during the day, peaking in the early evening (Edwards 1997).
- **Drugs.** Alcohol diminishes perception of cold, impairs shivering and causes vasodilation, thus predisposing to a lowered body temperature. Sedative and narcotic drugs may reduce perception of cold, and thus the likelihood of appropriate behavioural responses (Marieb 2006).
- **Infection.** One of the body's responses to infection is to raise body temperature; the thermostat of the hypothalamus is reset, causing increased heat production and inhibition of heat loss (Marieb 2006).
- **Menstrual cycle.** Many women have higher body temperature around ovulation (Childs 2006).
- **Eating.** The process of digesting and metabolising food can produce enough heat to raise body temperature slightly (Childs 2006).

Nurses must take all these factors into account when interpreting temperature measurements.

ACTIVITY

Identify reasons why you might record the person's temperature in each of the scenarios.

You would measure Anne's temperature during her initial patient assessment and as a baseline for future recordings. Also she may have become hypothermic if she was lying on the ground outside in very cold weather. Ken's temperature would be recorded as part of his general assessment, particularly if he feels hot or cold to touch. He may have an infection causing him to feel unwell. Natalie's temperature would have been recorded during her admission assessment which acts as a baseline against which future measurements can be compared. Her body temperature may be lower due to alcohol consumption.

Body temperature is routinely recorded when a person is admitted to hospital, pre- and postoperatively, following invasive procedures and during various treatments. For people with learning disabilities, recording body temperature can help identify whether behavioural changes are due to a physical health problem. Also, recording temperature regularly for people with learning disabilities, perhaps during routine health check-ups, promotes familiarity with the equipment and procedure so temperature measurement should not cause undue distress during ill-health.

Frequency of measurements may range from just one recording on admission, to hourly in a person with a high temperature. Mooney (2007) warns of the limitation of one-off readings, suggesting that a range of several readings is best practice.

Learning outcome 2: Identify the sites and equipment used for measuring temperature

Ideally the same site and method should be used for temperature measurement each time to promote greater consistency. Different sites and methods are appropriate in different circumstances.

ACTIVITY	From your experience in practice, as well as personal experience of having your temperature taken, list the equipment and sites that can be used to record body temperature.

There are advantages and disadvantages to using the different sites and equipment.

Sites

You are likely to have seen the following sites used:

- mouth
- axilla (armpit)
- tympanic membrane (in the ear).

The rectum can also be used to measure temperature but this site is rarely used, except in a few special circumstances. Taking temperatures rectally is invasive and can cause patients embarrassment. Oral measurements are unsuitable for people who are confused, unconscious or breathless. A breathless person tends to mouth breathe so oral temperature measurement would then be both distressing and inaccurate. Axillary temperature measurement requires good contact between the two skin surfaces so this site will probably be inaccurate with very thin people. The person must be able to keep the arm still by the side of the chest. The axillary temperature is not an accurate indicator of core body temperature if the person is vasoconstricted or chilled (Casey 2000), as Anne may be if she has been outside for a prolonged period. The tympanic membrane is a convenient site for temperature recording and can be used with most people if the equipment is available.

ACTIVITY	When you are next in the practice setting, observe which routes are used for temperature measurement for different people and identify the rationale for their choice.

Equipment

You may have seen chemical disposable, electronic and infrared light reflectance thermometers and in some clinical settings mercury-in-glass thermometers.

Mercury-in-glass thermometers

Over recent years, there have been concerns about the potential risks to nurses and clients of mercury spillage from broken glass thermometers. The Medicines and Healthcare products Regulatory Agency (MHRA) (2003a) advises that these devices can still be used if there is no available substitute. However, staff must be trained

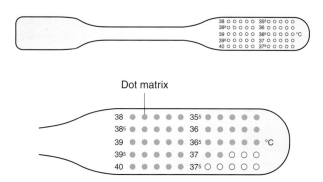

Figure 4.1: A chemical dot matrix thermometer, showing 37.1°C.

in safe handling of them and procedures for mercury spillage and disposal (MHRA 2003a). Farnell *et al.* (2005) highlights how mercury-in-glass thermometers are still used in some clinical areas. You should seek local training in these devices if relevant.

Chemical disposable thermometers

These thin plastic strips have 50 small dots of thermosensitive chemicals that change colour with increasing temperature (Torrance and Semple 1998a) and may be used in the mouth or axilla; see Fig. 4.1. They are disposed of after use so there is no cross-infection risk. Accuracy depends on correct technique in relation to timing and positioning. If the thermometer is left in the mouth for longer than two minutes or the axilla longer than five minutes, it must be re-recorded with a new thermometer (3M undated). Research suggests this method is as reliable as mercury-in-glass and tympanic thermometers (Molton *et al.* 2001). They must be stored at under 30°C.

Electronic thermometers

These consist of a probe, which is placed in the mouth, the axilla or the rectum, usually connected to a power supply and display unit. The purchase cost is significant, as are the ongoing costs of probe covers needed for each use. Most produce an auditory signal after a preset time or when maximum temperature is reached (Carroll 2000), so the user does not determine the timing.

Infrared-light reflectance thermometers

These detect heat radiated as infrared energy from the tympanic membrane; see Fig. 4.2. The temperature registers within a few seconds, causing little inconvenience or discomfort (Edwards 1997). Inaccurate readings from these devices mainly result from incorrect placement of the thermometer probe (Casey 2000). The thermometers are designed to detect heat from the tympanic membrane but will also detect heat from the ear canal (which may be 2°C lower) if not correctly placed to provide a snug fit (MHRA 2003b). In a study on a neonatal unit, Leick-Rude and Bloom (1998) found that tympanic thermometers were influenced by environmental factors, such as overhead heaters. However, Schmitz *et al.* (1995) suggest that their use is effective in pyrexial people, and they highlight their accuracy in measuring temperatures of 38°C and above. The use of disposable probe covers prevents cross-infection but adds to ongoing costs.

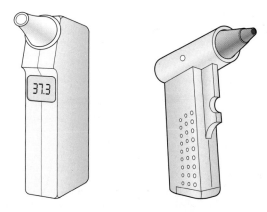

Figure 4.2: An infra red tympanic thermometer.

ACTIVITY

Which method and site is most appropriate for each of the people in the scenarios, and why?

Compare your answers with the points below:

- *Adult* – For Anne, a tympanic thermometer would probably be used. The oral route is not appropriate as she is disorientated, and she may be in pain, anxious and receiving oxygen via a mask. A tympanic thermometer would record her temperature without affecting her other treatments and observations.
- *Learning disability* – Ken's temperature could be measured in the axilla using either a disposable or an electronic thermometer. A tympanic thermometer could be used if the equipment is available. Ken may have preferences about the type of equipment used and method and these should be respected if at all possible. The nurse should explain carefully first if equipment used is unfamiliar to him.
- *Mental health* – Natalie's temperature could be recorded tympanically if a tympanic thermometer is available. The oral route is not suitable as she is not fully conscious. The axilla route could be used, using a disposable thermometer or electronic thermometer. The nurse would need to help her keep her arm by her side for the required length of time.

Learning outcome 3: Accurately measure a person's temperature

Oral measurements

ACTIVITY

Find a willing volunteer with whom to practise this activity. You will need a chemical disposable thermometer. Carefully work through the instructions in Box 4.1.

Factors that might affect the oral temperature measurement include:

- eating or drinking hot or cold substances shortly before the procedure;
- smoking;
- talking;
- breathing through the mouth;
- incorrect positioning of the thermometer;
- thermometer in the mouth for too short a time.

Box 4.1 Oral temperature measurement using chemical disposable thermometer

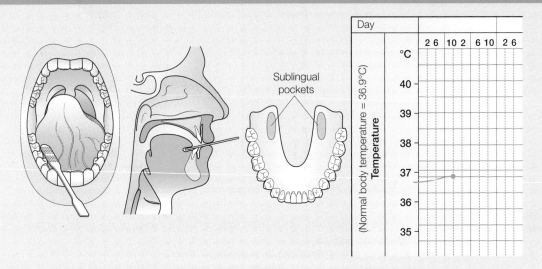

- Explain the procedure to the person, including the need to keep lips closed while the thermometer is in position.
- Position the plastic strip in the person's mouth under the person's tongue to the side; see the diagram for correct positioning. The face with the dots on (dot matrix) can be placed either way up and must be left in for 1 minute (Torrance and Semple 1998b).
- Remove the thermometer. Wait ten seconds and read the last blue dot, ignoring any dots in between that have not changed colour (3M undated). Dispose of the thermometer.
- Record the measurement on an observation chart, as per example, of a temperature of 36.8°C. Report abnormal temperatures.

An oral temperature should not be recorded within 15 minutes of the patient eating, drinking or smoking (Torrance and Semple 1998b).

Axilla measurements

ACTIVITY

Now try using a chemical disposable thermometer to measure axillary temperature using the instructions in Box 4.2. Compare this reading with the previous oral measurement.

Electronic devices

Instructions for using electronic thermometers are given in Box 4.3. You may be able to practise these if the equipment is available. Note that the tympanic temperature should not be taken with a hearing aid in place, in an ear that is infected or following ear surgery (Molton *et al.* 2001).

Box 4.2 Measurement of a temperature in the axilla, using a chemical, disposable thermometer

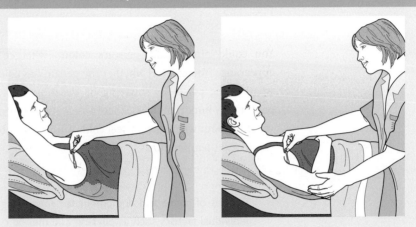

- Explain the procedure to the person, including the need to remain still while the thermometer is in position.
- Raise the person's arm. Place the thermometer in the centre of the person's axilla (see the diagram), positioning it with the dot matrix against the torso (Torrance and Semple 1998b).
- Check to ensure there is good contact with the skin when the arm is lowered.
- Rest the person's arm across the chest and maintain the thermometer in position for a minimum of 3 minutes (Torrance and Semple 1998b).
- Remove the thermometer, read and record the result as in Box 4.1.
- Dispose of the chemical thermometer.
- Report abnormal temperatures.

Box 4.3 Temperature measurement using electronic devices

Using an electronic thermometer to record oral or axilla temperature

- The positioning of electronic probes in the mouth or the axilla is the same as for chemical disposable thermometers (see Boxes 4.1 and 4.2).
- A new probe cover should be used for each person.
- Devices have either an auditory (e.g. bleeping sound) or visual (e.g. flashing) indicator when maximum temperature is reached; the probe should remain in place until this is heard.

Using an infrared tympanic membrane thermometer

- The speculum is covered with a disposable cover.
- The ear is pulled gently but firmly to straighten the ear canal, pulling the ear up and back (MHRA 2003b).
- The speculum is inserted gently into the ear canal, ensuring a snug fit.
- The start button is pressed.
- The reading is obtained within 1–2 seconds, indicated by a bleeping sound.

Using a thermometer will give you an accurate measurement of temperature, but what other observations could help you to assess body temperature?

You could observe the person's colour, whether they are pale or flushed in appearance. You can feel whether the person has cold extremities or is hot to touch, whether the person is shivering or sweating, and ask them how they feel. It is particularly important to use these observations if people are unable to communicate verbally about whether they feel cold or hot. Your observations may prompt you to record their temperature.

Summary

- Choice of route and equipment for measuring temperature should consider individual factors such as physical and mental condition, as well as the devices available in the particular practice setting.
- For each route and device used, the measurement should be conducted and recorded carefully and accurately.
- Abnormal measurements should be reported and action taken, for example administration of anti-pyretic medication (e.g. paracetamol).
- As temperature can vary between body sites, the measurement site should be recorded and the same site used for subsequent recordings whenever possible.

MEASURING AND RECORDING THE PULSE

When the left ventricle of the heart pumps blood into the already full aorta and out into the arterial system, this causes a wave of expansion throughout the arteries. Where arteries are near the surface of the body, this expansion – the pulse – can be felt when lightly pressing (palpating) the artery against bone. The pulse thus represents each ventricular contraction of the heart and in the healthy heart one heart beat corresponds to one pulse beat.

Disease can affect the cardiac cycle, leading to a difference between the heart rate and the pulse rate. The pulse rate is the number of heart beats in a 60-second period. Pulse measurement provides very useful information about health status. As with temperature, it will be recorded on admission to hospital as a baseline and subsequent measurements may be performed for monitoring purposes.

LEARNING OUTCOMES

By the end of this section you will be able to:
1 explain the rationale for monitoring pulse rate and the normal values of the pulse;
2 locate pulses in different areas of the body and identify which might be palpated in specific situations;
3 accurately measure a person's pulse rate.

Learning outcome 1: Explain the rationale for monitoring pulse rate and the normal values of the pulse

ACTIVITY

Look again at the definition of a pulse, and then identify what a person's pulse might actually tell you about their body.

The pulse is measured to identify the rate and strength of the ventricular contraction, and to gain information regarding a person's health. For example, in the case of trauma and severe bleeding, the pulse rate might be weak and fast. When measuring a pulse, the following should be observed:

- **The frequency of the pulse.** This indicates the rate of contraction of the left ventricle. It is affected by numerous factors, including age, exercise, stress, injury and disease. The normal adult heart rate ranges from 60 to 100 beats per minute (bpm), but at rest is usually between 60 and 80 bpm (Waugh and Grant 2006). The heart rate diminishes by 10–20 bpm during sleep (Herbert and Alison 1996). An abnormally slow pulse is termed **bradycardia**; in an adult this would usually be a pulse rate below 60 bpm. An abnormally fast pulse is termed **tachycardia** – usually a pulse rate above 100 bpm in an adult. There are many reasons for a fast pulse – for example, a fever, an overactive thyroid gland, and certain drugs speed up the pulse. An underactive thyroid gland, hypothermia and some drugs slow the pulse. The thickness and tension of a patient's arteriole walls influences the pulse. Atherosclerosis develops in many people over the age of 40 years and can lead to structural changes in the arteries, thus altering the pulse rate.

- **The volume.** This indicates the strength of the ventricular contraction. A weak contraction produces a pulse that feels weak, or it may not be strong enough to produce a pulse at the periphery – such as the wrist – at all. A lack of blood volume also leads to a weak pulse.

- **The rhythm.** This helps to establish whether the heart is beating regularly. An irregular pulse indicates a possible abnormality in the heart's conduction system. The National Institute for Health and Clinical Excellence (NICE) (2006) recommends that manual pulse palpation should be performed to identify an irregular pulse, which can indicate atrial fibrillation.

> Atrial fibrillation
> Fibrillation of the atria leading to irregular and often fast ventricular contraction and thus a highly irregular pulse rate.

Learning outcome 2: Locate pulses in different areas of the body, and identify which might be palpated in specific situations

It is important to know the sites where a pulse can be found.

ACTIVITY

Here is a list of pulses that can be palpated (see Fig. 4.3). How many can you find on yourself?
- temporal artery – on the side of the forehead
- facial artery – on the side of the face
- carotid artery – at the neck
- brachial artery – in the antecubital fossa of the arm
- radial artery – at the wrist

- femoral artery – in the groin
- popliteal artery – behind the knee
- posterior tibial artery – at the inner side of each ankle.

Note that the apex beat can be listened to with a stethoscope, and is located to the left side of the sternum over the heart.

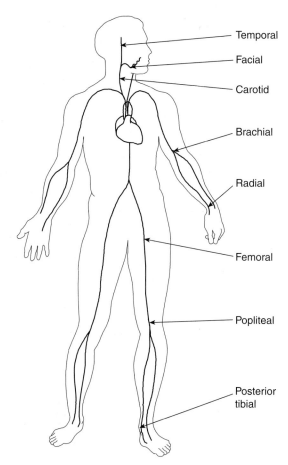

Temporal

Facial

Carotid

Brachial

Radial

Femoral

Popliteal

Posterior tibial

Figure 4.3: Location of pulses within the body.

Some pulses are easier to palpate and more accessible than others. Choice of site for pulse measurement depends on the individual and the situation. For adults in a non-emergency situation, the radial pulse is usually recorded because this site is non-invasive and easily accessible. Anne, Ken and Natalie could all have their radial pulses taken.

In an emergency situation when a person has collapsed it is often difficult to locate peripheral pulses (including the radial pulse), so the carotid or femoral pulse may be checked. However, the Resuscitation Council UK (2005) guidelines specify that only staff who are trained and experienced in clinical assessment should check the carotid pulse when assessing signs of life in a collapsed person. It may be difficult to palpate some pulse sites in people with contractures. Pulses in the lower legs are usually only palpated when assessing the presence of circulation to the limbs which might be after trauma or surgery.

Learning outcome 3: Accurately measure a person's pulse rate

With all individuals, the person's psychological state needs to be considered, and cooperation sought, prior to measuring the pulse. This involves explaining why the pulse needs to be measured.

ACTIVITY

You need a willing volunteer, a watch with a second hand or a digital watch, and an observation chart from your skills laboratory. Now follow the steps in Box 4.4 to measure and record the radial pulse.

When measuring the pulse rate, nurses often count the pulse for 30 seconds and multiply by two. With a regular pulse this gives a reasonably accurate measurement, but an irregular pulse should always be counted for a full minute – and the word 'irregular' should be written by the recorded rate.

ACTIVITY

Now ask your volunteer to jog on the spot for 1 minute and then record the pulse rate again. You will probably find that their pulse rate has risen, due to the extra oxygen demands caused by exercise. Can you remember any other reasons why the pulse may be faster in a healthy person?

Box 4.4 Measuring a radial pulse

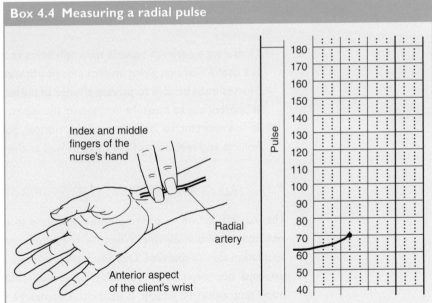

- Identify the radial artery. This is found with the palm of the hand facing upwards and gently pressing at the wrist region at the thumb side (see the diagram).
- Press the artery gently against the bone with your fingers (not your thumb, which itself has a pulse) and feel the pulse bounding.
- Using your watch, count the beats of the pulse for 1 minute. The number of beats corresponds to the pulse rate. For example, 70 beats indicates the person's pulse rate is 70.
- Using the example, which shows a pulse rate of 70 beats per minute (bpm), record the pulse on the observation chart.

Anxiety or stress raise the pulse rate. Thus Anne's pulse rate could be raised due to the anxiety about her situation. As discussed earlier, you need to put people at ease when recording vital signs, thus relieving anxiety and gaining an accurate measurement.

Electronic measurement of the pulse rate

Devices that can electronically record the pulse rate include:

- **Oscillometer** for blood pressure measurement (discussed later in this chapter). The pulse rate is usually displayed too.
- **Pulse oximeter** (discussed later in this chapter). As well as measuring oxygen saturation, the pulse rate is usually displayed.
- **Cardiac monitor.** This displays the heart rate as well as the rhythm of the person's heart. Chapter 11 discusses cardiac monitoring.

While these devices provide a pulse rate, they will not all indicate either the volume of the pulse or its regularity. With the pulse oximeter and cardiac monitor, movement may cause an artefact, leading to an inaccurate figure being displayed. Ensure that the pulse rate accurately represents your patient's physical appearance and your own assessment. If you doubt the accuracy of any observation, re-record it and inform a qualified member of the healthcare team.

Summary

- Measuring a person's pulse is minimally invasive and uses little equipment but is a useful vital sign giving insights into health status.
- Nurses must be able to palpate a range of pulses and be aware of which pulse is appropriate to measure in different situations.
- It is important to be aware of the normal pulse range and to assess the volume and regularity of the pulse as well as the rate.

MEASURING AND RECORDING RESPIRATIONS

The major function of the respiratory system is to supply the body with oxygen and remove carbon dioxide. When the respiratory rate is measured, it is the act of ventilation that is observed. One respiration consists of one inspiration (breathing in), and one expiration (breathing out). Respiratory rate measurement is an important aspect of patient assessment. Chapter 11 provides further detail about respiratory assessment.

LEARNING OUTCOMES

By the end of this section you will be able to:

1 discuss when and why observation of respiration is performed and state the range of normal respiratory rates for adults;
2 discuss other aspects of breathing to observe when measuring respiratory rates;
3 accurately measure and record the respiratory rate.

ACTIVITY

Why would a person's respiration be observed? The practice scenarios will give you some clues. List the possible reasons.

You may have thought of the following situations:

- admission to hospital or preoperatively, providing a baseline for future comparison;
- when a person in hospital or in the community is unwell or injured – for example, loss of consciousness, chest injury, difficulty with breathing, chest pain (so Anne, Ken and Natalie should all have their respiration rates measured);
- to monitor a patient's condition – for example after surgery, or during treatment, such as a morphine infusion;
- to monitor a patient's response to treatments or medication that affects the respiratory system.

When assessing respiratory rate you should know the expected normal rate, and if a baseline reading is available you can make a comparison with this. There is considerable individual variation in respiratory rates (Blows 2001). The respiratory rate varies according to age, size and gender and can also fluctuate in well people, for example if metabolic demands change.

The normal adult respiratory rate is about 12–20 breaths per minute (Wilkins *et al.* 2005). Exercise, stress and fear all increase the respiratory rate; this is a normal bodily response. If you count people's respiratory rates when they have just arrived at hospital, anxiety may lead to a raised respiratory rate, which would not be an accurate baseline. In deep (referred to as 'stage 4') sleep, respiratory rate drops to its lowest normal level. Knowledge of normal biological functioning will help you to recognise abnormalities and causes for concern.

An increased respiratory rate is termed **tachypnoea.** Ken's respiratory rate may increase due to his chest infection. A decreased respiratory rate is termed **bradypnoea.** Natalie's respiratory rate may decrease owing to the drugs she has taken. A serious side-effect of opioid drugs, such as morphine, is a depressed respiratory rate.

In healthy people, the relationship between pulse and respiration is fairly constant, being a ratio of one respiration to every four or five heart beats. Very rapid respirations, such as over 40 per minute in an adult (in the absence of exercise), or very slow respirations, such as 8 per minute, are cause for alarm and should be reported promptly.

ACTIVITY

When you are counting the respiratory rates of the people in the scenarios, what else about their respiration should you observe?

You should observe the difficulty, sound, depth and pattern of breathing, as discussed below.

Difficulty in breathing

Respirations are normally effortless and you should therefore observe whether breathing is difficult (termed **dyspnoea**). Dyspnoeic patients may use accessory muscles of respiration such as their neck and abdominal muscles. When Ken has a chest infection, he is likely to experience dyspnoea. People with dyspnoea often mouth breathe because there is less resistance to airflow through the mouth than the nose, and this can cause drying of the oral mucosa (Stocks 1996). Oral hygiene (discussed in Chapter 8) is therefore essential.

People with dyspnoea need to sit up, either in an armchair, or in bed well supported by pillows, to optimise ventilation. **Orthopnoea** is the term used when people cannot breathe unless they are upright. Dyspnoea is frightening and psychological support is essential.

Sound of breathing

You should also observe the sound of breathing, which is normally quiet. You may hear a variety of abnormal breath sounds. A **wheeze,** often heard in people with asthma, is a high-pitched sound occurring when air is forced through narrowed respiratory passages. A wheeze may also occur with chest infections. A **stridor** is a harsh, high-pitched sound that is heard during respiration when the larynx is obstructed.

Asthma
A respiratory disorder characterised by recurrent episodes of difficulty in breathing, wheezing on expiration, coughing and viscous mucoid bronchial secretions.

Depth of breathing

Depth of breathing should be observed. This relates to the volume of air moving in and out of the respiratory tract with each breath – the **tidal volume.** An adult's tidal volume should be about 500 mL (Blows 2001). The term **hyperventilation** refers to prolonged, rapid and deep ventilations which can occur during an anxiety attack, causing dizziness and fainting as the resulting low carbon dioxide level causes cerebral vasoconstriction.

Hypoventilation is the term used for slow and shallow breathing, which could lead to inadequate gaseous exchange. You should also observe whether the chest expands equally on both sides, particularly if there is a history of chest injury.

Pattern of breathing

The pattern of breathing should be observed. Terms are given to certain abnormalities.

- **Apnoea.** This is a period without breathing. It could occur during hypoventilation, with another breath only occurring when arterial carbon dioxide levels rise and breathing is stimulated.
- **Cheyne–Stokes respirations.** These are when there is a gradual increase in the depth of respirations leading to an episode of hyperventilation, followed by a gradual decrease in the depth of respirations, and then a period of apnoea lasting about 15–20 seconds.

- **Kussmaul's respiration.** This is very deep and laboured breathing sometimes associated with patients in a diabetic coma. The deep breathing is due to metabolic acidosis.

The person's respiratory rate should be equal between each breath, with a short pause at the end of inspiration and expiration. Irregularities of breathing rate may indicate respiratory disease.

Learning outcome 3: Accurately measure and record the respiratory rate

For the following activities you need a willing volunteer. If a colleague is not available, another friend or family member may oblige!

ACTIVITY

Measure your volunteer's respiratory rate, using the instructions in Box 4.5.

Respiratory rates, particularly on admission, may be recorded simply as a number (the number of respirations per minute). If the person's respiratory rate is recorded regularly over a period of time an observation chart is used. Frequency of recordings varies but may be quarter-hourly (for a patient with acute breathing difficulties), hourly, 4-hourly or daily.

ACTIVITY

Ask your volunteer to spend a couple of minutes exercising (e.g. jogging on the spot) and then count their respiratory rate again. Using the example in Fig. 4.4 as a guide, record on an observation chart the two respiratory rates which you have taken.

> ### Box 4.5 Measuring respiratory rate
> - Note the placement of the second hand of your watch.
> - Count each rise and fall of the chest for 1 minute.
> In practice you should do this when people are unaware that they are being observed, as otherwise they may alter their breathing pattern. For an unresponsive person, this precaution is not relevant.
> *Tip:* In an alert individual the respiratory rate may be counted directly after the pulse, while still outwardly counting the pulse.

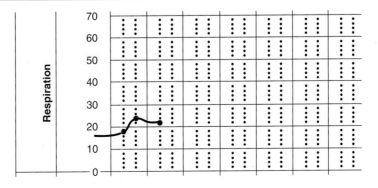

Figure 4.4: Observation chart, showing how respirations could be recorded.

Summary

- Respirations are measured as part of an acutely ill person's assessment, as a baseline for future comparison, and to monitor and evaluate a person's condition and response to treatment.
- It is important to be aware of normal respiratory rates, and of possible abnormalities that can occur.

MEASURING AND RECORDING BLOOD PRESSURE

Blood pressure results from the combination of heart output, circulating blood volume and peripheral *resistance,* which is the opposition to blood flow from friction between blood and blood vessel walls (Marieb 2006). Blood pressure is regulated by complex neural and hormonal systems (Tortora and Grabowski 2003). Currently blood pressure is measured in millimetres of mercury (mmHg) using a sphygmomanometer or electronic device (O'Brien *et al.* 2003).

According to Williams *et al.* (2004), blood pressure recording should be carried out routinely at least every five years until the age of 80, but people with high blood pressure should have more frequent measurements – at least annually. For people with learning disabilities, regular health checks should be carried out as part of their health promotion and these should include blood pressure measurement. This will lead to familiarity with the procedure and the establishment of a sound baseline. Ken's **Health Action Plan** should include his blood pressure measurements.

> **Blood pressure**
> The pressure that the blood exerts on the walls of the blood vessels (Waugh and Grant 2006). Blood pressure is different in different blood vessels, but in everyday clinical practice the term 'blood pressure' is used to mean *systemic arterial blood pressure* (Webster and Thompson 2006).

> **Health Action Plan**
> A personal action plan developed for each individual with a learning disability, containing details of their health interventions, medication taken, screening tests, etc. See *Valuing People* (DH 2001).

LEARNING OUTCOMES

By the end of this section you will be able to:

1 discuss the equipment used for blood pressure measurements and the meaning of the reading obtained;
2 identify the normal values for blood pressure and factors affecting blood pressure recordings;
3 accurately measure a person's blood pressure using manual equipment.

Learning outcome 1: Discuss the equipment used for blood pressure measurements and the meaning of the reading obtained

ACTIVITY

What equipment have you seen used to measure blood pressure? If you are not familiar with the sphygmomanometer ('sphygmo'), try to access one in the skills laboratory or the practice setting. If possible, look at electronic equipment too.

There are two main ways of measuring blood pressure:

- **Indirectly, using electronic equipment** – for example, oscillometry. An oscillometer is a machine that is attached to the patient's arm by means of a cuff. The cuff is inflated by the machine, which then reads the pressure within the artery. The result is displayed as two readings – the *systolic* and the *diastolic.* Some machines also display mean (average) blood pressure (MAP) during the reading, as well as the pulse rate.

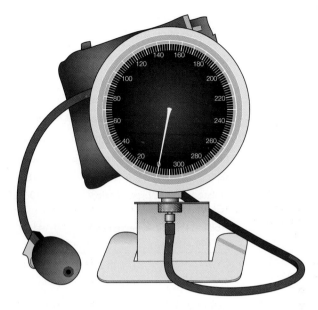

Figure 4.5: An aneroid sphygmomanometer.

- **Non-invasive auscultation method.** The pressure is taken manually by using a sphygmomanometer and stethoscope.

Blood pressure was traditionally recorded manually but is increasingly recorded electronically. Mercury sphygmomanometer usage is discouraged due to the risks of mercury spillage (MHRA 2005). They have been largely replaced with aneroid sphygmomanometers (see Fig. 4.5) but there is debate about their accuracy; these devices must be calibrated and serviced as per manufacturer's guidelines. Nurses need to learn how to record a blood pressure manually, as electronic devices are not always available, particularly in community and non-acute settings.

A blood pressure reading has two values, systolic and diastolic.

- **The systolic** occurs during ventricular contraction and is the maximum pressure of the blood against the wall of the artery. This is recorded as the top figure when documenting the blood pressure.
- **The diastolic** is the minimum pressure of the blood against the wall of the artery, which occurs following closure of the aortic valve. This measurement assesses the pressure when the ventricles are at rest and is recorded as the bottom figure.

Thus a blood pressure recorded as 120/70 means that the systolic pressure is 120 mmHg and the diastolic pressure is 70 mmHg. *The measurements of systolic and diastolic should be judged as one reading.* The difference between systolic and diastolic readings is termed the 'pulse pressure' (Webster and Thompson 2006).

Learning outcome 2: Identify the normal values for blood pressure and factors affecting blood pressure recordings

When measuring blood pressure, as with any other vital signs, you should be aware of expected normal ranges. O'Brien *et al.* (2003) highlight the variability in blood

Table 4.1: The British Hypertension Society's classification of blood pressure levels (Williams *et al.* 2004).

Category	Systolic BP (mmHg)	Diastolic BP (mmHg)
Optimal BP	<120	<80
Normal BP	<130	<85
High normal BP	130–139	85–89
Grade 1 hypertension (mild)	140–159	90–99
Grade 2 hypertension (moderate)	160–179	100–109
Grade 3 hypertension (severe)	⩾180	⩾110
Isolated systolic hypertension (Grade 1)	140–159	<90
Isolated systolic hypertension (Grade 2)	⩾160	<90

pressure from person to person. Normal adult blood pressure is generally considered to range from 100/60 to 140/90 (Mallet and Dougherty 2004). However, the British Hypertension Society guidelines for hypertension offer a more detailed classification of blood pressure levels (Williams *et al.* 2004) to indicate acceptable/unacceptable parameters (see Table 4.1).

ACTIVITY

Consider the people in the scenarios at the start of this chapter. What factors might affect their blood pressure recordings?

The term used for high blood pressure is **hypertension** and the term used for low blood pressure is **hypotension.** The physiological changes that occur during hypotension and hypertension are outlined by Marieb (2006).

Age, disease, injury and medicines all influence blood pressure and could be factors relevant to all three scenarios.

- **Blood volume.** The regulatory mechanisms can cope with minor fluctuations in circulating blood volume, but losses of 10 per cent or more – due to trauma, haemorrhage or severe dehydration – result in a fall in blood pressure (Tortora and Grabowski 2003).
- **Age.** Blood pressure increases from birth and throughout life (Marieb 2006). Anne and Ken may have a higher blood pressure than Natalie, who is a younger adult.
- **Disease.** Elasticity of the arteries is affected directly by diseases such as atherosclerosis (Webster and Thompson 2006). Many other diseases can raise blood pressure, including heart disease, kidney disease, endocrine disorders and neurological conditions (Marieb 2006). In these instances high blood pressure is termed **secondary hypertension.**
- **Posture and gravity.** A decrease in blood pressure may occur from lying to sitting or standing position, but O'Brien *et al.* (2003) assert that this is unlikely to lead to significant error in recording provided the arm is supported at the patient's heart level. Some people's blood pressure falls more significantly on standing (termed

orthostatic hypotension). This is more common in older people (Marieb 2006) and is a complication of immobility (see Chapter 6).

- **Drug use.** Some prescribed drugs affect blood pressure; examples are diuretics and tranquillisers (Tortora and Grabowski 2003). If Natalie has taken an overdose of tranquilliser, depending on the quantity, this could lower her blood pressure.
- **Emotional factors.** Stress, fear and anxiety all increase blood pressure. Failing to explain the procedure, rushing the procedure and anxiety about the outcome can all affect the reading (O'Brien *et al.* 2003). Relaxation techniques such as yoga and meditation can lower blood pressure (Everly and Sobelman 1987, cited by Smith and Fawcett 2006).
- **Weight.** An obese person's heart has to work harder and so the blood pressure may be higher (Marieb 2006).
- **Diet.** High salt and low calcium dietary intakes may lead to a rise in blood pressure (Marieb 2006).
- **Exercise.** People who take regular exercise may have a lower blood pressure (O'Brien *et al.* 2003).
- **Arm support and position.** Diastolic blood pressure may increase by 10 per cent if the arm is left unsupported (O'Brien *et al.* 2003). An overestimation of blood pressure can result if the arm is placed below the heart level.
- **Which arm?** It is recommended that, during a patient's initial assessment, bilateral blood pressure measurements are recorded to identify any clinical differences in the readings (Lane *et al.* 2002).
- **'White coat hypertension'.** This term is used when a person's blood pressure is consistently higher when recorded in a medical situation, such as a hospital, clinic or GP's surgery, than at home (O'Brien *et al.* 2003). It is a common phenomenon, affecting up to 25 per cent of those who appear to have hypertension (O'Brien 2001).

Learning outcome 3: Accurately measure a person's blood pressure using manual equipment

Although blood pressure can be measured at several sites, in most clinical situations the **brachial artery** is used as it is convenient for patients and easily accessible, so it is the artery you are most likely to have seen used in practice. Some electronic devices measure blood pressure at the **radial artery.** It is advisable to avoid recording the blood pressure on an arm that is affected by disability (e.g. weakness due to a stroke), or where an intravenous infusion is in place. When a person has suffered trauma or surgery affecting both arms, the **thigh** can be used. In this instance, a larger cuff is needed.

Faulty equipment and poor technique can also affect blood pressure measurements (see next section).

Recording korotkoff sounds

The Korotkoff sounds are heard through the stethoscope when you manually record a blood pressure (see Table 4.2). They are named after Nikolai Korotkoff, who first

Table 4.2: Korotkoff sounds (Korotkoff 1905, cited by O'Brien *et al.* 1999).

Phase	Sound	When they are normally heard
1	Clear tapping	Usually above 120 mmHg
2	Blowing or whistling	Around 110 mmHg
3	Soft thud	Around 100 mmHg
4	Low-pitched, muffled sound	Around 90 mmHg
5	Disappearance of all sounds	Around 80 mmHg

identified the audible sounds of blood pressure in 1905 (Korotkoff 1905, cited by O'Brien *et al.* 1999). There may be a period between phase 2 and 3 where no sounds are audible, yet they become audible again at a lower pressure. This phenomenon is known as an **auscultatory gap** (O'Brien *et al.* 2003) and is the reason that correct procedure involves palpation to find systolic blood pressure before using the sphygmomanometer. This technique is explained later.

There is debate about whether the diastolic pressure should be recorded at phase 4 or phase 5. Generally guidelines recommend phase 5 as the point of diastolic pressure (O'Brien *et al.* 2003). Phase 4 should be used to record diastolic blood pressure *only* if sounds are heard to virtually 0 mmHg, which can occur in pregnancy and states of high cardiac output (Armstrong 2002).

Steps in recording blood pressure

Blood pressure recording is frequently carried out by nurses and is a common experience for most people, but remember that for some people it will be their first time. Always give adequate explanation, warning about the tightness of the cuff, which some people find quite uncomfortable.

ACTIVITY

If you can access manual blood pressure recording equipment – a sphygmomanometer and a stethoscope – practise measuring and recording a blood pressure with a colleague, using the guidance in Box 4.6.

Errors in blood pressure measurement

Errors in blood pressure measurement, including equipment failure and operator error, can significantly affect a person's investigations and treatment. Nurses should be aware of the potential pitfalls in recording and overcome the risk of errors. However, Armstrong's research (2002) suggests that nurses have poor knowledge of some aspects of correct technique. Table 4.3 lists possible problems you may encounter and how to resolve them.

Ambulatory blood pressure monitoring

O'Brien *et al.* (2003), in the European Society of Hypertension recommendations for conventional, ambulatory and home blood pressure measurement, report that

Box 4.6 Steps in recording a blood pressure manually (adapted from O'Brien *et al.* 2003)

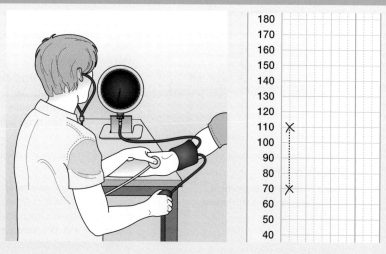

Use a properly maintained, calibrated and validated device. All equipment should be clean.
- Remove tight clothing and support the arm at heart level (see the diagram).
- Allow the person to sit down and relax, for 5–15 minutes if possible, prior to the recording. Measure sitting blood pressure routinely. Standing blood pressure should be recorded initially in older people and people with diabetes.
- Explain what you are going to do, to allay anxiety, and try to promote comfort and privacy.
- Select the correct size cuff. The cuff bladder (the insert of the cuff, made of rubber) should cover 80 per cent of the circumference of the upper arm. The average arm circumference is 30 cm. The cuff size should be clearly visible on those you use in practice. The following sizes are suggested as a guide only:
  – a standard bladder 12 cm by 26 cm is suitable for the majority of adults
  – an obese bladder 12 cm by 40 cm for obese arms
  – a small bladder measuring 10 cm by 18 cm for lean adults and older children.

Note: Each person's arm measurements are different and it is important that you seek the advice of a qualified nurse to ensure the correct choice. The sizes indicate the size of the bladder within the Velcro fastening or wrap-around cuff.
- Locate the brachial artery with your fingers and palpate to identify the pulse.
- Place the cuff on the arm 2.5 cm above the antecubital fossa with the mid-point of the cuff bladder in line with the brachial artery. This point may be marked on the cuff. The tubes from the bladder are best placed at the top of cuff (see diagram).
- Ensure that the cuff fits snugly to the arm and is secured.
- While palpating the radial pulse, inflate the cuff until the pulse disappears. Note the level at which this occurs, as this equates to the *systolic* pressure.
- Deflate the cuff fully and wait 1 minute to allow the circulation to recover.
- Place the stethoscope head over the brachial pulse.
- Inflate the cuff, to 30 mmHg above your estimated systolic measurement, and then open the valve so the cuff deflates slowly (approximately 2 mm per second), listening carefully.
- When you hear the first sound, note the measurement on the sphygmomanometer. This is the *systolic* blood pressure – the top number. Record this to the nearest 2 mmHg.
- Continue listening whilst deflating the cuff slowly and evenly. Note the changing sounds. When the sound disappears completely, phase V, this is the *diastolic* blood pressure – the bottom number.
- Record the results on your observation chart (as shown) and interpret the results, i.e. consider whether the blood pressure is high (hypertension) or low (hypotension) or within the normal range for the person.

O'Brien *et al.* (2003) warn of the dangers of treating a person on the grounds of an isolated reading and advise taking the mean of at least two readings, or more if there are marked differences in the two readings.

Table 4.3: Common problems with blood pressure measurement, and suggested solutions (O'Brien *et al.* 1999).

Problem	Solution
Incorrect blood pressure reading	Ensure that the measurement is made to the nearest 2 mmHg
Incorrect size and position of cuff for the patient	Use the appropriate size of cuff for the individual: the cuff bladder should cover 80% of the arm's circumference A too large or too small cuff will give a false reading
Confusion about diastolic blood pressure reading	Diastolic measurement taken at cessation of sounds
Poorly maintained equipment causing errors in measurement	Ensure that the manometer starts at zero and that the machine is calibrated according to the manufacturer's instructions The tubing and all connections should be carefully checked before use

ambulatory blood pressure devices are becoming more common to measure a person's blood pressure reading over several hours or days.

Ambulatory blood pressure devices consist of an electronic device which is worn on the person's arm for 24 hours while they continue their normal daily routines. This allows the healthcare team to review the person's blood pressure over a longer period than their hospital visit, providing a more accurate view of their blood pressure measurement. Ambulatory devices are used in people with an unusual variability of readings, possible 'white coat hypertension', to decide treatment regimes, review drug therapy effectiveness, review hypertension treatment in pregnancy and evaluate symptomatic hypotension.

Electronic pulse, blood pressure and oxygen saturation measurement

In many clinical areas, measuring the pulse, blood pressure and oxygen saturation are all carried out using electronic monitoring devices. Preparation of patients for blood pressure measurement (relaxation, explanation, arm support, correct cuff size selection) follows the steps in Box 4.6.

Connect the electronic device to the mains supply and allow the machine to carry out its checking and calibration testing. Place the blood pressure cuff on the patient's arm with the midpoint of the cuff's bladder (often indicated by an arrow on the cuff) over the patient's brachial pulse, 2.5 centimetres above the antecubital fossa. Press the start button on the monitor and advise the patient to keep still and that the cuff may feel tight around their arm for a short while. Allow the machine to measure the blood pressure and record the displayed systolic and diastolic blood pressure on the patient's observation chart. Read and record the patient's pulse rate. Place the oxygen saturation probe on the other hand and record the patient's oxygen saturation level (see next section for details). Once you have recorded all the observations, the machine will return to standby. If appropriate, set the timer to record regular observations – for example at 15-minute intervals. You should advise the patient that you are doing this, so that they are aware that the machine will constantly monitor their vital signs. If you are recording one set of vital signs, remove the cuff and oxygen saturation probe and return the monitoring device to its storage place, ensuring that you plug the machine in to recharge it.

During any vital signs monitoring, some people have difficulty in straightening their arms, or may have pulses that are not easy to find. Always ask for supervision when needed. Also, if you have any doubt about the accuracy of electronic recordings of blood pressure and pulse, do check them manually.

Summary

- Blood pressure measurements can be affected by psychological, physical and environmental factors, but technique and equipment are also important aspects.
- Electronic devices are increasingly used for recording pulse, blood pressure and oxygen saturation. However, an understanding of how to use manual equipment accurately remains important for nurses.

MEASURING OXYGEN SATURATION BY PULSE OXIMETRY

Pulse oximetry enables continuous non-invasive monitoring of the oxygen saturation of haemoglobin (SpO_2) in arterial blood, updated with each pulse wave, via a microprocessor with a probe attached to the patient. Haemoglobin (Hb) is a molecule, present in erythrocytes (red blood cells), which transports gases – especially oxygen – around the body. About 98 per cent of the oxygen in the blood is transported attached to these haemoglobin molecules (then called oxyhaemoglobin, HbO_2), while about 2 per cent is carried dissolved in the plasma. Pulse oximetry measures how saturated with oxygen are the haemoglobin molecules.

LEARNING OUTCOMES

By the end of this section you will be able to:

1 explain how pulse oximetry works and how it is used;
2 identify when pulse oximetry is used, its advantages and limitations.

You may be able to access a pulse oximeter in the skills laboratory or your practice setting.

Learning outcome 1: Explain how pulse oximetry works and how it is used

ACTIVITY

Have you seen pulse oximetry used in practice? If so, can you remember what the equipment looked like, and do you know how it works? What is a normal reading?

Pulse oximeters range from small hand-held devices displaying the percentage of oxygen saturation and the pulse rate, to more substantial devices that also show the pulsatile waveform (see Fig. 4.6). The box has a wire leading to the sensor or probe – a clip or sleeve which is placed on a finger, toe or earlobe. Probes can be disposable or reusable and are available in different sizes. The diagram in Fig. 4.7 shows how the sensor works.

Pulse oximeters monitor only light absorption from tissue with a pulsatile flow, so preventing false readings from fat, bone, connective tissue and venous blood. A good arterial blood flow is therefore needed for a reliable reading (Carroll 1997a).

ACTIVITY

If you have access to a pulse oximeter, measure your oxygen saturation using the instructions in Box 4.7.

The normal value of oxygen saturation is 95–100 per cent, so hopefully your reading was within that range. This figure refers to the percentage of haemoglobin molecules fully saturated with oxygen. **SpO_2 readings below 90 per cent give cause for concern** (Hill and Stoneham 2000) and must be reported. Repositioning the person to a more upright position, if not contraindicated, may provide significant improvement. Pulse oximeters have alarm systems, which sound if the measurement falls below a normal level.

Box 4.7   Use of pulse oximeter (adapted from Hill and Stoneham 2000)

- Turn the pulse oximeter on and allow the device to go through its checking and calibration procedure.
- Select the appropriate probe; ensure correct fitting and positioning on the digit. Avoid placing probe on false nails, or nail polished fingernails.
- Allow several seconds for the oximeter to detect your pulse and calculate your reading.
- Look at the waveform displayed.
- Read percentage (%) displayed – this is your own oxygen saturation. Record this on the observation chart.
- In practice you should record whether the patient is receiving oxygen (and if so, the percentage) or breathing air.

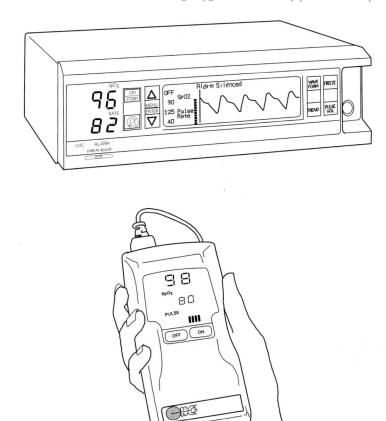

Figure 4.6: Examples of pulse oximeters.

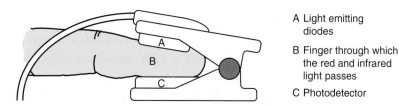

A Light emitting
   diodes

B Finger through which
   the red and infrared
   light passes

C Photodetector

Figure 4.7: Diagram showing how a pulse oximeter works.

Most manufacturers claim that their devices are accurate to plus or minus 2 per cent, at oxygen saturations of 70–99 per cent. The ability of pulse oximeters to detect **hypoxaemia** (insufficient oxygenation of blood) was confirmed by a systematic review (Pedersen *et al.* 2003). However, as hypoxaemia rises, pulse oximetry becomes less accurate and at 80–85 per cent a more detailed assessment is necessary. If there is any doubt about the accuracy of pulse oximetry, blood gas analysis (analysis of a sample of arterial blood) should be performed (see Chapter 11, Box 11.3). If the peripheral pulse is weak or absent, pulse oximetry readings will not be precise (Carroll 1997a). Cardiac arrythmias such as atrial fibrillation can interfere with capture of the pulsatile signal and thus reduce accuracy.

If possible the sensor should be attached to a part of the body which the patient is most likely to keep still. If digits are used, they should be supported rather than held in the air (Cowan 1997). Carroll (1997a) recommends that using the ear often reduces problems of movement.

Learning outcome 2: Identify when pulse oximetry is used, its advantages and limitations

O'Driscoll *et al.* (2008) recommend that oxygen saturation should be checked by pulse oximetry for all breathless and acutely ill patients, and that pulse oximetry should be available wherever emergency oxygen is used. Assessing hypoxaemia through observation is notoriously inaccurate and unreliable (Le Grand and Peters 1999; Sinex 1999) but it can rapidly lead to tissue damage. The brain is very sensitive to oxygen depletion, and visual and cognitive changes can occur when oxygen saturation falls to 80–85 per cent. Other signs of hypoxaemia include restlessness, agitation, hypotension and tachycardia. However, all these signs can be missed or wrongly interpreted.

Cyanosis is the visible sign of hypoxaemia, but is only detected at a saturation of about 75 per cent in normally perfused patients (Hanning and Alexander-Williams 1995). Pulse oximetry should therefore be a more accurate and objective measure of hypoxaemia, alerting health professionals at an early stage. It is cheap and non-invasive and can be easily measured during transfer of a patient.

> **Cyanosis**
> A bluish, greyish or purple discoloration of the skin due to presence of abnormal amounts of reduced haemoglobin in the blood.

ACTIVITY

Have you seen pulse oximetry used in practice? If so, what care situations was it used in?

- **Acute illness.** Pulse oximetry is part of the assessment of anyone who is acutely ill, particularly during initial assessment and management. Therefore, Anne will have a pulse oximeter attached. Summers *et al.* (1998) found that incorporating pulse oximetry into emergency assessment identified a small, but statistically significant, group whose hypoxia would otherwise have been missed. Currently pulse oximeters are not widely available outside acute hospital settings, so it is less likely that Ken or Natalie's oxygen saturations would be monitored, although they would provide a useful indication of their oxygenation adequacy.
- **During investigations and surgery.** Pulse oximetry is used during and after procedures and investigations involving general anaesthesia, or sedation.
- **Inpatients with respiratory and circulatory problems.** Patients with respiratory disease, particularly if receiving oxygen therapy, will have SpO_2 monitoring. The amount of oxygen administered may be adjusted according to the SpO_2. O'Driscoll *et al.* (2008) recommend that O_2 should be prescribed to achieve 94–98 per cent oxygen saturations for most acutely ill patients, or 88–92 per cent for those at risk of hypercapnic respiratory failure – and the target saturation should be written on the drug chart. Any patients who are at risk of hypoxaemia – such as

> **Hypoxia**
> A condition in which inadequate oxygen is available to the tissues to allow normal function.

> **Hypercapnic respiratory failure**
> Inadequate gas exchange by the respiratory system where there is a build-up of carbon dioxide.

Chronic obstructive
pulmonary disease.
A chronic disease, which
includes conditions such
as emphysema, chronic
bronchitis and chronic
asthma. It causes debillitating
breathlessness which affects
day-to-day living.

Cystic fibrosis
A genetic disease causing
oversecretion of a viscous
mucus predisposing to
respiratory infections.

those with pneumonia, congestive heart failure, chronic obstructive pulmonary disease (COPD) exacerbation or acute lung injury – may have continuous SpO_2 monitoring via a pulse oximeter (Rodriguez and Light 1998). Patients whose cardiorespiratory status is unstable, and are undergoing transfer, often have pulse oximetry *in situ*.

- **In the community.** Pulse oximetry can be used in the community with people who are at risk of hypoxaemia, for example with chronically ill patients such as those with cystic fibrosis. Carroll (1997b) notes the increasing use of pulse oximetry by community nurses.

Limitations of pulse oximetry

Pulse oximetry complements measurement of other vital signs but it does not replace them (Lowton 1999); oxygen saturations are only a single physiological variable and should not be over-relied upon. Pulse oximeters cannot differentiate between different forms of saturated haemoglobin (Carroll 1997a). When carbon monoxide is inhaled, carboxyhaemoglobin (COHb) is formed and is absorbed and registered as oxyhaemoglobin, leading to overestimation of oxygen saturation. Thus for people who have been involved in accidents where there was smoke, or who are affected by carbon monoxide poisoning, pulse oximetry is not recommended. COHb readings are also high in tobacco smokers (Moyle 1996).

Stoddart *et al.* (1997) note that it is the quality of oxygen delivery to the tissues that is of most importance – which depends on cardiac output, tissue perfusion and haemoglobin concentration – not just oxygen saturation of arterial blood. Oxyhaemoglobin saturation could be 99 per cent, but this is of no value if the heart cannot deliver it to the tissues.

ACTIVITY

What signs and symptoms might indicate a lack of oxygen to the tissues (hypoxia)?

Signs which you could observe for include the warmth of peripheral areas of the body, colour of skin and tongue, urine output and mental state (Place 1998).

Summary

- Pulse oximetry is widely used and has many applications.
- Pulse oximetry is non-invasive, easy to apply and provides a continuous measurement.
- It is important to understand the limitations of pulse oximetry and to be aware of its role as complementary to the overall clinical picture.

NEUROLOGICAL ASSESSMENT

Neurological assessment is performed to assess a person's neurological status and is appropriate whenever there is impaired consciousness, a history of loss

AVPU scale

A = Alert
V = (responds to) Voice
P = (responds to) Pain
U = Unresponsive

of consciousness, or a risk that the level of consciousness might deteriorate. Neurological assessment consists of either a quick review of a patient's neurological state using the AVPU scale, or an evaluation of the level of consciousness using the **Glasgow Coma Scale** (GCS), pupil size and reaction, motor and sensory function and vital signs. The GCS is now included in many clinical areas as part of the physiological track and trigger assessment or early-warning score process in the care of acutely ill people, as recommended by NICE (2007a). See Chapter 11 for more information.

LEARNING OUTCOMES

By the end of this section you will be able to:
1 understand why a neurological assessment would be needed and what instruments are used;
2 accurately perform and record an assessment of an adult's neurological status.

Learning outcome 1: Understand why a neurological assessment would be needed and what instruments are used

ACTIVITY

For which of the people in the scenarios would a neurological assessment be appropriate, and why?

Neurological assessment would be particularly important for Anne and Natalie as they have histories of impaired consciousness. Anne has a head injury and was unconscious briefly. Natalie is not fully alert and she has ingested an unknown quantity and variety of drugs that may affect her neurological function.

A head injury (as in Anne's case) is a particularly important reason for performing neurological assessment. In 2007, NICE published guidelines for assessing and managing people who have head injuries. These guidelines (available from www.nice.org.uk) should be referred to for further guidance. Neurological observations should be conducted only by professionals competent in assessment of head injury (NICE 2007b). The GCS, which forms part of this assessment, directly affects subsequent investigations and management for such patients.

Accurate neurological assessment is particularly important where there is a concern about the development of raised intracranial pressure (see Box 4.8). Being a rigid vault, the skull (cranium) cannot accommodate any swelling without the function of the brain being impaired. In disease or injury, the brain tissue, blood or cerebral spinal fluid (CSF) can increase in volume or size, causing a rise in intracranial pressure. This adversely affects cerebral blood flow (Winkelman 1995).

In some situations, particularly with a head injury where an extradural or subdural haematoma can develop, detection of deteriorating consciousness level

---

Extradural haematoma

This is an accumulation of blood between the dura and the skull. The meningeal artery passes through the extradural space, and can become torn after a head injury, resulting in an arterial bleed into the extradural space. The brain then becomes compressed and displaced. This is a serious life-threatening condition, requiring urgent treatment.

Subdural haematoma

Blood accumulates in the subdural space and gradually builds up to produce a haematoma. This can lead to compression of the brain, which in turn can result in loss of brain function.

> **Box 4.8 Signs of raised intracranial pressure (Winkelman 1995)**
>
> - Level of consciousness (decrease in arousal and awareness) – this is the most sensitive indicator of neurological function
> - Increasing headache
> - Pupils (enlargement, asymmetry, oval shape, decreased reaction) – a new unilateral, dilated fixed pupil is a medical emergency
> - Slowing of the pulse rate – this is a late sign
> - Respirations – abnormal or irregular pattern
> - Raised systolic blood pressure
> - Limb movements – variable responses.
>
> If any of the above changes occur it is extremely important that you report these immediately to a qualified nurse or doctor.

is paramount, as life-saving treatment could be needed. Neurological observations should be carried out under supervision of a registered nurse and any concerns reported immediately.

Instruments used to assess neurological status

The GCS was developed by Jennett and Teasdale (1974) and is widely used and recognised, often being incorporated into trauma assessment charts (Skinner *et al.* 2002). Hickey (2003) reports that the GCS is the most commonly used neurological assessment tool.

ACTIVITY

Access a neurological observation scale from your local practice setting. Look at the sections and how they are laid out. They should include the GCS, pupil reactions and limb movements and a section for charting vital signs.

The GCS is used to assist nurses in providing a consistent and standard measurement of people's neurological status (NICE 2007b). Scoring using the GCS is done in three sections: eye opening, motor response and verbal response (see Fig. 4.8). Each section is given a score and these are totalled to give a score ranging from 15 (best) to 3 (worst). As a person's neurological condition improves, so their GCS score should improve.

The severity of a head injury can be indicated by the score attained (Jennett and Teasdale 1974; Jennett 2005). A score of 8 or less indicates a severe head injury and the person will be in a coma. The rhyme 'If the Glasgow score is eight, then it's time to intubate' may help you to remember that a GCS of 8 or below is a serious clinical situation where the patient is unconscious. Maintenance of the patient's airway by intubation of the trachea or nasopharyngeal airway using an advanced airway is a specialised clinical skill, performed by advanced practitioners

	Score
Eye opening	
Spontaneous	4
To speech	3
To pain	2
None	1
Motor response	
Obeys commands	6
Localises to pain	5
Withdraws to pain	4
Abnormal flexion to pain	3
Extensor response to pain	2
No movement	1
Verbal response	
Oriented	5
Confused	4
Inappropriate words	3
Incomprehensible speech	2
None	1

Figure 4.8: Glasgow Coma Scale (adapted from Jennett 2005).

who have undergone training for this procedure. You may, however, be required to observe or assist with this skill in an emergency (see Chapter 11 for more information).

A score of more than 8 indicates that the person is conscious. People with a minor head injury might have a score between 13 and 15. Use of the GCS for people with head injuries is well documented, but it can be used for anyone who requires a neurological assessment, regardless of the underlying cause – so it may be relevant for Natalie and Ken, as well as for Anne.

Learning outcome 2: Accurately perform and record an assessment of an adult's neurological status

When assessing any person in your care the first priorities are to check responsiveness, ensure the patient has an open airway, check breathing, and maintain an adequate circulation following the basic life-support algorithms (Resuscitation Council UK 2005). Systematic assessment of acutely ill patients is discussed further in Chapter 11.

It should be quickly established whether the person lost consciousness at any stage and appears to be deteriorating, particularly following an accident (NICE 2007b). Thus the person and any bystanders should be asked about the incident. Bystanders are a valuable source of information regarding a person's head injury, fit or collapse (Walsh *et al.* 1999; Dolan and Holt 2000). Thus gaining a detailed history from Anne's husband about exactly what he observed is essential. The onset and duration of signs and symptoms, previous medical history and any recent illnesses are all useful to note. After taking a history, the person's neurological status can be assessed using the GCS. This assessment provides a quantitative score for assessing eye opening, verbal response and motor response.

ACTIVITY

Find a willing adult volunteer to help you to work through the GCS. Look at the scale in Fig. 4.8 and consider how you might assess whether your volunteer's GCS score was 15 – the best response.

A person with a GCS score of 15 will have airway, breathing and circulation that is present and normal, and will speak to you and answer questions appropriately. In brief, a talking, breathing, alert, coherent and orientated person will have a score of 15. We hope this applies to your volunteer!

Jennett (2005) and NICE (2007b) recommend that the scores for each of the three sections – eye opening (E), motor response (M) and verbal response (V) – should be documented separately to explain exactly what score has been awarded in each category. For example, if a person's score is 14 then you may see the score recorded as 'E = 4, M = 6, V = 4' (instead of 5, indicating that the patient is confused).

Each section of the scale will now be explained in more detail. This will be linked to how you might assess Anne, who has sustained a head injury.

Eye opening (E)

Assessment of Anne's eye opening response indicates the arousal mechanisms found within her brainstem. When observing her eye opening response, gently touch her arm when you ask a question. Touch is an important way of communicating non-verbally and is particularly important for people with hearing and visual deficits. Anne's husband could inform you if these apply to Anne. Some people with a head injury might have difficulty opening their eyes due to eyelid swelling, particularly if there is an accompanying facial injury.

- *Spontaneous* (scores 4). Anne will score 4 if she opens her eyes or already has her eyes open when you approach her.
- *To speech* (score 3). It is important to differentiate between a person sleeping and being unresponsive. This can be done by asking a simple question, such as 'Can you open your eyes?'
- *To pain* (score 2). If Anne does not open her eyes to speech, you should assess whether she responds to pain. How pain should be inflicted remains controversial.

You may only use appropriate touch and must take care not to cause damage such as bruising. One way is to squeeze the trapezius muscle. Use your thumb and two fingers and place them where the neck meets the shoulder and gently squeeze this muscle. Alternatively, you can apply supra-orbital pressure by pressing the skin just below the eyebrow, or apply the sternal rub by using the knuckles of a clenched fist to apply pressure to Anne's sternum. Underlying injuries must be taken into account when applying these techniques to avoid causing more pain or injury to people. Only the minimum stimulus to elicit a response should be used. For example, do not press over the sternum if you know the person has fractured ribs, and do not apply supra-orbital pressure if there is an injury in this area. You should discuss the accepted practice within your area with your supervising practitioner.

- *None* (score 1). This score is recorded where applying pain causes no eye opening response.

ACTIVITY

If your volunteer agrees, you could try out the different techniques for applying painful stimuli, or even try them on yourself!

Motor response (M)

When assessing motor response you should consider pre-existing disabilities and also any new injuries, which in Anne's case could have been sustained in her fall. The assessment of motor response is performed in relation to upper limbs, as lower limb responses can reflect spinal function (Aucken and Crawford 1998). **Note:** Assessment of limb movement (discussed later) is carried out on both upper and lower limbs.

- *Obeys commands* (score 6). When you are carrying out Anne's other observations you can assess whether she coordinates her actions in response to your requests. For example, you might ask Anne to roll up her sleeve for blood pressure measurement. Alternatives would be to ask her to close/open her eyes or stick out her tongue. If Anne were unable to obey commands, you would next apply painful stimuli (as discussed previously), and note her motor response to pain.
- *Localises* (score 5). Anne would move her hand towards the pain. For example, if you apply supra-orbital pressure she would try to push your hand away.
- *Withdraws* (score 4). If Anne's limb flexes normally to pain, this response scores a 4.
- *Abnormal flexion* (score 3). Anne's flexion to pain would be slow and abnormal.
- *Extensor response* (score 2). Anne would straighten her arm as a response to painful stimuli.
- *No movement* (score 1). Here no motor response to any painful stimulus is made.

Verbal responses (V)

The verbal response should be assessed in relation to a person's usual communication, so you need to be aware of how they would communicate normally. Anne's neurological status is being assessed by staff who do not know her and how she communicates, so her husband's input would be particularly helpful.

- *Orientated* (score 5). If Anne is fully orientated she should be able to answer your questions appropriately. She will tell you her name, where she is and the date.
- *Confused* (score 4). In this case, Anne can discuss something with you but may not give accurate information. For example, when asked 'Where are you?' she may respond: 'I'm in the town'.
- *Inappropriate words* (score 3). Here Anne will use words that do not make sense. She may appear agitated and at times aggressive when you ask questions.
- *Incomprehensible speech* (score 2). Anne will not use any understandable words but will make verbal noises such as mumbling, moaning or groaning.
- *None* (score 1). Anne will not respond verbally at all. If a person is intubated, they will be unable to talk and this should be recorded as: 'I'.

ACTIVITY	When assessing a person's GCS score, what factors could affect the accuracy of the assessment and how could you overcome these?

- **Hearing loss.** If the person has impaired hearing it may be difficult to communicate verbally, which could affect the accuracy of the result in all three categories. Sign language could be used or a communication board, provided that this is appropriate to the person's level of consciousness, and that their vision is not impaired. The person may lip-read and therefore be able to communicate effectively with you. Written responses are also valuable in this situation.
- **Language barrier.** If a person cannot understand or speak English, this could lead to difficulties with obtaining an accurate response, for example assessing orientation or whether commands are obeyed. A communication board may help, or interpretation via a relative or interpreter.
- **Speech difficulties or physical impairment.** A person with learning disabilities, for example, may communicate by a signing system, in which case information from their family or carers would be important.
- **Alcohol use.** If a person has ingested alcohol and has a suspected head injury, it is difficult to assess accurately. However, nurses should always err on the side of caution. A person's neurological assessment should never be assumed to be due to alcohol until other causes, for example a head injury, have been ruled out.

A nurse carrying out neurological assessment of any of the people in the scenarios would need to be aware of all the above factors. For example, any of them could have impaired hearing. Involvement by family or significant others who know the person's usual level of response is invaluable.

Pupil reaction

Assessment of pupil reaction usually forms part of neurological observation, as alteration in pupil sizes and reaction could indicate a rise in **intracranial pressure.** Look at the pupil sizes shown in Fig. 4.9: you will see that they are shown in varying sizes from 1 to 8 millimetres. The person should be examined in dim light as bright light affects pupil reactions to torchlight.

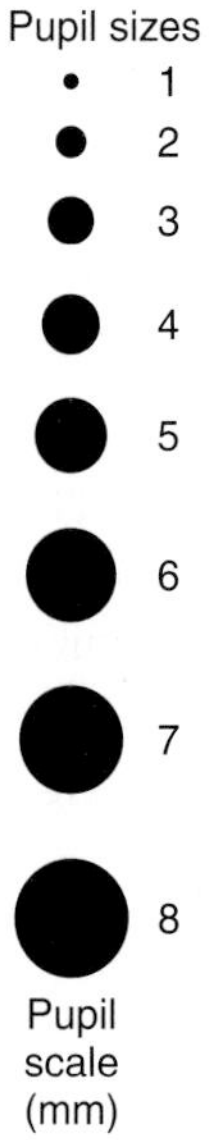

Pupil sizes

- 1
- 2
- 3
- 4
- 5
- 6
- 7
- 8

Pupil
scale
(mm)

Recording reactions:

B = Brisk reaction
SL = Sluggish reaction
– = No reaction
C = Closed

Pupils	Left	Size	4				
		Reaction	B				
	Right	Size	4				
		Reaction	B				

Figure 4.9: Pupil sizes and recording reactions.

ACTIVITY

Ask your willing volunteer to walk into a brightly lit room, and observe what happens to their pupils. Now observe the pupils in a dimly lit room. When did the pupil size appear the greatest?

When recording pupil reactions, the size and reaction of **each** eye is checked and recorded individually: L = left eye and R = right eye. A light beam (usually from a pen torch) is directed into the eye to assess the reaction to the light and the size of the pupil against the chart.

- **Pupil sizes and equality.** Before shining the light in the eyes consider: Are the pupils equal? Do they look between 2 and 5 mm? Do they look round?
- **Reaction.** What happens when a light is shone into the eyes? Are the reactions brisk? (If yes, record B.) Are they sluggish? (If yes, record SL.) Is there no reaction? (If yes, record None.) (Aucken and Crawford 1998).

Always note whether a person is wearing contact lenses or has a false eye as these will obviously affect the results. In Fig. 4.9 you will see that both the left and right pupils have been recorded as 4B, meaning that the pupils are approximately 4 mm in size and react to light briskly.

ACTIVITY

Now assess the size and reaction of your volunteer's pupils.

Glaucoma
An increase in the intraocular pressure of the eye causing reduced vision in the affected eye.

People with visual impairment and those who have had ocular surgery or disease may have altered pupil reactions, so you should establish what is normal for this person. For example, a person who has glaucoma may use eyedrops that constrict the pupil.

Box 4.9 Recording limb movements

L I M B	**M O V E M E N T S**	**A R M S**	Normal power	R		
			Mild weakness	L		
			Severe weakness			
			Flexion			
			Extension			
			No response			
		L E G S	Normal power	R/L		
			Mild weakness			
			Severe weakness			
			Flexion			
			Extension			
			No response			

Limb movements

A neurological chart contains a section for recording limb movements. There are different versions used in practice, but Box 4.9 gives one example. Verbal commands are used to examine these movements. For example, the nurse may ask the person to push and pull against them with each limb. The responses are recorded for arms and legs separately. If there is a difference between the limbs, they are recorded separately.

In Box 4.9 the assessment indicates normal power in both legs, a mild weakness in the left arm, and normal power in the right arm. *Normal power* is recorded when the person responds appropriately to commands and shows normal function and strength of the limb. *Mild weakness* implies that the limb can be moved but with reduced power. The arm weakness recorded on the chart shown may be due to a stroke or other pre-existing condition, such as cerebral palsy. *Severe weakness* implies movement is possible but with no real strength. **Flexion** is recorded when the knee or elbow is bent, and **extension** is recorded when the arm or leg straightens, when a painful stimulus is applied. 'No response' is recorded when no stimulus (as used in best motor response) obtains any motor response from the person.

ACTIVITY

Practise all the skills included in this chapter by recording a full set of neurological observations with your willing volunteer. This should include vital signs as well as level of consciousness, pupil reactions and limb movements.

The complexity and importance of neurological observations

Neurological assessment is complex and requires practice in the clinical setting (NICE 2007b). You should first observe a qualified nurse recording a neurological assessment and then take part under supervision, according to local policy. The first set of neurological observations forms the baseline for future assessment.

Ingram (1994) warned that people perform neurological observations differently, thus leading to unreliable results. To improve reliability before a new nurse takes over the care of the person, the previous nurse should demonstrate a neurological assessment.

Neurological observations should be carried out and recorded on a half-hourly basis until a GCS score equal to 15 has been achieved. The minimum frequency of observations for patients with a GCS score equal to 15 should be half-hourly for 2 hours, then hourly for 4 hours and 2-hourly thereafter (NICE 2007b).

Summary

- Neurological observations are frequently performed by nurses, and are very important when monitoring the condition of a person with actual or potential neurological impairment.
- The GCS has been developed to promote consistency in assessment. Nevertheless, slight variations of terminology in the categories of eye opening, motor responses and vocal responses varies as does how the scale is used in practice. To promote reliability between readings, one nurse should carry out the observations, and demonstrate how they were carried out to any other nurse who is taking over the care.
- The GCS score can be highly influential in terms of treatment , further investigation and predicting a patient's eventual outcome. Therefore students carrying out these observations should be working under supervision and report immediately any concerns.
- Most head injuries are mild, but a small number of patients suffer serious injuries to their brain, resulting in severe disability or death. Nurses who observe, measure and record neurological observations must be aware that people who have experienced neurological trauma can deteriorate very quickly. Noticing any changes in neurological function and notifying senior nursing and medical personnel of these changes is imperative so that life-saving procedures can be carried out.

CHAPTER SUMMARY

This chapter aimed to help you develop your skills in assessing vital signs within the practice setting. These observations should not be considered in isolation but as part of a person's *holistic assessment,* which will include a range of other observations and gaining information from various sources.

Vital signs must be assessed and recorded accurately, using the appropriate equipment in the recommended manner. They must also be reported and guidance sought in their interpretation. Some vital signs can change quickly along with the person's level of consciousness, so they must be carried out at the required frequency. (Chapter 11 offers further guidance regarding the assessment of patients whose condition is deteriorating.) It can take considerable practice with a range of people in a variety of settings to become really confident and competent in these skills.

ACKNOWLEDGEMENT

This chapter has been revised and updated. The author acknowledges the work of Sue Higham on this chapter in the previous two editions of the book.

REFERENCES

3M undated. 3M Tempa DOT Single-use Clinical Thermometers: How to read 3M Tempa DOT thermometers. Available from http://products 3.3m.com

Armstrong, R. 2002. Nurses' knowledge of error in blood pressure measurement technique. *International Journal of Nursing Practice* **8,** 116–19.

Aucken, S. and Crawford, B. 1998. Neurological assessment. In Guerrero, D. (ed.) *Neuro Oncology for Nurses.* London: Whurr.

Blows, W.T. 2001. *The Biological Basis of Nursing: Clinical observations.* London: Routledge.

Brooker, C. 1998. *Human Structure and Function,* 2nd edn. London: Mosby.

Carroll, M. 2000. An evaluation of temperature measurement. *Nursing Standard* **14**(4), 1174–8.

Carroll, P. 1997a. Pulse oximetry – at your fingertips. *RN* **60**(2), 22–7, 43.

Carroll, P. 1997b. Using pulse oximetry in the home. *Home Healthcare Nurse* **15,** 88–97.

Casey, G. 2000. Fever management in children. *Nursing Standard* **14**(40), 36–42.

Childs, C. 2006. Temperature control. In Alexander, M., Fawcett, J. and Runciman, P. (eds) *Nursing Practice Hospital and Home: The adult,* 3rd edn. Edinburgh: Churchill Livingstone, 813–31.

Cowan, T. 1997. Pulse oximeters. *Professional Nurse* **12,** 744–5, 747–8, 750.

Department of Health 2001. *Valuing People: A new strategy for learning disability for the 21st century.* London.

Dolan, B. and Holt, L. 2000. *Accident and Emergency Theory into Practice.* London: Baillière Tindall.

Edwards, S. 1997. Measuring temperature. *Professional Nurse* **13**(2), s5–7.

Farnell, S., Maxwell, L., Tan, S. *et al.* 2005. Temperature measurement: comparison of non-invasive methods used in adult critical care *Journal of Clinical Nursing* **14,** 632–9.

Hanning, C.D. and Alexander-Williams, J.M. 1995. Pulse oximetry: a practical review. *British Medical Journal* **311,** 367–70.

Herbert, R.A. and Alison, J.A. 1996. Cardiovascular function. In Hinchliff, S.M., Montague, S.E. and Watson, R. (eds) *Physiology for Nursing Practice,* 2nd edn. London: Baillière Tindall, 374–451.

Hickey, J.V. 2003. *The Clinical Practice of Neurological and Neurosurgical Nursing,* 5th edn. New York: Lippincott.

Hill, E. and Stoneham, M. 2000. *Practical Applications of Pulse Oximetry.* Available from www.nda.ox.ac.uk. Accessed 25 November 2007.

Ingram, N. 1994. Knowledge and level of consciousness: application to nursing. *Journal of Advanced Nursing* **20**, 881–4.

Jennett, B. and Teasdale, G. 1974. Assessment of the coma and impaired consciousness. *Lancet* **2**, 81–4.

Jennett, B. 2005. Development of Glasgow coma and outcome scales *Nepal Journal of Neuroscience* **2**(1), 24–8. Available from www.neuroscienceforum.org.np/14j.pdf.

Lane, D. Beevera, M. Barnes, N. *et al.* 2002. Interarm differences in blood pressure: when are they clinically significant? *Journal of Hypertension* **20**, 1089–95.

Le Grand, T.S. and Peters, J.I. 1999. Pulse oximetry: advantages and pitfalls. *Journal of Respiratory Diseases* **20**, 195–200, 206.

Leick-Rude, M. and Bloom, L. 1998. A comparison of temperature taking methods in neonates *Neonatal Network* **17**(5), 21–37.

Lowton, K. 1999. Pulse oximeters for the detection of hypoxaemia. *Professional Nurse* **14**, 343–50.

Mallett, J., and Dougherty, L. (eds) 2004. *The Royal Marsden Hospital Manual of Clinical Nursing Procedures,* 6th edn. Oxford: Blackwell Science.

Marieb, E. 2006. *Human Anatomy and Physiology and Brief Atlas of the Human Body,* 7th edn. San Francisco: Benjamin Cummings.

Medicines and Healthcare Products Regulatory Agency 2003a. *Medical Devices Containing Mercury.* Available from www. mhra. gov.uk. Accessed 28 May 2008.

— 2003b. *Infra-red Ear Thermometer for Home Use.* Ref.MDA/2003/010. Available from www. mhra. gov.uk. Accessed 28 May 2008.

— 2005. *Report of the Independent Advisory Group on Blood Pressure Monitoring in Clinical Practice.* Available from www.mhra.gov.uk. Accessed 28 May 2008.

Montague, S.E., Watson, R. and Herbert, R. 2005. *Physiology for Nursing Practice,* 3rd edn. Edinburgh: Elsevier.

Mooney, G. 2007. *Temperature.* Available from www.nursingtimes.net. Accessed 18 December 2007.

Molton, A., Blacktop, J. and Hall, C. 2001. Temperature taking in children. *Journal of Child Health Care* **5**(1), 5–10.

Moyle, J. 1996. How to Guides: Pulse oximetry. *Care of the Critically Ill* **12**(6), insert.

National Institute for Health and Clinical Excellence (NICE) 2006. *Atrial fibrillation. The management of atrial fibrillation.* London: NICE. Available from www.nice.org.uk Accessed 27 November 2008

National Institute for Health and Clinical Excellence (NICE) 2007a. *Quick Reference Guide. Acutely Ill Patients in Hospital:Recognition of and response to acute illness in adults in hospital.* London: NICE. Available from www.nice.org.uk. Accessed 18 December 2007.

National Institute for Health and Clinical Excellence (NICE) 2007b. *Head Injury: triage, assessment, investigation and early management of head injury in infants, children and adults.* London: NICE. Available from www.nice.org.uk. Accessed 27 November 2008.

Nursing and Midwifery Council (NMC) 2007. *Introduction of Essential Skills Clusters for Pre-registration Nursing Programmes.* NMC circular 07/2007.

O'Brien, E. 2001. Blood pressure measurement is changing! *Heart* **85**(1), 3–5.

O'Brien, E., Petrie, J., Littler, W. *et al.* 1999. *Blood Pressure Measurement Recommendations of the British Hypertension Society.* London: BMJ Publications.

O'Brien, E. Asmar, R., Beilin, L., *et al.* 2003. European Society of Hypertension recommendations for conventional, ambulatory and home blood pressure measurement. *Journal of Hypertension* **21**, 821–48.

O'Driscoll, B.R., Howard, L.S. and Davison, A.G. 2008. BTS Guideline for emergency oxygen use in adult patients. *Thorax* **63** (Suppl VI), vi1–vi68.

Pedersen, T., Dyrlund Pedersen, B. and Møller, A.M. 2003. Pulse oximetry for perioperative monitoring. *Cochrane Database of Systematic Reviews,* Issue 2.

Place, B. 1998. Pulse oximetry in adults. *Nursing Times* **94**(50), 48–9.

Resuscitation Council (UK) 2005. *Resuscitation Guidelines.* Available from www.resus.org.uk. Accessed 28 May 2008.

Rodriguez, R.M. and Light, R.W. 1998. Pulse oximetry in the ICU: uses, benefits, limitations. *Journal of Critical Illness* **13,** 247–52.

Salvage, J. 2000. Go slow on quicksilver. *Nursing Times* **96**(45), 22.

Schmitz, T., Bair, N., Falk, N. and Levine, C. 1995. A comparison of five methods of temperature measurement devices in febrile intensive care patients. *American Journal of Critical Care* **4,** 286–96.

Sinex, J.E. 1999. Pulse oximetry: principles and limitations. *American Journal of Emergency Medicine* **17,** 59–66.

Skinner, D., Driscoll, P. and Earlam, P. 2002. *ABC of Major Trauma,* 3rd edn. London: BMJ Publications.

Smith, G.D. and Fawcett, J. 2006. Stress. In Alexander, M., Fawcett, J. and Runciman, P. (eds) *Nursing Practice Hospital and Home: The adult,* 3rd edn. Edinburgh: Churchill Livingstone, 693–713.

Stocks, J. 1996. Respiration. In Hinchliff, S.M., Montague, S.E. and Watson, R. *Physiology for Nursing Practice,* 2nd edn. London: Baillière Tindall, 530–81.

Stoddart, S., Summers, L. and Platt, M.W. 1997. Pulse oximetry: what it is and how to use it. *Journal of Neonatal Nursing* **3**(4), 10, 12–14.

Summers, R.L., Anders, R.M., Woodward, L.H. *et al.* 1998. Effect of routine pulse oximetry measurements on ED triage classification. *American Journal of Emergency Medicine* **16**(1), 5–7.

Torrance, C. and Semple, M.C. 1998a. Recording temperature. *Nursing Times* **94**(2), Practical Procedures for Nurses Suppl.

Torrance, C. and Semple, M.C. 1998b. Recording temperature. *Nursing Times* **94**(3), Practical Procedures for Nurses Suppl.

Tortora, G. and Grabowski, S. 2003. *Principles of Anatomy and Physiology,* 10th edn. New York: John Wiley.

Walsh, M., Crumbie, A. and Reveley, S. 1999. *Nurse Practitioners: Clinical skills and professional issues.* Oxford: Butterworth–Heinemann.

Waugh, A. and Grant, A. 2006. *Ross and Wilson's Anatomy and Physiology in Health and Illness,* 10th edn. London: Churchill Livingstone.

Webster, R. and Thompson, D. 2006. The cardiovascular system. In Alexander, M., Fawcett, J. and Runciman, P. (eds) *Nursing Practice Hospital and Home: The adult,* 3rd edn. Edinburgh: Churchill Livingstone, 7–71.

Wilkins, R.L., Sheldon, R.L. and Krider, S.J. 2005. *Clinical Assessment in Respiratory Care,* 5th edn. St Louis: Elsevier Mosby.

Williams, B., Poulter, N.R., Brown, M.J. *et al.* 2004. British Hypertension Society guidelines for hypertension management: summary. *British Medical Journal* **328,** 7440–634.

Winkelman, C. 1995. Increased intracranial pressure. In Urban, N.A., Greenlee, K.K., Krumberger, J.M. and Winkelman, C. (eds) *Guidelines for Critical Care Nursing.* St Louis: Mosby, 3–11.

Administering Medicines

Veronica Corben

In almost every practice setting, nurses administer medicines or supervise their administration. To do this safely, nurses require a breadth of knowledge, including pharmacology, legal and policy issues, how to administer medicines via a variety of routes, and how to do calculations. Nurses must also have the skills to work in partnership with patients and colleagues (such as the pharmacist). Only a registered nurse can administer medicines unsupervised, but to develop competence requires considerable experience and practice. Therefore students should take every opportunity to develop their knowledge and skills during the pre-registration nursing programme. The Nursing and Midwifery Council's (NMC) (2007a) Essential Skills Clusters for medicines management are represented in this chapter's content.

This chapter includes:
- Legal and professional issues in medicine administration
- Safety, storage and general principles of medicine administration
- Administering oral medication
- Applying topical medication
- Administering medication by injection routes
- Administering inhaled and nebulised medication
- Intravenous fluid and blood administration
- Calculating medicine and intravenous fluid administration doses
- Preventing and managing anaphylaxis

Note: Administration of rectal medication (via suppositories or enemas) is covered in Chapter 9, 'Meeting elimination needs'. Administration of medicines via the enteral tube route is covered in Chapter 10 'Assessing and Meeting Nutritional Needs'.

Recommended biology reading

It is important that you have an understanding of how medicines are absorbed, and how they reach the site where their action is required. The following questions will help you to focus on the biology underpinning this chapter's skills. Use your recommended textbook to find out:
- What are medicines? What do they do? How do they know where to act?
- How do they achieve their effects?
- What are placebos? When might they be used?

- What do the terms 'bioavailability', 'agonist' and 'antagonist' mean?
- Which routes of administration would be described as enteral and which as parenteral?
- What factors affect the absorption rate of orally administered medicines?
- What is the first-pass effect?
- Medicines often have unwanted side-effects. What do the terms 'nephrotoxic' and 'hepatotoxic' mean?
- In order to be effective, medication levels must be within the therapeutic range. What could happen following the administration of a wrong dose?
- Drugs must be metabolised in order to be eliminated from the body. Where does drug metabolism occur?
- How are drugs excreted from the body?
- What factors will affect the absorption, distribution, metabolism and elimination of drugs?
- What do the terms 'drug interactions', 'drug toxicity', 'drug tolerance', 'drug dependence' and 'drug addiction' mean?

It will also be useful to revise:
- the structure of the skin (for the section on medication by injection);
- vein structures and blood groups (for the section on intravenous fluid and blood administration);
- immunity and antibody–antigen reactions (for the section on preventing and managing anaphylaxis).

There are pharmacology books available that are applied to nursing and healthcare practice and you may find these helpful. Examples are:
- Greenstein, B. (2004) *Trounce's Clinical Pharmacology for Nurses,* 17th edn, Edinburgh: Churchill Livingstone.
- McGavock, H. (2007) *How Drugs Work: Basic pharmacology for health care professionals,* 2nd edn. Radcliffe: Oxford.

PRACTICE SCENARIOS

The following practice scenarios illustrate situations where medicines are being administered via several different routes, and where nurses require knowledge of these drugs' actions and side-effects, as well as how to store and administer them safely. These scenarios will be referred to throughout the chapter.

Adult

Mercy Makumbe is 72 years old. She has recently had a below-knee amputation of her leg, has a long history of cardiovascular disease, and has now been transferred to her local community hospital, where she is currently receiving subcutaneous (SC) heparin, as well as oral morphine solution for pain. For years she has taken diuretics and other medication for her cardiac problems and she is concerned about having to take regular strong pain-relieving medicines too. She has had

Heparin
An anticoagulant that works by prolonging the anticoagulation time. It is not absorbed orally and is given either subcutaneously or intravenously.

Diuretic
Drug that causes increased excretion of urine by the kidneys. There are many types of diuretic medicine.

Fucidin

A topical antibiotic cream used for treatment of a wide variety of infected skin conditions.

Dementia

A chronic and progressive condition that has many causes and commonly presents with memory and language impairment, decline in self-care ability, and behavioural and personality changes (Jacques and Jackson 2000).

Dosett box system

An aid to support medication compliance. A pre-prepared box of medication with identified doses for each day. 'Nomad' is another similar system.

a known penicillin allergy for some time. She has also been prescribed fucidin cream for a small infected area behind one ear. A recent urinalysis showed blood in her urine.

Learning disability

Carol Lee is a 57-year-old woman who has mild learning disability and has been diagnosed as having symptoms of early-onset dementia. She lives with one other person with a learning disability and they are now supported by a sleep-in support worker. Over the last year she has experienced two 'seizure'-like episodes and has been prescribed anticonvulsant medication. She wishes to maintain her independence and self-medicate. The community learning disability nurse is working with her and her support worker to enable her to manage this. They are using a dosett box system and pictures as prompts. They are also helping her to record any side-effects.

Mental health

Malcolm Barber is 49 years old and has a long history of schizophrenia. His main carer is his wife. His condition was stabilised on oral medication, until he experienced side-effects of weight gain and akathesia (an inability to sit still). Because of these side-effects he stopped taking the medication, began to neglect himself and developed symptoms of psychosis. This deterioration led to his admission to an acute mental health unit as a voluntary patient. On admission he was given a test dose of a depot, which is a slow-release injection of an antipyschotic drug. This led to an improvement in his mental state, with minimal side-effects. The plan is for him to continue with these injections administered twice-monthly by his community mental health nurse. Malcolm also has mild asthma and has a salbutamol inhaler which he uses occasionally.

LEGAL AND PROFESSIONAL ISSUES IN MEDICINE ADMINISTRATION

Nurses must adhere to a number of legal and professional issues relating to safe medicine administration.

LEARNING OUTCOMES

By the end of this section you will be able to:
1 identify key aspects of legislation, policies and professional issues governing medicine administration;
2 discuss important professional issues for nurses who are administering medicines;
3 discuss the importance of working in partnership with patients;
4 understand what Patient Group Directions are and how they are used in practice.

Learning outcome 1: Identify key aspects of legislation, policies and professional issues governing medicine administration

ACTIVITY

Who do you think might provide rules about medicine administration? Discuss this with one of your colleagues. Consider abuse of drugs and who regulates this. What have you seen about drug safety in the media?

All major issues related to managing the prescribing and safety of medicines are regulated by government legislation. Therefore all issues connected with medicines management involve legal as well as professional issues (Griffith and Griffiths 2003). The National Patient Safety Agency (NPSA) monitors and advises on many issues related to medicines administration. Have a look on their website (www.npsa.nhs. uk) for news of recent advice.

Traditionally medicines were prescribed only by doctors. Recent legislation (DH 1999) permits non-medical staff, including nurses, to prescribe from the *British National Formulary* if they have received special training. This is called **non-medical prescribing** (Griffith and Griffiths 2003).

ACTIVITY

See if you can find a nurse who is able to prescribe and ask him/her about what this involves. You will probably be doing it one day!

You are probably aware that there is government legislation covering abuse of drugs, sale of medicines over the counter, labelling of medicines and pharmacies in supermarkets. Two important Acts of Parliament provide public protection in this and related matters and infringement of these is a criminal offence. There are other related Acts and reports too. The main ones are introduced below.

* The *Misuse of Drugs (Safe Custody) Regulations 1973* identify drug schedules for controlled drugs, and control the storage, sale and administration of controlled (addictive) drugs.
* The *Medicines Act 1968* controls the labelling, sale and distribution of all medicines and establishes a licensing system.
* The *Mental Capacity Act 2005* defines and advises on a patient's capacity to understand treatment, including medicine administration. It also covers the role of professionals in protecting such patients. It would be useful to read this summary especially if you work with vulnerable adults.
* The recently revised *Duthie Report* (Royal Pharmaceutical Society of Great Britain 2005) provides further guidance on storage and administration of medicines.

Categories of medicines defined in the Medicines Act 1968
* **Prescription-only medicines (POM).** These can be obtained only on prescription. In hospitals almost all medicines are POM, so each patient has a prescription chart. If you have any medicines prescribed by your GP, in many cases you will see POM printed on the packet.
* **Pharmacy-only medicines (P).** These can be sold only in the presence of a pharmacist, but do not require a prescription.

- **General sale list (GSL).** This is a restricted list of simple medicines that can be freely sold through almost any outlet, for example garages and supermarkets. However, in hospital settings there is control over these drugs too.

Can you think of an example for each of the above three categories of medicines?

Suggested examples are antibiotics (POM), cough mixtures (P) and aspirin (GSL). There are many other examples of course. Note that the category into which a drug is placed can change; for example, ibuprofen was a pharmacy-only medicine but is now a GSL medicine.

Controlled drugs

Controlled drugs were mentioned briefly above. Why would a drug need to be controlled in some special way? What might make a drug particularly dangerous if people could access it easily?

A 'controlled' drug is addictive, because of the dependency that could result. These drugs may not be as toxic to the body as others that are more easily available. For example, taking an overdose of just ten paracetamol tablets can be fatal but the drug is not 'controlled'. However, access to pethidine, morphine or any other drugs of the opiate family (derived from opium) can cause addiction, with all its consequences, very quickly if taken for non-therapeutic reasons. These medicines are therefore dangerous and their sale is controlled because of their addictiveness, not their toxicity. They are controlled under the Misuse of Drugs Regulations 1973, already mentioned.

Since the Shipman Inquiry (2005), their control has been tightened still further, including electronic prescribing only in many acute settings. Anyone collecting controlled drugs also now has to provide official identity before collection. Mercy, like many other patients, may be anxious about taking morphine because of this view of potentially addictive drugs. This issue is considered in Chapter 12, in a discussion about analgesics.

The Royal Pharmaceutical Society of Great Britain (RPSGB) (2005) identifies five categories of controlled drugs – category 1 being those requiring most control because of their serious addictive qualities, category 5 requiring the least. It also underlines that controlled drugs must be kept in a separate locked cupboard with no other medicines in them, and supplied with a key that is different from any other key in that setting. It does *not* stipulate the need for a locked cupboard within a locked cupboard.

In people's homes, too, drugs must be kept very securely, with decisions based on an assessment of local risk (NMC 2007b). The level of safety has to be negotiated with the person concerned, because it is within their property. Carol's nurse will have to consider this.

Controlled drugs can be ordered only by a registered nurse. They must be administered by a registered nurse with a second checker, who fits the local drug policy criteria for a checker. This may vary in community settings and where people are self-medicating. You should check these details in every setting you work in, and try to access the appropriate medicines policy (RPSGB 2005). Checking administration of controlled drugs requires an understanding of the gravity of the issue, as detailed above. For this reason, student nurses may be able to check these medicines, but in some areas this may not be permitted. Your local medicines policy may direct that you can be a checker once you enter the branch.

Checking during administration involves the whole procedure from preparing the medicine, each checker individually calculating the dose, administration of the medicine and disposal of any remaining medicine and equipment (NMC 2007b). Therefore if you were the second checker when Mercy receives her morphine, you would have to accompany the registered nurse throughout the procedure. As a student nurse, you need to feel confident to check and give such drugs. You may decide that you need more observational practice and knowledge before being prepared to take on this role.

Controlled drugs registers must include details of stock and drugs administered and must be signed by both persons providing such detail. They should be kept for at least two years (Hopkins 1999). Electronic ordering records are now kept permanently (RPSGB 2005).

ACTIVITY

As you are now aware, there are laws that govern medicine administration. What other organisations may be involved in medicine regulation?

You should have included professional bodies and employers.

Professional bodies

Professional bodies involved in medicine regulation in the UK include the British Medical Association (BMA), the RPSGB and the NMC.

Pharmacists provide expert knowledge about drugs and often have an information adviser who can provide instant and accurate advice. Initiatives to expand the role of community pharmacists and to improve GP collaboration are developing (Pilling *et al.* 1998). The NMC issues guidance via statements of principles on many issues, including administration of medicines, to all its registered nurses in all branches. It is vital that nurses read these and abide by them, to protect patients/clients and themselves professionally. The booklet *Standards for Medicines Management* (NMC 2007b) clarifies that administration is about thought and judgement as well as a task, and that registered nurses must take personal accountability for their actions.

Did you know that 20 per cent of all clinical negligence litigation arises from errors linked to prescribed medicines (Audit Commission 2002)? See how important it is that nurses know what they are doing!

ACTIVITY Access and familiarise yourself with the NMC's (2007b) *Standards for Medicines Management* and the NMC's (2008) *The Code: Standards of conduct, performance and ethics for nurses and midwives* (both downloadable from www.nmc-uk.org).

Employers

Employers, both private healthcare employers (e.g. care homes) and NHS Trusts, produce medicine policies. Social Services also have policies about medicine administration, which Carol's community nurse must comply with. Similarly Malcolm's Mental Health Trust will have a policy about patients' mental capacity to understand and adhere to prescribed treatments.

Staff must work to the regulations set out in their particular employer's policy. These policies contain useful information in a usually readable format. They refer to the student role and other issues too. They are particularly useful where administration is not straightforward, as in all three scenarios in this chapter. They should always be accessible in practice areas, even if you do not have your own copy. It is one of the most important documents in all areas of practice!

ACTIVITY Find out where the medicines policy is kept in your current, or next, practice placement.

Learning outcome 2: Discuss important professional issues for nurses who are administering medicines

Professional issues of particular relevance are personal accountability, knowledge and honesty.

Personal accountability

When administering medicines a registered nurse takes personal accountability for his or her actions, as with all interventions carried out by registered nurses (NMC 2008). Therefore if you as a student give out medication under supervision, the registered nurse is accountable for what you do, as well as their own actions. RPSGB (2005) states that the person administering medication (e.g. Carol's sleep-in support worker) can be someone suitably trained.

ACTIVITY Consider who takes accountability for Carol's medication arrangements.

This may vary according to local policy and arrangements. Carol's support worker is likely to have operational responsibility for supervising her self-medication, understanding medication use and side-effects, reporting to the community nurse or senior support worker. The NMC (2007b) recommends that ideally compliance aids (e.g. Dosett or Nomad boxes) should be dispensed, labelled and sealed by a pharmacist, who then takes accountability for this aspect. The community learning disabilities nurse is likely to be accountable for educating Carol and the support worker about her medication, using the picture prompts. She also has overall responsibility as the registered nurse for ensuring processes are carried out properly, according to Carol's level of capacity (Mental Capacity Act 2005), in view of her dementia.

Although as a student you are not professionally accountable you should consider these issues in preparation for becoming a registered nurse (NMC 2007b).

Knowledge of medicines

Nurses need a working understanding of medicines administered, therapeutic dosages and side-effects (Watt 2003), coupled with due thought and professional judgement (Watkinson and Seewoodhary 2008). As a student, you need basic knowledge of the medicines you are involved in administering, continuing to develop this throughout your pre-registration programme and after registration. New medicines are constantly being developed and knowledge about existing medicines is expanding.

ACTIVITY

Review the scenarios. Are there any particular issues about side-effects of medicines? Why should nurses know about side-effects of the medicines they administer? Where can you find out about these?

The side-effects from Malcolm's oral medication were so unpleasant that he stopped taking these medicines, leading to a recurrence of his mental health symptoms. A urinalysis showed blood in Mercy's urine (haematuria). Nurses caring for her should be aware that this could be a side-effect of her prescribed heparin, which is an anticoagulant. Morphine has various unpleasant side-effects, including constipation, so these might cause Mercy's reluctance to take them. People with learning disabilities like Carol may be hypersensitive to medication or may experience side-effects different from those commonly expected. Staff like Carol's support worker should be extra vigilant for any unusual effects when medication is prescribed.

There is a compendium called the *British National Formulary* (BNF) which provides up-to-date information about all aspects of medicines, including side-effects. This book should be available in all clinical settings, but it can also be accessed at www.bnf. org. This would help you understand why Malcolm's medication has been changed. This compendium would also assist in Mercy's case; she is taking various medicines together so you need to know about their interactions.

Honesty about possible errors

If you suspect a medicine administration error, always report it immediately to the nurse in charge. Similarly, if you do not agree with a dosage or any other aspect of a prescription, always have the courage to speak up. Errors cannot be retracted and the patient is the one who ultimately suffers. An atmosphere of openness and honesty is now being positively encouraged in this respect at all times (NMC 2007b).

Learning outcome 3: Discuss the importance of working in partnership with patients

The NMC (2007a) Essential Skills Clusters for medicines management include the requirement for nurses 'to work in partnership with patient/clients and carers in relation to concordance and managing their medicines'. **'The Medicines Partnership'** is a Department of Health-supported initiative which aims to enable patients to get the most out of medicines, by involving them as partners in decisions about treatment and supporting them in medicine taking. The Medicines Partnership (see http://www.npc.co.uk/med_partnership/about-us/concordance.html) defines concordance as 'a process of prescribing and medicine taking, based on partnership', comprising these components:

* that patients have enough knowledge to participate as partners, including information about their condition, treatment options and their risks and benefits, and the confidence to discuss their medication;
* that health professionals are prepared for partnership which includes having the skills to engage with patients and being committed to giving the necessary time to reach agreements.
* that prescribing consultations involve patients as partners: patients are asked to talk about taking their medicines and professionals fully explain treatments, reach a joint understanding with patients and check their ability to follow the treatment;
* that patients are supported in taking their medicines, including regular medication review, addressing practical difficulties and sharing of information between professionals.

The term 'adherence' is also a relevant concept to medicines management. Banning (2008) identifies that adherence can be considered as the aim of medicine prescribing while concordance is the process used.

ACTIVITY

Re-read the scenarios: What signs are there that health care professionals are working in partnership with Mercy, Malcolm and Carol, in relation to their medicines?

There is no obvious indication of partnership working with Mercy from the scenario provided; in particular it does not appear that pain management methods were discussed with her and an agreement reached as she apparently remains concerned about taking opiates. As with any medication prescribing, Mercy should be encouraged to discuss her values and beliefs about her medicines. Banning (2008) reviewed the literature about patients' beliefs, perceptions and views in relation to medication adherence, highlighting the need for shared decision-making between older people and prescribers. With Carol, partnership working seems much more evident as the community learning disability nurse is working with her and her support worker. There are booklets available for people with learning disabilities to complete about their medication (see http://www.npc.co.uk/med_partnership/resource/patients-and-public/learning-disability.html). Carol could insert these into her **Health Action Plan**. In Malcolm's scenario, a lack of partnership working could have underpinned his decision to stop taking his oral anti-psychotic medication, when he experienced side-effects, rather than an alternative treatment plan being developed with him. Hopefully, this time, the acute mental health unit staff have worked in partnership with Malcolm in relation to his depot injections, so that medication adherence is more likely.

As you read above, regular medication review is one of the components of concordance and would be important for all the patients in this chapter's scenarios. For example, Malcolm's community mental health nurse should review his medication with him when administering his injections. Like many older people, Mercy is taking a number of medications concurrently and her medication must be regularly reviewed in partnership with her. Clyne *et al.* (2008) provide a comprehensive guide to medication review including the different types of reviews and engaging with patients.

Learning outcome 4: Understand what Patient Group Directions are and how they are used in practice

Although as a student you cannot administer Patient Group Directions (PGDs), you should understand what these entail. *In certain circumstances* healthcare professionals can administer prescription-only drugs without a prescription, using a PGD; see National Prescribing Centre (NPC) (2004). This is a legal framework allowing certain healthcare professionals (e.g. nurses and therapists) to supply and administer medicines to groups of patients who fit certain criteria, laid down in a previously agreed PGD.

For example, certain travel vaccines can be administered to groups of people who fit certain criteria – those who are medically fit, blood pressure within normal limits, no known allergies etc. The medicine does not need to be prescribed by a doctor or a non-medical prescriber, but can be given by someone trained in the use of PGDs and related pharmacology, for a particular patient group. PGDs are often used in areas where there is not always a doctor, such as clinics or some emergency settings.

ACTIVITY

Consider what would be needed for safety in PGDs?

You may have thought of:
- a clear framework that identifies who can be given the medicine, and in what circumstances;
- extra training for the professional in pharmacology, understanding the patient group;
- ongoing effective monitoring of processes and personal competency.

You might wonder about the difference between PGDs and non-medical prescribing. The non-medical prescriber assesses an individual's suitability and issues a medicine prescription for them. PGDs are in a legal framework where a specific medicine can be given to a group of patients who fit certain criteria, without the need for a prescription.

Summary

- Medicine administration by a student must be under the direct supervision of a registered nurse.
- Medicine administration must comply with both legal and professional requirements. Therefore nurses must be familiar with the relevant legislation and NMC guidance and work within their employers' policies.
- Nurses must take responsibility for developing their knowledge about the medicines they are administering, recognising their personal accountability in relation to medicine administration.
- Nurses and other professionals must work in partnership with patients for effective medicine management.
- Appropriately trained nurses can initiate medicine administration using PGDs and non-medical prescribing.

SAFETY, STORAGE AND GENERAL PRINCIPLES OF MEDICINE ADMINISTRATION

LEARNING OUTCOMES

By the end of this section you will be able to:
1 discuss issues concerning the safety and storage of medicines;
2 understand the general principles of medicine administration.

Learning outcome 1: Discuss issues concerning the safety and storage of medicines

The revised Duthie Report (RPSGB 2005) reaffirms safety procedures for storing and handling medicines.

ACTIVITY

When you are next in practice, ask a practitioner what these safety procedures are and check them with the points below.

Safe storage

This varies depending on the setting. In a hospital there will be a locked cupboard or immobilised medicine trolley. In a person's home it could be the kitchen table, if a patient is immobile and lives alone. Even lotions and cleaning agents must be stored like medicines, in a locked or safe place, especially where there are children around. The RPSGB (2005) states that in care settings there should be separate locked cupboards for controlled drugs, internal and external medicines.

In some settings, for example community hospitals, where Mercy is a patient, patients may have their own locked receptacles, where they can access their medication themselves (NMC 2007b). These must not be readily portable (RPSGB 2005). Continuous assessment of patients' competency to self-medicate must be performed and appropriate documentation completed.

A cool place

Medicines are often quite unstable chemically and may even be manufactured with a stabiliser included in the chemical compound. They generally become more unstable if warm; hence a cool dark place, away from direct sunlight, is most suitable for storage. This is why medicines are usually stored in dark bottles. Some medicines must be stored in a refrigerator, for example insulin. In residential settings of any kind, a separate locked drugs fridge should be used which has a visible temperature gauge on the outside; the temperature is regulated to 8°C (Greenstein 2004).

Stock rotation

As with food storage, medicines should be kept in chronological order, with new items put to the back, and the older ones used first. Where the expiry date is given as a month and year, the medicine can be used until the last day of that month.

Labelling of medicines

Most UK medicines have an approved (non-proprietary) name and a brand (proprietary) name. The approved name is the chemical name, and is used by all prescribers. The brand name may be different, depending on the company who produced it. For example, cold remedies may contain the same constituents, but be marketed under different names. This can cause confusion, so all prescriptions should display the approved name, especially in hospital settings (Sexton and Braidwood 1999) – and this is strictly controlled under the Medicines Act 1968.

European law now requires use of the recommended International Non-proprietary Name (**rINN**) for medicines (available in *BNF* 2008). Most British approved names (**BANs**) are the same as the rINNs, but a few BANs have had to be altered and are listed in the *BNF*. For example, frusemide, a commonly prescribed diuretic, is now known as furosemide.

Medicine containers are labelled with a number specific to a batch of medicines produced at the same time. For this reason medicines should never be transferred from one container to another. Labels could also be misread and different medicines be mixed in the same container.

Holding drugs keys

Keys should always be held by a registered nurse, preferably the nurse in charge (NMC 2007b). As a student you should never hold the drug keys.

In areas where there is no registered nurse, as in some settings for people with learning disabilities (like Carol), you may be advised not to be involved in medicine administration. This is because staff will be unable to comply with professional regulations – although, as discussed earlier, there will be a different policy in place. Talk to your lecturers about this.

Learning outcome 2: Understand the general principles of medicine administration

Medicine administration must be under direct supervision of a registered nurse until you qualify. Good patient/client assessment is vital before administering medicines of any kind.

ACTIVITY

What precautions and preparations should you consider before giving medication to patients/clients by any route? A prescription chart may help you with your answer.

The National Patient Safety Agency has produced a useful procedural guide to giving oral medication (NPSA 2007a). Box 5.1 outlines the points you should have considered and these are discussed below.

Patient/client identity

How do you know that this is the correct person for the medicine? For hospital inpatients in acute hospitals, identity bands are recommended (NPSA 2005). However, the person may not have a name band, for example in outpatient settings, when a patient is newly admitted, or long-term residents in settings for older people or people with a learning disability (like Carol). You will need to ask the person, or a friend or relative to tell you their name and date of birth, where possible as well. If you merely ask the person to acknowledge what you think their name is, they may agree regardless, because of their developmental level of functioning or if they are too unwell to think clearly. Up-to-date photos may be used for identity in some settings, attached to the prescription chart (NMC 2007b).

Allergies

Does the person have any allergies? For example Mercy is allergic to penicillin. An allergic reaction to a medicine could produce a serious local or systemic reaction – anaphylaxis. Anaphylaxis is a potentially life-threatening condition and is discussed later in this chapter. Allergies should always be written on the identity band (NPSA 2005), as well as in patient records and the medicine chart.

Consent

Does the person (e.g. Carol) understand what the medicine is for and agree to it being given? Only in rare circumstances does consent not need to be given – for example, if the medicine is considered essential (e.g. life-saving) and the person is unconscious, very unwell, or unable to understand for developmental reasons.

Box 5.1 Medicine administration: checks that should be made

- Patient/client identity
- Allergies
- Consent
- Time
- Route
- Prescription
- Dose

The Mental Capacity Act 2005 states that, when working with potentially incapacitated people for whatever reason, the healthcare professional must assess their individual capacity at that moment when making decisions on their behalf regarding their care, which includes medicine administration. In some instances it is necessary to organise a meeting to discuss what medication is in the person's best interests. If Carol's dementia increased and she eventually lacked capacity to make decisions about her medication, the community learning disability nurse would coordinate such a meeting, ensuring the relevant people are invited (e.g. Carol's GP, a family member or advocate).

People who are detained under Section 3 of the Mental Health Act 1983 may be administered medicines to treat their mental health condition without consent, even if they have declined this treatment, for up to three months. However, it is only the medication required for their mental health condition, as specified on their section papers, which can be given without consent. A clear explanation about the medicine and rationale for its prescription is essential – see earlier discussion about working in partnership with patients. The explanation should take into account level of understanding and developmental stage, as in Carol's case using picture prompts.

Time

Is the medicine due now or is it prescribed only if required by the person? Malcolm and his wife need to understand the importance of him receiving his depot injection on exactly the correct day. Some medicines should be taken with food if they need an acid medium in which to be metabolised, whereas others (e.g. the antibiotic flucloxacillin) should be taken on an empty stomach because an acid medium would break the medicine down before it can be absorbed in its useful form.

Mercy is taking diuretics, which are usually prescribed in the morning to prevent a diuresis late in the day or at night. She needs to understand that it is preferable to take morphine at regular intervals, instead of waiting until the pain is already severe. Paracetamol can be as effective as stronger painkillers when taken regularly rather than only 'when necessary'.

Never leave drugs out anywhere (except in the patient's own home), if they are not to be taken immediately (RPSGB 2005).

Route

How is the medicine to be given and is this the most appropriate route? For example, an oral route may not be appropriate if the person is feeling nauseated. Some medicines are given only by injection because they are destroyed by the gut; an example is heparin, as prescribed for Mercy.

Prescription

Is this written clearly throughout, including the medicine itself (using the approved name), the date and signature of the doctor, and the route and time of administration? Are the person's name and any special instructions (e.g. '30 minutes before food') clearly written? If any of this information is unclear or missing, the registered nurse must not give the medicine (NMC 2007b). Any alteration to a prescription must be signed and dated by the doctor.

In an emergency, verbal messages may be taken over the phone by a registered nurse (NMC 2007b), but the prescription chart must be signed by the prescribing doctor within 24 hours. Many employers request that the prescription be repeated to two nurses over the phone. Student nurses should *not* become involved in verbal messages; always check local medicines policy on these issues.

You may find that abbreviations are used on prescription charts. The *BNF* (2008) states that, while generally directions on prescriptions should be written in English without abbreviations, it is recognised that some Latin abbreviations are used. Increasingly frequently, you will see electronic prescribing and administration used in hospital settings. However facilities must still exist to do this manually if technological breakdown occurs.

ACTIVITY

The *BNF* 'recognises' all the following abbreviations. Do you know what they mean? Answers are at the end of the chapter.

b.d., o.d., o.m., o.n., q.d.s., t.d.s., stat, e/c, i/m, m/r, mL, p.r.n.

Enteral
Absorption via the gastrointestinal tract only, which includes all forms of administration by mouth.

Parenteral
The administration of medication by a route other than via the gastrointestinal tract, thus including all injections and topical routes.

Dose

Nurses must decide or advise how much of a medicine to give to a patient if the prescription gives a varied dose (e.g. 5–10 mg), thus exercising professional judgement. The nurse should consider whether the dose seems correct for the person. Oral doses will often be larger than intravenous doses, because oral medicines have to pass through the gut and liver before entering the circulation, and some of the medicine may be lost here, rather than entering the circulation directly. This is called the **first-pass effect** and is why enteral medicines take longer to work than parenteral medicines, which do not have to pass via the liver first.

You must also consider whether the dose involves a complex calculation, as then two nurses will be needed. If a calculation has to be done, both nurses need to work it out separately and then compare their answers, otherwise it is really only one calculation (NMC 2007b).

ACTIVITY

Check with your local medicines policy about your role as a student in being a checker for medicine calculations.

Summary

- Nurses need to be familiar with legislation and local policies concerning medicine storage and be aware of issues that could affect safe storage.
- It is crucial that medicines are stored safely, whether in a hospital or in the community, and in appropriate conditions, thus maintaining their effectiveness.
- There are a number of key safety principles that apply to medicine administration by any route to any individual, and it is very important to adhere to these, to uphold safety of patients/clients.

ADMINISTERING ORAL MEDICATION

By the end of this section you will be able to:
1 identify the different types of oral medication available;
2 discuss how to administer oral medication safely.

Learning outcome 1: Identify the different types of oral medication available

ACTIVITY

What types of oral medication have you seen? Devise a list with a colleague.

- **Tablets.** These are convenient, are accurately dosed and relatively cheap. They often contain additives to prevent disintegration in the gastrointestinal tract.
- **Capsules.** These are oval-shaped, with a coat of hard gelatin. They are useful for bitter drugs, and for unpleasant liquid like chlormethiazole. Remember: never open capsules as they are made to be swallowed whole (Greenstein 2004).
- **Elixirs and syrups.** These flavoured and sweetened liquids are particularly useful for children and many are sugar-free.
- **Emulsions.** These are a mixture of two liquids, one dispersed through the other (Greenstein 2004), for example oil and water. They need to be shaken well to mix the contents.
- **Linctus.** This is a sweet syrupy preparation, for example cough linctus (Greenstein 2004).

There are two other forms of medicines which, although taken into the mouth, are not swallowed:

- **Sublingual medication.** These are produced as sprays or as tablets and are absorbed through the mucosa under the tongue. As the sublingual area is very vascular, absorption and effect of the drug occur rapidly.
- **Buccal medication.** These medicines are usually produced as tablets, and are put on to the gum under the lip. Again, the effect of the drug is rapid.

When these routes are used, careful instructions should be given so that the person understands that sublingual and buccal tablets should not be swallowed straight away.

Learning outcome 2: Discuss how to administer oral medication safely

Before administering any medicine, you should know:
- what the medicine is;
- how it works;
- the normal dosage;
- any known side-effects;
- any extra precautions you should tell the person.

We are now going to look at how you would administer oral medication to a patient. What should you always do before any intervention with patients? You should, of course, perform hand hygiene (covered in Chapter 3) and gain consent, as discussed earlier. You should identify the appropriate bottle or packet of medicine that corresponds with the prescription. Check all the prescription details with the medicine label, the expiry date and any special instructions. Think about the person's positioning before administering, as sitting up well (if not contraindicated) makes swallowing easier and safer.

Liquids

For people with swallowing difficulties, which includes some people with learning disabilities, most oral medicines prescribed will be in liquid form. Liquids are much more quickly absorbed than tablets because the gastrointestinal transit time is reduced. Many suspensions are sold with a double-ended spoon, which can measure 2.5 mL and 5 mL volumes, but 5 mL special oral medicine syringes can be obtained from chemists.

First shake the bottle for even distribution, then hold the bottle with the label uppermost, so that the medicine cannot flow over the label and deface it. Now carefully pour into a measuring glass, at eye level for accuracy.

If the dose is 1 mL or less, use a 1 mL syringe and aspirate it directly from the bottle or via a quill, and then put the lid back on the bottle. It may be useful to use a syringe for withdrawing larger quantities too, as they are more accurate than medicine pots. This would be appropriate for measuring Mercy's morphine. The *BNF* (2008) recommends that, for any oral medication prescribed in doses other than multiples of 5 mL, an oral syringe should be used (see www.bnf.org). Oral syringes have a different appearance from usual syringes, and they should be used for all oral liquid medication, to reduce risk of mistakes (NPSA 2007a). They are often coloured, well labelled and have a different connection, preventing them from being attached to intravenous cannulae.

If an oral medication is given intravenously in error, this could have serious or even fatal consequences.

Tablets

If the tablets are in a bottle, tip the correct amount into the lid and then tip into a medicine glass or spoon. The lid is as clean as the inside of the medicine bottle. Many tablets are supplied in blister packs, so that they can be individually sealed and then pushed out through a foil backing into a medicine pot without being touched (Hopkins 1999).

ACTIVITY

Consider the following scenario: a patient has difficulty swallowing her tablets. A colleague suggests to you that the tablets could be crushed and given to the patient in food. How might you respond and why?

Crushing tablets is **not recommended** as:

• Crushing tablets could alter the medicine's therapeutic action, making it ineffective or causing adverse effects. For example, slow release tablets which are crushed will no longer be released in the way intended. Crushing enteric-coated tablets (e.g. prednisolone) would remove the protective coating and could cause tissue damage. Particles of crushed tablets might be inhaled.

- Crushing tablets has legal consequences as it changes the product's licence – if an adverse action resulted then the person crushing the tablet will be responsible. Crushing must only occur if underwritten by a pharmacist who has determined that the medicine will not be compromised by crushing and that crushing is in the patient's best interest (NMC 2007b).

Putting medicines in food is also not recommended as:

- It can be difficult to know how much of the tablets have been taken, when given in food.
- The food might affect the medicine's actions.
- Patients may not realise they are taking medication if it is given in food or drink.

So what should you do? Having explained to your colleague that you cannot crush tablets to be put in food for the above reasons, you should discuss the situation with the pharmacist. Most medicines are now available in liquid form or there may be another alternative such as the topical route.

Administering the medicine

Next consider how to administer the medicine. Can the person self-administer or do you need to administer it on a spoon? Is the medicine best put into the mouth from a syringe? For obvious reasons (prevention of cross-infection) never touch medication with your hand. If the person cannot self-administer, put it into their mouth using a utensil. Gentle downward stroking motions over the larynx may help with swallowing. Always provide adequate fluids, about 50 mL for an adult, to ensure medication has been swallowed, and offer a choice of fluid. Ensure that the person has swallowed all the medication before documenting. A patient may pocket tablets, spit them out when you have gone or be unable to totally clear them from the mouth.

ACTIVITY

For this exercise you need a tube of Smarties, a small cup, a bottle of water and a syringe. You should be able to access a syringe in the skills laboratory, but you may need permission – do check. Practise tipping a Smartie out into the lid and then into the cup without touching it. Now try feeding the Smartie on a spoon from the cup to a willing volunteer, taking care not to touch the sweet. Repeat, putting the liquid from the syringe into a volunteer's mouth. Ask them what it feels like.

When documenting medicine administration, the registered nurse must countersign the signature of any student they are supervising (NMC 2007b). If you are the second checker for a controlled drug you should sign the register, along with the registered nurse. If any prescribed medicine is not given for some reason (e.g. refusal) this must be documented and further action taken as necessary. After medicine administration, clear away all equipment, and wash your hands again.

Medicines not used should be disposed of immediately, for whatever reason, in accordance with standard operating procedures for the organisation (RPSGB 2005). In both community and hospital settings, unwanted medicines should be returned to the pharmacy.

Medicines should never be disposed of in a waste bin where someone else could have access to them.

ACTIVITY

Look in your local medicines policy: what is the guidance for disposal of medicines?

Note: Nurses/carers need to evaluate whether the medication has been effective and whether side-effects have occurred, as in Mercy's case, and document this.

Summary

- Both preparation and administration of oral medicines should be performed systematically, ensuring that policy is adhered to, promoting safety and prevention of cross-infection.
- Careful assessment should ensure that the oral medicine administration is performed in an acceptable and appropriate manner for each individual, taking into account factors such as swallowing ability.
- Useful tip! Once you have a good set process for medicine checking, always stick to it as it will help to ensure you don't leave anything out in the checking process.

APPLYING TOPICAL MEDICATION

The topical route consists of medicine administration via the epidermis (outer layer of the skin) and external mucous membranes, therefore including administration into eyes and ears. These preparations may also affect the patient systemically, so they must be treated as all other medicines (Watkinson and Seewoodhary 2008). In hospital and care home settings, these medicines must be kept in locked bedside lockers, medicine cupboards or trolleys and some must be kept in the medicine refrigerator.

LEARNING OUTCOMES

By the end of this section you will be able to:
1 understand the indications and preparations used for the topical route;
2 show awareness of how topical medication is administered and the particular precautions that are necessary.

Learning outcome 1: Understand the indications and preparations used for the topical route

ACTIVITY	Mercy is prescribed fucidin cream for the small infected area behind her ear. Why might a topical antibiotic cream have been prescribed for her?

The topical route permits local rather than systemic absorption of the medicine and reduces its side-effects on the body generally. In Mercy's case it would have been considered appropriate as the lesion is small and superficial.

Medications are increasingly available in topical form. Common examples are patches applied to the skin being used for pain relief (fentanyl) or angina (glyceryl trinitrate). Many topical medications are designed to give a 24-hour slow release of the drug and therefore continuous action. Topical preparations also include drops into eyes and ears, where absorption occurs through the mucous membranes. Topical preparations reduce, but do not eliminate, unwanted systemic side-effects (Marsden and Shaw 2003). There must be enough absorption from the site of application to be effective.

Topical preparations

- **Pastes.** These contain a large amount of powder and a little water in their composition, and are therefore fairly stiff and may be difficult to spread. Lids must be carefully secured to prevent drying when exposed to the air, which would make them even drier in texture.
- **Creams.** These are easier to spread and less prone to solidification as they are emulsions – either oil dispersed in water (e.g. aqueous cream) or water dispersed in oil.
- **Ointments.** These may be water- or oil-based, are semi-solid and are usually available in a tube. They are more occlusive and therefore better for dry lesions (Selli 1995). Creams and ointments should be applied exactly as prescribed; for example, steroid creams are always applied very sparingly. Sometimes directions are given as a weight in grams, and as a rough guide 2 g is a 10 cm length from a standard nozzle (Greenstein 2004).
- **Patches.** Medication in this form is sealed in a small patch, with a peel-off sheet, which exposes the adherent part to be placed on the skin. You must follow the instructions for where it should be placed, but most are applied to the abdomen or chest, in a relatively hairless region if possible. The site is alternated each time the patch is changed, usually every 24 hours. The skin needs to be sufficiently permeable to allow absorption, so areas with good vascularity, like the trunk, are preferable (Greenstein 2004).
- **Drops.** Drops are presented in solution in either single-use containers called minims, or in a larger bottle with a pipette-type end or dropper. Care must be taken to ensure that they are used for one person only, that the expiry time once opened is observed, usually 28 days (Kelly 1994), and that they are refrigerated if indicated. Patients must be aware of these instructions, and never to stop drops without consulting a doctor, and to use one minim for each eye each time unless a bottle

is provided. Drops facilitate relatively rapid absorption compared with ointment, which provides a more sustained drug action and less systemic toxicity (Kelly 1994).

- **Sprays.** These are produced in containers under pressure and enable a fine spray to be directed on to the area requiring it, for example nasally.

ACTIVITY	If you have access to a dropper, you could practise this skill on to a target on a piece of paper.

Learning outcome 2: Show awareness of how topical medication is administered, and the particular precautions that are necessary

ACTIVITY	Many principles that we have already discussed – for example, explanation and consent, infection control and safety issues – apply to topical medication as well. Can you think of any extra precautions that might be necessary when administering topical medications?

While infection control is necessary when administering medication by any route, there are specific aspects relating to topical medication. Eyes in particular are highly susceptible to infection, which can have a devastating effect on sight. Creams and ointments must be applied to skin without risk to nurses or patients. Attention to hand decontamination is therefore essential, before and after application of topical medication. The patient's position when topical medication is applied needs careful consideration, too.

Applying medication to eyes, ears and nose

Eyedrops and eye ointments should be applied with the face horizontal, the person preferably lying flat. Looking up reduces the blink reflex (Kelly 1994), as well as making it easier to apply the drops or ointment into the correct place.

Slowly squeeze the bulb when applying drops and drop vertically, from as near to the patient as possible, without actually touching the eye. Always put the drop inside the lower lid (see Fig. 5.1) (Watkinson and Seewoodhary 2008). This holds the drops for approximately three times longer than the globe of the eye (Kelly 1994). Eyedrops can sting and some leave an after-taste at the back of the throat (Marsden 1998).

Ensure the eye is kept shut for 60 seconds after application, and always instil drops before an ointment (Marsden and Shaw 2003), if both are being used, as the ointment leaves a film over the eye, preventing the drops being absorbed. Eye ointment should be applied to the inside of the lower lid (see Fig. 5.2), and the eye held closed afterwards for a short time, where possible, enabling the ointment to settle. Applications of ointment to the eye are therefore usually applied at night. Vision may be blurred afterwards for a while. Excess medication should be wiped away with a clean tissue. Applicators are now available for administering eye ointment (Watkinson and Seewoodhary 2008).

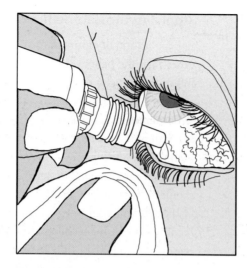

Figure 5.1: Administration of eyedrops.

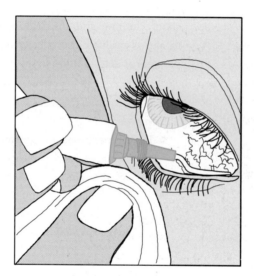

Figure 5.2: Administration of eye ointment.

If eye medication is being applied to both eyes, use separate products for each eye, ensuring bottles and tubes are labelled R and L (Watkinson and Seewoodhary 2008). Apply to the least affected eye first, to reduce the risk of spreading the infection. If more than one medication is being used, leave at least 3–5 minutes between applications (Watkinson and Seewoodhary 2008).

For application into ears, lying with the ear to be treated uppermost is most effective. For nasal sprays, the person should be upright. Nasal medication should be administered 20 minutes before food so that the nasal passages are clear, which makes eating easier. Ensure the patient has blown their nose or cleared their mouth or throat before administration; and follow closely any special instructions accompanying the spray.

Applying topical medication to the skin

For application of ointment or cream to the skin, gloves should be worn if someone other than the patient is applying the medication. This is partly to prevent cross-infection from you to the patient and vice versa, but also to prevent you absorbing any of the medication applied into your own skin.

Encourage people to apply topical medication themselves to promote independence and reduce the risk of cross-infection, although this will not always be possible. For example, in Mercy's case it might be difficult with the sore area being behind her ear. Often some manual dexterity is necessary to apply topical medication, so people should be assessed for their ability to manage this treatment themselves. All stages of the skill will need to be taught, with handwashing explained carefully so that the medicine is not inadvertently transferred to other parts of the body. Creams and ointments should be gently massaged in the direction of the hair flow (Selli 1995). Steroid creams thin the skin, so apply them sparingly.

Following application, the patient should remain still for several minutes and the type of covering to be applied, if any, must be considered. People may require advice about clothing and instructions about possible staining or soiling. Remember to always evaluate the effectiveness of the treatment and report and document progress or deterioration to the doctor or nurse in charge.

Summary

● Topical medicines are prepared in many different formats and have a number of advantages, such as direct action on the affected area, and slow absorption through the skin.
● Specific instructions should be followed carefully.
● Measures to prevent cross-infection when administering topical medication are particularly important.

ADMINISTERING MEDICATION BY INJECTION ROUTES

Nurses in most settings give injections sometimes and it is therefore a practical skill that you need to acquire during your pre-registration programme. However, intramuscular injections are being used less often nowadays so you should make the most of any opportunity to gain this experience (Hemsworth 2000).

Note that **parenteral** means the administration of medication by a route other than via the gastrointestinal tract, thus including all injections and topical routes too. **Enteral** means absorption via the gastrointestinal tract only, which includes all forms of oral administration.

Useful reading: The number of errors reported when giving injectables is increasing. The NPSA (2007b) has produced a detailed procedure for giving injections safely, which is well worth reading.

By the end of this section you will be able to:
1 understand the rationale for using the injection route;
2 outline the principles of, and issues relating to, administering medicine by injection;
3 discuss health and safety issues, especially for nurses, when giving injections;
4 identify key principles of practice for administering intramuscular and subcutaneous injections.

Learning outcome 1: Understand the rationale for using the injection route

ACTIVITY

What injection routes have you seen used, and where do you think the point of the needle rested on administration? Why do you think these routes were chosen?

You may have seen injections into muscle (**intramuscular**), into the fat layer under the skin (**subcutaneous**), into veins through a cannula (**intravenous**), or under the skin (**intradermal**). Injections can also be given into joints, into the epidural space or directly into the heart. As a student nurse you can give only intramuscular and subcutaneous injections and this must be under direct supervision. Injections must always be given by the person who has drawn them up (NMC 2007b) – this includes you as a student nurse. When more than one injection is being given at the same time, syringes must be labelled (NPSA 2007b).

To use the intravenous route you will require further training and supervised practice as a registered nurse. The intradermal route is used mainly for local anaesthetic prior to invasive procedures. It is also used for some vaccines, for example the BCG against tuberculosis (DH 1996). Registered nurses in some specialities undergo preparation to give intradermal injections. The other injection routes mentioned are mainly used by medical staff.

Note: Evidence-based literature related to injection technique is very limited, so you should keep your reading up to date and abide by local policies. The Vaccination Administration Taskforce (VAT) (2001), when investigating all aspects of vaccine administration, thoroughly reviewed the literature relating to injection administration, and will be referred to where appropriate in this section. Malkin's (2008) review of the evidence underpinning intramuscular injection is also useful.

Rationale for injections

Here are some situations in which an injection will be used rather than other routes for medicine administration:
- when speed of effect is required – medicines are more rapidly absorbed into the circulation when they avoid the gastrointestinal tract completely (Rodger and King 2000);

- when patients are 'nil by mouth';
- when the drug is destroyed by digestive enzymes in the gut – for example insulin;
- when long-term release of a drug is required – for example depot injections for mental health clients, as in Malcolm's case (Wynaden *et al.* 2006).

Key features of the intramuscular route

- The effects are more rapid than the subcutaneous route because of the good blood supply to skeletal muscles, so it takes approximately 10 minutes for the effect to begin (Rodger and King 2000).
- Absorption can last for 2–5 weeks if desired, using oil-based, slow-release preparations, as in Malcolm's scenario.

Key features of the subcutaneous route

- A large variety of sites are available as any subcutaneous tissue can be used (Greenstein 2004).
- The speed of action is slower than with the IM route because of the poorer blood supply. The medication administered therefore has a longer duration, which can be useful.
- The person's ability to absorb needs to be considered. If peripheral circulation is poor, the drug may stay in the subcutaneous region and not be absorbed.

Learning outcome 2: Outline the principles of, and issues relating to, administering medicine by injection

Remember, all safety procedures for the oral route apply to injections too.

ACTIVITY

Consider the following issues in relation to IM and SC injections. What have you seen in practice regarding: skin cleaning, injection sites, syringe and needle selection? Compare what you have observed with the points made below.

Skin cleaning

Views vary considerably about this (Hemsworth 2000). Lawrence *et al.*'s study (1994) indicated that a 5-second disinfection time using alcohol-based swabs results in a 97 per cent reduction in all bacteria except spore-forming bacteria. Other studies have suggested that social cleanliness is sufficient (Koivisto and Felig 1978; Royal College of Paediatrics and Child Health 2002). Skin cleaning prior to injections for patients who are immunocompromised and thus susceptible to infection continues to be recommended.

VAT (2001) advised that skin cleansing is unnecessary in socially clean patients and that, if cleansing is required, soap and water is adequate. They warn that if spirit swabs are used the site must be left to dry as vaccines can be inactivated by alcohol. The Royal College of Paediatrics and Child Health (2002) estimated the rate of abscess formation to be 1 per 1–2 million injections. They commented that skin preparation has been largely abandoned with no sudden increase in abscess

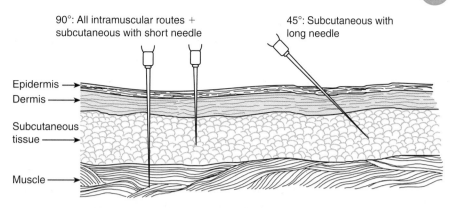

90°: All intramuscular routes +
subcutaneous with short needle

45°: Subcutaneous with
long needle

Epidermis →

Dermis →

Subcutaneous
tissue →

Muscle →

Figure 5.3: Subcutaneous and intramuscular injections: diagram to show skin, subcutaneous and muscle layers, and needle insertion.

occurrence and that formal skin preparation is not necessary prior to injection administration. Thus in practice, alcohol swabs are now rarely used prior to injections, with apparently no adverse effects, but you should check your local policy on this issue. Always allow to dry for 30 seconds if used (DH 2007). Alcohol swabs are always contraindicated when subcutaneous insulin and heparin are administered, as alcohol interferes with the medicines' action and hardens the skin (King 2003).

Injection sites

The site used is influenced by such factors as age, medication to be injected and general client condition. Figure 5.3 shows skin, subcutaneous and muscle layers, and needle insertion.

Intramuscular sites

Intramuscular sites are shown in Fig. 5.4. In adults, up to 4–5 mL can be given into most sites, but only 1–2 mL in deltoid muscle.

The *gluteus maximus* muscle has the slowest uptake of medication, whereas the *deltoid* has the fastest (Greenstein 2004). The deltoid is excellent for small volumes as the site area is small and minimal undressing is required; VAT (2001) recommended this site for vaccines in children over one year and adults. The antero-lateral aspect of the thigh, the *vastus lateralis*, is easy to access, has few major blood vessels in the area and is suitable for all age groups. The *rectus femoris* muscle is useful for self-administration, but can leave considerable discomfort (Rodger and King 2000). The *ventrogluteal* site is a fairly new area to be used for injections, but is free of penetrating blood vessels and nerves and contains a large muscle mass, making it a good site to use for adults (Donaldson and Green 2005). However, though seen as the site of choice, it is infrequently used by UK nurses.

If the gluteus maximus muscle in the buttock is used, it is important to quarter the buttock first and then administer in the upper outer quarter, thus avoiding the **sciatic nerve** totally. Any other quarter could cause nerve injury. When injecting intramuscularly, spreading the skin 2–3 cm sideways (see Fig. 5.5) to provide a Z-track reduces the chance of leakage and pain (Cocoman and Murray 2006).

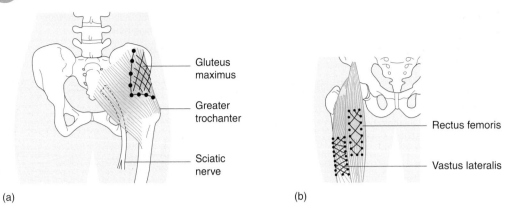

(a)

(b)

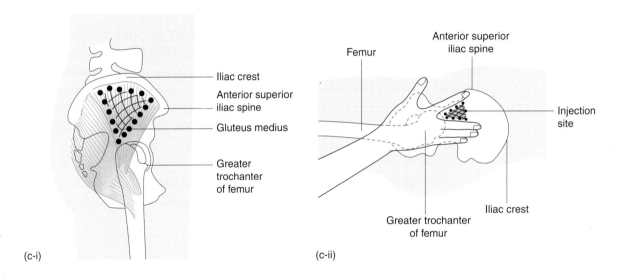

(c-i)

(c-ii)

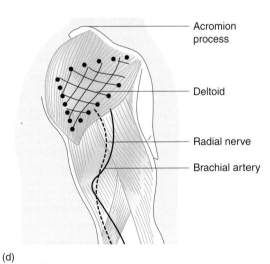

(d)

Figure 5.4: Intramuscular injection sites: (a) gluteus maximus site (upper outer quadrant of buttock); (b) quadriceps sites – vastus lateralis (outer middle third of thigh), rectus femoris (anterior middle third of thigh); (c-i) ventrogluteal site (hip); (c-ii) locating the ventrogluteal site; (d) deltoid site (upper arm).

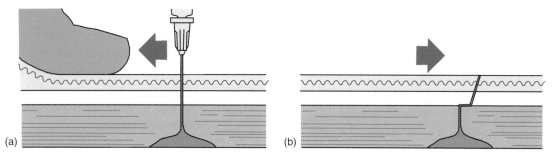

Figure 5.5: The Z-track technique: (a) skin spread to the left on administration of intramuscular medication; (b) skin released afterwards, showing formation of Z-track as a result.

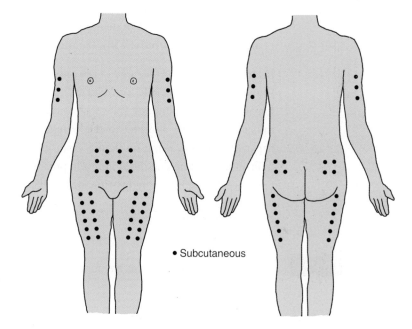

Figure 5.6: Subcutaneous sites for injection.

This method will be advantageous when giving Malcolm his injection, as depot injections can cause discomfort.

Subcutaneous sites

Subcutaneous sites are numerous, but the main ones are shown in Fig. 5.6. When administering by this route, ensure a skin fold is gently pinched to free the adipose tissue from the underlying muscle (King 2003). Patients should always be encouraged to give their own injections when possible. This is particularly applicable to people with diabetes who take insulin and have been admitted to hospital.

Syringe and needle selection

Syringes are selected according to the volume to be given. Volumes of 1 mL and under must be given in a 1 mL syringe, because of the smaller units of graduation, usually 0.1 mL. Some drugs require a special syringe. For example insulin needs a syringe that is marked in units, which is how insulin is prescribed. Insulin syringes incorporate a needle as well. Some injections (e.g. low-molecular-weight heparin) are pre-prepared and these also have a needle attached.

Otherwise needles are selected according to the route and sometimes according to the body adipose of the person. For example, for an intramuscular injection, if there is a large amount of adipose a longer needle will be required to ensure the drug enters the muscle. Nurses sometimes underestimate the required needle length by trying to be kind to patients, but using too short a needle means that the drug does not enter the muscle (Zaybak *et al.* 2007).

Needles are colour-coded according to their gauge (G); the higher the gauge the narrower the lumen of the needle. VAT (2001) identifies standard UK sizes as:

- **green**: 21G and 38 mm (1½ in) length;
- **blue**: 23G and 25 mm (1 in) length;
- **orange**: 25G and 10 mm (⅜ in), 16 mm (⅝ in) or 25 mm (1 in) length.

In general, green needles (21G) are used for adult IM injections, so the nurse should use a green needle for Malcolm's depot injection. Orange needles are used for SC injections, although the most commonly given SC injections have a short thin needle already attached to the syringe (for insulin or low-molecular-weight heparin). When drawing up liquids from glass ampoules, use a needle that has a built-in filter where possible, to prevent possible particles of glass being withdrawn. Filter needles are increasingly being used (NPSA 2007b).

Learning outcome 3: Discuss health and safety issues, especially for nurses, when giving injections

ACTIVITY   What hazards might nurses encounter when administering injections?

Drug contamination

There can be a danger of **contact dermatitis,** particularly if there is frequent exposure to a certain drug. For example, a nurse preparing a penicillin solution for injection could contaminate his or her hands with the drug. Repeated contact can cause skin sensitisation and so gloves should be worn.

Needlestick injury

The Infection Control Nurses Association (ICNA) (2003) reported that 3.4 per cent of recorded sharps injuries happen to student nurses. Remember that you should never re-sheath used needles. These are contaminated and should be left uncovered on the injection tray and disposed of immediately into a designated sharps container. Also put all syringes, needles and glass ampoules into the sharps container. Never overfill the sharps box.

Despite these precautions, needlestick injuries can still occur (particularly when sharps boxes are overloaded), so what should you do if this happens?

- Remove the needle from your skin quickly.
- Encourage the wound to bleed by applying *indirect* pressure.

- Then place the injured area under cold running water.
- Cover with a dressing or plaster if required.
- Complete an incident form.

The Occupational Health Department policy will advise you about further action. Chapter 3 in this book, 'Preventing cross-infection', covers these issues in detail. Further guidance can be found in your local Infection Control Policy, and the ICNA (2003) guidelines.

Note: Unless the syringe is prepared beside the person to be injected, you will need to re-sheath the needle carefully after drawing up the drug, to prevent the needle becoming contaminated on exposure to air. This can be done using a **non-touch technique,** by placing the needle cover on the injection tray and re-sheathing. Alternatively, the needle can be changed to a new, sheathed needle after drawing up, using a non-touch technique. Follow local policy on this issue.

Learning outcome 4: Identify key principles of practice for administering intramuscular and subcutaneous injections

You may have the opportunity to access equipment in the skills laboratory so that you can practise drawing up an injection. There may be an artificial injection pad (showing the layers of the skin, the subcutaneous tissue and muscle) available into which you can practise injecting. This can help you to become familiar with the equipment and technical aspects of the skill, thus increasing your confidence.

ACTIVITY

Discuss with a colleague or lecturer any anxieties you may have about giving injections and how this could affect your ability to administer safely. Remember that although injections can be uncomfortable, they have been prescribed to enhance recovery or relieve symptoms.

The steps to take when giving an intramuscular or subcutaneous injection are set out in points 1–16 below.

1. Ensure that the injection is *due* to be given, is written up correctly, and that the patient has given consent. Look back to the section on consent earlier in this chapter if necessary. Appropriate explanation must be given taking into account ability to understand.
2. Perform hand hygiene and put on disposable gloves (NPSA 2007b).
3. Assemble equipment: cleaned reusable injection tray (DH 2007), or equivalent, appropriate syringe and needle, cotton-wool swab (or alcohol swab if local policy), medication and diluent if required.
4. Check details of the medication, then draw it up either directly from the vial or, if powder, by mixing according to the manufacturer's instructions. Use a filter needle for drawing up from a glass ampoule where possible. Some injections are

supplied with a separate diluent and very specific instructions for preparation, so check carefully.

- Always use the exact volume and diluent recommended to provide the most therapeutic concentration. Holding the syringe at eye level ensures you get the exact volume.
- Remember to check the vial for cracks, precipitation or cloudiness.
- Clean the rubber septum on vials with an alcohol wipe and allow to dry for 30 seconds. Inject an equal volume of air to that of the volume being withdrawn, to make withdrawal easier (NPSA 2007b). It may help to pierce the septum with a second needle if the volume is large, to make withdrawal easier.
- Use an ampoule snapper if available (NPSA 2007b) to reduce injury from glass ampoules.

5. Recheck the person's details and medication, consent and name band if appropriate. Your approach to the person is very important in developing rapport and reducing anxiety about the injection. It is better not to state, nervously, that this is your first injection! Some form of simple distraction may be appropriate.

6. Position the person comfortably, supporting the limbs if necessary. Depot injections like Malcolm's can be very uncomfortable.

7. Identify the site. For intramuscular sites look again at Fig. 5.3. Take into account the volume to be administered and convenience to the person when choosing the site. Some large injections need to be divided and given into two sites. An example is pabrinex, given to people undergoing alcohol detoxification, which is 7 mL – too large for any site. You should also rotate sites if repeated injections are being given. It helps to look at the muscle itself, and check whether it is of a large enough size to take the volume.

8. Check that the skin is socially clean, and clean the skin if required to do so by local policy (see earlier section 'Skin cleaning').

9. For intramuscular injections, spread the skin in a Z-track fashion to prevent seepage (see Fig. 5.5). For subcutaneous injections, bunch the skin to release the subcutaneous tissue from the muscle. Hold the needle at approximately 90 degrees for all IM and most SC injections (as for insulin or low-molecular-weight heparin) (Katsma and Katsma 2000). Having first warned the patient, gently insert two-thirds of the needle into the skin.

10. With intramuscular injections, pull back on the plunger. If blood appears in the syringe, support the skin, withdraw the needle and recommence the process (Hemsworth 2000). This is because the needle must have entered a capillary and the route would then be intravenous rather than intramuscularly. If no blood appears, administer the injection slowly (especially when giving a depot as with Malcolm). Use the recommended rate if one is given, or at 1 mL per 10 seconds.

11. Observe the person carefully throughout the procedure, providing reassurance as necessary.

12. Quickly withdraw the needle, supporting the skin with the swab and apply gentle pressure over the site. Do not rub the skin (Rodger and King 2000) as you will cause local irritation and may alter the drug absorption rate.

13. Ensure the person is comfortable. Check that there is no untoward form of reaction, either systemic or local. All nurses should be aware of signs of anaphylaxis, a severe allergic reaction (see later section). Some drugs are known to be more likely to cause a severe allergic reaction, for example pabrinex (Greenstein 2004).

14. Dispose of equipment according to local policy. Chapter 3 in this book discusses sharps disposal and waste disposal.

15. Document on the prescription chart and in the person's notes or wherever is required.

16. Return to the patient about 15 minutes later to check the effectiveness of the drug. The site itself should be checked 2–4 hours after administration (Rodger and King 2000).

ACTIVITY	What would be the IM sites of choice for: (a) a fully dressed woman who is prescribed an IM tetanus injection (0.5 mL); and (b) a patient lying on his back in bed, who has abdominal pain that is worse on movement, and is prescribed an IM injection of 100 mg of pethidine (2 mL) and 10 mg of metoclopramide (2 mL)?

For case (a) the obvious site would be the deltoid muscle, as this can take an injection of 1–2 mL and is less intrusive for this woman, who need only roll her sleeve up. You will remember from earlier that this is the preferred site for vaccinations. In case (b) the volume for injection is too great for the deltoid. As this man has pain on movement, it would be better to inject into his thigh (vastus lateralis) or the ventrogluteal site so that he does not have to move.

ACTIVITY	You yourself will have experienced receiving injections. What do you think are the main problems associated with them?

Main problems associated with injections

Pain

This may be unavoidable but can be reduced by using distraction techniques. Applying a local anaesthetic cream (EMLA) will reduce the pain. However, VAT (2001) advises that generally using local anaesthetic cream prior to vaccinations is impractical but can be used if needle phobia is preventing vaccination. Keeping the skin taut helps to reduce pain as it stretches the small nerves and reduces sensitivity (Greenway *et al.* 2006). Ice packs may be similarly useful. With an IM injection, try to encourage the person to relax by choosing a comfortable position for them, as injecting into a tense muscle will be more painful.

Tissue damage

Damage can be caused by the drug being administered. This can be avoided by ensuring correct dilution according to the manufacturer's instructions, and by using the appropriate technique; for example, always use the Z-track technique for depot injections like Malcolm's. Bruising may sometimes be unavoidable especially when giving subcutaneous anticoagulants. The nurses administering Mercy's injections

EMLA cream

EMLA (eutectic mixture of local anaesthetics) contains local anaesthetic and when applied to the skin enables an intravenous cannula to be inserted or blood to be taken (venepuncture) without causing pain. It is used extensively with children but can also be used for adults with needle phobia. At least 45 minutes must be allowed after application to produce adequate analgesia.

should rotate the site to prevent local damage. You should never inject into an already bruised area.

Infection

Using an aseptic technique (see Chapter 3) in the preparation and administration of an injection should render this very rare. Making sure the skin is socially clean will help reduce the risk.

Hypersensitivity

It is important to obtain a clear allergic history from patients before giving a medicine for the first time. Observe the patient/client carefully during administration and after, especially during the first few doses. Because of the first-pass effect, the action and therefore reaction to the drug will be faster than when it is given orally.

Staining of the skin

This may occur with pigmented drugs like iron. Using the Z-track method should leave intact tissue above the injected material in an indirect line, thereby preventing leakage to the surface tissue (Cocoman and Murray 2006).

Summary

- Student nurses can give intramuscular and subcutaneous injections under supervision. It is advisable to take opportunities to observe and then practise injection administration, so that skill and confidence develops.
- It is important to understand the sites, equipment and hazards involved in intramuscular and subcutaneous injections, and to be aware of how complications can be avoided.

ADMINISTERING INHALED AND NEBULISED MEDICATION

The inhaled route permits medication to go directly to where it is needed in the mucous membranes of the bronchioles, providing an effective method of absorption. As less drug is required, side-effects can be reduced. Examples of drugs commonly inhaled are bronchodilators, and steroids for their anti-inflammatory effect.

The nebulised route is the passage of medication to the bronchioles directly, as with inhalers, but by vaporising the particles in a stream of air or oxygen. Nebulised particles are much smaller in diameter than inhaled particles (British Thoracic Society 1997). Medication for nebulisers is normally supplied in solution in single-use plastic sealed containers called **nebules.** As with inhalers, the most common drugs given by nebuliser are bronchodilators and steroids.

LEARNING OUTCOMES

By the end of this section you will be able to:
1 understand why inhalers are used and how they can be used effectively;
2 demonstrate knowledge of various types of inhaler;
3 identify indications for nebulised rather than inhaled therapy;
4 administer nebulised therapy safely and effectively.

You may be able to look at different inhalers within the practice setting. Placebo inhalers may be available in the skills laboratory. A nebuliser with mouthpiece and mask attachments should be available in the skills laboratory or you might find them in your practice setting.

Learning outcome 1: Understand why inhalers are used and how they can be used effectively

| ACTIVITY |

For what reasons, and by whom, have you seen inhalers used?

Chronic obstructive pulmonary disease
A chronic respiratory disease, including conditions such as emphysema, chronic bronchitis and chronic asthma. It causes debilitating breathlessness.

Allergen
A foreign substance that initiates an allergic response.

You have probably seen inhalers used by both children and adults. Asthma is probably the commonest reason for inhaler use: 1 in 5 households has someone with asthma (Asthma UK 2008). Inhalers are also used in **chronic obstructive pulmonary disease (COPD)**. Inhalers may be used as maintenance therapy (often brown ones and called **preventers**), as well as in emergency situations where acute breathlessness occurs (usually blue ones called **relievers**). Malcolm's inhaler is therefore a reliever. Inhalers can be used as prophylactic (preventative) treatment, for example before coming into contact with animal fur, grass, pollen, etc., which may be **allergens** to people with asthma, or before taking strenuous activity where extra oxygen is needed. If steroid inhalers are being used, they need to be taken first, then bronchodilators.

| ACTIVITY |

Instructions for using an inhaler are listed in Box 5.2. Think about how you would actually explain this to somebody.

To ensure concordance and maximum benefit, take into account the patient's ability to understand instructions (Leyshon 2007). This is especially relevant if your client has a learning disability. Demonstration is a useful teaching strategy and can be used for people of all ages. The commonest errors have been found to be failure to shake the device, poor coordination of actuation and inhalation, and absence

---

Box 5.2 Instructions for inhaler use

The person should be sitting or preferably standing, to maximise lung expansion, with their head slightly tilted to give them a clear airway. They should clear the respiratory tract by coughing if necessary, and then inhale and exhale deeply before commencing.

- Check inhaler details (medication and dose) and prescription.
- Remove the cap and shake the inhaler.
- Place the mouthpiece into mouth and at the start of a slow deep inspiration, press the canister down, and continue to inhale deeply.
- Remove the inhaler from mouth and hold breath for 10 seconds, or as long as possible (Vines *et al.* 2000).
- Wait several seconds before repeating for a second time if prescribed (note that most people are prescribed two puffs at a time).
- Record administration on the prescription chart.
- Wash and dry mouthpiece twice weekly (Vines *et al.* 2000).

of breath holding (Dow *et al.* 2001). Duerden and Price (2001) propose that frequent re-assessments and re-education are needed as correct technique usually deteriorates over time. This has implications for all healthcare practitioners in contact with people using inhalers.

Remember that inhaled medication must always be prescribed and patient details checked as per the medicines policy. In inpatient settings, the drug should be signed for on the medicine administration sheet in the usual way.

Did you know?

* Fifty per cent of people using inhalers do not do so correctly, and even after instruction this rises to just 60 per cent (University of York 2003).
* An inhaler and spacer, used correctly, are cheaper and more convenient than nebulisers, and can be as effective (Jennings 2002).
* You can now get a haleraid device from pharmacists, which fits over the traditional inhaler, so that a squeezing rather than pushing-down action can be used (Leyshon 2007).

Measuring the effectiveness of inhalers

Peak flow measurements can be helpful in monitoring effects of inhaled medication (see Chapter 11). Observation of respiration, including difficulty, rate and sound, are important indicators of whether the medication has been effective. You can also ask the person how they are feeling and observe their colour, mental state and how well they are able to talk.

Learning outcome 2: Demonstrate knowledge of various types of inhaler

ACTIVITY   Think back to inhalers that you have seen and identify different types of devices currently in use.

The most commonly used is the **pressurised metered dose inhaler** (pMDI), which contains liquid medication under pressure. This is released in the form of a mist when the inhaler is used. pMDIs are widely available and comparatively cheap. Other examples you might have remembered include the **diskhaler** and the **rotohaler.** With a diskhaler the inhaled particles are contained within a disk, and with a rotohaler the particles are enclosed in a capsule. The disk or capsule is then inserted into the inhaler to deliver a metered amount, and activated by inspiration. Patient preference regarding device is crucial, so a good assessment is very important. **Autohalers** and the **Easi-breathe** are alternative types, which are both breath activated, removing the need for good coordination; but the range of drugs is restricted in these devices (Leyshon 2007). Another device you have probably seen is a spacer (see Fig. 5.7).

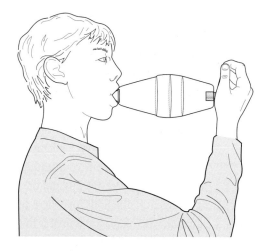

Figure 5.7: The volumatic inhaler.

Spacers

Spacers, sometimes referred to as a holding device, can be large (e.g. the Volumatic), or small (e.g. the Aerochamber). They are often more effective than any other hand-held inhaler (BTS/SIGN guidelines 2007) and preferred by many patients (Leyshon 2007). The spacer holds the medication that has been released, allowing time for the drug to be inhaled through a mouthpiece by activating a one-way valve.

The large chamber in the spacer device slows down the speed of the drug leaving the inhaler from 70 to 40 mph and permits the larger particles to stick to the chamber walls (Fink 2000) instead of the mouth, where they may cause *Candida* infections (Leyshon 2007). The smaller particles in the middle of the chamber then travel on into the trachea and bronchioles for absorption. By filling the chamber with inhaled particles of drug, the person can then breathe these in at their own rate, usually two breaths per inhaled dose, and the particles are less likely to be lost into the atmosphere. The manufacturers supply detailed instructions for using spacers. It is important that only one puff is squirted into the spacer at a time.

Large doses of inhaled bronchodilators can be given via a pMDI and spacer for emergency treatment of an asthma attack (Olinsky and Marks 2000). Spacers can also be used for older people or those with learning disabilities, if they are unable to coordinate breathing and using the canister (Leyshon 2007).

Spacers need replacing every 6–12 months, and should be washed in mild detergent, rinsed and allowed to dry naturally on a regular basis (BTS/SIGN 2007). As with any other equipment, you should check manufacturer's instructions for advice about usage and maintenance.

Learning outcome 3: Identify indications for nebulised rather than inhaled therapy

ACTIVITY   Can you identify the advantages of nebulised therapy over inhaled therapy?

The nebulised route enables bronchodilators to be transported more effectively than inhalers to the bronchioles because the oxygen or air in which it is converted into a vapour reduces the size of the particles, preventing them from sticking to the oral mucosa, and therefore being lost to the respiratory tract (Booker 2007). The smaller particles can also travel more easily into the respiratory tract.

Nebulisers are useful for people who cannot manage to hold and coordinate a metered-dose inhaler, such as some people with learning disabilities who have asthma, and unconscious patients. Nebulised medication can be delivered without a high degree of patient cooperation, for example by a mask, or holding a nebuliser mouthpiece between the lips and breathing normally. Thus nebulisers tend to be given in emergency situations, or where high doses of drug need to be administered in a situation where a person is unable to use other forms of inhaler device (Pearce 1998).

Jet nebulisers release the atomised medication through a tiny hole under pressure, called a Venturi. Breath-assisted nebulisers are a further refinement, and boost nebulisation during inhalation and reduce it during exhalation (Booker 2007).

Learning outcome 4: Administer nebulised therapy safely and effectively

ACTIVITY

Are there any special instructions you would need to give a patient receiving nebulised therapy?

The following points are all important:
- sitting upright to ensure an optimum position for ventilation;
- safety measures if oxygen is being used (see Chapter 11 for detail);
- the need to explain the noise of the nebuliser and the sensation within the mouth.

Nebulisers are mainly used during acute episodes to treat those who do not respond to inhalers, and for severe exacerbations (BTS/SIGN guidelines 2007).

ACTIVITY

If you can access nebuliser equipment in the skills laboratory, try fitting the elements together. You need to find a nebuliser unit including a mouthpiece or mask and tubing. Assemble the equipment as in Fig. 5.8 or follow the manufacturer's instructions. Remember that before assembling the equipment for a patient you should perform hand hygiene to reduce the risk of infection (DH 2007).

Nebulised medication must always be prescribed and patient details checked as per the medicines policy, and the drug signed for in the usual way. At home people will not need to do this, but just check the medication before administration.

ACTIVITY

Before administering a nebuliser, what questions would you need to ask yourself?

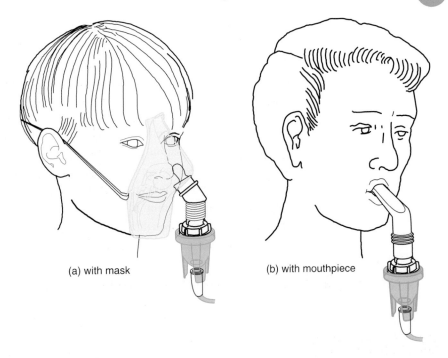

(a) with mask   (b) with mouthpiece

Figure 5.8: Nebuliser equipment.

Does the peak flow need to be measured first?

This would serve as a baseline for comparison afterwards. Chapter 11 explains peak flow measurement.

Should the person use a mouthpiece or a mask?

Mouthpieces are used where patients are physically and cognitively able to cooperate with holding it in the mouth. They should sit with their chest in a vertical position to ensure good ventilation, and mouth breathe to gain maximum effect. A very breathless patient may find this too difficult and prefer to use a mask. However, masks can be distressing to patients. There is no difference in effectiveness when applied correctly.

If using a cylinder (either air or oxygen) or piped oxygen/air, what flow rate would be set on the flow meter?

The flow rate must at least 6 L per minute (BTS/SIGN 2007), otherwise the particles will not be reduced to the appropriate size for inhalation.

Should the nebuliser be administered via air or oxygen?

Some patients with chronic respiratory disease continually have a high level of carbon dioxide in their blood and their breathing is only stimulated by lack of oxygen. These patients should carry an oxygen alert card (O'Driscoll *et al.* 2008). Nebulisers for such patients should therefore be administered via air (Jevon 2007), either through an air cylinder (which is grey, rather than the black with white shoulders oxygen cylinder), a piped air outlet, or by using an air compressor if available. If a patient requires ongoing nebulisers at home, these portable air compressor machines are much more convenient. They extract air from the atmosphere and are available on prescription. When you are working in a community setting make sure you observe for these.

What instructions would I need to give to the person?

The person will need to understand that the mouthpiece or mask must be kept in place and that nebulisation only occurs on inhalation, so it is important to inhale well. There is no need to remove to exhale. The nebuliser unit must be kept vertical throughout administration, and continued until all the liquid disappears from the unit, usually within 10 minutes (Booker 2007). It is worth telling the patient to tap the chamber halfway through, to ensure all the solution is nebulised and not left on the chamber wall.

ACTIVITY   After administering a nebuliser, what questions might you ask yourself?

What should be done with the equipment?

You need to check the manufacturer's instructions as to whether the equipment is 'single-use only' or 'single-patient use'. If it is 'single-use only' it is not suitable for re-using (Gallagher 2002). However, if it is 'single-patient use', and the nebuliser unit and mouthpiece or mask are washed in warm tap water at least once daily, dried well and kept covered in a clean place, the set can last for a maximum of three months (Booker 2007). Tubing should not be washed as it cannot be dried properly. It is now possible to purchase durable nebulisers which, if boiled once weekly in washing up liquid for 10 minutes, will last for one year (BTS/SIGN 2007).

How can I evaluate the nebuliser's effectiveness?

You can observe whether the person is still breathless, whether their colour has improved, and whether peak flow readings have increased. You should also consider whether there are any apparent side-effects. Nebulised therapy can produce unpleasant side-effects.

ACTIVITY   If you know anyone who has used nebulisers, ask them to describe any side-effects they encountered.

Adverse side-effects can include giddiness, tremor, palpitations, wheeziness and irritable coughing. These may be related to the drugs and then dosage may need adjustment. It is also important that the nebules are not too cold as this would cause bronchoconstriction. Mouth infections (e.g. candidiasis) may occur after prolonged use of steroid inhaled drugs, so rinsing the mouth after use is beneficial in this case. If a nebulised steroid is being administered, delivery via a mask may cause irritation to the eyes and skin. Ipratropium bromide, a quite commonly prescribed bronchodilator, can also be irritating to the eyes when given via a mask, so washing the face afterwards may help.

Summary

- Inhaled medication is frequently prescribed, particularly for people with chronic obstructive pulmonary disease and asthma. A number of different devices are available.
- Inhaled medication is taken both prophylactically and as an emergency measure.
- Inhalers act directly on the respiratory tract, so doses can be lower than when medication is taken systemically.
- Inhaler technique must be effective so that the correct dose of medication is inhaled.
- Nebulised therapy is widely used, particularly for people with acute respiratory disease.
- Appropriate decisions must be made as to whether to administer a nebuliser with a mask or a mouthpiece, and via air or oxygen.
- Nurses should be aware of side-effects, and how these can be prevented or reduced.

INTRAVENOUS FLUID AND BLOOD ADMINISTRATION

Do you think intravenous fluids and blood are forms of medicine? Yes they are, as they are prescribed products used in the treatment of patients. As a student or healthcare assistant you are not allowed to administer these fluids in any way. This means you cannot connect up a bag of infusion fluid, or alter the flow rate, as both actions mean you are administering the intravenous fluid. However, if a drip has run through, or in certain emergency situations – for example, if a patient is possibly having a violent reaction to a drug – it would be acceptable to turn the infusion off. As always, abide by your local policy.

So what do you think you need to know about infusions of fluid and blood? You may well be caring for patients receiving infusions, so you need to know how to care for them safely, general precautions (e.g. how to ensure the infusion site is kept clean), signs to look for if the infusion is causing the patient problems etc. The RCN's (2005a) *Standards for Infusion Therapy* is useful reading.

LEARNING OUTCOMES

By the end of this section you will be able to:

1 understand the main indications for administration of intravenous fluids and medicines;
2 know how to care for a patient with an infusion or transfusion;
3 recognise some of the common problems and safety issues surrounding intravenous fluid and blood administration;
4 understand the limitations of your role in managing patients with intravenous infusions and blood transfusions in progess.

Learning outcome 1: Understand the main indications for administration of intravenous fluids and medicines

Intravenous infusions can be given *peripherally* into a vein (Dougherty and Lamb 2008) or *centrally* into the right atrium.

ACTIVITY

Why do you think fluids and medicines are administered intravenously? Think back to patients you have cared for in practice.

You might have identified that they are used to:
- provide large volumes of fluid, blood or other nutritional supplements;
- provide fluids when other routes are not appropriate, as with patients who are 'nil by mouth';
- provide a route for certain drugs (e.g. chemotherapy, drugs destroyed by the gut).

Whole blood is now rarely given to patients, as there are alternative products that can be used that are less difficult and costly to collect but are just as effective. So, packed cells, plasma, platelets etc. are given where there is a specific need (e.g. a patient with low platelets following chemotherapy), but if the patient has lost blood but is still medically stable, intravenous fluids may provide sufficient replacement while their body manufactures more blood cells.

Learning outcome 2: Know how to care for a patient with an infusion or transfusion

ACTIVITY

Ask a patient what it feels like to have an intravenous infusion. Imagine what it feels like to have a tube in your arm and be physically attached via it to a drip stand. It reduces your mobility and independence considerably. So care involves more than just managing the line – remember there is a patient at the end of the line!

Cannulae should be sited in the non-dominant arm where possible (RCN 2005a; Dougherty and Lamb 2008) and not in the antecubital fossa unless necessary. Where the infusion is connected to a drip stand, make sure the stand is lightweight and has wheels that run smoothly, to preserve independence of mobile patients. Ensure that clothing worn is loose, and that tubing is fed through sleeves etc. to provide maximum normality. This would have helped maintain some of Mercy's independence following surgery.

Useful tip: When putting on clothing, put the bag and tubing through the sleeve, followed by the affected arm. Reverse this when removing clothing.

Ensure the patient understands why they have an infusion and to be careful not to knock it. A lightweight bandage to secure the site may help. Patients will have a prescription chart with details of their regime and a fluid chart to monitor fluid balance.

Learning outcome 3: Recognise some of the common problems and safety issues surrounding intravenous fluid and blood administration

ACTIVITY What problems and safety issues are you aware of relating to intravenous and blood transfusion?

Key problems relate to infection risk and systemic reactions.

Infection risk

One of the main risks of infusions is infection, particularly at the site of cannula insertion (NICE 2003; DH 2006). The Department of Health's Saving Lives campaign (2007) focuses on issues of safe care, especially infection prevention in line management (see Box 5.2).

Systemic reactions and care

Patients may have more central or systemic reactions to infusion management, so you need to observe for these and report them to a registered nurse. Reactions include breathlessness, which could indicate either an over-infusion of fluid (i.e. a bag that has been administered too quickly, causing some cardiac failure) or an allergic reaction to an infusion fluid (e.g. blood or a drug). Postoperatively, while receiving intravenous infusions, Mercy should have been observed carefully for breathlessness because of her previous cardiac history. Also, watch and report alarms sounding on pumps and any untoward discomfort, including rashes (Dougherty and Lamb 2008), which could be a sign of an allergic reaction too.

Ensure that you document observations or care provided and report any changes. Many patients with infusions will have their intake and output monitored on a fluid balance chart, so then ensure all oral input and all forms of output, including vomit, are measured.

Box 5.2   Infection prevention in intravenous line management (adapted from DH 2007)

- Always wash hands and put on gloves before and after each patient contact.
- Check the cannula site locally at least daily for local inflammation (erythema), swelling around site (extravasation), and any inflammation along the line of the blood vessel (phlebitis) – and document this.
- Ensure that a dry adherent transparent dressing is intact over the insertion site.
- Ensure trained staff change administration sets at least every 72 hours – and document this.
- Cannulae should be changed at least every 72 hours by trained staff, who should be encouraging discontinuation as soon as possible, to reduce infection risks.

Safety issues regarding blood transfusions

Blood cells are very fragile, so bags need careful handling, and some such as platelets are therefore never put through a pump which would crush them further. They are all infused through filtered giving sets, and blood products must also be used within 30 minutes of removal from the designated blood fridges they are kept in, otherwise the cells start to become damaged; see British Committee for Standards in Haematology (BCSH) (1999).

The main problem with blood products is that they carry different antigens on their cell surfaces, which are described by the different blood groups (A, B, AB and O) and by the rhesus factor. This means that, if the patient is not matched or given the correct blood group (incompatibility) the patient will quickly become ill with a haemolytic reaction and could die if not treated fast (Serious Hazards Of Transfusion 2004).

ACTIVITY

You may have observed the process involved in administering blood. When do you think the main errors in the process are likely to occur?

You may not have been aware that these occur when the blood is collected from the designated blood fridge and also when the bedside checks are done immediately before administering the blood (BCSH 1999). The NPSA (2008) has produced a new competency assessment, which is now part of all hospitals' policies on blood administration, and it recommends that all NHS Trusts have a designated Transfusion Nurse or team.

ACTIVITY

Find out whether your Trust has a designated Transfusion Nurse or team.

It is important that the patient's identity is checked properly before administering blood products, both by the person collecting the blood and by two people before administration (SHOT 2004). This is when most mistakes are made, especially during emergency situations (BCSH 1999).

The person's temperature, pulse and blood pressure must be taken before administration and every 15 minutes for the first 30 minutes during administration (RCN 2005b), as this is when reaction is most likely to occur (see later section on anaphylaxis). You must report any rise in temperature, pulse or drop in blood pressure immediately to a registered nurse.

You must monitor the patient for shivering, breathlessness, loin pain, rashes, fever etc., as these are all signs of reaction. If you see any of these signs, tell the nurse in charge immediately who will stop the transfusion, change it to saline and call the doctor. The patient will need close observation and possibly oxygen. Be prepared to resuscitate if anaphylaxis occurs. See the UK Blood Transfusion and Tissue Transplantation Services (www.transfusionguidelines.org.uk) for detailed information on all aspects of blood transfusion.

Learning outcome 4: Understand the limitations of your role in managing patients with intravenous infusions and blood transfusions

As a student nurse or healthcare assistant, you cannot administer any fluid, blood or drug intravenously. However, you may well be the person caring for patients undergoing these therapies at the bedside, so you need to know how to recognise and report unusual signs and symptoms, while providing them with as much safe independence as possible.

Do check your own organisation's transfusion policy on this, but generally you will not be permitted to collect blood. This is done by staff, often porters, who have been signed as competent to do it. You cannot be a second checker, as it has to be two qualified nurses, but you may take observations during the transfusion, as long as you understand the importance of reporting (NMC 2005). You can clearly also provide all other care to patients while the transfusion is in progress.

Summary

- Students and healthcare assistants are not permitted to administer intravenous fluids, blood or drugs.
- There is guidance from the NPSA and RCN which describes how to safely manage patients requiring intravenous therapy.
- Good intravenous care requires holistic care of patients.

CALCULATING MEDICINE AND INTRAVENOUS FLUID ADMINISTRATION DOSES

Nurses often worry about their ability to calculate medicine doses. However, if you follow the simple rules and standard formulae you cannot go wrong! One of the commonest issues is the ability of nurses to do basic maths, like understanding decimals. Therefore if you have a problem with basic maths, talk to a friend or family member, and ask them to help you solve it and/or access maths support sessions in your university. The application of the formulae is for most people the easy part. Computer-assisted learning packages are available and are valuable to some students. With increasing technology, the maths required is often more complex and critical (Weeks 2000).

Tip: Try to be involved in doing calculations in the clinical setting whenever possible. Many nurses find this easier than doing calculations from a book or in the classroom (Wilson 2003).

For further explanations and more practice exercises, there are many books specifically focusing on this topic. An example is Lapham, R.W. and Agar, H. (2003) *Drugs Calculations for Nurses: A step-by-step approach*, 2nd edn. London: Hodder Arnold.

LEARNING OUTCOMES

By the end of this section you will be able to:
1 show insight into the need for effective numeracy skills in practice;
2 handle fractions and decimals in calculations;
3 understand conversion of units within medicine calculations;
4 use a formula to calculate medication;
5 use a formula to calculate intravenous administration rates for pumps and giving sets.

Learning outcome 1: Show insight into the need for effective numeracy skills in practice

ACTIVITY

Consider what the outcome of occasionally getting a calculation slightly wrong would be. Can you ever be justified in giving a person an inaccurate dose?

The answer must always be no. You have to be 100 per cent accurate all the time. Even a small discrepancy will mean that the patient will not receive the prescribed dose, which could be very harmful. Not understanding the full implications of decimals could mean that a patient receives ten times more or less than the prescribed dose if the decimal point is one place wrong.

ACTIVITY

Discuss with your colleagues the advantages and disadvantages of using calculators to calculate drug doses. Should these be allowed? They are now commonplace in schools and are freely available to all.

There is great debate about this. They can increase accuracy and are certainly useful for complex calculations. However, there may be occasions when a calculator is unavailable or not working. It is also only as good as its operator, hence if the wrong numbers are put in by mistake, the answer will be wrong. Also, if you are totally unable to work without a calculator, you cannot estimate easily what the right answer will be and therefore have no way of checking that the calculator answer is about right (Lumsden and Doodson 2003). The NMC (2007b) advises that using calculators should not act as a substitute for arithmetical knowledge and skill.

It is therefore sensible to be able to calculate medicine doses manually and by calculator, to prevent any chance of error.

Learning outcome 2: Handle fractions and decimals in calculations

Converting fractions to decimals

In a fraction, for example ⅜, the lower figure tells you how many times the whole has been divided, in this case into eighths. If the lower figure were 4, this would tell you that the whole had been divided into quarters. The top number tells us how many of that division there are, so in this fraction there are three-eighths.

Try to think of the line between the two numbers as a dividing line. To convert the fraction into a decimal, you need to divide the top number by the bottom number. Thus ⅜, is 3 divided by 8. This obviously will not result in a whole number, so the answer is going to be 0. something.

The figures after the decimal point indicate a different type of fraction, this time expressed in tenths or decimals. These are the units we use in fractions of drug doses. Most calculations will divide into relatively easy numbers, because nurses have to be able to give that proportion of the drug without dividing into complicated amounts; for example, a dose of ⅓ tablet or 0.0065 mL etc. would, of course, be unrealistic and unsafe. In the fraction ⅜ we have been looking at, 3 divided by 8 equals 0.375. This answer has three figures past the decimal point and may be *rounded up* to 0.38.

Calculation exercise I

Try the following conversions into decimals, to two figures past the decimal point only (round up if 5 or above, or down if below 5). Answers are at the end of the chapter.

(a) $\frac{3}{9} =$ (d) $\frac{4}{20} =$

(b) $\frac{6}{12} =$ (e) $\frac{7}{10} =$

(c) $\frac{25}{75} =$ (f) $\frac{6}{30} =$

To divide and multiply decimals

Your calculations will always involve multiplying and dividing by units of 10 (see next section). Because decimals represent fractions in tenths, this makes these processes very easy.

- To multiply by 10, move the decimal point one place to the right. For example, $0.05 \times 10 = 0.5; 5.8 \times 10 = 58$.
- If you want to multiply by a different unit of ten (e.g. 1000), move the decimal point to the right by the number of 0s – in the case of 1000, three places, in the case of 100, two places. For example, $0.06 \times 1000 = 60; 5 \times 1000 = 5000; 0.67 \times 100 = 67$.
- If there are no more figures to move the point over, add 0 to fill the spaces. For example, $5.8 \times 100 = 580$.
- To divide by 10, or multiples of, do the reverse. For example, $\frac{500}{10} = 50; \frac{6.3}{100} = 0.063; \frac{25}{1000} = 0.025$.

Calculation exercise 2

Answers are at the end of the chapter.

(a) $2.5 \times 100 =$ (d) $\frac{36}{100} =$

(b) $0.3 \times 1000 =$ (e) $\frac{125}{1000} =$

(c) $54 \times 10 =$ (f) $\frac{5.5}{1000} =$

Learning outcome 3: Understand conversion of units within medicine calculations

It is essential to use the same units throughout a medicine calculation – you cannot work with both micrograms and milligrams, or millilitres and litres. Therefore you need to convert the medicine doses in the calculation into the same units. It does not matter which unit you change them into. However, most people find whole numbers easier to work with, even if they are very large (Lumsden and Doodson 2003). There is a simple rule for conversion which is the rule of thousands: everything that needs converting is achieved by either dividing or multiplying by a thousand. This is because:

- 1000 micrograms = 1 milligram
- 1000 milligrams = 1 gram
- 1000 grams = 1 kilogram
- 1000 millilitres = 1 litre.

With a few exceptions, these are the units used in medicine prescriptions. So, to convert 5 milligrams (mg) into micrograms (mcg), you need to multiply by 1000 (equals 5000 micrograms).

To convert the other way, you need to divide by 1000. For example, 50 micrograms to milligrams equals 0.05 mg.

In essence, to convert to a larger unit, you need to divide the figure, so there will be less of them. To convert to a smaller unit you need to multiply, so there will be more of them.

Calculation exercise 3

Answers are at the end of the chapter.

(a) 2000 mg = __ g   (d) 3 mg = __ mcg
(b) 2 L = __ mL   (e) 3500 mL = __ L
(c) 50 mg = __ g   (f) 125 mg = __ g

Learning outcome 4: Use a formula to calculate medication

Remember: There is one magic formula for all calculations! There are no exceptions and it can be used for tablets and liquids for oral doses or injections. The formula is:

$$\frac{\text{Dose prescribed}}{\text{Stock dose}} \times \text{Stock volume (if liquid)} = \text{Dose to be given}$$

For example, 80 mg of furosemide (a diuretic) is needed for Mercy, and the stock dose is 40 mg tablets. Thus, to follow the formula:

Dose prescribed = 80 mg

Stock dose = 40 mg

$\frac{80}{40}$ = 2 tablets.

Now try Exercise 4. Remember that in each calculation you must ensure that the medicines are in the same units before you apply the formula.

Calculation exercise 4

Answers are at the end of the chapter.

(a) 200 mg trimethoprin required; stock dose is 100 mg tablet
(b) 100 mg chlorpromazine required; stock dose is 25 mg tablet

(c) 10 mg diazepam elixir required; stock dose is 5 mg per 5 mL
(d) 1.2 g augmentin required; stock dose is 600 mg tablet
(e) 240 mg paracetamol elixir required; stock dose is 120 mg per 5 mL
(f) 50 mg morphine elixir required; stock dose is 10 mg per 5 mL
(g) 40 mg pethidine required; stock ampoule contains 50 mg per mL
(h) 6 mg morphine is required; stock ampoule contains 10 mg per mL
(i) heparin 2000 units required; stock ampoule contains 5000 units per mL

Learning outcome 5: Use a formula to calculate intravenous administration rates for pumps and giving sets

Try to stay calm when reading this section, as these calculations often cause students anxiety. If you think logically, it's easy! Always round up 0.5 and above to the nearest whole number on the rates.

Pump rates

Look at a pump and see how fluid rates are measured. They are all in millilitres (mL) per hour. 'Per' means divided by, so you need to divide the total volume prescribed by the number of hours it has been prescribed over, and that will give you the pump *rate*.

Example
Prescribed: 1 litre (1000 mL) of normal saline over 8 hours:

$$\frac{\text{Total volume in mL}}{\text{Time in hours}} = \frac{1000}{8} = 125 \, \text{mL per hour}$$

Calculation exercise 5
Answers are at the end of the chapter.
(a) 500 mL of normal saline in 6 hours
(b) 1 litre of dextrose in 10 hours
(c) 50 mL of normal saline in 2 hours

Manual giving set rates

What are these measured in? The answer is 'drops per minute'. This means drops divided by minutes. So, we need:

$$\frac{\text{Total volume in drops}}{\text{Time in minutes}} = \text{Drops per minute}$$

We need to know the drop factor (number of drops in 1 mL) for the giving set. This is usually 20, but you will need to check on each type of set.

Example
1 litre in 6 hours, with a drop factor of 20 drops per mL:

$$\frac{\text{Total volume (mL)} \times \text{drop factor}}{\text{Time (mins)}} = \frac{1000 \times 20}{6 \times 60} = \frac{20000}{360} = 55.5 \, \text{drops/min}$$

The answer is therefore (rounded up to) 56 drops per minute.

Calculation exercise 6

Calculate these rates in drops per minute, all with a drop factor of 20 drops per mL. Answers are at the end of the chapter.

(a) 500 mL in 4 hours
(b) 1 litre in 10 hours
(c) 1000 mL in 12 hours

Summary

- All nurses must be able to calculate medicine doses accurately. For this a basic understanding of fractions and decimals is needed.
- There are formulae that can be used when a calculation is required and it is important to develop skill in their application.
- Students do not carry out medicine calculations unsupervised. However, it is advisable to start working on this skill at an early stage, in preparation for registration, and because students may be asked to be second checkers for a calculation at some stage during the pre-registration programme.

PREVENTING AND MANAGING ANAPHYLAXIS

Anaphylaxis is a severe allergic reaction, which is potentially fatal (Bryant 2007) and therefore requires rapid recognition and treatment (Resuscitation Council UK 2008). The allergen which is the substance causing the reaction may be a drug, so it is important that when medicines are being administered (especially straight into a vein) nurses observe the patient closely. It often occurs after the second dose rather than the first, when the body has already become sensitised to the drug. Such allergic reactions may also be caused by plaster, tape, dressings, food, etc.

Useful reading: The Resuscitation Council UK (2008) detailed guidelines on the emergency treatment of anaphylactic reactions (available from www.resus.org.uk).

LEARNING OUTCOMES

By the end of this section you will be able to:
1 identify how to prevent anaphylaxis;
2 know how to recognise and manage anaphylaxis.

Learning outcome 1: Identify how to prevent anaphylaxis

When you assess a new patient, always ask about any allergies they may have. Mercy should be asked regarding this because of her penicillin allergy. These must be written clearly on the patient's identity band (NPSA 2005) and checked before any medicine is given. Knowing how to recognise anaphylaxis and when it is most likely to occur will help you prevent it from worsening.

People with known allergies often carry an auto-injector (e.g. Epi-pen), which contains a measured dose of epinephrine (adrenaline), an emergency treatment for anaphylaxis. They must self-administer it. See www.anaphylaxis.org.uk for more details.

> **Box 5.3 Recognising and managing anaphylaxis (adapted from Resuscitation Council (UK) 2008)**
>
> Recognition of symptoms
> - Early call for help
> - Airway problems – swelling, stridor
> - Breathing problems – shortness of breath, wheeze, cyanosis
> - Circulation – shock, blood pressure drop, pulse raised, consciousness reduced
> - Disability – neurological status – confusion, agitation, loss of consciousness
> - Exposure – skin colour: flushing, facial swelling etc.
>
> Management
> - Positioning – *airway/breathing problems:* sit-up; *low blood pressure:* lie down and raise legs where possible; *unconscious:* recovery position.
> - Remove triggering source where possible, e.g. stop infusion of medication.
> - Give high-concentration oxygen.
> - Get intramuscular epinephrine ready, or get patient to administer their Epi-pen.
> - Be prepared to resuscitate.

ACTIVITY

Find someone who carries an auto-injector and talk with them about its use.

Learning outcome 2: Know how to recognise and manage anaphylaxis

Recognition is often difficult because the symptoms can vary so much. With drugs, the speed of onset is usually linked to the route; for example, if intravenous it will be much quicker (10 minutes) than if oral (several hours) (Finney and Rushton 2007). The body's reaction to an allergen is to produce histamine in large quantities, which can induce severe bronchospasm and swelling of the bronchioles and face.

Chapter 11 focuses on deteriorating patients and the ABCDE assessment process. Box 5.3 summarises the Resuscitation Council's guidelines for recognising and managing anaphylaxis; you can read these in detail on the website.

> **Summary**
> - All patients/clients must be asked about allergies and the information recorded.
> - Anaphylaxis can be rapidly fatal, so be sure you know how to recognise it.
> - The body may react more severely to a second dose of a drug where the antibodies remember the allergen.
> - Epinephrine (adrenaline) is the main medicine used to correct anaphylaxis, but be prepared to resuscitate too. Medical help will be needed.

CHAPTER SUMMARY

This chapter has explained the importance of having a basic understanding of the laws concerning medicine administration and of ensuring that local drugs policies are adhered to in practice. You should now be able to understand the need for a working knowledge of the medicines you are giving, and be able to calculate doses accurately. The chapter has stressed the importance of safe practice with regard to medicine administration and the student role and should have helped you to understand the reasons for different routes of administration. It should have prepared you to administer medicines safely in a variety of clinical settings.

Remember: The golden rule in medicine administration is to be honest to yourself. If you do not understand or agree with what is being given for any reason, you must challenge the situation you find yourself in.

ANSWERS TO EXERCISES

Abbreviations (source: www.bnf.org)

b.d. = twice daily; o.d. = daily; o.m. = every morning; o.n. = every night; q.d.s. = to be taken 4 times daily; t.d.s. = to be taken 3 times daily; stat = immediately; e/c = enteric-coated; i/m = intramuscular; m/r = modified release; mL = millilitre; p.r.n. = when required.

Drug calculation exercises

Exercise 1

(a) $\frac{3}{9} = 0.33$ (d) $\frac{4}{20} = 0.2$

(b) $\frac{6}{12} = 0.5$ (e) $\frac{7}{10} = 0.7$

(c) $\frac{25}{75} = 0.33$ (f) $\frac{6}{30} = 0.2$

Exercise 2

(a) $2.5 \times 100 = 250$ (d) $\frac{36}{100} = 0.36$

(b) $0.3 \times 1000 = 300$ (e) $\frac{125}{1000} = 0.125$

(c) $54 \times 10 = 540$ (f) $\frac{5.5}{1000} = 0.0055$

Exercise 3

(a) 2000 mg = 2 g   (d) 3 mg = 3000 mcg
(b) 2 L = 2000 mL   (e) 3500 mL = 3.5 L
(c) 50 mg = 0.05 g   (f) 125 mg = 0.125 g

Exercise 4

(a) 2 tablets   (d) 2 tablets   (g) 0.8 mL
(b) 4 tablets   (e) 10 mL   (h) 0.6 mL
(c) 10 mL   (f) 25 mL   (i) 0.4 mL

Exercise 5

(a) 83 mL per hour   (c) 25 mL per hour
(b) 100 mL per hour

Exercise 6

(a) 42 drops per minute   (c) 28 drops per minute
(b) 33 drops per minute

REFERENCES

Asthma UK 2008. *Home page.* Available from www.asthma.org.uk. Accessed 23 March 2008.

Audit Commission 2002. *Acute Hospital Portfolio. Review of National Findings on Medicines Management.* London: Audit Commission.

Banning, M. 2008. Older people and adherence with medication: a review of the literature. *International Journal of Nursing Studies* **45**, 1550–61.

Booker, R. 2007. Correct use of nebulisers, *Nursing Standard* **22**(8), 39–41.

British Committee for Standards in Haematology (BCSH) 1999. *Guidelines for the Administration of Blood and Blood Components and the Management of Transfused Patients.* Available from www.bschguidelines.com. Accessed 23 March 2008.

British National Formulary 2008. Available from www.bnf.org. Accessed 7 January 2008.

British Thoracic Society and Scottish Intercollegiate Guidelines Network 2007. *British Guidelines on the Management of Asthma.* SIGN Publication 63, revised edn. Edinburgh: BTS/SIGN. Available from www.brit-thoracic.org.uk. Accessed 23 March 2008.

Bryant, H. 2007. Anaphylaxis: recognition, treatment and education. *Emergency Nurse* **15**(2), 24–8.

Clyne, W., Blenkinsopp, A. and Seal, R. 2008. *A Guide to Medication Review 2008.* National Prescribing Centre. Available from www.npc.co.uk

Cocoman, A. and Murray, J. 2006. IM injections: How's your technique? *World of Irish Nursing,* **14**(4), 50–1.

Department for Constitutional Affairs 2005. *Mental Capacity Act for England and Wales.* London: DCA. Available from www.dca.gov.uk/legal-policy/mental-capacity. Accessed 14 March 2008.

Department of Health (DH) 1996. *Immunisation against Infectious Disease.* London: HMSO.

— 1999. *Final Report on Review of Prescribing, Supply and Administration of Medicines.* London.

— 2001. *Valuing People.* London.

— 2005. *Shipman Inquiry.* London. Available from www.the-shipman-inquiry.org.uk/home/asp. Accessed 4 March 2008.

— 2006. *The Health Act 2006: Code of practice for the prevention and control of healthcare associated infections.* London. Available from www.dh.gov.uk/assetRoot/04/13/93/37/04139337.pdf. Accessed 31 March 2008.

— 2007. *Saving Lives: Reducing infection, delivering clean and safe care.* London. Available from www.dh.gov.uk. Accessed 21 March 2008.

Donaldson, C. and Green, J. 2005. Using the ventrogluteal site for intramuscular injections. *Nursing Times* **101**(16), 36–8.

Dougherty, L. and Lamb, J. 2008. *Intravenous Therapy in Nursing Practice,* 2nd edn. Oxford: Blackwell.

Dow, L., Fowler, L., Lamb, H. and Hall, G.H. 2001. Elderly people's technique in using dry powder inhalers. *British Medical Journal* **323**, 49–50.

Duerden, M. and Price, D. 2001. Training issues in the use of inhalers. *Disease Management Health Outcomes* **9**, 75–87.

Fink, J.B. 2000. Aerosol device selection: evidence to practice. *Respiratory Care* **45**(7), 874–85.

Finney, A. and Rushton, C. 2007. Recognition and managements of patients with anaphylaxis. *Nursing Standard* **27**(37), 50–9.

Gallagher, C. 2002. When once is enough. *Nursing Times* **98**(38), 22–5.

Greenstein, B. 2004. *Trounce's Clinical Pharmacology for Nurses,* 17th edn. Edinburgh: Churchill Livingstone.

Greenway, K., Merriman, C. and Statham, D. 2006. Using the ventrogluteal site for intramuscular injections. *Learning Disability Practice* **9**(8), 34–7.

Griffith, R. and Griffiths, H. 2003. Administration of medicines. Part 1: The law. *Nursing Standard* **18**(2), 47–53.

Hemsworth, S. 2000. Injection technique. *Paediatric Nursing* **12**(9), 17–20.

Hopkins, S.J. 1999. *Drugs and Pharmacology for Nurses,* 13th edn. Edinburgh: Churchill Livingstone.

Infection Control Nurses Association 2003. *Reducing Sharps Injuries by Prevention and Risk Management.* Bathgate: ICNA.

Jacques, A. and Jackson, G.A. 2000. *Understanding Dementia,* 3rd edn. Edinburgh: Churchill Livingstone.

Jennings, J. 2002. Revisiting nebulisers: cleaning and use. *Practice Nursing* **13**(4), 173.

Jevon, P. 2007. Respiratory procedures. Part 3: Use of a nebuliser. *Nursing Times* **103** (34), 24–5.

Katsma, D.L. and Katsma, R.P.E. 2000. The myth of the 90-degree angle: intramuscular injection. *Nurse Educator* **25**(1), 34–7.

Kelly, J.S. 1994. Topical ophthalmic drug administration: a practical guide. *British Journal of Nursing* **3**(10), 518–20.

King, L. 2003. Continuing professional development: injection management. *Nursing Standard.* **17**(34), 45–52.

Koivisto, V.A. and Felig, P. 1978. Is skin preparation necessary before insulin injection? *Lancet* **1,** 1072–3.

Lapham, R.W. and Agar, H. 2003. *Drugs Calculations for Nurses: A step-by-step approach,* 2nd edn. London: Hodder Arnold.

Lawrence, J.C., Lilly, H.A. and Kidson, A. 1994. The use of alcoholic wipes for disinfection of injection sites. *Journal of Wound Care* **3**(1), 11–14.

Leyshon, J. 2007. Correct technique for using aerosol inhaler devices. *Nursing Standard* **21**(52), 38–40.

Lumsden, H. and Doodson, M. 2003. Neonatal drug calculations: a practical approach. *Journal of Neonatal Nursing* **9**(1), 14–18.

Malkin, B. 2008. Are techniques used for intramuscular injection based on research evidence? *Nursing Times* **104**(50/51), 48–51.

Marsden, J. 1998. Use of eye drops and ointments in A&E. *Emergency Nurse* **6**(8), 17–22.

Marsden, J. and Shaw, M. 2003. Correct administration of topical eye ointment. *Nursing Standard* **17**(30), 42–44.

Medicines Act 1968. London: HMSO.

Misuse of Drugs (Safe Custody) Regulations 1973. London: HMSO.

Misuse of Drugs Regulations 2001. London: The Stationery Office.

National Institute for Health and Clinical Excellence (NICE) 2003. *Infection Control: Prevention of healthcare-associated infection in primary and community care.* London: NICE.

National Patient Safety Agency (NPSA) 2005. *Safer Practice Note Wristbands for hospital inpatients improves safety.* Available from www.npsa.nhs.uk/advice. Accessed 26 May 2008.

— 2007a. *Oral and Enteral Syringes.* Available from www.npsa.nhs.uk. Accessed 12 January 2008.

— 2007b. *Promoting Safer Use of Injectable Medicines: NPSA template standard operating procedure for use of injectable medicines.* London. Available from www.npsa.nhs.uk/health/ alerts. Accessed 31 March 2008.

— 2008. *Right Patient, Right Blood: New advice for safer blood transfusion.* Available from www.npsa.nhs.uk/advice. Accessed 20 April 2008.

National Prescribing Centre (NPC) 2004. *A Practical Guide and Framework of Competencies for all Professionals using Patient Group Directions.* London. Available from www. groupprotocols.org.uk. Accessed 31 March 2008.

Nursing and Midwifery Council (NMC) 2005. *Guidelines for Records and Record Keeping.* London.

— 2007a. *Introduction of Essential Skills Clusters for Pre-registration Nursing Programmes.* NMC circular 07/2007.

— 2007b. *Standards for Medicines Management.* London.

— 2008. *Code: Standards of conduct, performance and ethics for nurses and midwives.* Available from www.nmc-org.uk. Accessed 24 April 2008.

O'Driscoll, B.R., Howard, L.S. and Davison, A.G. 2008. BTS Guideline for emergency oxygen use in adult patients. *Thorax* 63(Suppl VI) vi1–vi68.

Olinsky, A. and Marks, M. 2000. Respiratory conditions. In Smart, J. and Nolan, T. (eds) *Paediatric Handbook.* Oxford: Blackwell Science.

Pearce, L. 1998. Know-how: asthma inhalers. *Nursing Times* **94**(9) Suppl.

Pilling, M., Geoghegan, M., Wolfson, D.J. and Holden, J.D. 1998. The St Helens and Knowsley Prescribing Initiative: a model for pharmacists-led meetings with GPs. *Pharmacy Journal* **260**, 100–2.

Resuscitation Council (UK) 2008. *Emergency Treatment of Anaphylactic Reactions: Guidelines for healthcare providers.* Available from www.resus.org.uk/pages/reaction.pdf. Accessed 12 April 2008.

Rodger, M.A. and King, L. 2000. Drawing up and administering intra-muscular injections: a review of the literature. *Journal of Advanced Nursing* **31**, 574–82.

Royal College of Nursing (RCN) 2005a. *Standards for Infusion Therapy.* London. Available from www.rcn.org.uk. Accessed 7 March 2008.

— 2005b. *Right Blood, Right Patient, Right Time.* London.

Royal College of Paediatrics and Child Health (RCPCH) 2002. *Position Statement on Injection Technique.* London: RCPCH.

Royal Pharmaceutical Society of Great Britain (RPSGB) 2005. *The Safe and Secure Handling of Medicines: A team approach* (revised Duthie report). London: RPSGB.

Selli, R. 1995. Which topical steroid? *Community Nurse* **1**(3), 36–8.

Serious Hazards Of Transfusion (SHOT) 2004. *Introduction to the SHOT Toolkit.* Available from www.shotuk.org. Accessed 27 March 2008.

Sexton, J.A. and Braidwood, C.C. 1999. The nurse's role in medicines administration: Operational and practical consideration. In Luker, K. and Wolfson, D.J. (eds) *Medicines Management for Clinical Nurses.* Oxford: Blackwell Science, pp. 237–57.

University of York 2003. *Inhaler Devices for the Management of Asthma and COPD.* NHS Centre for Reviews and Dissemination 8(1), 1–11.

Vaccination Administration Taskforce 2001. *UK Guidance on Best Practice in Vaccine Administration.* London: Shirehall Communications.

Vines, D.L., Shelledy, D.C. and Peters, J. 2000. Questions and answers about inhalers. *Journal of Critical Illness* **15**, 563–4.

Watkinson S. and Seewoodhary R. 2008. Administering eye medications. *Nursing Standard* **22**(18), 42–8.

Watt, S. 2003. Safe administration of medicines to children: Part 1. *Paediatric Nursing* **15**(4), 40–3.

Weeks, K. 2000. Written drug dosage errors made by students: the threat to clinical effectiveness and the need for a new approach. *Clinical Effectiveness in Nursing* **4**(4), 20–9.

Wilson, A. 2003. Nurses' maths: researching a practical approach. *Nursing Standard* **17**(47), 33–6.

Wynaden, D., Landsborough, I., McGowan, S. *et al.* 2006. Best-practice guidelines for the administration of intramuscular injections in the mental health setting. *International Journal of Mental Health Nursing* **15**(3), 195–200.

Zaybak, A., Gunes, Y., Tamsel, S., Khorshid, L. and Eser, I. 2007. Does obesity prevent the needle from reaching the muscle in intramuscular injections? *Journal of Advanced Nursing* **58**(6), 552–6.

Caring for People with Impaired Mobility

Glynis Pellatt

The World Health Organization (WHO 2001) describes mobility as:

> moving by changing body position or location or by transferring from one place to another, by carrying, moving or manipulating objects, by walking, running or climbing and by using various forms of transport.

Mobility is a multidimensional concept, encompassing physical, cognitive, emotional and social dimensions.

Impaired mobility affects not only the ability to move about. It impacts also on self-esteem and quality of life by restricting participation in activities and life situations (Weaver 2005). Nurses in many healthcare settings encounter people who have impaired mobility and are therefore susceptible to complications. Nurses have an important role, therefore, in actively preventing complications as well as promoting mobility safely whenever possible.

Correct moving and handling techniques are necessary when caring for people with impaired mobility, and some key principles are highlighted in this chapter. You must remain up to date with these techniques and attend organised sessions. As a registered nurse, you will also need yearly updates. The Nursing and Midwifery Council (NMC) (2007) endorses the engagement of patients/clients as partners in care, so when caring for people with mobility problems nurses should actively involve patients/clients in the assessment process and care planning.

This chapter includes:
- Pressure ulcer risk assessment
- Pressure ulcer prevention
- Prevention of other complications of immobility
- Key principles of moving and handling patients
- Assisting with mobilisation and preventing falls

Note: You should also revise the layers of the skin.

PRACTICE SCENARIOS

The following scenarios illustrate situations where nurses need to assist with and promote mobility, and implement measures to prevent complications of impaired mobility.

Adult

Diane Beck is a 50-year-old woman with multiple sclerosis who lives at home with her husband and two teenaged children. She has difficulty walking. She has tingling and burning pains, and spasms in her legs, so she uses walking sticks or a wheelchair. She has a suprapubic catheter for her bladder problems.

Learning disability

Marion Pearce is a 42-year-old woman with a severe learning disability who lives in a community home. Due to accompanying physical disabilities she uses a wheelchair for mobilising. She is underweight and incontinent of urine and faeces; her skin tends to be dry. Joint deformities make it very difficult to position her comfortably in the wheelchair. She has a poor appetite and is unable to eat independently or manage her own hygiene needs. Marion's health facilitator is the community nurse for learning disabilities. She acts to coordinate her Health Action Plan, which includes input from a number of different health professionals including the general practitioner, the occupational therapist and the physiotherapist. She has also been assessed by the speech and language therapist.

Multiple sclerosis
A condition where the autoimmune system attacks the myelin sheath (nerve coating) in the central nervous system. This demyelination causes transmission of impulses along the nerves to become slow and erratic.

Spasm
Stiff muscles that resist passive movement.

Health facilitator
A member of the community learning disabilities team (often a nurse) who supports a person with learning disabilities to access the healthcare they need. See *Valuing People* (DH 2001a).

Health Action Plan
A personal action plan developed for each individual with a learning disability, containing details of their health interventions, medication taken, screening tests etc. See *Valuing People* (DH 2001a).

Mental health

John Barnes, aged 52 years, is a client on an acute mental health admission ward. He has severe depression and also has a history of limited mobility and chronic pain following an accident ten years ago. He needs a walking frame for support but unfortunately fell on the ward recently and sustained a fractured wrist, which is now in a plaster cast.

PRESSURE ULCER RISK ASSESSMENT

A **pressure ulcer** (sometimes termed a bedsore, pressure sore or decubitus ulcer) is defined by the National Pressure Ulcer Advisory Panel (NPUAP) as *an area of localised injury to the skin and underlying tissue, usually over a bony prominence, as a result of pressure, or pressure in combination with shear and/or friction.* A number of contributing or confounding factors are also associated with pressure ulcers, but the significance of these factors 'is yet to be elucidated' (NPUAP 2007). Although pressure ulcers most commonly occur over bony prominences (Anton 2006; Dinsdale 2007) pressure damage can occur in other areas in some circumstances. *The Essence of Care* (DH 2001b) identified benchmarks of best practice for pressure ulcer risk assessment and prevention.

LEARNING OUTCOMES

By the end of this section you will be able to:
1 identify how pressure ulcers are formed and the areas of the body that are most at risk;
2 discuss why some people are more likely to develop pressure ulcers;
3 use a pressure ulcer risk calculator to identify people at risk of pressure ulcers;
4 discuss the importance of accurate documentation of pressure ulcer risk assessment.

Learning outcome 1: Identify how pressure ulcers are formed and the areas of the body that are most at risk

ACTIVITY

Hold a clear plastic tumbler in your hand using your fingertips. Press with your fingers and notice how your fingertips have become very pale. Now release the pressure and look at your fingertips: they will have a red flush.

The red flush, called **reactive hyperaemia,** is one of the first signs of pressure damage when skin and other tissues are compressed between bone and another surface. Body cells die if the blood flow in the capillary bed is insufficient to supply oxygen, carbohydrates and amino acids for metabolism and to remove carbon dioxide and the products of catabolism (Anton 2006). Capillary closing pressure is the degree of external pressure required to occlude blood vessels. External pressures above the mean capillary blood pressure can cause capillary closure. The average mean capillary blood pressure in healthy people is 16–32 mmHg, but can be much lower in ill-health (Hampton and Collins 2005). If the pressure is not relieved, vessels become inflamed and micro-thrombi form in the capillaries (Hampton 2003).

The time taken for irreversible changes to occur, leading to tissue death, varies. If the pressure is relieved while the capillary and lymphatic circulation are intact, there is a sudden increase in blood flow to the area as the build-up of metabolites acts on the arteriole sphincters. However, if the capillaries and lymphatic circulation have been irreversibly damaged the hyperaemia will be non-blanching. The reddening is then caused by blood leaking from damaged capillaries. In patients with darker skin, warmth, oedema or hardness can indicate non-blanching hyperaemia (Anton 2006; Vanderwee *et al.* 2007).

There is an inverse relationship between time and pressure. A person can endure a large amount of pressure during a short amount of time or a low amount of pressure over a longer time without sustaining tissue damage (Armstrong and Bortz 2001).

> **Non-blanching hyperaemia**
> The term 'non-blanching' means that when you apply light finger pressure to the red area it remains red rather than whitening, as in blanching hyperaemia where the micro-circulation remains intact. The damage present in non-blanching hyperaemia progresses to deeper layers if the pressure is not relieved.

ACTIVITY

What areas of the body are most at risk of developing pressure ulcers? Which of these sites are risk areas for the people in the scenarios?

The skin over bony prominences is particularly at risk of pressure ulcers (see Fig. 6.1).

The sacrum, hips, heels, elbows, knees and malleoli are at risk for patients who are confined to bed, visiting the X-ray department, or undergoing surgery. Lying on a trolley, X-ray table or operating table adds to the risk to vulnerable areas due to immobility, and people who are being operated on will be unable to feel the pain caused by pressure and shearing forces (Schoonhoven *et al.* 2002). Anaesthetic agents lower blood pressure and alter tissue perfusion, also increasing risk of tissue damage (Armstrong and Bortz 2001).

When seated, 75 per cent of body weight is supported by the areas at or near the ischial tuberosities (buttocks and thighs) (Collins 2002). Marion and Diane use wheelchairs, therefore the skin areas over their ischial tuberosities and the inner aspects of their knees are vulnerable. Patients who are immobile in the seated position have a more rounded shape, allowing them to rock backwards on to the sacrum – posterior pelvic tilt – creating friction and shear forces (Collins 2002).

The shoulder blades, iliac crests, sides of feet, ears and spine are also at risk. However, pressure ulcers can occur anywhere there is pressure exerted by equipment or clothing – such as tight clothes, shoes, splints, ill-fitting plaster casts, oxygen masks, intravenous lines or catheters (RCN 2001). Nurses caring for John should be aware that his plaster cast could rub, particularly if it becomes too loose or too tight, and so should advise him to report any discomfort. Skin covered by anti-embolic stockings is also vulnerable (NICE 2005).

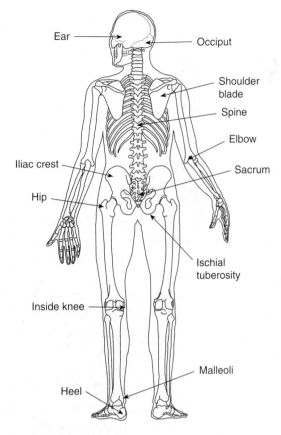

Figure 6.1: Skin areas particularly at risk of pressure ulcer formation.

Box 6.1 Signs of early pressure ulcer development (NPUAP 2007)

- Non-blanching redness of a localised area usually over a bony prominence.
- Darkly pigmented skin may not have visible blanching. Its colour may differ from the surrounding area.
- The area may be painful, firm, soft, warmer or cooler compared with adjacent tissues.

Inspection of vulnerable areas

Areas of the body at risk of pressure ulcers are usually termed 'pressure areas'; nurses should be vigilant about checking these for early signs of pressure. Vulnerable areas of risk for each patient should be inspected regularly. People can also be taught to inspect their own skin, using a mirror where necessary. See Box 6.1 for signs of early pressure ulcers.

Learning outcome 2: Discuss why some people are more likely to develop pressure ulcers

ACTIVITY

Sit in a straight-backed chair. Now see how long you can sit there without moving.

How long did you manage: 5 minutes, 10 minutes or longer? What made you move? You probably found that your pressure areas became uncomfortable and eventually you had to move position. Immobility is the most important factor in the development of pressure ulcers (Lindgren *et al.* 2004). The body's defence against pressure is to shift weight frequently, whether asleep or awake, in response to sensory stimulation. Therefore anyone with reduced mobility, including people with impaired consciousness, have an increased risk of developing pressure ulcers.

Some people have reduced sensation to pressure and pain neurologically induced by medical conditions such as multiple sclerosis (like Diane), spinal cord injury or stroke. Some medication, such as sedatives, may cause chemically induced reduction in sensitivity to pressure and pain. Sedation from hypnotic and psychotropic drugs can cause people to be too drowsy to move around (Dinsdale 2007). John is depressed and could lack motivation to move, or pain may prevent him moving. Some people (e.g. those with dementia) are unable to respond to pressure stimuli and cannot spontaneously alter their position (Fletcher 1996). Patients receiving epidural analgesia for postoperative pain management may have leg weakness or complete motor block, or there may be some sensory loss without motor block. Maternity clients with sensory loss due to epidural analgesia both during and shortly after labour may be at risk. Patients should therefore be encouraged to change position regularly (RCN 2004; Weetman and Allison 2006).

Factors that render people at increased risk of pressure ulcers are often classified as **extrinsic** (outside the person, e.g. environmental) or **intrinsic** (to do with individuals themselves). Reduced mobility and sensation are therefore intrinsic factors.

> **Spinal cord injury**
> Damage to the spinal cord, causing paralysis and loss of sensation below the injury.

> **Stroke**
> Cerebral damage caused either by decreased blood flow or haemorrhage. Effects vary but it often causes paralysis down one side of the body (hemiplegia) and speech and swallowing difficulty.

ACTIVITY

Think about factors other than reduced sensation and mobility that may make people susceptible to pressure ulcers. Try to think of some extrinsic factors and some other intrinsic factors.

Box 6.2 lists the main factors contributing to pressure ulcer formation; these will now be discussed.

Extrinsic factors

We have already considered the role of pressure in causing pressure ulcers. *Shear* occurs when a person begins to move or slide due to gravity, but the skin under pressure remains stationary. Tissues are then wrenched in opposite directions, resulting in disruption or angulation of capillary blood vessels causing them to be starved of oxygen and nutrients. The pressure level needed to reduce blood flow can be halved in the presence of shear (Hampton 2003), thus making skin more vulnerable. *Friction* damage is caused by skin rubbing against a support surface (Fernandez 2007). Diane has spasm which may cause uncontrolled movement of

> ## Box 6.2 Factors contributing to pressure ulcer formation
>
> Extrinsic
> - Pressure
> - Shearing
> - Friction
>
> Intrinsic
> - Reduced mobility
> - Reduced sensation
> - Moisture
> - Acute illness – pyrexia, infection
> - Severe chronic or terminal illness
> - Ageing
> - Body weight – emaciation, obesity
> - Poor nutrition
> - Pain
> - Poor oxygen perfusion

limbs, thus causing friction. Friction damage often occurs due to poor moving and handling techniques (RCN 2001). Shear and friction could be a problem for Marion and Diane because they may slide if not properly positioned in their chairs.

Intrinsic factors

Moisture

Moisture makes skin more vulnerable due to greater risk from maceration, friction and shearing (RCN 2001). Contamination by urine and faeces adds to the vulnerability, so Marion is particularly at risk. The risk of pressure ulcer development can be increased five-fold by the presence of even small amounts of moisture (Dealey 1997). Chapter 9 has further discussion of how incontinence affects skin integrity.

Acute illness

Acutely ill people are vulnerable to pressure ulcer formation for various reasons. Pyrexia increases the metabolic rate, particularly the demand for oxygen, which endangers ischaemic areas. Severe infection can also cause nutritional disturbances, with bacteria increasing demand on local metabolism by both their own requirements and the response of the body's defence mechanism (Simpson *et al.* 1996).

Metabolic rate
The overall rate at which heat is produced in the body.

Severe chronic or terminal illness

Patients are at risk of pressure ulcers due to multi-organ failure, poor perfusion and immobility.

Ageing

Pressure ulcers are more common in older people for a number of reasons. The skin contains collagen to give it tensile strength. Collagen contains thin strands of elastin that provides flexibility. As people age the strength of the collagen and the elasticity of the elastin decrease. This leads to sagging and wrinkling of skin and greater risk of damage due to trauma (Penzer and Finch 2001). Loss of sweat and sebaceous glands may make older people more vulnerable to pressure ulcer development (Lindgren *et al.* 2004).

Bodyweight

Weight status and weight loss are associated with pressure ulcer development and poor healing of pressure ulcers (Ferguson *et al.* 2000). People who are underweight have less cushioning over bony prominences (Fletcher 1996), so this is a further risk factor for Marion who is underweight. Obese people may not be able to lift clear and experience friction when moving in the bed. Obesity also makes wheelchair transfers more difficult (Liou *et al.* 2005). 'Morbidly' obese people, 'bariatric' patients (Palmer 2004) are those whose body mass index (BMI) exceeds 40.

Poor nutrition

Malnutrition and dehydration are recognised risk factors for pressure ulcers (NICE 2005); many people are already malnourished on admission to hospital (Strachan-Bennett 2003). Marion has a poor appetite, and nutrition – including adequate hydration – is important in pressure ulcer prevention (Ferguson *et al.* 2000). Lewis (1998) suggests that protein, zinc, vitamin C and iron contribute to preventing pressure ulcers. Fractured neck of femur is a common injury in older people and the fracture increases nutritional requirements as well as reducing mobility.

Pain

Pain prevents patients from repositioning themselves, particularly at night. John has chronic pain and could have difficulty moving, especially with his arm in a plaster cast. Diane has burning pains in her legs.

Poor oxygen perfusion

Patients who have poor oxygen perfusion due to conditions such as heart disease, respiratory disease, anaemia and diabetes have a lower peripheral capillary pressure (RCN 2001). Evidence suggests that smoking reduces the hyperaemic response to pressure (Noble *et al.* 2003).

Learning outcome 3: Use a pressure ulcer risk calculator to identify people at risk of pressure ulcers

NICE (2005) recommends that patients should be assessed for pressure ulcer risk using both formal and informal procedures, and that assessment should take place within 6 hours of admission to a care episode. Pressure ulcer risk calculators can help identify people at risk of developing pressure ulcers. They use scoring systems based on risk factors for pressure ulcers, as discussed earlier.

Obese
People who weigh 20 per cent or more above their normal body weight.

Body mass index (BMI)
Measure of body fat based on height and weight – see Fig. 10.1, which discusses BMI in more detail.

Anaemia
Reduced haemoglobin concentration in the blood, or abnormal haemoglobin, resulting in reduced oxygen-carrying capacity.

Diabetes (mellitus)
A disease caused by deficient insulin release leading to inability of the body cells to use carbohydrates, and an elevated blood glucose.

ACTIVITY

Have you seen any pressure ulcer risk calculators used in the practice setting? If so, which ones have you seen?

There are many pressure ulcer risk calculators in use, including those listed below. The calculator used should be appropriate to the clinical setting and research with a similar care group should support the calculator's accuracy.

- **The Norton score.** This was developed in 1962 (Norton *et al.* 1962) in a unit for the care of older people. It consists of five headings, each giving a numerical score. A score under 14 indicates a patient is at risk of pressure ulcer development. The scale's predictive value is derived from it being based on factors known to predispose patients to pressure ulcers (Smith *et al.* 1995).
- **The Waterlow scale.** The Waterlow risk assessment card was developed for use with general adult populations (Waterlow 1985, 1988). It identifies three degrees of risk status: 'at risk', 'high risk' and 'very high risk'. The tool also provides guidelines on nursing care, preventive aids and equipment, wound assessment and dressings (Waterlow 2005). It is widely used in the UK, sometimes in adapted forms; the revised 2005 version can be seen in Fig. 6.2. The developer of this tool emphasises that education to accompany its use is essential and has set up a web page (www.judy-waterlow.co.uk) and developed a *Pressure Ulcer Prevention Manual* – the 'Waterlow Manual' – for this purpose.
- **Pressure sore prediction score.** This was developed at the Royal National Orthopaedic Hospital for orthopaedic, trauma and spine injury patients (Lowthian 1987). The scale consists of six questions with 'yes', 'yes but', 'no', 'no but' answers; a score of 6 or more indicates risk of pressure ulcer development.
- **The Braden scale.** This was developed to predict pressure ulcer risk due to intrinsic factors (Bergstrom *et al.* 1987). It comprises six subscales; the first three reflect primary factors (sensory perception, activity, mobility) contributing to pressure. The other three subscales (moisture, nutritional status, friction and shear) reflect factors contributing to diminished tissue tolerance.

ACTIVITY

Use either the Waterlow scale in Fig. 6.2 or the pressure ulcer risk assessment tool used in your practice setting to assess the people in the scenarios for pressure ulcer risk. Ask a colleague to undertake the same exercise and compare your answers. Did you both arrive at the same score for each person?

In the above activity you were assessing reliability of the tool, which concerns whether different people using the tool arrive at the same score. The many risk calculators are all based on factors known to predispose people to pressure ulcer formation. Many studies have reviewed these scales. To be accurate, risk calculators need to demonstrate predictive validity – that is, **sensitivity** (the ability to predict patients who will develop pressure ulcers) and **specificity** (the ability to predict patients who will not develop pressure ulcers) (Papanikolaou *et al.* 2007). Some calculators may over-predict pressure ulcer risk, which has cost implications when pressure-relieving equipment is provided. However, if a scale under-predicts, there is the human cost of pain and suffering from a pressure ulcer as well as cost implications if a patient's stay in hospital is prolonged.

WATERLOW PRESSURE ULCER PREVENTION/TREATMENT POLICY
RING SCORES IN TABLE, ADD TOTAL. MORE THAN 1 SCORE/CATEGORY CAN BE USED

BUILD/WEIGHT FOR HEIGHT		SKIN TYPE VISUAL RISK AREAS		SEX AGE		MALNUTRITION SCREENING TOOL(MST) (Nutrition Vol.15, No.6 1999 – Australia)			
AVERAGE		HEALTHY	0	MALE	0	A–HAS PATIENT LOST WEIGHT RECENTLY		B –WEIGHTLOSS SCORE	
BMI = 20–24.9	0	TISSUE PAPER	1	FEMALE	2	YES – GO TO B		0.5 – 5kg = 1	
ABOVE AVERAGE		DRY	1	14 – 49	1	NO – GO TO C		5 – 10kg = 2	
BMI = 25–29.9	1	OEDEMATOUS	1	50 – 64	2	UNSURE – GO TO C		10 – 15kg = 3	
OBESE		CLAMMY, PYREXIA	1	65 – 74	3	AND		> 15kg = 4	
BMI > 30	2	DISCOLOURED GRADE 1	2	75 – 80	4	SCORE 2		unsure = 2	
BELOW AVERAGE		BROKEN/SPOTS		81+	5	C – PATIENT EATING POORLY OR LACK OF APPETITE 'NO' = 0; 'YES' SCORE = 1		NUTRITION SCORE If > 2 refer for nutrition assessment/intervention	
BMI < 20	3	GRADE 2 – 4	3						
BMI = Wt(Kg)/Ht(m)^2									

CONTINENCE		MOBILITY		SPECIAL RISKS				
COMPLETE/ CATHETERISED	0	FULLY	0	TISSUE MALNUTRITION		NEUROLOGICAL DEFICIT		
URINE INCONT.	1	RESTLESS/FIDGETY	1	TERMINAL CACHEXIA	8	DIABETES, MS, CVA		4 – 6
FAECA INCONT.	2	APATHETIC	2	MULTIPLE ORGAN FAILURE	8	MOTOR/SENSORY		4 – 6
URINARY+ FAECAL INCONTINENCE	3	RESTRICTED	3	SINGLE ORGAN FAILURE (RESP, RENAL, CARDIAC,)	5	PARAPLEGIA(MAX OF 6)		4 – 6
		BEDBOUND e.g. TRACTION	4	PERIPHERAL VASCULAR DISEASE	5	MAJOR SURGERY or TRAUMA		
		CHAIRBOUND e.g. WHEELCHAIR	5	ANAEMIA (Hb < 8)	2	ORTHOPAEDIC/SPINAL		5
SCORE				SMOKING	1	ON TABLE > 2 HR#		5
10+ AT RISK						ON TABLE > 6 HR#		8
15+ HIGH RISK				MEDICATION – CYTOTOXICS, LONG TERM/HIGH DOSE STEROIDS, ANTI–INFLAMMATORY MAX OF 4				
20+ VERY HIGH RISK				# Scores can be discounted after 48 hours provided patient is recovering normally				

©J Waterlow 1985 Revised 2005*
Obtainable from the Nook, Stoke Road, Henlade TAUNTON TA3 5LX
*The 2005 revision incorporates the research undertaken by Queensland Health.

www.judy–waterlow.co.uk

REMEMBER **TISSUE DAMAGE MAY START PRIOR TO ADMISSION, IN CASUALTY. A SEATED PATIENT IS AT RISK**
ASSESSMENT (See Over) IF THE PATIENT FALLS INTO ANY OF THE RISK CATEGORIES, THEN PREVENTATIVE NURSING IS REQUIRED A COMBINATION OF GOOD NURSING TECHNIQUES AND PREVENTATIVE AIDS WILL BE NECESSARY
ALL ACTIONS MUST BE DOCUMENTED

PREVENTION
PRESSURE REDUCING AIDS
Special Mattress/beds: 10+ Overlays or specialist foam mattresses.
15+ Alternating pressure overlays, mattresses and bed systems
20+ Bed systems: Fluidised bead, low air loss and alternating pressure mattresses
Note: Preventative aids cover a wide spectrum of specialist features. Efficacy should be judged, if possible, on the basis of independent evidence.

Cushions: No person should sit in a wheelchair without some form of cushioning. If nothing else is available - use the person's own pillow. (Consider infection risk)
10+ 100mm foam cushion
15+ Specialist Gell and/or foam cushion
20+ Specialised cushion, adjustable to individual person.

Bed clothing: Avoid plastic draw sheets, inco pads and tightly tucked in sheet/sheet covers, especially when using specialist bed and mattress overlay systems
Use duvet - plus vapour permeable membrane.

NURSING CARE
General HAND WASHING, frequent changes of position, lying, sitting. Use of pillows
Pain Appropriate pain control
Nutrition High protein, vitamins and minerals
Patient Handling Correct lifting technique - hoists - monkey poles Transfer devices
Patient Comfort Aids Real Sheepskin - bed cradle
Operating Table
Theatre/A&E Trolley 100mm(4ins) cover plus adequate protection

Skin Care General hygene, NO rubbing, cover with an appropriate dressing

WOUND GUIDELINES
Assessment odour, exudate, measure/photograph position

WOUND CLASSIFICATION - EPUAP
GRADE 1 Discolouration of intact skin not affected by light finger pressure (non-blanching erythema)
This may be difficult to identify in darkly pigmented skin
GRADE 2 Partial thickness skin loss or damage involving epidermis and/or dermis
The pressure ulcer is superficial and presents clinically as an abrasion, blister or shallow crater
GRADE 3 Full thickness skin loss involving damage of subcutaneous tissue but not extending to the underlying fascia
The pressure ulcer presents clinically as a deep crater with or without undermining of adjacent tissue
GRADE 4 Full thickness skin loss with extensive destruction and necrosis extending to underlying tissue.

Dressing Guide Use Local dressings formulary and/or www.worldwidewounds

IF TREATMENT IS REQUIRED, FIRST REMOVE PRESSURE

Figure 6.2: The Waterlow card (revised version 2005). Reproduced with kind permission of Judy Waterlow (www.judy-waterlow.co.uk).

Both the RCN (2001) and NICE (2005) advise that pressure ulcer risk calculators should be used only as an *aide-memoire* and should not be a substitute for clinical judgement. Papanikolaou *et al.* (2007) argue that, if assessment scales have such limitations, they may have little to offer and more reliable tools need to be developed. Kelly (2005) suggests that, if risk assessment tools are used only as *aides-memoire*, then perhaps they should only identify a patient's 'at risk' status rather than the degree of risk. The RCN (2001) also advises that risk assessment tools selected for use in practice should have been tested in the same care speciality. Papanikolaou *et al.* (2007) add that all staff carrying out pressure ulcer risk assessment should be properly trained in the factors to be considered in their particular clinical setting.

Learning outcome 4: Discuss the importance of accurate documentation of pressure ulcer risk assessment

ACTIVITY

Consider why it is important to record information relating to pressure ulcer risk in nursing documentation.

The care plan is the principal means of communication between the nurses caring for a patient and other healthcare professionals. What is written or omitted may seriously affect the care a patient receives (Taylor 2003), which has important implications for patient safety.

Pressure ulcer development may be construed as medical negligence and is an increasing cause of compensation claims (Walsh and Bennett 2000). There are regular cases and complaints involving poor standards of communication which include inadequate documentation and non-reflective practice (Stephens and Bick 2002). Therefore, evidence of risk assessment and pressure ulcer prevention must be recorded in patient records. NICE (2005) highlighted that all formal risk assessments should be documented and readily available to all members of the multidisciplinary team and patients, and carers and relatives where appropriate should be involved in care decisions.

Summary

- There are many factors rendering people vulnerable to pressure ulcer formation.
- Pressure ulcer risk calculators may help nurses to identify those at risk but should not replace clinical judgement.
- There are a range of pressure ulcer risk calculators available. Nurses need to choose one suitable for their patient/client group after considering available evidence.
- Documentation of pressure ulcer risk assessment is essential for medico-legal reasons and to promote good communication.

PRESSURE ULCER PREVENTION

It is estimated that 95 per cent of pressure ulcers are preventable; the 5 per cent that are not are due to pre-admission problems such as lying on the floor for a long period following a fall (Hampton 1998). However, the drive towards early hospital discharge, expansion in day care, and technologies that lengthen the survival of patients who previously would not have survived has resulted in more very ill hospital patients (Gould *et al.* 2000). Therefore comparisons between the incidence rate and prevalence rate of pressure ulcers made several years apart are not valid.

LEARNING OUTCOMES

By the end of this section you will be able to:
1 discuss why pressure ulcer prevention is an important aspect of the nurse's role;
2 identify ways of preventing pressure ulcers in people at risk.

Learning outcome 1: Discuss why pressure ulcer prevention is an important aspect of the nurse's role

ACTIVITY

Why is it important that pressure ulcer prevention is implemented for people identified at risk of pressure ulcers?

You may have thought of some or all of the following points.

- Pressure ulcers can have serious physical effects. They can lead to infections including osteomyelitis (infection of bone) (Culley 1998), which can result in amputation, and they can be life-threatening (Fernandez 2007). The scar tissue resulting from pressure ulcers predisposes patients to further pressure ulcers owing to the reduced tissue strength.
- Pressure ulcers can markedly affect health-related quality of life (Clark 2002). They can cause pain, depression, loss of independence and social isolation with severe effects on people's relationships. They are chronic wounds and can adversely affect body image and self-esteem (Fox 2002; Hopkins *et al.* 2006).
- Patients with pressure ulcers remain in acute settings on average 5 days longer than patients without pressure ulcers (Hampton 1998).
- Pressure ulcers are a financial drain on the National Health Service with an estimated cost in the UK of at least £750 million a year (Stephens and Bick 2002). There has been considerable government pressure to reduce the incidence of pressure ulcers, and guidelines developed to inform prevention and treatment (Stephen-Haynes 2006).
- Pressure ulcers have been identified as a key indicator of quality of care and an important parameter in clinical audit and quality (Walsh and Bennett 2000).

There are therefore many reasons why pressure ulcers must be prevented. This has always been a nursing role – Florence Nightingale believed that good nursing care could prevent pressure ulcers. However, there must also be a multidisciplinary approach, which requires the whole organisation's commitment (RCN 2001), a view also supported by *The Essence of Care* (DH 2001b). Nevertheless, as nurses assess, plan, implement and evaluate care to meet all aspects of patients/clients' needs, they are in a key position to minimise pressure ulcers.

Learning outcome 2: Identify ways of preventing pressure ulcers in people at risk

ACTIVITY

List some methods of pressure ulcer prevention that you have observed in practice. Consider which might be suitable for patients/clients in the scenarios.

Pressure ulcer prevention can take several forms. It includes maintaining and improving tissue tolerance to pressure, protection against pressure, shear and friction forces, and education of staff, patients/clients and carers.

Pain control

Uncontrolled pain will prevent patients from moving, so adequate pain control is essential. Diane has tingling and burning pains in her legs, and John has chronic pain from his previous injury and acute pain from his newly fractured wrist. Nurses caring for them, in conjunction with the multidisciplinary team, must implement appropriate pain management strategies and promote their comfort. You can read more about this in Chapter 12.

Nutrition

Nutritional status should be assessed and if the patient seems to be at risk then a more detailed screening should be undertaken, with referral to a dietician (RCN 2001). This may be necessary for Marion; the staff who are caring for her need to understand the importance of nutrition in maintaining her skin integrity. Some people's dietary intake may need to be supplemented, particularly to increase vitamin and trace elements. Chapter 10 focuses on assessing and meeting nutritional needs in detail.

Promotion of continence and skin care

Marion is incontinent. Skin that is in contact with urine or faeces for long periods is at risk of maceration and breakdown, so her skin must be kept clean and dry. As constant washing with soap removes the body's natural protective oil (sebum), foam skin cleansers containing a moisturiser are preferable (Nazarko 2007). Super-absorbent incontinence pads help to keep skin dry and faecal incontinence must be dealt with promptly. Chapter 9 explores this topic in detail.

Patient handling techniques and repositioning

The patient handling sessions you attend will prepare you to employ good moving and handling techniques which prevent people being dragged up the bed, thus avoiding friction and shear. Patient handling education aims to teach the principles of good practice and problem-solving skills so that you have the flexibility to apply, modify and adapt the principles to different situations (Pellatt 2005). There is a vast range of patient handling equipment available which is designed either to help a patient move independently or, with help, to move a patient who is totally dependent. Equipment includes transfer boards, sliding sheets and hoists (Collins 2004). Specialised equipment is required for bariatric patients as most beds, mattresses, hoists and other equipment are not safe for use by very heavy patients (Palmer 2004). Marion's carers need instruction on correct patient handling techniques and how to use the necessary equipment.

Pressure damage can be avoided by repositioning patients regularly to ensure tissue perfusion. This will be necessary for Marion, who has a high risk of pressure ulcers. However, the exact time limits for particular point pressures in most patient situations, and therefore the required frequency for patient repositioning, are unknown (Lowthian 1997). *The Essence of Care* benchmark for best practice recommends that patients/clients' needs for repositioning should be assessed and documented, and that there should be ongoing reassessment (DH 2001b). NICE (2005) advises that turning schedules should be devised on an individual basis rather than ritualistically.

Repositioning schedules must consider a range of patient factors, such as their breathing and the patient's total care management (e.g. treatment by other healthcare professionals, meal times etc.). Some patients develop their own routines to prevent pressure ulcers, which should be appreciated by healthcare professionals (RCN 2001). For example, Diane has probably been living with her condition for some years and developed her own routine.

Regular turning of patients also helps to prevent chest infections, osteoporosis, deep vein thrombosis (DVT) and contractures (Pellatt 2007a). Therefore repositioning should occur even when patients are on pressure relieving devices (RCN 2004). It has been suggested that positioning patients in bed using a 30-degree tilt rather than at a 90-degree angle when they are on their back or sides disperses pressure away from bony prominences. However, Young (2004) found that the 30-degree tilt did not reduce pressure damage in a sample of acute medical hospital inpatients, and patients found it difficult to assume and maintain the position.

Pressure-relieving devices

A wide range of pressure-relieving devices has been developed to assist in protecting skin against pressure damage. *The Essence of Care* benchmark for best practice states that 'Patients at risk of developing pressure ulcers are cared for on pressure redistributing support surfaces that meet their individual needs (including comfort)' (DH, 2001b). The NICE-commissioned guidelines (RCN 2004) use the term 'pressure relieving' for all types of devices and support systems.

Devices are available as mattresses, bed systems, overlays and seat cushions and are designed to either reduce or redistribute pressure.

Seat cushions

Marion and Diane spend a lot of time in their wheelchairs and need appropriate wheelchair cushions that will relieve pressure. Sitting time in wheelchairs may need to be restricted to less than 2 hours for people with a high risk of pressure ulcers (NICE 2005). However, this is not always possible, especially in the community, where there may be a lack of available carers (Collins 2002).

Wheelchair cushions should fit the seat and the user, be at the right height, be stable, promote symmetrical posture and positioning and be comfortable. The cushion's ability to reduce the interface pressure and promote the ideal sitting posture is equally important. No one seat cushion has been shown to perform better than another (Collins 2004). The patient or carer should be able to maintain the cushion (Collins 2001). There are different types of cushion:

> **Interface pressure**
> The pressure between a hard surface and weight-bearing bony prominences (Hampton and Collins 2005).

- Foams, in a variety of densities, reduce friction and shear by acting as a barrier between the skin and the chair. They are lightweight and can be cut or contoured but will deteriorate if exposed to heat or ultraviolet light. Foam can act as an insulator and increase skin temperature, making the skin more susceptible to damage.
- Gel cushions provide even distribution of weight and conform to body shape, stabilising the pelvis and supporting the thighs, enhancing comfort. They conduct heat away from the body. However gel can be heavy and may leak if punctured.
- Air-filled cushions distribute pressure evenly, but care must be taken when inflating them. If under-filled they will not relieve pressure, and if over-filled they can be unstable. An alternative means of positioning is to use a moulded chair to fit the person's body shape (Collins 2002; Fernandez 2007).

Marion and Diane need to be correctly positioned in their chairs. The joints of the lower limbs should be in the mid-range of movement. The weight of the upper body should be supported evenly by both ischial tuberosities with the pelvis in a slight anterior tilt. The pelvis should rest at 90 degrees of flexion, the knees should be flexed to 90 degrees and the feet placed flat on the footplates. The head should be directly over the pelvis to encourage normal spinal curvature (Collins 2002).

Mattresses

A standard foam mattress will not be a suitable surface for Marion, and may not be appropriate for Diane or John either. The minimum provision for people assessed as vulnerable to pressure ulcers should be a high-specification foam mattress with pressure-relieving properties; this should be instigated for patients undergoing surgery too (Cullum *et al.* 2003; NICE 2005). There are two main categories of pressure-relieving mattress systems:

- *Systems that increase the area of the body in contact with the support surface.* They use materials that mould or contour to the body shape, distributing the load more widely and reducing pressure at bony prominences. These are also known as static or 'low-tech' equipment. Examples include foam mattresses and get or air-filled mattresses.

- *Systems that relieve the source of pressure from the surface of the body.* They do this by alternately inflating cells in a cyclical manner so that the body is supported on one set of cells while the remaining cells deflate away from the body. These are also known as dynamic or 'high-tech' equipment (Collins 2004; RCN 2004). Examples include alternating pressure, air fluidised or low air loss devices and turning beds.

There is little good-quality data to support the selection of any one particular piece of equipment and more research is needed (NICE 2005). However, 'high-tech' devices are recommended for people who are at high risk of pressure ulcers, where the individual's previous history of pressure ulcer prevention and/or clinical condition suggests they are best nursed on a high-tech device, or where low-tech devices have failed, on the basis of professional consensus (RCN 2004). Air-fluidised and low-air-loss beds have been found to promote pressure ulcer healing better than standard beds.

When choosing a surface, other criteria need to be considered too. Patient acceptability is very important. If the equipment is uncomfortable, increases pain or disturbs sleep then its use must be reconsidered. Hopkins *et al.*'s (2006) small study found that alternating-pressure air mattresses increased their patients' pain.

Another vital consideration is effects on **mobility.** The goal is to increase mobility, so using a support system that reduces mobility is inappropriate. Reduced mobility may occur for a number of reasons:

- Lack of a firm edge to the bed gives insufficient support for people transferring in and out of bed. Lack of stability can make transferring on and off surfaces difficult. The person needs to push down on the surface to obtain leverage; the contents will move when the body weight is lifted and support disappears.
- Increased height of the bed or chair may reduce access, particularly for wheelchair users.
- Loss of balance can occur with alternating-pressure systems, low-air-loss and fluidisation beds. A hoist may be needed to transfer on/off these beds (DLF 2006).

Other criteria when choosing a support system include the size and weight of the equipment, the patient's weight, the patient's lifestyle, cost implications, availability of carers/healthcare professionals to reposition the patient, and ease of use (NICE 2005).

Some people may need joint protectors for comfort, protection and pressure relief. Examples are fleece joint protectors or booties, polyester fibre, air-filled, fluid-filled or foam joint protectors. Pads are available for walking equipment and to line prostheses to protect the skin (DLF 2006); their fastenings must not exert pressure.

NICE (2005) has produced evidence-based clinical guidelines for pressure ulcer prevention; they can be accessed from www.nice.org.uk. However, many organisations have developed their own evidence-based local guidelines. Clinical guidelines are gaining increased support from the NHS Executive and other healthcare organisations. There is a legal duty for nurses to keep up to date with current pressure ulcer guidelines (Mckeeney 2002).

ACTIVITY

In your clinical setting, find out about:
- any local guidelines for pressure ulcer prevention;
- whether there are locally based tissue viability specialist nurses and how they can be contacted for advice;
- how pressure-relieving equipment is ordered locally.

Summary

- Pressure ulcers can have serious consequences. When a patient/client has been identified as being at risk of pressure ulcers, effective measures must be taken to prevent pressure ulcer formation.
- Appropriate preventive measures for people at risk of pressure ulcers must be planned. These should include providing a suitable support surface that does not impair mobility, using correct moving and handling techniques, promoting adequate nutrition, carer/patient education, pain management, and appropriate skin care.
- Patients/carers should be involved in decision-making processes about pressure ulcer prevention.

PREVENTION OF OTHER COMPLICATIONS OF IMMOBILITY

Pressure ulcers are a significant potential problem for people with impaired mobility, but there are a number of other possible complications.

LEARNING OUTCOMES

By the end of this section you will be able to:
1 identify physical and psychosocial problems arising from impaired mobility;
2 identify ways in which nurses can prevent complications of immobility.

Learning outcome 1: Identify physical and psychosocial problems arising from impaired mobility

ACTIVITY

Think of people you have cared for whose mobility was reduced for some reason. They may have been confined to bed or were dependent on a wheelchair, or physical or psychological problems may have made walking difficult. What problems did their limited mobility cause them?

> **Box 6.3 Physical and psychosocial problems caused by reduced mobility**
>
> - Circulatory – deep vein thrombosis, pulmonary embolus, orthostatic hypotension
> - Respiratory – chest infection
> - Gastrointestinal – loss of appetite, constipation
> - Urinary – renal calculi, urinary tract infection, incontinence
> - Musculoskeletal – osteoporosis, muscle wasting, contractures
> - Psychosocial – loss of self-esteem, frustration, boredom, isolation

Compare your answers with the list of problems in Box 6.3. You may observe that immobility affects many bodily functions, as well as having psychosocial effects; this highlights the multidimensional nature of immobility. Some of the problems are discussed below.

Circulatory and respiratory problems

Formation of a **DVT** can occur due to three predisposing factors (known as Virchow's Triad):

- trauma – for example from surgical procedures;
- blood coagulation changes – causes include dehydration, the ageing process, and any disease that affects blood clotting, such as inflammatory bowel disease;
- stasis of venous circulation – due to immobility or conditions such as heart failure (Van Wicklin *et al.* 2006).

Normally, movement of the legs contracts the muscles, which press on the veins and cause them to empty. Legs that are not mobile cannot maintain this pumping action, so the venous blood pools, causing a DVT. There may be no indication that there is a problem until the clot becomes detached and enters the pulmonary circulation into the lungs, causing a fatal pulmonary embolus (Breen 2000; Nutescu 2007). The risk of DVT in patients who have had a stroke is high owing to the underlying vascular disorder (Gibbon 2002). The **Autar DVT scale** is available to identify people at risk of DVT (Autar 1996).

Orthostatic hypotension (when blood pressure falls on moving to an upright position) can quickly develop in patients confined to bed or chair. Marion, for example, may feel faint and dizzy when she is transferred from bed to wheelchair. Normally, about 30 per cent of circulating blood volume is in the thoracic cavity. When moving to an upright position, the effect of gravity causes a volume drop of about one-third, reducing venous return to the heart and consequently reducing blood pressure. This triggers physiological responses to return the blood pressure to normal. Certain conditions – such as spinal cord injury, diabetes mellitus, ageing and prolonged bedrest – can prevent normal compensatory mechanisms from functioning adequately (Grubb *et al.* 2003; Clayden *et al.* 2006).

Decreased cardiac output and **reduced tissue perfusion** related to immobility can cause venous leg ulcers, particularly if there is associated poor calf muscle function or venous obstruction (Tyrrell 2002). Leg ulcers will limit a person's mobility as standing and walking may cause pain. Wound dressings, swollen legs, leakage and the need to wear large shoes compromise mobility too (Persoon *et al.* 2004).

Impaired mobility can cause **reduced ventilation of the lungs** and **reduced stimulation for coughing,** leading to a build-up of secretions in the bronchi and bronchioles, which can become infected. Oxygen uptake is reduced, with the danger of pneumonia (Markey and Brown 2002; Lindgren *et al.* 2004). Marion could be at risk of chest infections. Patients with paralysis of their abdominal and intercostal muscles, such as patients with spinal cord injury, will have reduced lung ventilation affecting their ability to cough, putting them at risk of a chest infection.

Gastrointestinal problems

Impaired mobility can predispose to **constipation** as exercise stimulates digestion and the movement of the gastrointestinal system (Weaver 2005), and can also affect diet and fluid intake, further increasing the risk. Immobility may also cause weakening of the abdominal wall muscles, making straining and therefore defecation difficult (Kyle 2006). Immobility can impair **appetite,** and people with reduced mobility may find it difficult to pour out their own drinks or eat independently.

Constipation not only causes discomfort but can also cause urinary tract infection, acute urinary retention or incontinence due to pressure of impacted faeces on the bladder (Pellatt 2007b).

Urinary problems

Urinary stasis may be caused by reduced mobility, which can cause **urinary tract infection** or **renal calculi** ('stones'). Stones consist of calcium and/or oxalate and uric acid (Pellatt 2007c). People who are immobile rely on staff to take them to the toilet or provide bedpans, urinals or commodes. Impaired mobility may also cause difficulties removing or adjusting clothing, which could be an issue for all the patients/clients in the scenarios.

Having to be dependent on staff to assist with elimination can threaten dignity. Some people can experience incontinence due to inability to get to the toilet quickly because of impaired mobility.

Musculoskeletal problems

In immobile parts of the body, **muscle wasting** commences and this muscle degeneration will deplete the capacity for movement, leading to further impairment. It is estimated that 10–15 per cent of muscle strength can be lost each week (Markey and Brown 2002). The lack of muscle activity causes degenerative changes involving the release of calcium from the bones (**osteoporosis**), with loss of bone density. A study of ten healthy men found that deconditioning of the muscles and bone loss occurred after five weeks of bedrest and was not fully reversed after four weeks of active weight-bearing, which highlights the importance of exercise and early mobilisation (Berg *et al.* 2007).

If joints remain in one position too long, the muscle fibres around the joint shorten and the collagen within the joint becomes tightly packed. This combined process causes a **contracture** (Nussbaum 2000). For patients with paralysed limbs, a range of positions should be adopted to discourage the development of abnormal tone and contractures (Gibbon 2002), but Marion already has some joint deformities. Joints particularly at risk are the shoulders, elbows, wrists, neck, fingers, hips, knees, ankles and toes. Diane has spasm in her legs which leads to a restricted range of joint movement due to muscle shortening or contractures. Contractures are associated with reduced mobility, pain, decreased function and pressure ulcers (Currie 2001; Jones 2004). Contractures reduce stability and increase the risk of falls, thus restricting mobility further.

Psychosocial problems

Loss of mobility can cause people to experience **loss of self-esteem** and they may feel frustration at being dependent on others. Older people who are admitted to hospital for an acute medical episode may become functionally impaired, not only because of the disease process but also from the hospitalisation process, becoming confused and disorientated. They may become depressed and apathetic. Up to 75 per cent of functionally independent older people admitted into an acute hospital are no longer independent on being discharged (Markey and Brown 2002). People with profound learning and multiple disabilities (like Marion) may experience frustration at having to rely on carers for moving and having to make needs known with limited communication ability.

Impaired mobility can also affect the ability and opportunity to socialise and communicate with others, leading to **isolation,** boredom and sensory deprivation. John has had impaired mobility resulting from his accident for some time and this could have contributed to his **depression.** People can experience despair, loneliness and isolation as family and friends withdraw (Moore and McLaughlin 2003). Diane may be frustrated that her mobility problems limit her ability to actively participate in activities with her family.

Learning outcome 2: Identify ways in which nurses can prevent complications of immobility

Roper *et al.* (2000) suggest that when planning care the objective is:
* to prevent identified potential problems from becoming actual ones;
* to solve actual problems;
* where possible to alleviate problems that cannot be solved;
* to prevent reoccurrence of problems that have been resolved;
* to help the person to cope positively with those problems that cannot be alleviated or solved.

ACTIVITY

We have identified a number of potential and actual problems related to impaired mobility in our three patients/clients. Consider the nursing interventions that could be implemented to prevent or solve these problems.

A few points which you may have considered are discussed below.

Deep vein thrombosis/pulmonary embolus

> **Passive and active exercises**
> Passive exercises are where another person moves a client/patient's limb through a range of movements. Active exercises are when people carry out exercises by themselves.

Observation for signs and symptoms of DVT (painful, swollen calf), and of pulmonary embolus (chest pain, cough etc.), are all part of nursing assessment. Nurses, in liaison with physiotherapists, can help people with passive and active exercises of the legs. These activities help to break the cycle of immobility and increase circulation (Van Wicklin *et al.* 2006).

Graduated compression stockings, intermittent pneumatic compression pumps and venous foot pumps are other preventive measures; these enhance venous return and blood flow. When using these devices it is essential that the correct size is chosen, they are applied correctly and are removed only for a short time each day (Mathias 2007). Anticoagulants such as heparin and/or oral anticoagulants may be prescribed for those at high risk (Nutescu 2007). NICE (2007) has published guidelines for reducing the risk of venous thromboembolism in patients who are having surgery.

Orthostatic hypotension

For Marion, this can be alleviated by gradually sitting her up in bed before she is transferred into her chair. Marion's carers should be aware of the signs and symptoms of orthostatic hypotension as Marion may not be able to verbally communicate if she feels dizzy. It is also important to explain to Marion what is happening to reduce any anxiety relating to these symptoms.

Chest infection

Frequent repositioning and encouragement to do deep breathing exercises can help to prevent chest infection. The person can also be encouraged to cough to clear secretions and prevent them pooling in the lungs. Chapter 11 has a section on observation of sputum, which includes tips on how expectoration of sputum can be encouraged.

Loss of appetite and constipation

An adequate fluid and diet intake should be provided, taking individual preferences into account and ensuring that sufficient fibre is included. Patients' food and drinks should be positioned so that they can reach them. Patients with hemiplegia need to be provided with a non-slip mat to prevent the plate moving, a plate guard to help keep the food on the plate, and an appropriate cup for drinking from. John's dominant arm is in plaster, making it difficult to cut up his food. People with profound learning and multiple physical disabilities, like Marion, may have difficulty with eating and drinking; carers should aim to enhance the quality of their mealtime experience. Chapter 10 has more detail about these issues.

Urinary tract infection and incontinence

People who are at risk of urinary tract infection should be observed for signs such as cloudy, foul-smelling urine. Chapter 9 has a section on urinalysis and explains how urinary tract infection might be suspected and when a specimen of urine should be sent for microscopy, culture and sensitivity. Marion would require continence aids, but consideration must be given to body image, comfort and skin care, and as to how continence can be promoted, rather than only contained.

Patients with impaired mobility (e.g. following a stroke) should be positioned within a short walking distance from the toilet when they start to mobilise. People who are confused may need guidance to get to the toilet; making toilets easily identifiable by using colour, signs and pictures can help (Nazarko 1997). Diane will need to learn how to manage a suprapubic catheter as blockage, leakage and infection can be a problem (Bardsley 2000). Chapter 9 explores these issues and will help you to develop your skills to assist people who need help with elimination.

Muscle wasting and contractures

As muscle contraction increases, joint movement becomes further limited, which is an issue for Marion and Diane. People with profound learning disabilities who are immobile are particularly at risk of developing deformities. Diane's spasms can be helped by careful positioning. Pillows, T-rolls or wedges positioned under the legs to put them in flexion can reduce extensor and adductor spasm (Pellatt 2007a). Splints may be prescribed, and physiotherapy and occupational therapy plays an important role in preventing contractures.

Botulinum toxin can be used to reduce muscle tone and increase the range of movements in a joint. It can be targeted to individual muscles (Gibbon 2002). Antispasmodic drugs such as Baclofen are commonly used to reduce spasm (Currie 2001). However, some spasm can help to maintain blood circulation and aid transfers and walking, by acting as a splint to limbs, so treatment of spasticity should be selected carefully and regularly reviewed to maintain function (Jones 2004).

Loss of self-esteem, frustration, boredom and isolation

As discussed in Chapter 1, how nurses carry out care may affect how people feel about themselves. A caring and empathetic approach from nurses can assist in reducing the psychosocial effects of impaired mobility. Chapter 2 looks at the approach of nurses when carrying out practical skills, and emphasises self-awareness. Family and friends have an important role in providing support too.

Summary

- People who have reduced mobility are at risk of a number of physical and psychosocial complications.
- Nurses have an important role in identifying potential complications and implementing preventive care.

KEY PRINCIPLES OF MOVING AND HANDLING PATIENTS

Many patients require help with moving on an individual basis which may change over the duration of their treatment and care. For example, Diane does not currently need help with moving but if her condition deteriorates this situation may change. Patient handling practice is governed by legislation and NHS Trust policies. The principles of safe handling must be learned by all nurses. Smith's (2005) *Guide to the Handling of People* is a very useful resource for safe handling of patients and should be available in your organisation.

LEARNING OUTCOMES

By the end of this section you will be able to:
1 carry out a moving and handling risk assessment;
2 identify appropriate equipment for individual patients' needs;
3 discuss the importance of communication in patient handling;
4 understand the legal implications of patient handling.

Learning outcome 1: Carry out a moving and handling risk assessment

ACTIVITY

Find out about the moving and handling assessment tools in use in your clinical area.

You will probably have seen moving and handling assessment tools being used in practice for carrying out and documenting a systematic assessment. They are likely to include sections relating to task, individual capability, load and environment.

- **Task.** What exactly is the manoeuvre to be carried out? For example, the task might be to move Marion out of bed and into her wheelchair.
- **Individual capability.** Here nurses need to assess their own ability, physical fitness and what they are capable of.
- **Load.** How much can the person do? A person who is fit and has no communication problems with support and training may eventually be able to transfer from bed to wheelchair using a lateral transfer board. Marion, although not particularly heavy, is unable to move and therefore needs a hoist to move her out of bed.
- **Environment.** Is there enough room for you and the person to work in? Slippery floors are a danger for people like Diane and John who have difficulty walking or who are unsteady on their feet.

If people cannot move themselves then equipment must be used. You will be able to practise using different equipment in your moving and handling sessions.

Learning outcome 2: Identify appropriate equipment for individual patient's needs

ACTIVITY

What patient handling equipment is commonly in use in your clinical area?

If you are working in a clinical area that has very dependent patients/clients, you may have a wide range of equipment available. Hignett (2003) suggests that the minimum equipment list for a clinical environment where patient handling activities occur on a regular basis includes hoists, standaids, sliding sheets, lateral transfer boards, walking belts and height-adjustable beds and baths.

Nurses will need to use a hoist to move Marion from a height-adjustable bed to wheelchair and back, and in and out of a height-adjustable bath. They will also need to use a sliding sheet to move her around in bed. You may be working in an area where patient/clients are mostly independent – such as an acute mental health unit – but staff must have access to equipment if it becomes necessary and staff must keep their skills up to date. For example, if a patient like John falls and is unable to get himself up from the floor, a hoist will be needed.

Learning outcome 3: Discuss the importance of communication in patient handling

ACTIVITY

Why is it important to communicate with your colleagues and patients involved in handling manoeuvres?

When moving and handling, both patient and carers are working as a team. It is vital that one person leads and coordinates the activity. Patients need to know exactly what to expect and how they can help when equipment is being used (Palmer 2004). The team leader must communicate the command to the team, and when everyone is ready give the command clearly (e.g. 'ready ... brace ... move'). This means that the manoeuvre is smooth and coordinated.

Learning outcome 4: Understand the legal implications of patient handling

ACTIVITY

Identify some possible legal implications of patient handling.

Poor moving and handling practice has implications for patient safety. Moving patients in bed without using appropriate equipment can cause shear and friction to the skin. The 'drag lift' (whereby nurses hook their arms under the patient's armpits and drag them up the bed, or on to their feet from sitting) can cause bruising, fractures or dislocation of shoulders; this can be considered as abuse with associated legal consequences (Pellatt 2005).

Summary
- A risk assessment must be carried out before any manual handling activity takes place.
- It is important that appropriate patient handling equipment is available for patients who need it.

● Patient handling requires teamwork which includes the person being moved.
● Using inappropriate handling techniques compromises patient safety and can have legal consequences.

ASSISTING WITH MOBILISATION AND PREVENTING FALLS

Assisting with mobility is an important role of nurses in many settings, and involves overcoming barriers and working closely with the multidisciplinary team, particularly physiotherapists and occupational therapists.

LEARNING OUTCOMES

By the end of this section you will be able to:
1 identify barriers to mobilisation;
2 examine ways of preventing falls;
3 discuss how people can be assisted with mobilisation.

Learning outcome 1: Identify barriers to mobilisation

ACTIVITY

What barriers could prevent a person from mobilising? How might these apply to the people in the scenarios?

A few possibilities are listed below, but you may well have thought of others.

• Pain or fear of pain may prevent a person from mobilising and this is an important issue for John. Therefore pain must be assessed and controlled. Read more about this in Chapter 12.

• Lack of motivation, perhaps where people have depression or dementia, may lead to reluctance to mobilise. John's depression could therefore present a further barrier to mobilisation.

• Foot problems such as in-growing toenails, fungal nail infections, calluses, corns and bunions can impede mobility by causing pain and discomfort. Neurological diseases such as multiple sclerosis can alter gait, causing calluses and corns to develop (Tyrrell 2002; Nazarko 2006).

• Bunions and arthritic feet make it difficult to wear normal shoes, but unsuitable footwear makes mobilising difficult and dangerous. Slip-on shoes or slippers increase the tendency to shuffle (Woodrow *et al.* 2005). Shiny or plastic soles cause a frightened, small-step gait. Narrow shoes inhibit normal foot movement, reducing normal toe function and preventing normal toe 'push off', affecting gait pattern and weight transference. High heels put abnormal stress on knees, making the gait unstable (Godfrey 2006). Ill-fitting shoes can cause blisters, corns, calluses and bursae, which are painful and can lead to ulceration (Tyrrell 2002).

• Arthritic knees can cause instability and falls, which lead to loss of confidence.

• Shortening of one leg may occur after surgery for fractured neck of femur, making it difficult to put both feet on the ground together.

- Fear of falling is a common problem and can cause a fear of going outside, even leading to agoraphobia. When a person, like John, has already had one fall causing a significant injury, fear of another fall and a lack of confidence in mobilising are understandable.
- Fatigue is a common symptom of multiple sclerosis (Jones 2004) and can be an overwhelming feeling of exhaustion in response to minor exertion. Diane is able to walk with sticks sometimes but needs a wheelchair when she becomes severely fatigued.

Learning outcome 2: Examine ways of preventing falls

The prevention of falls is focused on in one of the sections in *The National Service Framework for Older People* (DH 2001c), and falls in older people are a problem that is being addressed nationally and internationally (Swift 2002). However, people in other age groups can, like Diane and John, be at risk of falling too. The effects of falls extend beyond physical injury and cost to the health services. Fear of subsequent falls can lead to restricted mobility and independence, contributing to functional decline and dependency, which in turn increases the risk of falling (McCarter-Bayer *et al.* 2005).

ACTIVITY

Consider people you have cared for in practice who were in hospital as the result of a fall, or perhaps fell while in hospital. List the reasons for their falls.

Parkinson's disease
There is a loss of dopamine-producing neurons within the brain, causing a chronic, progressive degenerative neurological disease with symptoms such as tremor, rigidity and bradykinesia (slow movement). It affects many activities including eating, with a risk of aspiration.

- *Physiological and psychosocial factors.* Both contribute to fear of falling. People may develop a morbid fear of falling (McCarter Bayer *et al.* 2005).
- *Poor vision.* This can be due to age-related deterioration or other visual problems (Lyons 2005). People may trip over objects in the dark, trip on carpets or uneven floors or miss stairs and fall.
- *Poor mobility with age-related changes in gait, posture and balance.* Neurological diseases, for example **Parkinson's disease**, causes people to stoop, lean forward and develop a short-stepped, shuffling gait. Multiple sclerosis (Diane) causes gait problems due to spasm, motor and sensory changes. Diabetes may cause decreased sensation in legs and feet. Stroke affects mobility and balance (Lyons 2005).
- *Changes in the inner ear.* This can affect a person's sense of balance.
- *Loss of muscle strength and flexibility.* This can cause difficulty in holding handrails or getting out of chairs.
- *Medications and alcohol.* These can cause dizziness, hypotension, blurred vision, weakness, poor balance and drowsiness (Jasniewski 2006). John's medication for his depression could have these effects. Diuretics and laxatives increase the number of trips to the toilet, often in a hurry. Taking more than four different medicines, especially centrally sedating or blood pressure lowering medicines, is a recognised predisposing factor in falls (DH 2001c).

- *Problems with bladder and bowels.* Falls can result from lack of control, such as with urge incontinence (McCarter-Bayer *et al.* 2005).
- *Dementia.* This causes cognitive impairment, memory loss and confusion which may contribute to the danger of falling (Chaābane 2007).

The National Service Framework for Older People recommends that older people who have fallen should be referred to a specialist falls service, which can carry out a comprehensive assessment (DH 2001c). NICE (2004) advise that this should be a multifactoral assessment (see www.nice.org for details). All nurses should understand risk factors for falls and be aware of the falls service and how referrals are made.

| ACTIVITY | Think of how falls can be *prevented* for people who are identified as being at risk. |

The following interventions can be effective in preventing falls:
- muscle strengthening, balance training and exercise;
- home hazard assessment and modifications to a person's home;
- review and possible withdrawal of psychotropic medications;
- cardiac pacing where appropriate (NICE 2004);
- regular eye examinations and provision of correct prescription lenses, walking sticks or frames;
- regular exercise to improve gait, posture and flexibility (Gatti 2002);
- continence promotion (Lyons 2005);
- hip protectors – may help to prevent hip fractures in older people who have a high risk of falling (Minns *et al.* 2004).

There is some evidence to suggest that Tai Chi exercises may help to prevent falls by improving balance and improve muscle and cardio-respiratory strength and fitness (Gallagher 2003).

Learning outcome 3: Discuss how people can be assisted with mobilisation

| ACTIVITY | Focus on the practice scenarios and identify strategies and equipment that might assist with mobilisation. |

You probably considered involvement of the multidisciplinary team, and will have encountered mobility aids. Helping a person to mobilise requires a multidisciplinary approach.

For example, the orthotist can supply walking sticks for Diane, callipers, shoes or knee braces to overcome some of the barriers to mobility. Physiotherapists will assess people for mobility aids such as crutches, or walking frames, both standard or wheeled ones for people who cannot lift a standard frame. Gutter frames can help people with arthritis. People who are unable to walk (Marion), or whose walking ability fluctuates (Diane), will be supplied with wheelchairs. Special chairs with

> **Box 6.4 Restoring or minimising loss of mobility in people with dementia (Logsdon *et al.* 2005)**
>
> - Caregivers are taught to guide the person with dementia in an individualised programme of endurance activities (walking, strength training, balance and flexibility)
> - Verbal and visual cues are given – e.g. walking with the person to illustrate the speed of walking and length or number of steps.
> - Use behavioural problem-solving strategies – e.g. identifying situations, time of day or behaviour of others that appear to trigger anxiety, agitation or reluctance and forming a plan such as walking at a different time of day.

cushions that rise slowly can help people who have difficulty getting up from a chair. For patients who have had a stroke, the physiotherapist will develop a plan; for example the Bobath technique prescribes how a patient should be handled and moved (Gibbon 2002). Aids and appliances must be cleaned and checked regularly as part of a regular maintenance programme to maintain patient safety (Swann 2007).

Restoring or minimising loss of mobility in people with dementia is challenging, but Logsdon *et al.* (2005) suggest an activity programme that uses both behavioural and exercise strategies (see Box 6.4). These strategies are enjoyable and help to improve physical and emotional health.

Dressing and undressing Marion, who has severe contractures, can be very difficult and the occupational therapist can advise about techniques and suitable clothing. Splints and braces can help to maintain body and limb posture. If considered in her best interests, arm gaiters could help to minimise involuntary muscle action so that she might be able to use an adapted motorised wheelchair, thus increasing her independence in mobilising. However, careful assessment will be needed to ensure that she can operate the wheelchair safely (Swann 2007).

Safety

When helping a person to mobilise, the safety of both the individual and the nurse is a major consideration. As we have already discussed, some people may be unsteady on their feet or have lost confidence. Therefore a risk assessment must be carried out before attempting to assist with mobilising. Risk assessment is a component of the Essential Skills Clusters (NMC 2007). You will have looked at risk assessment within moving and handling training sessions and will be aware of the importance of documentation.

Assisting a person to walk

When assisting a person to walk, you stand beside them, facing forward so you both move the same way. The use of a transfer belt around the person's waist gives you something to hold. For example, if someone has a slight weakness on the right side, you stand at their right side in a walk stance, with your left hand holding the belt

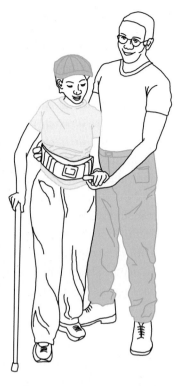

Figure 6.3: Helping a person to walk.

around their waist, and their right hand in your right hand, using a palm-to-palm grip (see Fig. 6.3).

On the command 'ready … brace … stand', you both move forward as you transfer your weight from the back leg to the front. You can now use this hold to give the person confidence to walk. You will have the opportunity to practise these techniques under supervision in the classroom. A very important aspect is not to hurry the person, maintaining a slow steady pace.

Summary

- Building people's confidence and self-esteem is an important aspect of mobilisation.
- Nurses have an important role in the multidisciplinary team, managing and caring for people with problems of mobility.
- Nurses should be aware of barriers to mobilisation, so that these can be addressed.
- Nurses should be aware of the people who are at risk of falling and implement interventions to prevent falls.
- When assisting with mobilising, risk assessment is essential and must be documented.
- Appropriate mobility aids should be provided for each individual. Nurses can give encouragement and support to people who are regaining mobility.

CHAPTER SUMMARY

There are many possible underlying reasons for impaired mobility, which can be temporary or permanent. The complications of impaired mobility can lead to much discomfort and further health problems, so nurses must take a proactive role to prevent these ill-effects.

Pressure ulcers were discussed in depth as their incidence remains widespread even though they are largely preventable. This chapter has emphasised the importance of identifying potential problems, so that effective preventive strategies for each individual can be implemented.

Promoting mobility wherever possible is key to preventing many problems and a multidisciplinary approach should be taken. Finally, when caring for people with impaired mobility, correct moving and handling techniques must be used to protect both clients and nurses. It was beyond the scope of the chapter to address this topic in depth. These techniques need to be learnt under supervision and attendance at moving and handling sessions is essential.

REFERENCES

Anton, L. 2006. Pressure ulcer prevention in older people who sit for long periods. *Nursing Older People* **18**(4) 29–36.

Armstrong, D. and Bortz, P. 2001. An integrative review of pressure relief in surgical patients. *AORN Journal* **73**, 645, 647–8.

Autar, R. 1996. Nursing assessment of clients at risk of deep vein thrombosis (DVT): the Autar DVT scale. *Journal of Advanced Nursing* **23**, 763–70.

Bardsley, A. 2000. The neurogenic bladder. *Nursing Standard* **14**(22), 39–41.

Berg, H., Eiken, O., Miklavic, L. and Mekjavic, I. 2007. Hip, thigh and calf muscle atrophy and bone loss after 5-week bedrest inactivity. *European Journal of Applied Physiology* **99**(3), 283–9.

Bergstrom, N., Braden, B.J., Laguzza, A. and Holman, V. 1987. The Braden scale for predicting pressure sore risk. *Nursing Research* **36**, 205–10.

Breen, P. 2000. DVT what every nurse should know. *RN* **63**(4), 58–61.

Chaābane, F. 2007. Falls prevention for older people with dementia. *Nursing Standard* **2**(6), 50–5.

Clark, M. 2002. Pressure ulcers and quality of life. *Nursing Standard* **16**(22), 74–8, 80.

Clayden, V., Steeves, J. and Krassiovikou, A. 2006. Orthostatic hypotension following spinal cord injury: understanding clinical pathology. *Spinal Cord* **44**(6), 341–51.

Collins, F. 2001. Sitting: pressure ulcer development. *Nursing Standard* **15**(22), 54–8.

Collins, F. 2002. Use of pressure reducing seats and cushions in a community setting. *British Journal of Community Nursing* **7**(10), 15–22.

Collins, F. 2004. Development and design of equipment over the last 15 years. *International Journal of Therapy and Rehabilitation* **11**(9), 411–16.

Culley, F. 1998. Nursing aspects of pressure sore prevention and therapy. *British Journal of Nursing* **7**(15), 879–80, 882, 884.

Cullum, N., Deeks, J., Song, F. and Fletcher, A.W. 2003. Beds, mattresses and cushions for pressure sore prevention and treatment (Cochrane review). In *The Cochrane Library*, issue 3. Oxford: Update Software.

Currie, R. 2001. Spasticity: a common symptom of multiple sclerosis. *Nursing Standard* **15**(33), 47–52, 54, 55.

Dealey, C. 1997. *Managing Pressure Sore Prevention*. Salisbury: Quay Books and Mark Allen Publishing.

Department of Health (DH) 2001a. *Valuing People: A new strategy for learning disability for the 21st century*. London.

— 2001b. *The Essence of Care: Patient-focused benchmarking for health care practitioners*. London.

— 2001c. *The National Service Framework for Older People*. London.

Dinsdale, P. 2007. Under pressure. *Nursing Older People* **19**(6), 18–24.

Disabled Living Foundation (DLF) 2006. *Choosing Pressure Relief Equipment*. London: DLF.

Ferguson, M., Cook, A., Rimmasch, H. *et al.* 2000. Pressure ulcer management: the importance of nutrition. *MEDSURG Nursing* **9**(4), 163–80.

Fernandez, T. 2007. Preventing pressure ulcers: selecting the right equipment. *International Journal of Therapy and Rehabilitation* **14**(5), 235–9.

Fletcher, J. 1996. The principles of pressure sore prevention. *Nursing Standard* **10**(39), 47–55.

Fox, C. 2002. Living with a pressure ulcer: a descriptive study of patients' experiences. *Wound Care* **11**(6), 10–22.

Gallagher, B. 2003. Tai Chi Chuan and Qigong: physical and mental practice for functional mobility. *Topics in Geriatric Rehabilitation* **19**(3), 172–82.

Gatti, J. 2002. Cochrane for clinicians: putting evidence into practice. Which interventions help to prevent falls in the elderly? *American Family Physician* **65,** 225–8.

Gibbon, B. 2002. Rehabilitation following stroke. *Nursing Standard* **16**(29), 47–52, 54–5.

Godfrey, J. 2006. Toward optimal health: D. Casey Kerrigan MD discusses the impact of footwear on the progression of osteoarthritis in women. *Journal of Women's Health* **15**(8), 894–7.

Gould, D., James, T., Tarpey, A. *et al.* 2000. Intervention studies to reduce the prevalence of pressure sores: a literature review. *Journal of Clinical Nursing* **9,** 163–78.

Grubb, B., Kosinski, D. and Kanjwal, Y. 2003. Orthostatic hypotension: causes, classification and treatment. *PACE* **26**(1), 892–901.

Hampton, S. 1998. Can electric beds aid pressure sore prevention in hospitals? *British Journal of Nursing* **7,** 1010–17.

Hampton, S. 2003. The complexities of heel ulcers. *Nursing Standard* **17**(31) 68, 70, 72, 74, 76, 79.

Hampton, S. and Collins, F. 2005. Reducing pressure ulcer incidence in a long-term setting. *British Journal of Nursing* **14**(15), S6–12.

Hignett, S. 2003. Systematic review of patient handling activities in lying, sitting and standing positions. *Journal of Advanced Nursing* **41**(6), 545–52.

Hopkins, A., Deeley, C., Bale, S., Defloor, T. and Worboys, F. 2006. Patient stories of living with a pressure ulcer. *Journal of Advanced Nursing* **56**(4), 345–53.

Jasniewski, J. 2006. Putting a lid on medication-related falls. *Nursing* **36**(6), 22–4.

Jones, C. 2004. Multiple sclerosis update. *Primary Health Care* **14**(2), 26–32.

Kelly, J. 2005. Inter-rater reliability and Waterlow's pressure ulcer risk assessment tool. *Nursing Standard* **19**(32), 86–92.

Kyle, G. 2006. Assessment and treatment of older patients with constipation. *Nursing Standard* **21**(8), 41–6.

Lewis, B. 1998. Nutrient intake and the risk of pressure sore development in older patients. *Journal of Wound Care* **7,** 31–5.

Lindgren, M., Unosson, M., Fredrikson, M. and Ek, A. 2004. Immobility: a major risk factor for development of pressure ulcers among adult hospitalised patients – a prospective study. *Scandinavian Journal of Caring Sciences* **18**(1), 57–64.

Liou, T., Pi-Sunyer, X. and Lafferrère, B. 2005. Physical disability and obesity. *Nutrition Reviews* **63**(10), 321–31.

Logsdon, R., McCurry, S. and Teri, L. 2005. A home health care approach to exercise for persons with Alzheimer's disease. *Care Management Journals* **6**(2), 90–7.

Lowthian, P. 1987. The practical assessment of pressure sore risk. *Care – Science and Practice* **5**(4), 3–7.

Lowthian, P. 1997. Notes on the pathogenesis of serious pressure sores. *British Journal of Nursing* **6**, 907–12.

Lyons, T. 2005. Fall prevention for older adults. *Journal of Gerontological Nursing* **32**(11), 9–14.

Markey, D. and Brown, R. 2002. An interdisciplinary approach to addressing patient activity and mobility in the medical-surgical patient. *Journal of Nursing Care Quality* **16**(4), 1–12.

Mathias, J. 2007. Preventing venous thromboembolism. *Supplement to OR Manager* **23**(3), 23–26.

McCarter-Bayer, A., Bayer, F. and Hall, K. 2005. Preventing falls in acute care: an innovative approach. *Journal of Gerontological Nursing* **31**(3), 25–33.

McKeeney, L. 2002. Legal issues for the prevention of pressure ulcers. *Journal of Community Nursing* **16**(7). Available from www.jcn.co.uk.

Minns, J., Dodd, C., Gardner, R. *et al.* 2004. Assessing the safety and effectiveness of hip protectors. *Nursing Standard* **18**(39), 33–8.

Moore, K. and McLaughlin, D. 2003. Depression: the challenge for health care professionals. *Nursing Standard* **17**(26), 45–52, 54–5.

National Institute for Health and Clinical Excellence (NICE) 2004. *The Assessment and Prevention of Falls in Older People*, Clinical Guideline 21. London. Available from http://www.nice.org.uk.

— 2005. *The Prevention and Treatment of Pressure Ulcers*, Clinical Guideline 29. London. Available from www.nice.org.uk.

— 2007. *Venous Thromboembolism: Reducing the risk of venous thromboembolism (deep vein thrombosis and pulmonary embolism) in inpatients undergoing surgery*, Clinical Guideline 46. Available from www.nice.org.uk.

National Pressure Ulcer Advisory Panel 2007. *Pressure Ulcer Stages*, revised by NPUAP. Available from www.npuap.org.

Nazarko, L. 1997. Continence: the whole story. *Nursing Times* **93**(43), 63–4, 66, 68.

Nazarko, L. 2006. Helping older people to care for their feet. *Nursing and Residential Care* **8**(3), 105–8.

Nazarko, L. 2007. Skin care: incontinence dermatitis. *Nursing and Residential Care* **9**(7), 310–13.

Noble, M., Voegeli, D., Clough, G., 2003. A comparison of cutaneous and vascular responses to transient pressure loading in smokers and non smokers. *Journal of Rehabilitation Research and Development* **40**(3), 283–8.

Norton, D., Exton-Smith, A. and McLaren, R. 1962. *An Investigation of Geriatric Nursing Problems in Hospital*. London: National Corporation for the Care of Old People.

Nursing and Midwifery Council (NMC) 2007. *Essential Skills Clusters (ESCs) for Pre-registration Nursing Programmes*. Annexe 2 to NMC circular 07/2007. Available from www.nmc-uk.org.

Nussbaum, S. 2000. Contracture management. In Nesathurai, S. (ed.) *The Rehabilitation of People with Spinal Cord Injury*, 2nd edn. Boston: Blackwell, 67–74.

Nutescu, E. 2007. Assessing, preventing and treating venous thromboembolism: evidence-based approaches. *American Journal Health-System Pharmacists* **64**(Suppl 7) S5–13.

Palmer, R. 2004. Moving and handling bariatric patients safely: a case study. *International Journal of Therapy and Rehabilitation* **11**(1), 31–3.

Papanikolaou, P., Lyne, P. and Anthony, D. 2007. Risk assessment scales for pressure ulcers: a methodological review. *International Journal of Nursing Studies* **44**(2), 285–96.

Pellatt, G. 2005. The safety and dignity of patients and nurses during patient handling. *British Journal of Nursing* **14**(21), 1150–6.

Pellatt, G. 2007a. Clinical skills: bed making and patient positioning. *British Journal of Nursing* **16**(5), 302–5.

Pellatt, G. 2007b. Urinary elimination. Part 2: Retention, incontinence and catheterisation. *British Journal of Nursing* **16**(8), 480–5.

Pellatt, G. 2007c. Anatomy and physiology of urinary elimination: Part 1. *British Journal of Nursing* **16**(7), 406–10.

Penzer, R. and Finch, M. 2001. Promoting healthy skin in older people. *Nursing Standard* **15**(34), 46–52, 54–5.

Persoon, A., Heinen, M., Carien, J.M. *et al.* 2004. Leg ulcers: a review of their impact on daily life. *Journal of Clinical Nursing* **13**(3) 341–54.

Roper, N., Logan, W. and Tierney, A.J. 2000. *The Roper–Logan–Tierney Model of Nursing.* Edinburgh: Churchill Livingstone.

Royal College of Nursing (RCN) 2001. *Pressure Ulcer Risk Assessment and Prevention: Recommendations.* London.

— 2004. *Guidelines Commissioned by the National Institute for Clinical Excellence: Use of pressure-relieving devices (beds, mattresses and overlays) for the prevention of pressure ulcers in primary and secondary care.* London.

Schoonhoven, L., Defloor, T. and Grypdonck, M. 2002. Incidence of pressure ulcers due to surgery. *Journal of Clinical Nursing* **11,** 479–87.

Simpson, A., Bowers, K. and Weir-Hughes, D. 1996. *Pressure Sore Prevention.* Gateshead: Athenaeum.

Smith, J. (ed.) 2005. *Guide to the Handling of People,* 5th edn. Teddington: BackCare.

Smith, L., Booth, N., Douglas, D. *et al.* 1995. A critique of 'at risk' pressure sore assessment tools. *Journal of Clinical Nursing* **4,** 153–9.

Stephens, F. and Bick, D. 2002. Organisational perspective: a pressure ulcer risk assessment and prevention audit: a pilot. *Nursing Management* **9**(3), 24–9.

Stephen-Haynes, J. 2006. Implementing the NICE pressure ulcer guideline. *Wound Care* **15**(9), 516–18.

Strachan-Bennett, S. 2003. Tool aims to standardise nurses' nutritional care. *Nursing Times* **99**(46), 7.

Swann, J. 2007. Keeping mobile: Part 2. *Nursing and Residential Care* **9**(1), 28–30.

Swift, C. 2002. The NHS English National Framework for Older People: opportunities and risks. *Clinical Medicine* **2,** 139–43.

Taylor, H. 2003. An exploration of the factors that affect nurses' record keeping. *British Journal of Nursing* **12**(12), 751–8.

Tyrrell, W. 2002. The causes and management of foot ulceration. *Nursing Standard* **16**(30), 53, 54, 56, 58, 60, 62.

Van Wicklin, S., Ward, K. and Cantrell, S. 2006. Implementing a research utilisation plan for prevention of deep vein thrombosis. *AORN* **83**(6), 1351–62.

Vanderwee, K., Grypdonck, M., Defloor, T. 2007. Non-blanching erythema as an indicator for the need for pressure ulcer prevention: a randomised controlled trial. *Journal of Clinical Nursing* **16**(2), 325–35.

Walsh, K. and Bennett, G. 2000. Pressure ulcers as indicators of neglect. *Nursing and Residential Care* **2**(11), 536–9.

Waterlow, J. 1985. Pressure sores: a risk assessment card. *Nursing Times* **81**(48), 49, 51, 55.

Waterlow, J. 1988. The Waterlow card for the prevention and management of pressure sores: toward a pocket policy. *Care – Science and Practice* **6**(1), 8–12.

Waterlow, J. 2005. *The Waterlow Score Card*. Available from www.judy-waterlow.co.uk. Accessed 3 December 2007.

Weaver, D. 2005 Helping individuals to maintain mobility. *Nursing and Residential Care* **7**(8), 343–8.

Weetman, C. and Allison, W. 2006. Use of epidural anaesthesia in post-operative pain management. *Nursing Standard* **20**(44), 54–64.

Woodrow, P., Dickson, N. and Wright, P. 2005. Foot care for non-diabetic older people. *Nursing Older People* **17**(8), 31–2.

World Health Organization 2001 *International Classification of Functioning Disability and Health*. Available from www.who.int/classifications/icf/en/index.html.

Young, T. 2004. The 30-degree tilt position versus the 90-degree lateral and supine positions in reducing the incidence of non-blanching erythema in a hospital inpatient population: a randomised controlled trial. *Journal of Tissue Viability* **14**(3), 88–96.

Principles of Wound Care

Janine Ashton

The maintenance of skin integrity and management of acute and chronic wounds is a major component of nursing care, relevant to all care settings (Bryant 2007). It is a developing field, with new technologies and research continually emerging (Gray *et al.* 2004). The nurse's role in wound care stretches from the initial holistic assessment of the wound and the patient, to making the correct decisions about treatment. Regular evaluation and setting of goals is essential to monitor the progress of the wound, and this should include the involvement of patients in the decision-making process. This chapter aims to assist you to develop knowledge and understanding of the breadth of issues involved with wound healing physiology, and to apply this to your practice.

Wound management is a vast topic with an ever-expanding and developing knowledge base, to which whole books and journals are dedicated. Therefore, while this chapter provides a foundation, further reading will be necessary, and you need to continually update your knowledge base. The Cochrane Library and the National Institute for Health and Clinical Excellence (NICE) – discussed in Chapter 1 – are good sources. When in the practice setting, there are specialist nurses (e.g. tissue viability, vascular and dermatology nurses) and other members of the multidisciplinary team (e.g. podiatrists) who will be valuable resources for your learning.

> This chapter includes:
> - The phases of wound healing
> - Classification of wounds and wound closure
> - Factors affecting wound healing
> - Wound assessment
> - Wound management

Although you can study this chapter at any stage of your learning programme, you will find it most relevant to work through the sections when based in a setting where you have patients/clients with different wounds. There is no substitute for looking at real wounds and applying theory to practice. Chapter 3, 'Preventing cross-infection', is essential prior reading, as when managing wounds an understanding of how microorganisms are transmitted, and adherence to standard precautions and aseptic technique, is paramount.

> **Recommended biology reading:**
>
> The following questions will help you to focus on the biology underpinning this chapter's skills. Use your recommended textbook to find out:
> - What characteristics must skin possess?
> - What are the major layers of the skin?
> - Which layer is avascular?
> - What are the major functions of the skin? What role does skin play in homeostasis?
> - How does the skin protect itself against damage and infection?
> - What factors can lead to a breakdown in skin integrity? What would the consequences be?
> - What is the goal of wound healing? What factors influence the degree of scarring?
> - How does age alter the skin's characteristics? Consider the skin at birth, adolescence, young adulthood and old age.
> - How does the appearance of skin change, during illness, injury or stress?
> - What factors are necessary to maintain normal healthy skin?

An understanding of the physiology of wound healing is essential when assessing and managing wounds, and is therefore included in this chapter.

PRACTICE SCENARIOS

The following practice scenarios illustrate different situations where wound care is required and are referred to throughout this chapter.

Adult

Type 2 diabetes
Develops when the body makes insufficient insulin, or when the insulin that is produced does not work effectively (known as insulin resistance). See www.diabetes.org.uk.

Mrs Warner is 78 years old, and has a history of **type 2 diabetes,** which is managed with oral hypoglycaemic medication. Since her husband died two years ago she has lived alone with her two cats and has been treated for depression. After falling in her kitchen she was unable to get off the floor, and was found by a neighbour some hours later. After assessment in the Emergency department she was diagnosed with a stable fracture of her pelvis. She was also found to have an ulcer (open sore) on one of her toes, which had an offensive discharge. Her blood glucose was high. She was transferred to a ward for rehabilitation and pain management. A few days later a large area of black necrotic (dead) tissue developed on her sacrum, and discoloured areas on both her elbows. These appeared to have been caused by the period of prolonged pressure on the kitchen floor. Mrs Warner is keen to get home as soon as possible as she is worried about her cats. She normally smokes ten cigarettes a day and is overweight. Her diet is high in fat and carbohydrates and she rarely eats fruit or vegetables.

Learning disability

Susan is 32 years old and has a moderate learning disability. She lives in a small group home and was recently in hospital having her acutely inflamed appendix

Health facilitator
A member of the community learning disabilities team (often a nurse) who supports a person with learning disabilities to access the healthcare they need. See *Valuing People* (DH 2001).

Clozapine
An atypical antipsychotic drug that has been proved to have efficacy in treatment-resistant schizophrenia and improving negative schizophrenic symptoms (King 1998).

Abscess
A localized collection of pus. Pus is a thick fluid containing leucocytes, bacteria and cellular debris, and indicates infection.

removed. She has been discharged home and has a small abdominal wound, which seems to be healing well. However, Susan is concerned about the wound and is worried about getting it wet when she showers, and drying and dressing afterwards in case she harms the wound. She is due to have her sutures removed by the practice nurse. The community nurse for learning disability, who is Susan's health facilitator, is visiting regularly to give some support in this situation.

Mental health

Colin is 28 years old, and is being treated as an inpatient in the acute mental health unit, after deterioration in his mental health, which has affected his self-care ability. He has a diagnosis of substance abuse and schizophrenia, which is currently being treated with clozapine. Colin requires careful blood monitoring, as clozapine can affect white blood cell levels. While on the unit he complained of pain in his left upper buttock. A large, hot, swollen area was found, which was diagnosed as being an abscess. Colin says that he has had several of these before. Incision and drainage took place in theatre and he has now returned to the unit, with a pack *in situ* in the wound. Antibiotics have been prescribed.

THE PHASES OF WOUND HEALING

A wound can be defined as (Lazarus *et al.* 1994):

> 'a disruption of normal anatomical structure and function which results from pathological processes beginning internally or externally to the involved organ.'

Different wounds do not necessarily follow the same pattern in the healing process. Doughty and Sparks-Defriese (2007) identify two ways in which wound repair occurs:
- Wounds confined to the epidermis and superficial dermal layers heal by regeneration.
- Wounds extending through the whole dermis heal by scar formation.

LEARNING OUTCOMES

By the end of this section you will be able to:
1 distinguish the phases of healing and recognise tissue appearance at each stage;
2 show awareness that healing does not in reality occur in a simple linear fashion.

Learning outcome 1: Distinguish the phases of healing and recognise tissue appearance at each stage

The process of wound healing is usually described in three distinct phases, but these descriptive models refer to the healing of acute wounds. Chronic wounds do not follow the normal sequence of events, so delays to the healing process are experienced (Timmons 2006). Williams and Young (1998) state that the wound healing phases are a false division – an attempt to simplify this very complex process. Some authors describe four or more phases/stages, but these variations are an expansion on the three phases described. You may also find different terminology being used to describe the phases. This chapter employs the approach that there are three *interdependent* phases during the wound healing process.

The inflammatory phase

This twofold phase prepares the tissue for repair. After wounding, blood loss is controlled by a complex series of events, known as **haemostasis.** This protective mechanism aims to minimise injury, whilst initiating the healing response through the release of growth factors, which then attract the migration of neutrophils, monocytes and macrophages to the wound bed (Timmons 2006). The cellular aspect of this phase occurs within hours of wounding (Krizek *et al.* 1997). The primary function of these cells is to attract phagocytes to the inflamed area to kill bacteria and remove debris from dead and dying cells within the tissue spaces (Timmons 2006). This process is known as **phagocytosis.** The five cardinal signs of inflammation are heat, redness, pain, swelling and loss of function.

The proliferative phase

This phase rebuilds the tissue through three separate processes.
- **Granulation** leads to the formation of new blood vessels (angiogenesis), which deliver oxygen and nutrients to the healing tissues. Fibroblasts and endothelial cells are the primary cells in this phase. Fibroblasts from the surrounding tissue become activated by growth factors released in the inflammatory phase, enabling them to replicate and produce a collagen-rich matrix which builds elasticity and strength into the wound (Timmons 2006). Granulation tissue is characterised by a reddish velvety carpet in the base of the wound. Unhealthy granulation tissue may be dark in colour and bleed easily, indicating possible infection and poor vascular supply to the tissue (Timmons 2006).
- **Contraction** is the approximation of the wound edges believed to be caused by the 'push' and 'pull' effect of the myofibroblasts (Timmons 2006).
- **Epithelialisation** resurfaces the wound by regeneration of epithelial cells.

In full-thickness wounds, regeneration occurs from wound margins, while in partial-thickness wounds remnants of partially ablated hair follicles also contribute to re-epithelialisation (Doughty and Sparks-Defriese 2007). Contraction and epithelialisation can be identified by a marginal zone of smooth tissue.

The maturation phase

This phase involves remodelling the tissue to form a **scar.** This can take a year or more as cellular activity reduces and the number of blood vessels in the wound decreases (Krizek *et al.* 1997).

ACTIVITY

Prepare notes on the phases of healing, which are outlined briefly above, from your recommended biology textbook. Focus your reading on the requirements for each phase of the healing process.

Your reading should have helped you to understand that the wound healing process is a complex interplay of events leading to complete healing.

Aim to observe an uncomplicated surgical wound, or a minor traumatic wound – this could even be a laceration on your own skin. Compare the appearance of the wound to the described criteria for different phases of healing. Discuss with a practitioner which phase of healing is predominant at present.

At different phases of wound healing, the tissue has a different appearance.

- When observed in the *inflammatory phase,* the wound appears swollen and red, and the surrounding tissue feels warm and can be painful. Recognising these signs (which occur due to local vasodilation) can be difficult at first. In the inflammatory phase, the wound is usually kept covered to prevent contamination.
- In the *proliferative phase,* signs of wound contraction commence. The appearance of tiny red buds is the first sign of primitive blood vessels emerging, acting as a transport system for nutrients, oxygen, cells and growth factors essential for connective tissue development (Timmons 2006). This friable tissue which fills the deficit at the wound bed is also referred to as granulation tissue. New epithelial cells divide and, using a leapfrog action, migrate from wound edges and any remaining islands of epidermal cells that may encompass sebaceous glands and hair follicles.
- A wound in the *maturation phase* may remain in this phase for up to two years. It will appear smaller, and may be white and hard (scar tissue) and fixed to surrounding tissue, or similar in appearance to surrounding tissue, indicating a healed mature wound. The maximum tensile strength after injury is 70–85 per cent (Levenson *et al.* 1965).

Gray *et al.* (2004) summarise the implications of the different colours of wounds as:

- **black**: necrotic (dead) tissue and therefore no healing has begun (Plate 1);
- **yellow**: slough (made up of dead cells) – occurs near the end of the inflammatory stage (Plate 2);
- **red**: granulation tissue (Plate 3);
- **pink**: epithelialisation (Plate 4).

Consider how the community nurse for learning disabilities might reduce Susan's anxiety about her wound, and prepare her for suture removal.

The community nurse will need to have assessed Susan's cognitive and physical ability to care for her wound and would then be able to help Susan to understand the wound's healing and the care it requires.

The nurse can use effective communication skills to ascertain Susan's understanding of the healing process, and her anxieties about this. Photos and pictures might be helpful. The nurse could encourage Susan to look at the wound and point out the signs of healing, explaining about the sutures being removed when the wound is healed.

Once Susan understands how the wound is healing, the nurse can then explain why she need not be afraid of showering, give her practical advice about drying herself without rubbing the wound itself, and about wearing clothing that will not rub the wound. The nurse must similarly ensure that Susan's carers understand these issues so they can reinforce the information and be consistent in their reassurance and explanation.

The nurse can prepare Susan for her suture removal and will be able to ensure that the practice nurse removing Susan's sutures knows how Susan communicates and how she has been prepared. If there is anyone who has a healed surgical wound, perhaps Susan could, with the person's permission, talk to them. Actually seeing a healed wound might help to allay her anxiety, if this is possible to arrange.

All the above aspects should be incorporated in Susan's Health Action Plan.

> **Health Action Plan**
> A personal action plan developed for each individual with a learning disability, containing details of their health interventions, medication taken, screening tests, etc. See *Valuing People* (DH 2001).

Learning outcome 2: Show awareness that healing does not in reality occur in a simple linear fashion

Owing to a number of factors, wound healing is not always a straightforward process. A review of wounds caused by trauma, pressure or ulceration illustrates these issues. These wounds are considered in further detail in the later section 'Classification of wounds and their management'.

ACTIVITY

If possible, select a patient with a wound caused by trauma, pressure or ulceration, in discussion with your practice mentor. Try to find out about the history of the wound and its healing process to date. Compare your investigations with the discussion below.

Trauma

Traumatic wounds vary greatly in nature. While minor wounds may heal in a straightforward manner, others involve extensive skin loss and contamination, which can affect the healing process and may require surgical intervention.

Pressure ulcers

Impaired circulation to the skin for even short periods is problematic in susceptible individuals, such as people who are frail, older or malnourished – consult Chapter 6 for a full discussion of pressure ulcers. Mrs Warner, as an older person who also has diabetes and had a period of immobility on a hard surface (the kitchen floor), was obviously a high-risk individual. The discoloured areas on Mrs Warner's elbows could potentially develop into necrotic ulcers similar to her sacral pressure ulcer.

Leg and foot ulceration

There are many causes of leg/foot ulceration, each having different distinguishing features, underlying pathology and treatment, but the majority are associated with circulatory problems (Nelson and Bradley 2007). For example:
- *diffusion* – problems arise when the distance between the capillary and tissue cells is increased (e.g. by oedema);
- *perfusion* – occurs when there is arterial or venous insufficiency.

Currently there are three national guidelines for leg ulcer care, produced by the Royal College of Nursing (RCN) (1998), the Clinical Resource Efficiency Support Team (CREST) (1998), and the Scottish Intercollegiate Guidelines Network (SIGN) (1998).

Ulcers are an increasingly common chronic wound and are often an extensive and longstanding problem (Anderson 2006). Plate 5 shows a large venous leg ulcer, which the patient concerned has had for many years. Briggs and Closs (2003) reviewed the literature relating to leg ulcer incidence and concluded that 0.11–0.18 per cent of the population have an open ulcer and that approximately 1–2 per cent of the population will suffer a leg ulcer at some point in their lives. It is estimated that 70 per cent of ulcers are venous in origin and 25 per cent are arterial (Nelson and Bradley 2007), but the ulcer can be of mixed aetiology too. Useful overviews of lower leg ulceration can be found in Doughty and Holbrook (2007) and Anderson (2006). There are also many books devoted entirely to leg ulcers and their management.

Diabetic ulcers can occur on the feet of people with diabetes; these are complex wounds and cause unacceptably high levels of morbidity and mortality (McIntosh 2006). Plate 1 shows how severe these ulcers can potentially be. A systematic review indicated that education of people with diabetes can reduce foot ulceration in high-risk patients (Valk *et al.* 2001). Additionally guidelines for patients and healthcare professionals have been developed by NICE (2004) and the International Working Group on the Diabetic Foot (1999) on how to prevent, detect and treat foot ulceration. However, Mrs Warner's depression could affect her ability to carry out this self-care (see Chapter 8, Box 8.2, 'Foot care').

You should now be aware that some wounds progress in a complicated fashion owing to underlying health problems. These complex wounds often necessitate a multidisciplinary team approach in diagnosis and management, with investigations performed to ensure accurate identification of the problem.

A scar is the end result of healing, but the formation of a mature scar can be a slow process. A scar is the product of many cells. However, specialist myofibroblast cells have a key role in healing, by shrinking the wound by contraction (Timmons 2006). Note that 75 per cent of normal wound healing is by contraction, which results in a smaller, less visible scar. A scar initially consists of raised vascularised tissue – hence the red colour. Gradually the redness disappears as the number of blood vessels reduces, and the colour changes to white. As noted earlier, the new tissue will not be as strong as previously and may predispose an individual such as Mrs Warner to increased risk of pressure ulcer damage.

Some individuals have problems with hypertrophic scars and keloids. While hypertrophic scars can regress, keloid scars do not. Management of both of these problems requires a specialist and multidisciplinary team approach, for both the physical and the psychological problems that may accompany them.

> **Hypertrophic scar**
> A raised, healed red scar that is uncomfortable and tight. This is caused by an increased deposition of collagen within the area of the original wound (Weiss 1995).

> **Keloid**
> A firm mass of scar caused by excessive collagen deposition, but it extends outside the wound boundaries (Weiss 1995).

Summary

- Wound healing is a complex process involving phases of healing through which the wound must pass in order to heal adequately.

- The process is theoretically sequential, but in reality parts of different phases occur concurrently.
- The end result is a scar of uncertain appearance and weakened structure in comparison to surrounding undamaged tissue.

CLASSIFICATION OF WOUNDS AND WOUND CLOSURE

Wounds are often divided into *acute* and *chronic*. Acute wounds result from surgery or trauma and usually heal relatively quickly with minimal need for external interventions, if no complications occur (Timmons 2006). Burns, due to the area of tissue damage, often behave more like chronic wounds (Timmons 2006).

Chronic wounds, such as leg ulcers, pressure ulcers, diabetic foot ulcers, malignant wounds and any non-healing acute wound, are usually caused by underlying health problems – so haemostasis may be absent from the process, and the individual's ability to heal is often impaired. Features of chronic wounds include their problematic and slow nature of healing, accompanied by other health, social and psychological problems. In chronic wounds, the inflammatory response is continually stimulated by the underlying disease process, resulting in a prolonged and excessive inflammatory phase of wound healing (Timmons 2006).

Learning to classify wounds will enable you to appreciate issues affecting their management, thus planning more effective care. There are a variety of ways of classifying wounds; this chapter uses a simple classification based on the cause.

LEARNING OUTCOMES

By the end of this section you will be able to:
1 distinguish between acute and chronic wounds;
2 discuss the principles of wound closure for different types of acute and chronic wounds.

Learning outcome 1: Distinguish between acute and chronic wounds

ACTIVITY

Table 7.1 shows a classification of wounds and Table 7.2 shows a classification of surgical wounds. Working from these tables, how would you classify the wounds of Mrs Warner, Susan and Colin?

You should have identified that Mrs Warner's sacral wound is a chronic pressure ulcer and her toe wound is probably a chronic diabetic foot ulcer. Susan and Colin both have acute surgical wounds. However, while Susan's is a clean contaminated wound, Colin's is a dirty wound as it contained pus. Plate 6 shows the wound of a man who had a hip replacement 10 days previously and has now had his skin closures removed. This wound would be categorised as a clean surgical wound. Now try using the table to classify wounds of patients/clients in the practice setting, in the following activity.

Table 7.1: Wound classification

Classification	Types of wound	Causes and features
Acute	Penetrating wounds	Causative objects include missiles (e.g. bullets, explosion debris) or hand-held objects (e.g. knives, billiard cues etc) High infection risk
Acute	Lacerations	Healing affected by the cause (whether it is a clean wound or is contaminated by dirt/debris), age of the wound and the individual Wounds involving the eyes and joints are priorities
Acute	Abrasions	Caused by the body being dragged against an abrasive surface, removing surface epithelium Can be very painful and sensitive as nerve endings are exposed If not meticulously cleaned, 'tattooing' results from dirt trapped in the dermis and epidermis, which is almost impossible to remove (Evans and Jones 1996)
Acute	Bites	Common cause of wounds; most are caused by dogs, but human bites are also common (Higgins et al. 1997) High infection risk owing to the large number of microorganisms found in mouths
Acute	Surgical	As these wounds are planned, risks (e.g. of infection) can be reduced to a minimum Infection rates vary according to the type of surgery (see Table 7.2) Mishriki et al. (1990) found an overall infection rate of 7.3% but this was affected by variables (e.g. age, surgeon) Bremmelgaard et al. (1989) found infection rates ranging from 2.3% (clean wounds) to 27.1% (dirty wounds)
Acute	Burns	Can be thermal (caused by flame, hot fluid or radiation), chemical (acid or alkali), or electrical. Can damage the epidermis only (superficial), the epidermis and the dermis (partial thickness) or extend into deeper tissue (full thickness). The extent of the burn is very important to assess, as fluid resuscitation may be needed.
Chronic	Venous leg ulcers	Caused by damage to the venous system in the leg, especially the valves, causing pooling and distending of vessels; byproducts of this process cause tissue death and ulcer formation Risk factors include varicose veins and rheumatoid arthritis Ulcers are usually shallow and situated in the gaiter area, with irregular edges (Doughty and Holbrook 2007) Pain may be severe, dull or aching
Chronic	Arterial leg ulcers	Occur when impaired blood supply due to various causes leads to areas of skin death, as the blood vessel supplying the area becomes occluded Ischaemic pain occurs and the ulcers tend to be small and deep with well-defined borders, situated at distal body locations (e.g. toes) (Doughty and Holbrook 2007)
Chronic	Diabetic neuropathic or neuro-ischaemic foot ulcers	Chronic hyperglycaemia causes impairment of the nerve supply to the foot and lower limb; the resulting loss of sensation can lead to pressure damage, repeated trauma and/or penetration by foreign bodies These ulcers are neuropathic in origin In neuro-ischaemic ulcers, the combination of neuropathy and arterial disease produces a very complex wound with a poor prognosis
Chronic	Pressure ulcers	Prolonged pressure on the skin produces obstruction of small vessels, resulting in death of skin, and sometimes deeper tissues, owing to lack of blood supply Shearing and friction also contribute to their development
Chronic	Infection-induced	Opportunistic organisms gain access through the skin via a small wound, and produce an ulcer Tropical ulcers are one of the most common forms
Chronic	Ulcers caused by cancer	Referred to as fungating wounds, these can complicate cancers in various areas of the body They present as a rapidly growing fungus or with a cauliflower-like appearance which may ulcerate (Goldberg and McGynn-Byer 2007)

Table 7.2: Classification of surgical wounds (Cruse and Foord 1980)

Type	Features	Infection rate
Clean	Surgery without infection present and no entry into hollow muscular organs. Appendicectomy, cholecystectomy and hysterectomy are included in this category if there is no acute inflammation	1.5%
Clean contaminated	Hollow muscular organ penetrated, but minimal spillage of contents occurred	7.7%
Contaminated	Hollow muscular organ opened with gross spillage of contents, or acute inflammation but no pus found. Traumatic wounds less than 4 hours of occurrence	15.2%
Dirty	Traumatic wound over 4 hours old. Surgery where there is presence of pus or a perforated viscus	40.0%

ACTIVITY

With reference to Tables 7.1 and 7.2, explore the nature and cause of wounds within your practice setting. Do all the wounds clearly fit into a category type? Are there any wounds that started as acute, and have ended up as chronic? If so, why?

Wounds are not always easy to categorise. Acute surgical wounds can break down and sometimes appear similar to pressure ulcers, thus starting as acute but becoming chronic. The underlying reasons are not always clearly understood, but often relate to the person's physical health. About 21000 surgical wounds per year in England and Wales become difficult to heal; that is, they do not heal in the normal way (NICE 2001). Plate 7 shows an abdominal wound, 5 days after surgery. The distal part has broken down due to infection and the clips have had to be removed early.

Learning outcome 2: Discuss the principles of wound closure for different types of acute and chronic wounds

Gottrup (1999) identified that wounds may be closed through:
• primary closure;
• early (delayed primary) closure, that is 4–6 days (performed before there is visible granulation tissue);
• late (secondary) closure, that is 10–14 days;
• grafting using skin or artificial skin products;
• no closure (leaving the wound to heal by granulation).

When wounds are closed (i.e. the skin edges are brought together), the wound is said to be healing by **primary intention.** Plate 6 shows a good example of a surgical wound that has healed by primary intention. When wounds are left open, this is termed healing by **secondary intention.** Although the wound in Plate 7 was planned to heal by primary intention, the lower part may have to heal by secondary intention unless the wound is reclosed after the infection has cleared. **Tertiary intention** consists of wound closure via surgical reconstruction techniques.

Try to find out how and when wounds are closed by observing in practice and asking practitioners. Consider:
- a surgical wound (such as Susan's abdominal wound);
- a traumatic wound
- a chronic wound (such as Mrs Warner's pressure ulcer).

Also find out how long closure materials (clips, staples or sutures), if present, are left in the wound before removal. Does the site of the wound have any effect on this?

Surgical wounds

Clean or clean–contaminated wounds are managed by primary closure, using sutures, staples or clips, at the end of surgery. The aim is to protect the wound from the bacteria circulating in a hospital environment (Chapter 3 has more information on preventing cross-infection) and promote the best cosmetic result. Thus Susan's wound will have been managed by primary closure at the end of her operation, as were the wounds shown in Plates 6 and 7.

With contaminated or dirty surgical wounds, delayed primary closure may be preferable. In some cases the wound may be left open, to heal by secondary intention. A dirty, infected wound, such as Colin's, will be left open to enable continuing drainage; closing the wound would allow build-up of pus and a further abscess.

Traumatic wounds

Management of traumatic wounds depends on the degree of contamination (taking into account where and how the wound occurred), the extent of skin damage/skin loss, the site of the wound, and how long ago the injury occurred. A clean incisional wound, with little tissue damage, that occurred less than 6 hours previously (caused by a knife for example) can be irrigated, debrided and managed by primary closure. However, if the injury is more than 6 hours old, or is heavily contaminated, for example by soil, then primary closure should be delayed (Niazi and Sacks 2005; Leaper 2006; Morris 2006).

There may be differing priorities though. Bites should usually be left to heal by secondary intention owing to their infection risk; exceptions are made where cosmetic effects are paramount, or restoring function takes priority (Mcheik *et al.* 2000). Facial wounds have an excellent blood supply and rarely become infected.

Incised wounds and lacerations can be closed with tapes, sutures or tissue adhesive, the choice depending on factors such as size, depth and site. Tissue adhesive could be suitable for a small scalp wound, due to decreased procedure time and less pain, but should not be used for lacerations of the nostril, mouth or eye, where suturing is preferable to ensure accuracy of alignment (Farion *et al.* 2001; Leaper 2006).

If a person with a traumatic wound has delayed seeking attention, then prolonged bacterial access will have occurred. Usually the wound will be cleansed with the aim of free drainage and/or detection of infection, followed by delayed primary closure by suturing at 4–6 days. Gottrup (1999) explains that secondary closure is used when a wound is heavily contaminated. Although this leaves a broader scar than after primary (early or delayed) closure, it is still cosmetically preferable to that achieved through the healing of an open granulating wound.

Chronic wounds

Chronic wounds are usually allowed to heal by secondary intention. Granulation tissue fills the defect and new epidermis covers the surface. This is slow and time-consuming and provides poor protection against risks such as repeated pressure and infection. It can, nevertheless, provide a successful outcome. Mrs Warner's pressure ulcer will need to heal by secondary intention. When surgical excision of necrotic tissue as in a pressure ulcer is performed, the aim is also for healing to occur by secondary intention. Attempts to directly close large defects by bringing the edges of the wound together have often been unsuccessful, since the tension on the suture line pulls the wound apart. An alternative is to use surgical techniques such as skin grafting and skin flaps, examples of tertiary intention. Beldon (2007) gives a brief overview of these techniques and their care.

When to remove skin closures

The decision on when to remove skin closures depends on various factors.

- Site. The face heals faster – sutures are often removed in 5 days. The feet heal more slowly, so sutures may be left *in situ* for 7–10 days.
- Factors such as ageing and diabetes can affect the rate of healing (see section on 'Factors affecting wound healing').

Patients being discharged from hospital with skin closures *in situ* must be informed of exactly when and where the skin closures will be removed. Susan's sutures would probably be ready for removal at 7 days, and she can attend her local health centre for their removal by the practice nurse. Sometimes it is necessary to arrange for the district nurse to visit a patient's home for skin closure removal, for example, if it is difficult for the person to leave the house due to poor general condition or lack of mobility. Adhesive glue has the advantage of not needing removal.

Summary

- Acute wounds usually heal uneventfully and quickly, but can in certain situations become chronic.
- Chronic wounds frequently fail to heal in a timely and orderly fashion.
- Different types of wound are managed in different ways. In general, clean surgical wounds heal by primary direct closure, contaminated traumatic wounds heal by delayed primary closure, and chronic wounds heal by secondary intention healing.

FACTORS AFFECTING WOUND HEALING

There are a wide range of biological, psychological and sociological factors that influence wound healing. It is important to identify factors that may affect wound healing for individuals, as a perpetuating wound will result if underlying causes are not addressed (Morris 2006; Troxler *et al.* 2006). A multidisciplinary approach may be needed to address these factors. Patients with acute wounds that are healing by primary intention usually require less input, but each individual should be assessed.

LEARNING OUTCOMES

On completion of this section you will be able to:
1 explore the range of factors that can affect wound healing;
2 identify how a multidisciplinary approach can address factors affecting wound healing;

Learning outcome 1: Explore the range of factors that can affect wound healing

Table 7.3 identifies general factors that can delay wound healing. When assessing a person with a wound, consider these questions:
- What underlying factors are interfering with wound healing?
- Does the patient have an underlying condition that is delaying wound healing?
- Does the wound require debridement?
- Is the wound infected?
- What needs to be changed to move the wound healing process forward?

The following exercise is based on this framework.

ACTIVITY

With the guidance of your practice mentor, identify a person who (like Mrs Warner) has a problematic wound. Carry out the activity below.
- Look at their assessment documentation. Identify any factors that could influence wound healing (Table 7.3 will give you clues). Remember to consider the person as a whole, as well as their wound.
- Then ask yourself, can these factors be altered/changed? What action could help?

Table 7.4 includes factors that might have been identified for Mrs Warner. Compare the list you prepared for your patient with this. You may well have identified a much

Table 7.3: General factors for delayed healing (Troxler *et al.* 2006). Reproduced with kind permission from World Wide Wounds.

Age	Immunosuppression
Anaemia	Microbes
Decreased oxygen	Necrotic tissue
Decreased perfusion	Nutrition (vitamins, minerals)
Dehydration	Oedema
Diabetes mellitus	Organ failure
Foreign body	Radiation
Malignancy	Smoking
Medication, such as corticosteroids, cytotoxics	Other wound-related factors

Table 7.4: Factors influencing Mrs Warner's wound healing.

Factor	Rationale for identification	Can be influenced?	Action required
Smoking	Serensen (2003) outlines effects of smoking on tissue function Smoking causes a compromised blood supply to the wound, and impairs the cardiovascular system, delaying healing It leads to inhibition of epithelialisation and a reduction in wound contraction	Potentially	Reduction in smoking balanced against quality of life issues
Diabetes mellitus and elevated blood glucose level	People with diabetes have impaired wound healing (NICE 2004) A wide range of underlying pathologies are responsible	Yes	Blood glucose monitoring, medication and dietary considerations
Depression	Depression affects ability to self-care, for example to manage her diabetes, relieve pressure, and care for her feet	Yes	Pharmacology and therapeutic approach
Poor nutritional intake	Adequate nutrients required for wound healing (see Table 7.5)	Yes	Promote nutritious and balanced diet
Ageing	The skin's ability to repair reduces with ageing (Pittman 2007) The disease processes that often accompany ageing may impair healing (Partridge 1998; Pittman 2007)	Indirectly by improving overall health	General health promotion
Stress and anxiety about being in hospital	Stress delays healing (Boore 1978; Kiecolt-Glaser et al. 1995; Jones 2003)	Potentially	Develop nurse–patient relationship, identify and address sources of anxiety
Infection in toe wound	Infection compromises healing, places stress on the body, and impairs diabetes stabilisation	Yes	Investigations (e.g. X-ray to identify whether there is bone infection) Wound management and antibiotics
Necrotic tissue in sacral ulcer	Necrotic tissue prevents wound healing	Yes	Debride necrotic tissue using suitable method

wider range of issues, depending on your individual patient (see also Miller 1999a; Partridge 1998).

You probably considered general health, age and nutrition. Other chronic conditions that affect wound healing include respiratory and cardiovascular disease, owing to their effect on tissue oxygenation (Williams and Young 1998). Plate 8 shows how a lack of blood supply affects skin and deeper tissues. This patient had heart failure and a lack of circulation to her feet, causing necrosis. An adequate blood supply to the skin and underlying tissues is essential, both to prevent wounds and to promote wound healing.

Are you aware of the effect of steroids on wound healing? The anti-inflammatory response of steroids reduces the inflammatory response, and affects the function of the macrophages, thus slowing healing (Williams and Young 1998).

Did you also identify stress and anxiety as a factor? This too can have a major influence on wound healing (Jones 2003); provision of information can contribute

Table 7.5: Nutrients required for wound healing and their function (adapted from Williams and Young 1998, pp. 26–7).

Nutrient	Function
Carbohydrate	Energy source for increased cellular activity during wound healing
Fat	Alternative energy source Fat-soluble vitamins are essential for the building of new cell membranes in wound repair
Protein	Essential for building the new wound bed (collagen formation) Patients already protein-depleted before wounding are worse effected
Vitamin A	Supports epithelial proliferation and consequent migration across granulation tissue More efficient when given prior to wounding
Vitamin B	Assists formation of collagen mesh which supports new blood vessels as they move into granulating tissue
Vitamin C	Assists formation of collagen mesh
Vitamin E	With vitamin C, attacks damaging oxygen free radicals that are present in infected wounds and during the inflammatory phase of wound healing
Minerals: zinc, copper, iron	Required for collagen formation Zinc also has an antibacterial effect, mainly against Gram-positive bacteria

to effective healing (Boore 1978). Colin has a longstanding mental health problem, and the discomfort associated with his wound may be a further source of stress. Susan, too, has been through a stressful experience. Now that she is back in her own environment with familiar staff members, it will be important to be supportive and reassuring. Thus nurses should aim to relieve their stress and anxieties and help them to relax (see Chapter 2).

Chapter 10 highlights the need for an increased nutritional intake for wound healing. However, many people with chronic wounds, such as pressure ulcers, have poor nutritional intake and risk factors for malnutrition (Williams and Leaper 2000; Gray and Cooper 2001). Williams and Young (1998) suggest that every patient with a wound should be assessed nutritionally. Table 7.5 outlines the key nutrients required for wound healing and their role in the process. Stotts (2007) extensively reviewed the literature linking nutrition and wound healing.

Finally, you may have identified factors to do with the condition of the wound and how it is being managed. Relevant factors include aspects to do with the wound itself, for example the presence of necrotic (dead) tissue or infection – both factors relevant to Mrs Warner. How the wound is being managed is also relevant. For example, frequent and excessive exposure of the wound causes a drop in temperature at the wound bed, and inappropriate use of antiseptics or certain wound products can damage fragile new tissue. All these factors could delay healing and are considered later in this chapter in the section 'Wound management'.

Learning outcome 2: Identify how a multidisciplinary approach can address factors affecting wound healing

Addressing factors affecting healing requires multidisciplinary team working, including relatives and the client, whose involvement is essential in the process of wound healing (Williams and Young 1998).

ACTIVITY Look back at Table 7.4 and list members of the multidisciplinary team who might be involved in addressing the factors affecting Mrs Warner's wound healing. Make a note of what their specific roles might be.

Mrs Warner, who has chronic wounds, would require considerable multidisciplinary teamwork to address the factors affecting her wound healing. Compare your list with Table 7.6, which gives some ideas; you may have thought of others.

If psychological adjustment relating to a wound is problematic, input from a psychologist is sometimes necessary. Voluntary organisations can also play a part in supporting individuals – Diabetes UK in Mrs Warner's case.

Summary

- A range of factors can potentially interfere with the healing process of a wound. These factors relate to the individual's general health status, the condition of the wound, and the care being received.
- Nurses should identify factors affecting wound healing in individuals and plan strategies to address them where possible, involving the multidisciplinary team appropriately.

Table 7.6: Addressing factors affecting wound healing: suggested multidisciplinary team (MDT) involvement for Mrs Warner.

MDT member	Role
Ward nurse	Blood glucose monitoring, improving nutritional status, relieving stress/anxiety etc., mobilisation, pressure relieving strategies, wound assessment and appropriate wound care, education of patient/carer and health promotion, support and information giving, liaison with other nurses, relatives and MDT
Specialist nurses: infection control, diabetes, nutritional support, tissue viability, dermatology, discharge liaison.	Specialist advice, education and support for patient and family, and ward team, to address the factors affecting wound healing and advise on appropriate strategies Equipment provision and resources
Physiotherapist	Promote mobility and correct positioning Education and advice
Occupational therapist	Positioning, mobility and dressing aids, seating, adaptations/equipment for home
Social worker	Discharge arrangements and support at home (e.g. home care, meals, day centre, financing of home adaptations/equipment)
Podiatrist	Foot care
Doctor	Blood glucose control, prescribing medication, surgical debridement of wounds (if needed), identifying and treating other health problems which may delay healing, liaison with GP
Pharmacist	Advice on wound care products
Dietician	Assessment and advice on dietary supplements
Primary Health Care Team: district nurse, health visitor, GP, practice nurse	Medical and nursing care in the community after discharge Assessment of health needs in the community
Chaplain	Spiritual needs and support

WOUND ASSESSMENT

As discussed in the previous section, when assessing a wound you must consider the whole person, so factors that could interfere with healing can be addressed wherever possible. This section now prepares you to assess the wound itself, based on your knowledge of the phases of wound healing, the ability to classify wounds and an awareness of wider issues that affect wound healing. All these aspects underpin the assessment process. Useful articles relating to wound assessment include Miller (1996, 1999b) and Gray *et al.* (2004).

LEARNING OUTCOMES

By the end of this section you will be able to:
1 discuss the features of a wound assessment and how wound assessment tools/charts can be used;
2 record key information in a useful format that can be used to plan appropriate interventions.

Learning outcome 1: Discuss the features of a wound assessment and how wound assessment tools/charts can be used

Wound grading tools provide information on the wound. For example, the *Pressure Ulcer Classification Guide* produced by EPUAP (European Pressure Ulcer Advisory Panel) is used to grade the degree of damage of pressure ulcers (see Box 7.1 and Fig. 7.1 for illustrations). Charts may include a diagram of the body for marking the location of the wound(s). The Red–Yellow–Black (RYB) system (Gray *et al.* 2004) is based on assessing the condition of the wound bed and has been incorporated in the wound assessment tool included in this chapter. Evaluating tissue type by a single variable such as colour has been described as limiting (Nix 2007), but it can be used as a basis for selecting a dressing. If you look at Plates 1–5,

Box 7.1 Pressure ulcer classification (EPUAP 1998)

- *Grade 1.* Non-blanchable erythema of intact skin. Discoloration of the skin, warmth, oedema, induration or hardness may also be used as indicators, particularly on individuals with darker skin.
- *Grade 2.* Partial-thickness skin loss involving epidermis, dermis, or both. The ulcer is superficial and presents clinically as an abrasion or blister.
- *Grade 3.* Full-thickness skin loss involving damage to, or necrosis of, subcutaneous tissue that may extend down to – but not through – underlying fascia.
- *Grade 4.* Extensive destruction, tissue necrosis, or damage to muscle, bone, or supporting structures with or without full-thickness skin loss.

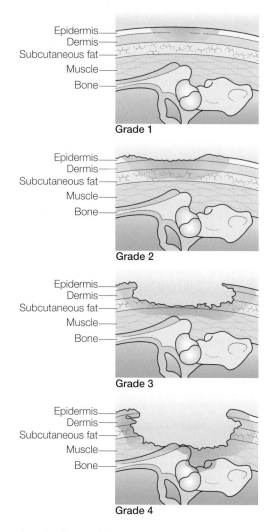

Figure 7.1: Pressure ulcer classification (EPUAP 1998).

you can see how the colours in the RYB system could be applied to these wounds (e.g. Plate 1: black).

Figure 7.2 gives an example of a wound assessment chart, which incorporates elements of both the Red–Yellow–Black and the EPUAP pressure ulcer classification systems. Its features are discussed below in relation to Mrs Warner's sacral pressure ulcer. Note that she would require a chart like this for each of her wounds as each must be assessed separately.

- *Wound site.* As stated earlier, a body map can be used to indicate this as well as writing 'sacrum' at the top of the chart.
- *Wound category.* This relates to the wound classification discussed earlier. Mrs Warner's sacral wound will be recorded as a pressure ulcer and then graded using the EPUAP pressure ulcer classification system (Box 7.1 and Figure 7.1).

Wound Assessment Record

Buckinghamshire Hospitals **NHS**

NHS Trust

WOUND SITE		

WOUND CATEGORY (please tick) Surgical Traumatic Burn Fistula/sinus Pressure Ulcer EPUAP 1 2 3 4 Leg ulcer Diabetic foot ulcer Fungating lesion Peg site	Patient Label		

	WARD	
	CONSULTANT	
MEDICATION (anti-inflammatory, steroids, cytoxic, anticoagulants)	**ALLERGIES**	

DATE OF ASSESSMENT			
PAIN - Site Intensity (circle score) Analgesics required?	1 2 3 4 5 6 7 8 9 10 Yes/No	1 2 3 4 5 6 7 8 9 10 Yes/No	1 2 3 4 5 6 7 8 9 10 Yes/No
PHOTOGRAPH (consent obtained)			
MEASUREMENT (cms) Width Length			
DEPTH (cms) partial/full thickness, tendon underlying structure exposed			
TYPE/COLOUR OF TISSUE (record %) necrotic (black) sloughy (yellow) granulating (red) epithelialising (pink) infected (green)			
SIGNS OF INFECTION (redness, purulent, inflammation, pyrexia, patient unwell)			
MALODOUR	Yes/No	Yes/No	Yes/No
SWAB TAKEN	Yes/No	Yes/No	Yes/No
EXUDATE (High, medium, low)			
COLOUR OF EXUDATE			
SURROUNDING SKIN healthy macerated erythema eczema cellulitis			
WOUND EDGES (shallow, rolled, punched out, undermined)			
DRESSING SELECTION			
FREQUENCY OF CHANGE			
ASSESSORS SIGNATURE			
DATE OF REASSESSMENT			

Figure 7.2: Example of a wound assessment chart. Reproduced with kind permission from Buckinghamshire Hospitals NHS Trust.

- *Medication.* Mrs Warner could be taking medication that will affect wound healing.
- *Allergies.* Mrs Warner could have a known allergy to a dressing product, which should be noted.

- *Pain.* Assessment of pain, using a number intensity scale where 1 is no pain and 10 is the worst pain imaginable, needs to occur prior to removing the dressing to establish if Mrs Warner requires any analgesics and whether the current pain management strategy is effective. If the pain only occurs during dressing removal, a different product may be required. If the pain has increased and is associated with other signs and symptoms such as malodour, inflammation, increased exudate, and delayed wound healing, a wound infection may be present (Kingsley *et al.* 2004).

- *Photograph.* Increasingly photos are used in wound assessment but consent from the patient must be obtained, preferably in writing. Often a ruler is placed by the side of the wound when taking the photograph, showing the wound's size as well as its appearance (see Plate 3). Clearly the sacral area would be a sensitive area to photograph and the reasons for doing so need careful explanation. However, the photos can be shown to Mrs Warner to help her to appreciate the nature of the wound, and how its healing is progressing.

- *Measurement.* The size is recorded in centimetres as width by length. Sometimes a tracing is made, which creates a record of shape as well as size and this can be attached.

- *Depth.* Depth is difficult to measure but a wound probe or sterile wound swab can be used and then measured against a ruler. The depth of the wound can also be assessed through the identification of exposed structures such as tendon or bone.

- *Type/colour of tissue.* This is where the RYB system has been incorporated into the tool to assist in identifying the type of tissue within the wound bed.
  - black = necrotic tissue
  - yellow = sloughy tissue
  - red = granulating tissue
  - pink = epithelialisation
  - green = infected tissue.

  The wound base may have several different types of tissue present. For example, Plate 5 shows a wound base that has both sloughy (yellow) areas and granulation tissue (red). Nurses assessing this wound would need to estimate the percentage of the wound bed covered with slough (yellow), and the percentage covered with granulation tissue (red) and record this on the chart. For Mrs Warner the recording will be 100 per cent necrotic (black), but in due course as the wound progresses there will be sloughy (yellow) areas, and then it is hoped some granulation tissue (red), and then areas that are epithelialising (pink). Necrotic tissue (black, as in Mrs Warner's sacral pressure ulcer and Plate 1) prevents or delays the healing process and therefore needs debriding to enable healing to progress.

- *Infection.* Several signs discussed so far will help to identify whether infection is present. This should be assessed at each dressing change as the presence of infection delays wound healing. See the European Wound Management Association's (2005) position statement for identifying a wound infection.

- *Malodour.* A slight odour can occur due to wound occlusion and is associated with some types of dressing. However, an offensive odour is often a sign of infection. Necrotic wounds (Mrs Warner's sacral pressure ulcer) and fungating wounds are often malodorous. Assessing odour can help to identify infection, as one of a range of criteria, but also helps with dressing choice as some dressings are deodorising.
- *Swab taken.* Wound swabs taken should be recorded but they have limitations. How and when to take wound swabs is discussed in Chapter 3. The nurses must remember to check the results and discuss with the medical staff whether it is appropriate to treat the wound with antibiotics or with an antibacterial dressing containing substances such as iodine, silver or honey.
- *Exudate.* This is fluid arising from the wound owing to increased permeability of capillaries. Estimating the amount of exudate (high, medium or low) is not easy. However, the presence and extent of exudate will influence your dressing choice. The production of large or increased amounts of exudate or pus could indicate infection, but other signs and symptoms (as discussed previously) should be taken into account too.
- *Colour of exudate.* The colour of the exudate will also indicate if infection is present in the wound.
- *Condition of surrounding skin.* This is important in considering the type of dressing to be used. For example, if the skin is moist/macerated a more absorbent dressing is needed. If erythema (redness) or eczema is present, great care will need to be taken in dressing choice and how it is secured. Cellulitis needs to be reported if it is a new feature as it indicates infection is present and systemic antibiotics are needed.
- *Wound edges.* In large and/or deep wounds, the edge of the wound may be undermined, whereby it is possible to reach underneath the edges of the wound. As the wound progresses towards the proliferative phase, a shallow white/pink almost transparent border appears. This new epidermal tissue is fragile and easily removed. Edges that are rolled in can delay healing time. In chronic wounds, the edges can have a punched-out appearance and small satellite wounds can be present. Wound edges that are hard and fibrous indicate a chronic wound.

> **Macerated skin**
> Macerated skin is soft and breaking down due to prolonged contact with excessive amounts of fluid, such as wound exudate (Cutting 1999).

As you can see in Fig. 7.2, the wound chart includes spaces for recording wound care, which is planned on the basis of the assessment.

Assessing a wound might also include any of the following considerations:

- *Is the wound open or closed?* Remember from earlier in this chapter: an open wound is one healing by secondary intention; a closed wound is predominantly healing by first intention. Thus Susan's wound is healing by first intention but Mrs Warner's sacral wound is healing by secondary intention. A dehisced wound is one where tissue has become separated from deeper tissue owing to the presence of infection; this complicates some surgical wounds.
- *Extent of tissue involvement.* Does the wound involve epidermis, dermis, fat, fascia, muscle and/or bone?
- *Presence of foreign bodies.* These delay the healing process. Foreign bodies like dirt or grit can also increase infection risk and lead to permanent marking (Leaper 2006).

- *Presence of a fistula or a sinus.* A fistula is an abnormal connection between two spaces such as skin surface and bowel. A sinus is a tract that ends in a blind cavity, and a sinus is frequently found in a deep pressure ulcer. A sinus should ideally heal from its base; if it heals first at the surface, fluid will accumulate within, promoting an abscess, which will subsequently break through to the surface. In Plate 7, the darkened central area of the dehisced part of the wound was found to be a sinus.
- *Wound drain and drain site.* Wound drains are inserted into some surgical wounds to promote the removal of fluid that would otherwise accumulate and form a potential growing medium for infection, or interfere with healing.

ACTIVITY

Find out whether there is a wound assessment tool/chart used in your local practice setting and try to access it. Otherwise use one from the literature or the one in Fig. 7.2. You also need a measuring instrument such as a ruler (disposable ones are available from wound product manufacturers) and good light. Under supervision, assess a patient's wound and document your assessment. After carrying out this exercise, consider the question: Should a wound assessment tool/chart be used for all wounds?

Minor straightforward wounds do not require a formal recorded assessment. If the wound is healing uneventfully, a record of this in the patient's notes will suffice. This would have been adequate for Susan's surgical wound when she was in hospital, and for the wound shown in Plate 6, which is a straightforward clean surgical wound which healed without complication. Judging when to use a tool/chart involves issues such as a wound that is not healing as expected, possibly reverting to a previous stage, wounds with problems, or where required as a legal record, for example after an assault or suspected neglect/abuse. The assessment of the patient's wound in Plate 7 should be documented on a wound assessment chart as it is complicated by infection causing dehiscence. Mrs Warner's pressure ulcer and ulcerated toe (which could, as a diabetic ulcer, deteriorate) are both chronic and problematic wounds and so the use of assessment tools/charts would be advantageous.

Leg ulcer assessment

All patients presenting with a leg ulcer should be screened for arterial disease by Doppler ultrasound measurement of ankle brachial pressure index (ABPI) by staff trained to carry out this investigation (CREST 1998; RCN 1998; SIGN 1998), alongside a thorough clinical investigation. Often a specific leg ulcer assessment chart is used to record this assessment, which includes documenting assessment of factors affecting wound healing (e.g. smoking, nutritional status) as discussed earlier. The ABPI is calculated by dividing the brachial systolic blood pressure by the ankle systolic blood pressure. A normal ABPI reading is about 1; and if the reading is 0.8 or above compression therapy can usually be applied (CREST 1998; RCN 1998: SIGN 1998). Compression therapy aims to provide graduated compression, with the highest pressure at the ankle and the lowest at the knee, thus returning blood from the lower limb and preventing pooling in distended lower leg veins. An arterial ulcer is caused by an inadequate arterial blood supply to the area, and a patient suspected of having an arterial ulcer may require vascular surgery.

Note: Applying compression to a limb with an arterial ulcer will have catastrophic results for the ulcer and the patient, potentially leading to loss of the limb affected. Thus accurate assessment is essential.

Learning outcome 2: Record key information in a useful format that can be used to plan appropriate interventions

ACTIVITY

Review the material that you recorded by using the wound assessment tool/chart earlier, and consider this question: Is it specific and comprehensive enough to help you to plan the wound's management, and to promote continuity of care?

- The tools employed are generally very wound-specific. They have to be simple to use, yet all-encompassing, but not so inclusive as to waste valuable time and deter usage.
- These are legal documents. Have you accurately described the wound environment? Have you avoided the use of colloquialisms, such as 'wound bed appears fine': what does 'fine' mean? Ensure that you use descriptive language that can be interpreted by anyone, not just yourself. This helps to promote continuity of care.
- A photograph of the wound can provide a more objective record of the wound's status, alleviating potential variation in the use of descriptive terms and their interpretation.
- Can the assessment help you to plan the wound management? Has it identified any problems with the current approach. For example, is the dressing allowing the wound to dry out, or the surrounding skin to become macerated? Was the dressing painful to remove?

Summary

- Wound assessment requires a holistic approach involving assessment of the whole person and the wound together.
- Wound assessment charts assist a systematic process and clear documentation of the wound's progress.
- Documentation is becoming increasingly important, for management as well as litigation reasons.
- Accuracy in recording assessment is an important skill to develop and does much to promote continuity of care, as well as a firm basis for planning interventions.

WOUND MANAGEMENT

You have already considered factors affecting wound healing and have identified that wound management must focus on both the wound and the patient as a whole.

It is important to be aware of the psychosocial effects of wounds, so that you can be supportive; this is relevant to both acute and chronic wounds. The effects on body image of acute wounds can result in a range of psychological reactions, including a grief response, anxiety and depression (Magan 1996; Jones 2003). Neil and Barrell (1998) point out that the skin is 'a major factor in a person's body image', with denial, anxiety, pain, immobility and altered body image experienced by people with chronic wounds. Being aware of this can help health professionals to be understanding, and effective assessment can promote helpful interventions, referrals and information provision (Neil and Barrell 1998).

In this section you will be focusing on care of the wound itself, using a concept called **wound-bed preparation** (WBP). The focus of WBP denotes the importance of removing non-viable tissue through cleansing/debridement, moisture balance, control of oedema and decreased bacterial burden (Falanga 2000; Fletcher 2003), in order to promote healing.

LEARNING OUTCOMES

By the end of this section you will be able to:
1 discuss how wound dressings are performed;
2 explain methods of debridement and cleansing;
3 identify a range of wound dressings, showing awareness of how they are selected for individuals;
4 outline ways of reducing pain and discomfort associated with wounds.

Learning outcome 1: Discuss how wound dressings are performed

For information on aseptic technique, applied to wound dressings, see Chapter 3. A sterile technique has traditionally been used for wound care but it may hold no advantage over a clean technique in some situations. Hollinworth and Kingston (1998) clarify that in both instances prevention of transmission of microorganisms is intended. In essence, when using sterile technique, equipment, fluids and dressings are sterile, while with a clean technique, clean but non-sterile single-use gloves can be used, with tapwater (that is safe enough to drink) used for cleansing.

ACTIVITY

How do you think you might identify when a sterile technique would be essential and when a clean technique might be sufficient?

Williams and Young (1998) suggest that risk to the individual patient should be assessed. Therefore, a sterile technique must be used if the patient is immunocompromised or has undergone surgery, which carries a high infection risk. However, chronic wounds are likely to be colonised with bacteria, so a clean rather than sterile procedure may be sufficient.

Effective handwashing and gloving techniques are essential, whether a sterile or clean technique is used for wound care, and aprons should be worn too (see Chapter 3). Some dressings are difficult to apply using gloves – hand hygiene and a non-touch technique is then essential to prevent contamination of the dressing (Williams and Young 1998). Wound dressings must always be sterile. Use of dressings from an opened pack, even if for the same patient, could introduce contamination and thus delay healing (Williams and Young 1998).

Learning outcome 2: Explain methods of debridement and cleansing

Debridement

Debridement is 'the removal of devitalised or infected tissue, fibrin, or foreign material from a wound' (NICE 2001). The body can naturally carry out debridement via autolytic debridement, but if large quantities of debris are present it delays healing and predisposes to infection. It was identified earlier that Mrs Warner's sacral wound requires debriding of its necrotic tissue. Debridement can be carried out in several ways (see Box 7.2). NICE (2001) reviewed the evidence on debridement for difficult-to-heal surgical wounds, concluding that no particular method could be supported. So the choice of debriding agent should be according to the individual and issues around comfort and odour control.

Dressings promoting autolysis and bio-surgical methods (sterile maggots) may be more acceptable to patients and less painful (NICE 2001). Sherman *et al.*'s (2001) study used maggots to debride non-healing wounds in outpatients, finding that maggot therapy was safe, effective and acceptable to most people. Plate 3 shows a deep sacral pressure ulcer the day after maggots had been removed after 3 days *in situ*. The ulcer, which was 60 per cent covered with slough, is now about 85 per cent granulation tissue. Vacuum-assisted closure uses negative pressure to remove slough and loosen necrotic tissue from the wound bed (Hampton 1999). The use of honey in wound care is also gaining interest. It has been found to have a debriding action as well as many other beneficial effects, for example antibacterial activity (Cooper *et al.* 2002; Morris 2006). However Fox (2002) found the current evidence base for honey to be weak.

Wound cleansing has sometimes been carried out ritualistically without sound rationale for practice.

ACTIVITY

You have probably seen wound cleansing carried out in practice. Think about the following: Why are wounds cleansed? How are wounds cleansed? What are wounds cleansed with? Compare your thoughts with the points below.

Purpose of wound cleansing

The aim of wound cleansing is to remove contaminated/foreign material from the wound bed, i.e. slough, necrotic tissue, exudate and dressing debris. Nurses must decide

Box 7.2 Methods of debridement

Autolytic

- Involves the body's own mechanisms of selective liquefaction, separation and digestion of necrotic tissue that occurs in wounds due to phagocytosis (Vowden and Vowden 2002).
- Enhanced through the presence of a moist wound environment, created by dressings such as hydrogels, hydrocolloids and hydrofiber.
- *Hydrogels* – designed to donate fluid to the wound bed through their high water content (Thomas 1994).
- *Hydrocolloids* – contain gel-forming agents combined with elastomers and an adhesive matrix, which in the presence of exudate forms a moist gel (Thomas 1994).
- *Hydrofiber dressings* – highly absorbent non-woven sheets or ribbon composed entirely of hydrocolloid fibre which in the presence of exudate converts to a soft moist gel (Stringfellow and Russell 2003).

Larvae therapy

Larvae act by moving over the surface of a wound bed and secreting powerful enzymes that break down dead tissue into a liquefied solution which they can then digest together with bacteria present in the wound (Thomas and Jones 1999, 2000; Thomas *et al.* 2002).

Sharp debridement

The removal of dead or foreign material just above the level of viable tissue using a scalpel, performed without anaesthetic by a doctor or an experienced nurse. It requires skill and knowledge of the anatomical structures and should be governed under strict local guidelines (Edwards 2000).

Surgical debridement

The excision or wide resection of necrotic tissue, often extending into the viable tissue. It is performed in the operating theatre by a surgeon (Fairbairn *et al.* 2002).

whether this can be achieved by cleansing or whether debridement, as discussed earlier, is needed. Williams and Young (1998) emphasise that cleansing should not be done unless it is clearly indicated. For example, if the wound is granulating, cleansing is not necessary and may even damage the new tissue; dressing renewal is all that is required. Surface exudate is beneficial to wound healing as it contains essential growth factors, but excessive exudate can macerate the surrounding skin (Fletcher 1997; Cutting 1999) and could provide a good culture medium for bacteria (Casey 1999).

Further reasons for wound cleansing are so that the wound can be assessed, and to maintain hygiene and enhance well-being, particularly when there is excessive exudate and malodour (Gouvela and Miguens 2007). When there is excessive production of exudate, as in infected sites or those with a large surface area, excess exudate should be removed to prevent maceration of surrounding skin, while leaving sufficient fluid in the wound bed to enhance the wound healing process (Gouvela and Miguens 2007).

Cleansing methods

There are a number of documented methods for wound cleansing (Gouvela and Miguens 2007). We will consider swabbing, irrigation and bathing/showering.

- **Swabbing.** Swabbing of wounds, using gloves or forceps and gauze swabs, is a traditional method of wound cleansing, but Thomlinson's (1987) study demonstrated that this merely led to redistribution of microorganisms.
- **Irrigation.** Irrigation of wounds is often considered preferable to swabbing. To irrigate you can use a syringe with a needle or quill, an aerosol spray, a showerhead, or simply pour the fluid over the wound from a sachet or capsule. You need to collect the fluid in a container such as a kidney bowl. The pressure of the irrigation may be difficult to measure or regulate. To dislodge debris from a wound, high-pressure irrigation can be achieved by using a 30 mL syringe with a large gauge needle, and pushing the plunger with maximum force from a distance of 2 cm above the wound (Young 1997). However, there is a risk of contamination to the patient, nurse or the environment should the needle detach (Gouvela and Miguens 2007), so care must be taken.
- **Bathing.** Williams and Young (1998) recommend that bathing a patient with a contaminated sacral pressure ulcer is the most efficient wound cleansing method, and is comforting for the patient. If there is no wound infection present, cleaning of the bath with normal detergent is adequate; but if the wound is infected, the bath should be cleaned with hypochlorite solution. This would be necessary, therefore, if Colin baths, which could well be a soothing method of wound cleansing for him.

How traumatic wounds should be cleansed depends on several factors. Young (1997) recommended that if a person presents with a low-energy traumatic wound within 6 hours of injury and has a clean, uncontaminated incision, it should be irrigated with tepid water or saline. However, a wound presenting more than 12 hours after injury with ragged edges and contamination, and caused by high-energy trauma, requires more extensive cleansing and debridement. Bites, in particular, need very thorough cleansing (Higgins *et al.* 1997).

Wound cleansing solutions

Drosou *et al.*'s (2003) review highlights the clinical controversy surrounding use of antiseptics in open wounds, particularly in relation to:

- whether these solutions are toxic to healing tissue;
- whether they actually promote healing.

Many of the studies to determine the effects of these solutions have been conducted in laboratories rather than clinical trials, and this evidence is therefore not necessarily applicable to the practice setting. However, while antiseptics are undoubtedly antibacterial, they have been found to be quickly inactivated when in contact with body tissues and fluids, pus and necrotic tissue (Hugo and Russell 1992, cited by Leaper 1996). A detailed review of the qualities of povidine–iodine identified that it can prevent colonisation of wounds with pathogenic bacteria, which could prevent

MRSA
A strain of *Staphylococcus aureus* which is highly resistant to many commonly used antibiotics (see Chapter 3).

some from becoming infected, which may be particularly important in the prevention of MRSA infections (Lawrence 1998). However, Young (2000) notes that there is no consensus on the use of antiseptics (e.g. povidine–iodine and chlorhexidine) for wounds containing MRSA. Casey (1999) suggests that, as healing tissue is very delicate, a good strategy is never to use an antiseptic that we would not wish used in our eyes.

While a wide selection of solutions have been used to cleanse wounds, normal saline is often considered the solution of choice, as it is isotonic and non-toxic to healing tissue (Gouvela and Miguens 2007). However, a study comparing tapwater with sterile saline for cleansing acute traumatic wounds found that tapwater appeared to be preferable (Angeras *et al.* 1992).

Williams and Young (1998) noted that chronic wounds always contain large numbers of bacteria, which do not delay wound healing; only systemic infection does this. They therefore suggest that tapwater is a satisfactory cleansing agent, and that for patients with leg ulcers it can be comforting, and psychologically enhancing, to bathe their legs in a bucket lined with a waterproof plastic bag, which can then be disposed of afterwards. Fernandez and Griffiths's (2008) review supported the use of tapwater for wound cleansing, noting that boiled and cooled water as well as distilled water can also be used as wound cleansing agents. However, they also noted that there is no evidence that wound cleansing in itself reduces infection or increases wound healing.

Solutions used for cleansing/irrigating should be used at body temperature if possible, thus reducing the cooling of the wound bed which adversely affects healing (Myers 1982).

Learning outcome 3: Identify a range of wound dressings, showing awareness of how they are selected for individuals

Before considering which dressing to apply, see Table 7.7 which gives an overview of the requirements of the ideal dressing (Thomas 2008). The table details whether each requirement is purely attributed to design and construction of the product (design) or can be influenced by the nature and condition of the wound (wound related) – for example, contributes to autolytic debridement. Thomas (2008) points out that 'it is unlikely that a single dressing or dressing system will possess all of these attributes'.

ACTIVITY

Study Table 7.7 and relate this to the range of products you have access to in the practice setting and/or the skills laboratory. Which of the criteria do they meet? How might you select a dressing? Discuss with a practitioner how a specific dressing is chosen for an individual. There may be local clinical guidelines and, if so, try to locate them.

Before asking which dressing to use, your question might sometimes be: Does the wound require a dressing at all? In an extensive study involving 3674 wounds, Weiss (1983) demonstrated that wound dressings are unnecessary for clean surgical wounds after 24 hours, and suggested that dressings are expensive, time-consuming, can interfere with breathing and cause discomfort. Susan's wound dressing could, therefore, have been removed after 24 hours and the wound left open. However,

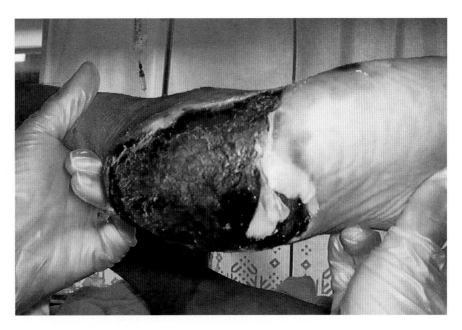

Plate 1: A diabetic ulcer that developed on this patient's heel due to a combination of poor circulation and unrelieved pressure. The tissue bed is covered in hard black necrotic tissue. The wound will not heal until this is removed. Unfortunately this ulcer eventually led to amputation of the patient's lower leg and foot.

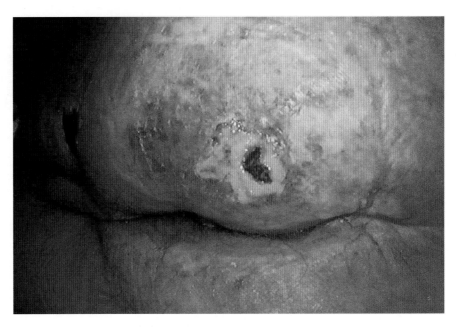

Plate 2: A pressure ulcer (EPUAP grade 3) that developed on the sacrum of a patient with multiple sclerosis. The wound bed is covered with yellow slough, except for a central necrotic area. Slough is soft necrotic tissue containing dead phagocytes, and the wound will not heal until it is removed. Surrounding this ulcer are other areas of pressure damage, evidenced by discoloration (EPUAP grade 1) and superficial ulceration (EPUAP grade 2).

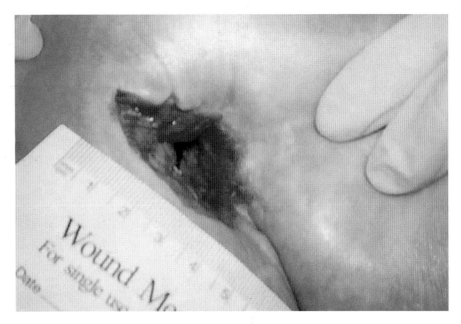

Plate 3: A pressure ulcer, which extends down to bone (EPUAP grade 4), that developed on the sacrum of a patient with a spinal injury. The ulcer was covered with 60 per cent slough prior to debridement by maggots. The wound is now almost filled with red granulation tissue. This photo also shows how a ruler placed by the side of a wound before the photo can provide a more accurate record of its dimensions.

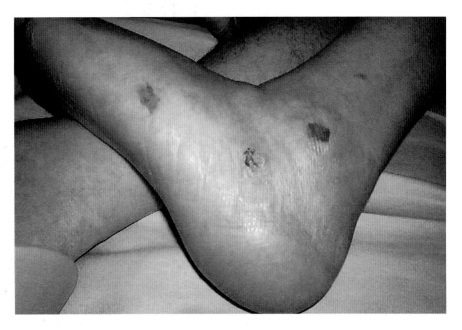

Plate 4: Pressure ulcers (EPUAP grade 2) on the side of the foot/ankle of a patient who has multiple sclerosis. They are now almost healed, with tissue beds showing mainly pink epithelialising tissue.

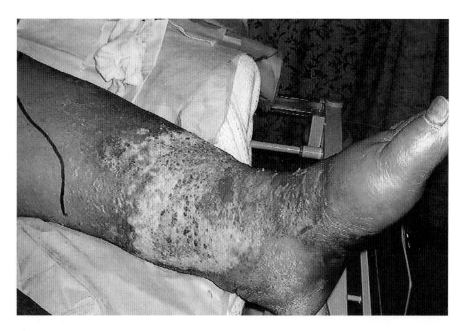

Plate 5: A venous leg ulcer that has been a longstanding problem for the patient concerned. There are large areas of yellow slough and areas of red granulation tissue covering the wound. The lower foot looks oedematous and there is hard scaly skin (hyperkeratosis) present. The surrounding skin also looks red, suggesting cellulitus.

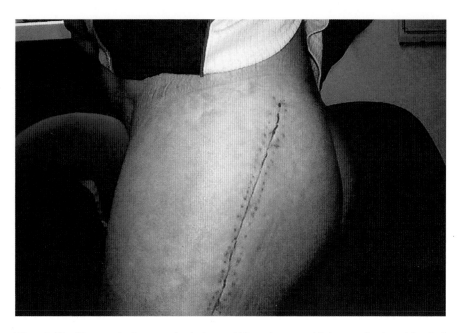

Plate 6: The hip wound of a man who had a total hip replacement, 10 days previously, and just had his skin closures (clips) removed. This is a good example of a clean surgical wound that has healed as planned by primary intention.

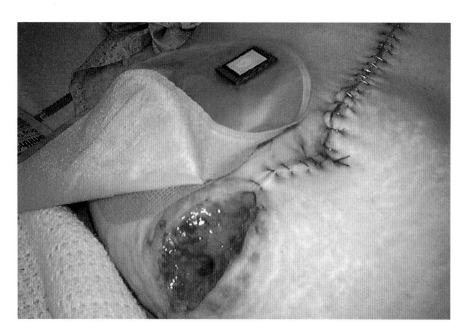

Plate 7: The abdominal wound of a woman who has had an abdominoperineal resection, with colostomy formation, for ulcerative colitis. The colostomy has been sited very close to the wound. The photo was taken on the fifth postoperative day. The wound had started to ooze pus from the distal part of the wound, and had dehisced. The clips from this area have been removed. Towards the top of the wound and the central area there is slight inflammation. In the dehisced area, small patches of red granulating tissue can be seen but other areas look unhealthy. There is a dark centre to this area, which was found to be a sinus.

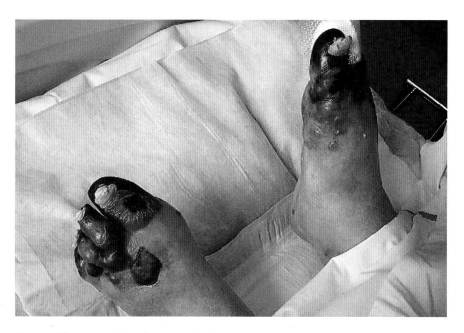

Plate 8: This patient, whose feet are shown here, had a history of heart surgery and heart failure. Over two weeks she developed black necrotic toes, and the condition spread to the distal area of her feet owing to the lack of arterial circulation.

Table 7.7: Performance requirements of the 'ideal dressing' (Thomas 2008). Reproduced with kind permission of World Wide Wounds.

Primary requirements	Type of feature
Free of toxins or irritants	Design feature
Does not release particles or non-biodegradable fibres into the wound	Design feature
Forms an effective bacterial barrier (effectively contains exudate or cellular debris to prevent the transmission of microorganisms into or out of the wound)	Design feature
If self-adhesive, forms an effective water-resistant seal to the periwound skin, but is easily removable without causing trauma or skin stripping	Design feature
Maintains the wound and the surrounding skin in an optimum state of hydration (implies the ability to function effectively under compression)	Design/wound related
Requires minimal disturbance or replacement	Design/wound related
Provides protection to the periwound skin from potentially irritant wound exudate and excess moisture	Design/wound related
Produces minimal pain during application or removal as a result of adherence to the wound surface	Design/wound related
Maintains the wound at the optimum temperature and pH	Design/wound related
Secondary requirements	Type of feature
Possesses antimicrobial activity: capable of combating localised infection	Design feature
Has odour absorbing/combating properties	Design feature
Has ability to remove or inactivate proteolytic enzymes in chronic wound fluid	Design feature
Possesses haemostatic activity	Design feature
Exhibits effective wound cleansing (debriding) activity	Design/wound related

Briggs' (1996) small study indicated that a film dressing left *in situ* until skin closure removal promotes pain relief. Susan might feel more comfortable and less worried about her wound if it is kept covered with a film dressing.

The Molndal dressing technique for managing wounds following orthopaedic surgery has become standard practice in the majority of orthopaedic centres in Sweden (Folestad 2002). The technique uses a hydrofiber dressing called AQUACEL covered with a film dressing. A comparative clinical study showed an increased wear time for the AQUACEL/film dressing combination due to delayed strike-through compared with a standard dressing (adhesive dressing and adsorbent pad secured by tape and adhesive net) (Folestad 2002). Leakage of blood and exudate out of the dressing were also reduced for the AQUACEL/film dressing combination, as was the incidence of skin problems including blistering (Folestad 2002). This technique has been adopted throughout many orthopaedic centres across the UK.

Your choice of dressing should relate to your wound assessment, taking into account the attributes of an effective wound care product. Consider the stage of wound healing, type and colour of tissue, site of wound, pain relief, and amount of exudate, but many other individual factors too. Key groups of dressings, and their uses, are summarised in Table 7.8, and Table 7.9 provides a wound dressing selection guide based on wound-bed tissue and exudate level.

Table 7.8: Wound dressings (based on Morris 2006 except where stated).

Dressing type	Examples	Description	Uses
Simple	Mepore	Simple wound covering providing protection from contamination and absorbs mild exudate	Wounds healing by primary intention (e.g. straightforward surgical wound)
Adhesive film dressings	Opsite Tegaderm Bioclusive	Transparent, vapour-permeable adhesive film dressing that acts as a barrier to bacteria and water Allows bathing/showering Allows observation of wound.	Primary wound closure (e.g. straightforward surgical wound) To protect skin susceptible to damage from shearing, abrasions
Tulles: medicated and non-medicated	Jelonet Bactigras Inadine	Open-weave cotton or rayon dressing impregnated with soft paraffin, antiseptics or antibiotics	Infected wounds healing by secondary intention; abrasions; minor burns
Hydrogels	Intrasite gel Purilon Aquaform Granugel	Dressing based on starch polymers, providing a moist wound environment, and promoting debridement	Dry, necrotic and granulating wounds; light to moderately exudating wounds; abrasions Requires a secondary dressing
Foam dressings	Allevyn Tielle Biatain Cavicare Flexipore Truform	Highly absorbent dressing made from polyurethane or silicone Available as a flat dressing and a cavity dressing	Heavily exudating wounds; full-thickness cavity wounds healing by secondary intention; granulating and epithelialising wounds
Hydrocolloids	Granuflex Duoderm Duoderm Signal Comfeel plus Tegasorb Hydrocol	Polyurethane foam sheet fixed on to a semi-permeable film Provides a moist environment, promotes debridement, granulation and epithelialisation	Moderately but not heavily exudating wounds; necrotic, infected, sloughy, granulating or epithelialising wounds; abrasions
Alginates	Kaltostat Sorbsan	Made from the sodium and calcium salts of alginic acid, a seaweed-derived polymer Reacts with wound exudate to form a gel which, it is believed, aids autolytic debridement and promotes wound healing	Moderately to heavily exudating wounds, including infected, sloughy and granulating wounds Can be used to pack puncture and cavity wounds Requires a secondary dressing
Hydrofiber dressings	Aquacel	Absorbent dressing that provides a moist wound healing environment	Moderately to heavily exudating wounds, including infected, sloughy and granulating wounds Can be used to pack puncture and cavity wounds Requires a secondary dressing
Cadexomer iodine dressings (Collier 2002)	Iodosorb Iodoflex	Dressings contain hydrophilic beads impregnated with iodine	Wounds with low to moderate exudates; infected wounds healing by secondary intention
Silver-impregnated products (Lansdown et al. 2003)	Acticoat Actisorb Silver 220 Aquagel Ag Contreet Advance	Metallic silver and its salts have antibacterial properties and bind DNA of the bacteria which then impairs cell production Effective broad-spectrum antimicrobial effect	Infected wounds

(Continued)

Table 7.8: (Continued)

Dressing type	Examples	Description	Uses
Honey dressings	Activon Mesitran	Honey has antibacterial, debriding and anti-inflammatory properties	Necrotic and sloughy wounds; infected wounds
Topical negative pressure (Birchall *et al.* 2002)	VAC	Applies localised sub-atmospheric negative pressure to a wound bed via a computerised therapy unit	Assists in the removal of excessive exudate, reduces oedema, improves circulation, stimulates granulation tissue formation and wound contraction, reduces bacterial loading

Table 7.9: Wound dressing selection guide. Reproduced with kind permission from Buckinghamshire Hospitals NHS Trust.

	Low Exudate	Medium Exudate	High Exudate
Necrotic (BLACK)			
Primary	HYDROGEL	HYDROGEL or HYDROFIBER	HYDROFIBER
Secondary	HYDROCOLLOID	HYDROCOLLOID	FOAM
Sloughy (YELLOW)			
Primary	HYDROGEL	HYDROFIBER	HYDROFIBER
Secondary	HYDROCOLLOID	FOAM	FOAM
Granulating (RED)			
Primary	HYDROCOLLOID	HYDROFIBER	HYDROFIBER
Secondary		HYDROCOLLOID	FOAM
Epithelialising (PINK)			
Primary	HYDROCOLLOID	HYDROCOLLOID or FOAM	HYDROFIBER
Secondary			HYDROCOLLOID or FOAM
Infected (GREEN)			
Primary	ANTIMICROBIAL DRESSING	ANTIMICROBIAL DRESSING	ANTIMICROBIAL DRESSING
Secondary	FOAM	FOAM	FOAM

The first line treatment for Diabetic Foot Ulcers is an antimicrobial or a low-adherent dressing

Foster and Moore (1999) note that, despite the vast range of dressings produced, many require more sound evidence for their use than is currently available as trials have often used insufficient numbers of people. A systematic review of wound care management found little evidence regarding which dressings or topical agents are the most effective in treating chronic wounds (Bradley *et al.* 1999). However, there was evidence to support the use of hydrocolloids for pressure ulcers, and that low-adherent dressings are as effective as hydrocolloids beneath compression bandaging for venous leg ulcers. Always consult the manufacturer's instructions when applying dressings.

Dressings for diabetic foot ulcers must be chosen with particular care (Foster 1999). Gill (1999) identifies that many dressing trials exclude people with diabetes, making it difficult to make evidence-based decisions on product choice. A systematic review

> ## Box 7.3 The ideal dressing for a diabetic foot ulcer (Foster et al. 1994)
>
> The ideal dressing should:
> - perform well in the enclosed environment of a shoe, and not take up too much space;
> - absorb large quantities of exudate but enable drainage;
> - withstand the pressures and shear of walking;
> - not be associated with side-effects;
> - not depend for its maximum effect on being left in place for long periods, as diabetic ulcers can deteriorate very rapidly;
> - be easy to remove/lift for inspection.

found much uncertainty over how to effectively prevent and treat diabetic foot ulcers (O'Meara *et al.* 2000). Hydrocolloid use for these wounds appears to be particularly controversial; but Gill (1999), in a critical review, suggests that this product has often been used incorrectly – left in place for too long a time without inspecting the wound. Box 7.3 provides criteria for an ideal dressing for a diabetic foot ulcer.

As noted at the start of this chapter, there are constantly new products being developed. This chapter has incorporated available systematic reviews and clinical guidelines but there are many more in progress; check the Cochrane Library and NICE for their latest publications.

All patients/clients need education about their wound care and dressings. This has already been discussed a little in relation to Susan and her wound.

ACTIVITY

If you were being discharged home with a dressing *in situ,* or had had a dressing applied by the community nurse, what sort of things would you want to know?

You would probably want to know some of the following:
- Can I get the dressing wet? If not, how can I manage activities such as washing?
- When should the dressing be redone, and by whom?
- What should I do if the dressing becomes loose, uncomfortable, too tight, falls off or soaks through?
- What should I expect of the wound? For example when will it heal?
- Will the wound be painful? If so, how can I deal with this?
- How will I know if the wound is becoming infected?
- Are there any special instructions I should follow?

Education should involve relatives and carers as applicable. For Susan, her carers should have been educated prior to her discharge, and explanations given to Susan using appropriate communication methods. This information is also important to people receiving inpatient care to allay anxiety, build confidence and promote self-care.

Written information can back up verbal instructions; it is difficult for people to retain a lot of new information, particularly when under stress. Written patient information should be readable, understandable and culturally relevant to be effective in promoting self-care and relieving anxiety (Wilson and McLemore 1997).

Leg ulcer bandaging

A systematic review by Cullum *et al.* (2001) concluded that compression increases venous ulcer healing rates when compared with no compression, that multilayered systems are more effective than single-layered systems, that high compression is more effective than low compression, but that there are no clear differences between different types of high compression.

In addition to the previously mentioned guidelines (CREST 1998; RCN 1998; SIGN 1998), the European Wound Management Association (2002) published an evidence-based pathway for the use of compression therapy in the treatment of venous leg ulcers (Ashton 2003). However, compression should be used only in the absence of significant arterial disease; so, as discussed earlier in this chapter, arterial blood supply must first be assessed.

Treatment needs to be continued after healing, as without compression the underlying problem – venous hypertension – will return, and a leg ulcer will form once more (Williams and Young 1998). When the ulcer is healed, continuing to use compression (of the strongest tolerable) is associated with reduced rates of recurrence (Nelson *et al.* 2000). Therefore patient education and involvement are essential.

Before selecting a compression bandage, each patient is assessed individually and lifestyle considered (Williams and Young 1998). Bandaging should extend from the base of the toes to the knee (Scully 1999). RCN guidelines (1998) state that leg ulcer bandaging should be applied by a trained practitioner, have adequate padding and be capable of sustaining compression for at least a week. You should get the opportunity to observe leg ulcer bandaging in practice, possibly at a clinic, or with the district nurse. Try to find out about a local leg ulcer clinic, and arrange a visit.

Learning outcome 4: Outline ways of reducing pain and discomfort associated with wounds

Unfortunately patients often associate their wounds with pain. A study of 694 patients with a variety of chronic wounds found that almost half experienced pain (Lindham *et al.* 1999). Any care relating to wounds can cause fear and distress, be this removal of a surgical drain, a dressing change or removal of skin-closing devices such as staples, clips or sutures. A person with a traumatic wound experienced pain when the injury occurred, so the thought of having a wound dressing could be distressing. A pain assessment should be completed for each patient; a numerical analogue scale is incorporated into the wound assessment tool (see Fig. 7.2).

Table 7.10 provides a summary of factors contributing to pain associated with wounds, and possible solutions. Chapter 12 considers assessment and management of pain in detail.

Analgesia prior to dressing changes may be required. Opiates are necessary if the pain is severe, but otherwise non-steroidal anti-inflammatory drugs or simple

Table 7.10: Causes of wound pain and measures to minimise pain and trauma to the tissues and the surrounding skin (adapted from Hollinworth 2005).

Wound cleansing and debridement

• Gentle irrigation of the wound with warm normal saline or tap water

• Restrict the use of antiseptics to contaminated traumatic wounds

• Plan and organise dressing changes to reduce prolonged exposure to air

• Avoid wiping gauze or cotton across the wound bed

Wound management products: areas to consider

• Select the correct dressing for the conditions at the wound bed, related to tissue type and level of exudate present. Does
• the dressing need to absorb exudate or donate fluid?

• Hydrogels and hydrocolloids will cause maceration to the peri-wound area if used on heavily exudating wounds, extending tissue damage and increasing pain levels

• Alginates and hydrofiber will adhere to wounds with low exudate, causing pain and trauma upon removal

• Avoid adhesive dressings on patients with very fragile skin, an excoriated peri-wound area or those on long-term steroid treatment

• Some dressings such as honey products can create an osmotic pull on the wound bed, which some patients find extremely painful

• Antibacterial dressings containing iodine and silver can cause increased pain

• Refrain from changing the dressing too frequently if not indicated

• Always remove dressings as per the manufacturer's instructions

Treatments

• Compression therapy can be extremely painful

• Negative-pressure therapy (VAC) can increase pain and can cause tissue trauma upon removal

• Larval therapy can increase pain

Emotional and social aspects

• Increased pain may be related to how the patient perceives their wound and the effect it has upon their lives, so nurses should empathise and help to alleviate their anxieties

• Malodour may contribute to these negative feelings

Disease processes

• Identify and treat clinical wound infection as this may cause the pain at the wound bed

• Associated diseases may contribute to the pain, such as peripheral vascular disease, ischaemia, rheumatoid arthritis, osteoarthritis, diabetic neuropathy, phantom limb pain, oedema, cellulitis, cancer, eczema

analgesics are suitable. Sufficient time should be allowed for them to take effect before the dressing change (Emflorgo 1999). Nitrous oxide (entonox) can also help some people. Other pain reduction strategies include use of relaxation and distraction.

ACTIVITY

Drawing on the material in this section, identify possible strategies for wound care for Mrs Warner, Colin and Susan. Remember to consider debridement, cleansing, wound dressing choice and pain management.

Points that you might have identified can be found in Table 7.11.

Table 7.11: A possible wound management strategy for Colin, Mrs Warner and Susan

	Colin	Mrs Warner	Susan
Wound type	Dirty surgical wound on buttock	(1) Necrotic sacral pressure ulcer (2) Infected diabetic neuropathic ulcer on toe	Clean contaminated surgical wound on abdomen
Debridement needed?	Was performed surgically	(1) Yes, identify an appropriate option for this individual (see Box 7.2)	Not required
Cleansing?	Yes: bathing, showering or irrigation with warm saline	Could bath or shower, or the wounds could be irrigated with warm saline when the dressings are renewed. Consider use of antiseptic for infected toe ulcer (Miller 1998)	Not required. Can bath or shower as she wishes
Which dressing?	Pack wound with alginate or hydrofiber, and cover with a foam dressing	(1) Sacrum: hydrogel with hydrocolloid as a secondary dressing (2) Toe: antimicrobial dressing with foam as a secondary dressing	Not necessary after first 24 hours (Weiss 1983), but Susan may find it more comfortable or acceptable if her wound is covered with a film dressing until her sutures are removed
Pain management	Assess pain. Information giving and explanations. Regular analgesics (e.g. non-steroidal anti-inflammatory drugs). The alginate or hydrofiber dressing should be comfortable to wear and painless to remove	Assess pain. Information giving and explanations. Hydrogel, hydrofiber, hydrocolloid and foam dressings are all comfortable to wear and their removal should be painless. Regular analgesics if needed (neuropathic ulcers are usually painless)	Assess pain. Information giving and explanations. Regular analgesics may be needed. Remove of film dressing with care. Removal of skin closures will need careful preparation, reassurance and support

Summary

- Wound assessment must precede effective wound management, which requires the application of suitable cleansing methods, the most appropriate dressing to cover the wound and pain-relieving strategies.
- Application of these skills in the care of each individual is the product of knowledge and experience.

CHAPTER SUMMARY

This chapter has aimed to introduce an understanding of how wounds heal, with an emphasis on the systemic nature of wound healing, and the range of factors that may impair wound healing. An awareness of how wounds can be assessed and managed, taking into account their underlying causes, has also been promoted. The chapter emphasised an individualistic and holistic approach to wound care, and discussed different options available for managing wounds.

You have been encouraged to take the opportunity to apply knowledge to practice and to start to gain experience in observing wounds and identifying their stage of healing. Involving patients/clients and their families, working with the multidisciplinary team, accessing expert knowledge, and being aware of the need to continually update have all been addressed. This chapter did not attempt to include specialist knowledge – further in-depth reading in relation to individual topics such as leg ulcers and burns should be undertaken where applicable.

To conclude, an understanding of wound care is important for all nurses. This chapter has aimed to introduce key principles to act as a foundation for future learning.

ACKNOWLEDGEMENT

This chapter has been revised and updated. The author acknowledges the contribution of Deirdre Thompson to this chapter in the second edition of this book.

REFERENCES

Anderson, I. 2006. Aetiology, assessment and management of leg ulcers. *Wound Essentials* **1,** 20–37.

Angeras, M.H., Brandberg, A., Falk, A. and Seeman, T. 1992. Comparison between sterile saline and tap water for the cleansing of acute traumatic soft tissue wounds. *European Journal of Surgery* **158,** 347–50.

Ashton, J. 2003. A review of a recommended management pathway in the treatment of venous leg ulcers. *Nurse2Nurse Magazine* **3**(3), 46–8.

Beldon, P. 2007. What you need to know about skin grafts and donor site wounds. *Wound Essentials UK* **2,** 149–55.

Birchall, L., Street, L. and Clift, H. 2002. Developing a trust-wide centralised approach to the use of TNP (topical negative pressure). *Journal of Wound Care* **11,** 311–14.

Boore, J. 1978. *Prescription for Recovery.* London: Royal College of Nursing.

Bradley, M., Cullum, N., Nelson, E.A. *et al.* 1999. Systematic reviews of wound management. Part 2: Dressings and topical agents used in the healing of chronic wounds. *Health Technology Assessment* **3**(17 Pt 2), 1–135.

Bremmelgaard, A., Raahave, D., Beier-Holgersen *et al.* 1989. Computer aided surveillance of surgical infections and identification of risk factors. *Journal of Hospital Infection* **13,** 1–18.

Briggs, M. 1996. Surgical wound pain: a trial of two treatments. *Journal of Wound Care* **5,** 456–60.

Briggs, M. and Closs, S.J. 2003. The prevalence of leg ulceration: a review of the literature. *EWMA Journal* **3**(2), 14–20.

Bryant, R.A. 2007. Preface. In Bryant, R.A. and Nix, D. (ed.) *Acute and Chronic Wounds: Current management options,* 3rd edn. St Louis: Mosby Elsevier, vii–ix.

Casey, G. 1999. Wound management in children. *Paediatric Nursing* **11**(5), 39–44.

Clinical Resource Efficiency Support Team (CREST) 1998. *Guidelines for the Assessment and Management of Leg Ulceration.* Northern Ireland.

Collier, M. 2002. Wound care. Wound bed preparation. *Nursing Times* **98**(2), 55–7.

Cooper, R., Halas, E. and Molan, P. 2002. The efficacy of honey in inhibiting strains of *Pseudomonas aeruginosa* from infected burns. *Journal of Burn Care and Rehabilitation* **23,** 366–70.

Cruse, P. and Foord, R. 1980. The epidemiology of wound infection: a ten-year prospective study of 62,939 wounds. *Surgical Clinics of North America* **60,** 27–40.

Cullum, N., Nelson, E.A., Fletcher, A.W. and Sheldon, T.A. 2001. Compression for venous leg ulcers. *Cochrane Database of Systematic Reviews,* Issue 2.

Cutting, K.F. 1999. The causes and prevention of maceration of the skin. *Journal of Wound Care* **8,** 200–1.

Cutting, K.F. and Harding, K.G. 1994. Criteria for identifying a wound infection. *Journal of Wound Care* **3,** 198–201.

Department of Health (DH) 2001. *Valuing People: A new strategy for learning disability for the 21st century.* London: DH.

Doughty, D.B. and Holbrook, R. 2007. Lower-extremity ulcers of vascular etiology. In Bryant, R.A. and Nix, D.P. (eds) *Acute and Chronic Wounds: Nursing management,* 3rd edn. St Louis: Mosby, 258–306.

Doughty, D.B. and Sparks-Defriese, B. 2007. Wound-healing physiology. In Bryant, R.A. and Nix, D.P. (eds) Acute and Chronic Wounds: *Nursing Management,* 3rd edn. St. Louis: Mosby, 56–81.

Drosou, A., Falabella, A. and Kirsner, R.S. 2003. Antiseptics on wounds: an area of controversy (part one). *Wounds* **15**(5), 149–66.

Edwards, J. 2000. Sharp debridement of wounds. *Journal of Community Nursing* **14,** 1.

Emflorgo, C.A. 1999. The assessment and treatment of wound pain. *Journal of Wound Care* **8,** 384–5.

European Pressure Ulcer Advisory Panel 1998. *Pressure Ulcer Treatment Guidelines.* Available from www.epuap.org. Accessed 1 May 2008.

European Wound Management Association. 2005. *Position Paper: Identifying criteria for wound infection.* London: Medical Education Partnership. Available from www.ewma.org

Evans, R.C. and Jones, N.L. 1996. The management of abrasions and bruises. *Journal of Wound Care* **5,** 465–8.

Fairbairn, K., Grier, J., Hunter, C, and Preece, J. 2002. A sharp debridement procedure devised by specialist nurses. *Journal of Wound Care* **11**(10), 371–5.

Falanga, V. 2000. Classification for wound bed preparation and stimulation of chronic wounds. *Wound, Repair and Regeneration* **8,** 347–52.

Farion, K., Osmond, M.H., Hartling, L. *et al.* 2001. Tissue adhesives for traumatic lacerations in children and adults. *Cochrane Database of Systematic Reviews,* Issue 4.

Fernandez, R., and Griffiths, R. 2008. Water for wound cleansing. *Cochrane Database of Systematic Reviews,* Issue 1.

Fletcher, J. 1997. Wound cleansing. *Professional Nurse* **12,** 793–6.

Fletcher, J. 2003. The benefits of applying wound bed preparation into practice. *Journal of Wound Care* **12**(9), 347–9.

Folestad, A. 2002. The management of wounds following orthopaedic surgery: the Molndal dressing. *European Othopaedic Product News,* March/April, 33.

Foster, A. 1999. Diabetic ulceration. In Miller, M. and Glover, D. (eds) *Wound Management: Theory and practice.* London: NT Books, 72–83.

Foster, L. and Moore, P. 1999. Acute surgical wound care. Part 3: Fitting the dressing to the wound. *British Journal of Nursing* **8,** 200, 202, 204, 206, 208–10.

Foster, A.V.M., Greenhill, M.T. and Edmonds, M.E. 1994. Comparing two dressings in the treatment of diabetic foot ulcers. *Journal of Wound Care* **3,** 224–8.

Fox, C. 2002. Honey as a dressing for chronic wounds in adults. *British Journal of Community Nursing* **7,** 530–4.

Gill, D. 1999. The use of hydrocolloids in the treatment of diabetic foot. *Journal of Wound Care* **8,** 204–6.

Goldberg, M.T. and McGynn-Byer, M. 2007. Oncology-related skin damage. In Bryant, R.A. and Nix, D.P. (eds) *Acute and Chronic Wounds: Nursing management,* 3rd edn. St Louis: Mosby, 471–89.

Gottrup, F. 1999. Wound closure techniques. *Journal of Wound Care* **8**, 397–400.

Gouvela, J.C. and Miguens, C. 2007. Is it safe to use saline solution to clean wounds. *EWMA Journal* **7**(2), 7–12.

Gray, D. and Cooper, P. 2001. Nutrition and wound healing: what is the link? *Journal of Wound Care* **10**(3), 86–9.

Gray, D., White, R., Cooper, P. and Kingsley, A. 2004. The wound healing continuum, an aid to clinical decision making and clinical audit. *Applied Wound Management Supplement. Wounds UK* **1**(1), 9–12. Available from www.wounds-uk.com.

Hampton, S. 1999. Choosing the right dressing. In Miller, M. and Glover, D. (eds) *Wound Management Theory and Practice.* London: NT Books, 116–28.

Higgins, M.A.G., Evans, R.C. and Evans, R.J. 1997. Managing animal bite wounds. *Journal of Wound Care* **6**, 377–80.

Hollinworth, H. and Kingston, J.E. 1998. Using a non-sterile technique in wound care. *Professional Nurse* **13**, 226–9.

Hollinworth, H. 2005. The management of patients' pain in wound care. *Nursing Standard.* **20**(7), 65–70.

International Working Group on the Diabetic Foot (IWGDF) 1999. *International Consensus on the Diabetic Foot.* Amsterdam: IWGDF.

Jones, J. 2003. Stress responses, pressure ulcer development and adaptation. *British Journal of Nursing* **12**(11 Suppl), s17–22.

Kiecolt-Glaser, J.K., Marucha, P.T., Malarkey, W.B. *et al.* 1995. Slowing of wound healing by psychological stress. *Lancet* **346**, 1194–6.

King, D.J. 1998. Atypical antipsychotics and the negative symptoms of schizophrenia. *Advances in Psychiatric Treatment* **4**, 53–61.

Kingsley, A., White, R. and Gray, D. 2004.The wound infection continuum: a revised perspective. *Applied Wound Management Supplement. Wounds UK* **1**(1), 13–18. Available from www.wounds-uk.com.

Krizek, T.J., Harries, R.H.C. and Robson, M.C. 1997. Biology of tissue injury and repair. In Georgiade, G.S., Riefkohl, R. and Scott-Levin, L. (eds) *Georgiade Plastic Maxillofacial and Reconstructive Surgery,* 3rd edn. London: Williams & Wilkins, 3–9.

Lansdown, A.B.G., Jensen, K. and Jensen, M.Q. 2003. Contreet foam and contreet hydrocolloid: an insight into two new silver-containing dressings. *Journal of Wound Care* **12**, 204–10.

Lawrence, J.C. 1998. The use of povidine iodine as an antiseptic agent. *Journal of Wound Care* **7**, 421–5.

Lazarus, G.S., Cooper, D.M., Knighton, D.R. *et al.* 1994. Definitions and guidelines for assessment of wounds and evaluation of healing. *Archives of Dermatology* **130**, 489–93.

Leaper, D. 1996. Antiseptics in wound healing. *Nursing Times* **92**(39), 63–64, 66.

Leaper, D. J. 2006. ABC of wound healing: traumatic and surgical wounds. *British Medical Journal.* **332**, 532–5.

Levenson, S.M., Geever, E.F. and Crowley, L.V. *et al.* 1965. The healing of rat skin wounds. *Annals of Surgery* **161**, 293.

Lindham, C., Bergsten, A. and Berglund, E. 1999. Chronic wounds and nursing care. *Journal of Wound Care* **9**, 5–10.

Magan, M.A. 1996. Psychological considerations for patients with acute wounds. *Critical Care Nursing Clinics of North America* **8**, 183–93.

Mcheik, J.N., Vergniss, P. and Bondonny, J.M. 2000. Treatment of facial dog bite injuries in children: a retrospective study. *Journal of Paediatric Surgery* **35**, 580–3.

McIntosh, C. 2006. Diabetic foot ulcers: what is the best practice in the UK? *Wound Essentials* **2**, 162–9.

Miller, M. 1996. Best practice in wound assessment. *Community Nurse* **2**(3), 41–2, 44, 47.

Miller, M. 1998. How do I diagnose and treat wound infection. *British Journal of Nursing* **7**, 335–8.

Miller, M. 1999a. Wound assessment. In Miller, M. and Glover, D. (eds) *Wound Management Theory and Practice.* London: NT Books, 23–36.

Miller, M. 1999b. Nursing assessment of patients with non-acute wounds. *British Journal of Nursing* **8**(10), 12–14.

Mishriki, S.F., Law, D.J. and Jeffrey, P.J. 1990. Factors affecting the incidence of post-operative infection. *Journal of Hospital Infection* **16**, 223–30.

Morris, A. 2005. Skin trauma. In White, R. (ed.) *Skin Care in Wound Mangement: Assessment, prevention and treatment.* Aberdeen: Wounds UK Publishing, 74–86.

Morris, C. 2006. Wound management and dressing selection. *Wound Essentials* **1**, 178–83.

Myers, J.A. 1982. Modern plastic surgical dressings. *Health and Social Service Journal* **92**, 336–7.

National Institute for Health and Clinical Excellence (NICE) 2001. *Guidance on the Use of Debriding Agents and Specialist Wound Care Clinics for Difficult to Heal Surgical Wounds.* London.

— 2004. *Clinical Guidelines for Type 2 Diabetes: Prevention and management of foot problems,* Clinical Guideline 10. London.

Neil, J.A. and Barrell, L.M. 1998. Transition theory and its relevance to patients with chronic wounds. *Rehabilitation Nursing* **23**, 295–9.

Nelson, E.A. and Bradley, M.D. 2007. Dressings and topical agents for arterial leg ulcers. *Cochrane Database of Systematic Reviews,* Issue 1.

Nelson, E.A., Bell-Syer, S.E.M. and Cullum, N.A. 2000. Compression for preventing recurrence of venous ulcers. *Cochrane Database of Systematic Reviews,* Issue 4.

Niazi, Z.B.M. and Sacks, J. 2005. Management of acute wounds. In Lee, B.Y. (ed.) *The Wound Management Manual.* New York: McGraw-Hill, Chapter 11.

Nix, D.P. 2007. Patient assessment and evaluation of wound healing. In Bryant, R.A. and Nix, D.P. (eds) *Acute and Chronic Wounds: Nursing management,* 3rd edn. St Louis: Mosby, 130–48.

O'Meara, S., Cullum, N., Majid, M. and Sheldon, T. 2000. Systematic reviews of wound care management. Part 3: Antimicrobial agents for chronic wounds; Part 4: Diabetic foot ulceration. *Health Technology Assessment* **4**(21).

Partridge, C. 1998. Influential factors in surgical wound healing. *Journal of Wound Care* **7**, 350–3.

Pittman, J. 2007. Effect of aging on wound healing: current concepts. *Wound Ostomy Continence Nursing* **34**(4), 412–15.

Royal College of Nursing (RCN) 1998. *The Management of Patients with Venous Leg Ulcers.* London: RCN.

Scully, C. 1999. In on a limb. *Nursing Times* **95**(27), 59–60, 62, 65.

Scottish Intercollegiate Guidelines Network (SIGN) 1998. *The Care of Patients with Chronic Leg Ulcers,* Guideline 26. Edinburgh: SIGN.

Serensen, L.T. 2003. Smoking and wound healing. *European Wound Management Association Journal* **3**(1), 13–15.

Sherman, R.A., Sherman, J., Gilead, L. *et al.* 2001. Maggot debridement in outpatients. *Archives of Physical Medicine and Rehabilitation* **82**, 1226–9.

Stotts, N.A. 2007. Nutritional support and assessment. In Bryant, R.A. and Nix, D.P. (eds) *Acute and Chronic Wounds: Nursing management,* 2nd edn. St Louis: Mosby, 149–60.

Stringfellow, S. and Russell, F. 2003. Modern wound management: an update of common wound products. *Nursing and Residential Care.* **7**(5), 322–33.

Thomas, S. 1994. Assessing the hydro-affinity of hydrogel dressings. *Journal of Wound Care* **3**(2), 89–91.

Thomas, S. 2008. The role of dressings in the treatment of moisture-related skin damage. *World Wide Wounds.* Available from www.worldwidewounds.com/2008/march/Thomas/Maceration-and-the-role-of-dressings.hmtl. Accessed 31 March 2008.

Thomas, S. and Jones, M. 1999. *The Use of Sterile Maggots in Wound Management.* Wound Care Society, Educational Leaflet 6(4).

Thomas, S. and Jones, M. 2000. Maggots can benefit patients with MRSA. *Practice Nurse* **20,** 101–4.

Thomas, S., Wynn, K., Fowler, T. and Jones, M. 2002. The effect of containment on the properties of sterile maggots. *British Journal of Nursing* **11**(12), 21–8.

Thomlinson, D. 1987. To clean or not to clean. *Nursing Times* **83**(9), 71, 73, 75.

Timmons, J. 2006. Skin function and wound healing physiology. *Wound Essentials* **1,** 8–17.

Troxler, M., Vowden, K. and Vowden, P. 2006. Integrating adjunctive therapy into practice: the importance of recognising 'hard to heal' wounds. *World Wide Wounds.* Available from www.worldwidewounds.com/2006/december/Troxler/Integrating-Adjunctive-Therapy-Into-Practice.hmtl. Accessed 28 March 2008.

Valk, G.D., Kriegsman, D.N.W. and Assendelft, W.J.J. 2001. Patient education for preventing diabetic foot ulceration. *Cochrane Database of Systematic Reviews,* Issue 4.

Vowden, K. and Vowden, P. 2002. Wound bed preparation. *World Wide Wounds.* Available from www.worldwidewounds.com/2002/april/Vowden/Wound-Bed-Preparation.html. Accessed 23 March 2008.

Weiss, E.L. 1995. Connective tissue in wound healing. In McCulloch, J.M., Luther, C., Kloth, L.C. and Feedar, J.A. (eds) *Wound Healing Alternatives in Management,* 2nd edn. Philadelphia: FA Davis, 16–31.

Weiss, Y. 1983. Simplified management of operative wounds by early exposure. *International Surgery* **68,** 237–40.

Williams, L. and Leaper, D. 2000. Nutrition and wound healing. *Clinical Nutrition Update* **5**(1), 3–5.

Williams, C. and Young, T. 1998. *Myth and Reality in Wound Care.* Dinton: Mark Allen Publishing.

Wilson, F.L. and McLemore, R. 1997. Patient literacy levels: a consideration when designing patient education programs. *Rehabilitation Nursing* **22,** 311–17.

Young, T. 1997. Wound care in the accident and emergency department. *British Journal of Nursing* **6,** 395–6, 398, 400–1.

Young, T. 2000. Managing MRSA wound infection and colonisation. *NTPlus* **96**(14), 14–16.

USEFUL WEBSITES

World Wide Wounds: www.worldwidewounds.com

Wounds UK: www.wounds-uk.com

Wounds Research: www.woundsresearch.com

European Wound Management Association: www.ewma.org

European Pressure Ulcer Advisory Panel: www.epuap.org

Meeting Hygiene Needs

Jenni Randall

Assisting patients to meet their fundamental hygiene needs has always been at the forefront of nursing care. This was reinforced by the inclusion of personal and oral hygiene in the Department of Health's *Essence of Care* benchmarks (DH 2001a). The Chief Nursing Officer's review of mental health nursing, *From Values to Action*, also highlighted personal and physical care as being important skills for mental health nurses (DH 2006a).

The ability to maintain one's own personal hygiene is a skill learnt early in life and is integral to a person's self-esteem, confidence and motivation (Holland and Hogg 2001). However, sometimes disability and/or physical and mental health problems lead to people needing assistance on either a temporary or a permanent basis. Henderson's definition of nursing emphasised this point, stating that the 'unique function of the nurse is to assist the individual ... in the performance of those activities contributing to health ... that he would perform unaided if he had necessary strength, will or knowledge'(Henderson 1960).

Meeting hygiene needs greatly contributes to comfort and the well-being of patients (Scott 2001), allowing the opportunity to build up a trusting relationship as well as assessing the individual physically and psychologically. As with any other skill/procedure, hygiene must be discussed fully with the person beforehand and verbal consent obtained. As this chapter focuses on the care of the body, last offices – care of the body after death – is also included.

The principles of care (e.g. observation, comfort, communication, safety and prevention of cross-infection) discussed in this chapter are generally relevant to anyone, but how they are carried out for each individual varies. It is also important to consider the religious and cultural needs of individuals when meeting hygiene needs.

This chapter includes:
- Rationale for meeting hygiene needs and potential hazards
- Bathing a person in bed
- Washing a person's hair in bed
- Bathing and showering in the bathroom
- Facial shaving
- Oral hygiene
- Last offices

> ### Recommended biology reading:
>
> You should revise the layers of the skin. In addition, these questions will help you to understand the biology underpinning this chapter's skills. Use your recommended textbook to find out:
>
> - The skin and oral cavity hosts a range of microorganisms. Which of these are potentially pathogenic?
> - What is saliva composed of? Where is it produced, and what is its role in maintaining a healthy mouth?
> - What protective mechanisms do eyes have that prevent them from infection?
> - Distinguish between transient and resident bacteria found on the skin. Which of these cannot be removed by handwashing? Chapter 3 will help you with this.
> - How does skin maintain its waterproof properties?
> - Why does the skin of the palms of the hands and soles of the feet wrinkle when soaked in water?
> - How does ageing affect the skin?
> - What part does nutrition play in maintaining a healthy skin, hair and nails?
> - Why do we sweat and what does sweat contain?
> - Why does stale sweat smell?
> - What is the 'acid mantle' and how can it be destroyed?

PRACTICE SCENARIOS

The following practice scenarios are referred to throughout this chapter in relation to meeting hygiene needs.

Adult

Metastases
Secondary deposits of cancer that have spread from the primary site, either directly or via blood or lymph.

Body mass index (BMI)
BMI is explained in Chapter 10 in the section 'Nutritional screening'. A BMI of 16 indicates a person is underweight.

William Newton, who likes to be called 'Bill', is a retired accountant aged 73. He is terminally ill with a history of oesophageal cancer and metastases in his lungs. He is cared for by his wife at home with the support of community nurses and the Macmillan nurse. He is taking regular oral morphine for pain control. He has a very low haemoglobin and has been admitted for a blood transfusion. He is weak, breathless and his general condition is poor. He has a body mass index (BMI) of 16. He can swallow only very small amounts of liquidised food and drink. He has some of his own teeth but also a partial denture which he likes to wear although it is now ill-fitting. His tongue appears coated and his mouth is dry.

Learning disability

Ellen Grey is a 47-year-old woman with a learning disability. She lives in sheltered accommodation in her own flat. There is a communal lounge. She has always managed her own personal hygiene adequately. However, recently she has developed an unpleasant smell and other residents have begun to avoid her because of this. The community nurse for learning disabilities has been asked to assess the situation and find out what has changed. She identifies that the reason Ellen's personal hygiene has become compromised is because of the recent development of nocturnal incontinence. As well as her bed-linen being wet, the situation has disrupted Ellen's usual hygiene routine.

Mental health

Miss Smith, aged 83 years, was admitted to an inpatient assessment unit for older people following concerns from her social worker and GP about her inability to cope at home due to severe depression. She lives on her own with only her pet dog for company. As she can no longer climb her stairs she has been sleeping in an armchair downstairs. Her poor mobility also prevented her from reaching the bathroom. Although Miss Smith is in reasonable physical health her clothing has obviously not been changed for many months and is encrusted with dirt and excrement. Her hair is badly knotted and matted and her skin is in poor condition. She also has poor oral hygiene, which she has obviously neglected for some time. Miss Smith was initially distrusting of staff and resisted all attempts to help her have a bath and clean clothes. Eventually she agreed to do this but remained hostile towards staff, accusing them of stealing her dog and her house. However nurses explained that her dog had been taken to the local RSPCA kennels and was in good health. Gradually Miss Smith became more accepting of her new surroundings and began to engage nurses in conversation without her previous hostility or suspicion.

RATIONALE FOR MEETING HYGIENE NEEDS AND POTENTIAL HAZARDS

LEARNING OUTCOMES

By the end of this section you will be able to:
1 identify why facilitating patients/clients to meet their hygiene needs is a beneficial nursing action;
2 discuss possible hazards and problems associated with meeting hygiene needs.

Learning outcome 1: Identify why facilitating patients/clients to meet their hygiene needs is a beneficial nursing action

ACTIVITY

Why is it important for nurses to assist with hygiene needs? Consider how you might feel if you were incapacitated mentally or physically and unable to meet your hygiene needs.

- Feeling clean and comfortable is an important social need for most people; to feel well groomed and not offensive to others can help to maintain self-esteem (Rader 1994; Henley and Schott 1999). Thus for Ellen to be aware that she has an unpleasant odour which others are discussing could cause her some distress. Miss Smith's poor mobility has prevented her maintaining her hygiene and this is probably upsetting for her.

- Cleanliness is also important within culture and religion (see later discussion). For example, for Muslims, cleanliness has both a spiritual and physical dimension (Rassool 2000). A study of older South Asian patients' experiences of culturally sensitive care highlighted that maintaining their hygiene was essential for dignity (Clegg 2003).

- The act of assisting people with personal hygiene needs allows nurses to build up a trusting relationship (Winkworth 2003). It is a private time where communication may be facilitated. Brawley (2002) points out that for people living in care homes bathtime may be one of the only opportunities for individual attention.

- Valuable observations can be made, for example the condition of the skin. This will be important for all the people in this chapter's scenarios.

- Cleansing the skin removes potentially harmful microorganisms and also sweat, dead skin cells and the bacteria which produce body odour.

- Washing stimulates the circulation; the movement associated with this and the effect of warm water on the skin is beneficial, both physiologically and psychologically (Sloane et al. 1995).

- Bathing has been described as one of the 'great pleasures in life' (Brawley 2002).

- For some patients, being washed or bathed by others can be humiliating so nurses must protect self-esteem and dignity as far as possible by adhering to individual wishes (Holland and Hogg 2001). The DH (2006b) has actively been promoting a Dignity in Care campaign encouraging all staff to consider patients' needs in relation to their dignity.

As identified above, observant nurses can learn a great deal about people when assisting with their hygiene needs.

ACTIVITY

What could you observe while assisting a patient/client with hygiene? Looking at the scenarios may give you some clues.

Oedematous
Swelling caused by the accumulation of fluid in the interstitial spaces

---

- **Condition of the skin.** Is there redness or bruising, and are there breaks in the skin? Is there any skin infection? Are there any old scars? This is important for Bill because of advancing disease, but is also relevant to Ellen and Miss Smith.

- **Hydration and nutrition.** Does the skin feel dry, loose or oedematous? Any of the people in this chapter's scenarios could become dehydrated due to poor fluid intake and their skin could become dry.

- **Mental state.** Is the person anxious, calm, restless, depressed, demotivated, cheerful, lethargic or confused?

- **Physical ability.** How much can the person do? Do they require prompting? With Ellen the nurse will be able to assess how much she can do for herself, what aspects she requires assistance with and what aids might be required. Does the activity cause them breathlessness, fatigue? This will affect Bill's ability to care for himself.

- **Condition of wounds, drains, intravenous sites** (IV). This could apply to Bill, for example inflammation of his IV site.

Learning outcome 2: Discuss the possible hazards and problems associated with meeting hygiene needs

As discussed above, meeting patients' hygiene needs should be a therapeutic intervention, yet there are several potential complications or difficulties.

<table>
<tr><td>ACTIVITY</td><td>What hazards or problems could be associated with meeting hygiene needs?</td></tr>
</table>

- *Access.* The person might be unable to get into a bathroom or the shower owing to mobility issues.
- *Environment.* Patients can become cold if left exposed for too long. There are health and safety aspects in relation to wet floors, and water being too hot/cold.
- *Cross-infection.* Some studies have shown that there were more bacteria on a patient's skin after a bed bath than before (Parker 2004).
- *Damage to skin.* The person might have allergies to particular soaps, or over-washing may remove essential oils.
- *Embarrassment.* Patients/clients may have a fear of their bodies being seen naked by others. Cultural or religious beliefs need to be considered.
- *Patient fatigue.* For example, meeting Bill's hygiene needs could exhaust him.

<table>
<tr><td>ACTIVITY</td><td>Consider the cultural and religious beliefs of the patients/clients you care for. What particular aspects are you aware of? The list that follows gives some examples.</td></tr>
</table>

- *African – Caribbean.* Hair type requires regular moisturising. The hair and scalp should be moistened every other day at least and the skin moistened once or twice a day (Christmas 2002).
- *Rastafarian.* The person might wear hair natural and uncut in obedience to God, who told the Nazarenes (a group of ancient Israelites) to do so. Some Rastafarians keep their hair covered. Modesty in dress is important. Hospital gowns may be viewed as immodest for women (Baxter 2002).
- *Sikhism.* Personal hygiene is very important. Hands and face must be washed and teeth brushed before eating. Showering is preferred to bathing (Gill 2002).
- *Islam.* A very high standard of hygiene is required (Rassool 2000). Muslims must wash before they pray (Holland and Hogg 2001).
- *Hinduism.* Handwashing is essential before and after eating. Washing in free flowing water is preferable.

Assessment and discussion with patients/clients on how they would like their hygiene needs met are key for this procedure to be therapeutic and will ensure any individual cultural/religious needs are met. *The Essence of Care* (DH 2001a) emphasises the need for assessment and re-assessment in order to maintain levels of hygiene.

Summary

- Assisting people to meet their hygiene needs can greatly increase comfort and provide an excellent opportunity for observation and assessment.
- Nurses must remember that not all patients/clients will enjoy the experience of being washed. They should therefore consider the key principles of care and comfort so care is delivered therapeutically.

BATHING A PERSON IN BED

Bathing a person in bed is necessary when people are unable to get out of bed for medical reasons (e.g. after certain surgery or injuries), or when they are too unwell or weak to be able to get out of bed. Bill may need this option at present. The procedure described in this section – bed-bathing – involves washing a patient's body while they are in bed, using a bowl of water and cloths. An alternative technique involves covering the face and body with warm towels that have been soaked in emollient/water solution in a plastic bag, referred to as a 'bag-bath' (Lentz 2003; Collins and Hampton 2003) or 'soft towel' method (Hancock *et al.* 2000). Hancock *et al.* found this method was preferred by patients and nurses; in particular the method kept patients warmer.

While this section focuses on bathing in bed, some patients who are unable to wash in the bathroom can sit out in a chair to wash, using a bowl. Nurses need to give assistance according to individual needs, based on assessment; the principles discussed in this section can be adapted to each situation.

LEARNING OUTCOMES

By the end of this section you will be able to:
1 discuss ways of maintaining patients' dignity and enhancing comfort when bathing a person in bed;
2 describe the procedure for carrying out bed-bathing.

Learning outcome 1: Discuss ways of maintaining patients' dignity and enhancing comfort when bathing a person in bed.

ACTIVITY

How might you maintain a patient's dignity and comfort while undertaking a bed-bath?

Points you may have considered include:
- ensuring that you have all necessary equipment before starting, to avoid leaving the patient during the procedure;
- ensuring privacy by drawing the curtains;
- ensuring windows are closed to avoid draughts;
- encouraging the patient to do as much as possible, allowing them the time to do this;
- asking the patient how they normally wash, what they use;

- covering the patient with a towel, only exposing areas of the body when necessary;
- using your communication skills – the atmosphere and relationship the nurse builds with the patient will do much to promote the patient's dignity;
- being aware that clothing may have special significance within some religions.

For example, in Sikhism there is a symbolic dress code – the five Ks: kesh (uncut hair), Kangha (wooden comb worn in the hair), Kara (steel bangle on right wrist), kirpan (small sword often secured in a cotton body-belt under clothes) and Kaccha (undershorts); these should not be removed unless absolutely necessary (Gill 2002).

The *National Service Framework for Older People* (DH 2001b) asserted that service users and carers should be able to expect that personal hygiene needs are carried out sensitively and in privacy.

Learning outcome 2: Describe the procedure for carrying out bed-bathing

Before commencing the bathing of a person in bed, you must assess the individual.

Assessment

ACTIVITY

Using one of the patient scenarios as a guide, what items should you include in your assessment? Compare your list with the following.

- What is the patient's normal hygiene routine? When do they normally wash/bathe? Can that be facilitated while they are in hospital?
- What toiletries do they use? Are they available?
- How does the patient feel today? Do they want a full wash or the bare minimum? This may change on a daily basis depending on how the patient is feeling.
- Does any care need to be given prior to the wash. For example, if the patient is due to have an enema it would be preferable to administer this prior to the wash.
- Does the patient require any analgesia prior to the bed-bath to ensure comfort when moving and turning?
- How much assistance is required? How much can the patient do? Does the nurse need to be present to prompt and guide, or does the patient want to be left alone to undertake some aspects?
- Does the patient want a member of the family to be involved in providing care? If yes, have they been asked? What is that person willing to do?
- How much time is needed to undertake this activity for this particular patient? What else is happening to the patient today: X-ray, theatre?
- How many staff are needed to undertake this activity for a particular patient?
- Are other healthcare professionals involved in the patient's care: occupational therapist, physiotherapist? Do they need to be involved to make a needs assessment?

Equipment

It is important to gather everything required prior to starting, to avoid having to leave the patient unattended; this will enhance the patient's privacy, dignity and

> ### Box 8.1 Preparing to bath a patient in bed: equipment required
>
> - Patient's own washing bowl
> - Soap, skin cleanser
> - Patient's own flannel or disposable flannel
> - Towels
> - Comb and/or brush
> - Toiletries as required, and may include shaving foam, razor, anti-perspirent, moisturiser
> - Clean bed linen and bed clothes
> - Linen bags and waste bag
> - Plastic apron and disposable gloves

comfort. Box 8.1 lists the equipment that you are likely to need, but always consider the patient's own individual requirements.

Procedure

Listed below is a suggested procedure for bathing a person in bed that is likely to maintain comfort and prevent the person from becoming cold. A sensitive and empathetic approach should be maintained throughout. Ensure that you have introduced yourself to the patient, and that you use the bed-bath as an opportunity to build further rapport. Patients you are bathing may be pleased to engage in conversation; but they may feel too weak and wish for a minimum of interaction, so be sensitive to non-verbal cues.

- Wash your hands and put on the plastic apron (and gloves if needed – see Chapter 3).
- Fill the bowl with comfortably warm water.
- Remove the top bedclothes, leaving the patient covered by a blanket, sheet or towels.
- Remove the pyjama jacket or nightdress. If the patient has a weak arm or has an intravenous infusion attached (as has Bill), remove this arm from the clothing last.

ACTIVITY

Practise with a friend or colleague, removing a jacket or cardigan from each other, while pretending that one arm's mobility is impaired. Now try replacing it, inserting the affected arm first.

- Can the patient wash his or her own face? Even quite unwell people often like to do this for themselves. Otherwise, wash the patient's face, using soap if wanted. Never poke inside ears. Rinse off soap, if used, and dry carefully. With eyes, take care to wash from the inner to outer corner of the eye, thus reducing the risk of contamination. Always approach any care relating to eyes with gentleness and cleanliness to avoid risk of trauma or cross-infection.

ACTIVITY

With a friend or colleague, practise washing and drying each other's face. How did it feel?

People who are unconscious or semi-conscious are at risk of their eyes becoming dry. Eyes need to be assessed regularly for signs of irritation, corneal drying, abrasions and oedema (Geraghty 2005).

ACTIVITY | Find out about the eye care policy in your current care setting.

The policy should include the following:
1. an eye assessment;
2. how to cleanse eyes;
3. what to use to cleanse eyes;
4. any ointments to be administered;
5. whether to maintain eyelid closure.

Having completed your patient's face wash, the bathing procedure should continue:
- Place a towel under the arm furthest away from you, and wash from the hand to the axilla. Rinse off the soap and dry thoroughly, taking care not to dislodge any cannulae or dressings. Repeat with the other arm.
- Uncover the chest and abdomen and wash and dry this area in the same way, again taking care not to dislodge dressings or attachments. Work gently but quickly to prevent the patient from becoming chilled. Pay special attention to skin folds and under the breasts, as these areas may be moist through sweat and therefore heavily colonised with microorganisms. A little talcum powder may be applied if liked; shake it into your hand rather than directly on to the patient, as the fine powder can be irritating if inhaled. Cover the chest and abdomen once this is completed. Other toiletries such as anti-perspirant or body spray can be applied as wished by the patient.
- Change the water at this point, or at any time if it feels cool or becomes excessively soiled. If water is not changed and the same washcloth is used for the whole body the water can become full of bacteria and be a potential hazard to patients with breaks in their skin (Ayliffe *et al.* 2001).
- Now remove any lower body clothing including anti-embolism stockings, cover the leg nearest you, and place the towel under the opposite leg. Wash the leg from toes to groin, rinse and dry. Apply moisturising lotion if the skin appears dry over the shins or feet. Repeat with the other leg.

ACTIVITY | What observations should you be making while washing arms, body and legs?

Your observations should include condition of the skin, checking for dryness, colour, bruises, abrasions, rashes, swelling or oedema. Nurses should apply skin moisturisers for patients as needed. You should also note any tenderness in the limbs, particularly the calves, which might indicate a deep vein thrombosis (see Chapter 6).

For some people, attention to foot care is particularly important. Those at risk of foot problems include older people and people with diabetes, peripheral vascular disease or peripheral neuropathy (Thompson 1999). Foot problems in people with diabetes are discussed in detail by many authors (e.g. Edwards 1998; Renwick *et al.* 1998; Foster 1999); see also Chapter 7 in this book. A systematic review indicated that patient education about foot care may reduce foot ulceration and amputations, especially in high-risk patients (Valk *et al.* 2001). When people are unable to self-care, nurses must carry out the foot care and observation required, and report any concerns immediately. In some circumstances, nurses can use this opportunity to educate people about foot care. Box 8.2 outlines the key principles.

The bathing procedure should continue:

- Using a disposable washcloth, wash the genitals and perineal area, working from front to back to prevent contamination of the urethra and/or vagina with faecal matter. Catheter care may be required at this point (see Chapter 9, section on 'Caring for people who have urinary catheters'). Change the water now – remember the rationale for this (see previous section, learning outcome 2).

ACTIVITY   Recall your earlier thoughts in learning outcome 1 and how you could maintain dignity during this intimate care. What might be Bill's specific needs?

Box 8.2 Advice about foot care for people with diabetes (adapted from NICE 2004)

- Wash feet daily, drying them carefully and thoroughly, particularly between the toes.
- Examine feet daily for problems (colour change, swelling, breaks in skin, pain or numbness). If they occur, report them to a healthcare professional. People with a foot care emergency (new ulceration, swelling, discoloration) should be seen by a multidisciplinary foot care team within 24 hours. Check the top of the foot, the sole of the foot (patients can be taught to use a mirror to do this), between the toes and pressure areas, i.e. tips of toes and heels.
- Check for signs of redness around nail areas, and ensure nails do not cut into adjacent toes. Cut immediately after bathing when nails are soft, following the shape of the toe and not down into tissue. If nails are thick and brittle, do not attempt to cut – refer to podiatrist.

Note: Follow local policies regarding nail-cutting.

- Make sure that shoes and hosiery fit well.
- Ensure that feet are assessed at least annually by trained personnel.

In addition, people at increased or high risk of foot ulcers (neuropathy, and/or absent pulses or other risk factor) should:

- Have feet reviewed by a foot protection team 3–6 monthly.
- Never walk barefoot.
- Realise that any break in the skin is potentially serious.
- Check bath temperatures carefully (numb feet cannot assess temperature).
- Avoid hot waterbottles, electric blankets, foot spas and sitting with feet too close to fires.
- Get help to deal with calluses and corns (avoid over-the-counter remedies).
- Regularly inspect footwear for rough areas, ripped linings, etc.

Most people, if at all able, would probably prefer to attend to this care themselves, but some people are too physically or mentally impaired to do so. Although Bill is weak, he might be able to do this for himself with some help.

- At this point, you need to assess how you can wash the patient's back. You can either sit the person forward or lie them on their side. Sitting Bill forward to wash his back would be best as he might become breathless if lying on his side for long, You can ask/assist him to lean forward, wash, rinse and dry his back, using a clean washcloth. The pillowcases can be changed, and he can be assisted into a clean pyjama jacket. For a woman, a clean nightdress can be put on at this point.

- To wash a person's back if they cannot sit forward, and to wash people's buttocks, you need to turn them on their side; you may require assistance to do this. The bottom sheet can be changed at this time. A slide sheet could be inserted to assist with turning and then moving the patient up the bed after completing the wash. If you feel assistance is not required, you need to raise the opposite bed side to provide security for the patient when rolling on to their side. Assist the patient to roll over, using the log roll method. Roll up the soiled bottom sheet lengthways, close to the patient. Place a towel along the patient's back, wash, rinse and dry the back and buttocks, noting any skin problems as previously outlined.

ACTIVITY Which areas of skin do you think you should pay most attention to while the patient is on their side?

You should observe the areas most at risk from pressure damage. These include the sacrum, trochanters, elbows and shoulder tips, base of the skull and heels. See Chapter 6 section on 'Pressure ulcer risk assessment' for more details; Box 6.1 outlines how to inspect skin for signs of early pressure damage.

- Now assist with putting on pyjama trousers or adjusting a nightdress. Some people prefer to wear underwear in bed, so then ensure you help them with this. Replace the anti-embolism stockings if worn and change the bottom sheet. To do this, roll or concertina fold a clean sheet close to the patient, taking care not to contaminate the clean sheet with the soiled one. Assist the patient to roll back towards you, and support them while your assistant removes the soiled sheet, pulls though the clean one and secures it.

ACTIVITY What might be the infection control issues when disposing of the soiled sheet?

Look back to the principles of preventing cross-infection outlined in Chapter 3. Used linen (soiled and foul) should be disposed of in white or off-white bags. Infected linen should be placed into a water-soluble bag and then into a red bag.

ACTIVITY You will need two friends/colleagues for this exercise, and access to a bed in the skills laboratory. Practise changing the bottom sheet, taking it in turns to be the 'patient'. Consider whether you felt vulnerable during this. What reassured you?

- Using safe moving and handling methods, assist the patient into an appropriate and comfortable position, according to their condition and care plan.
- Brush or comb the patient's hair into their preferred style. Carry out any other hair care needed at this stage – check the patient's personal requirements and what assistance they need.
- Assist with make-up if required by the patient, and with oral hygiene (see later section).
- Place the locker and call bell within reach.
- Wash and dry the bowl, and dispose of soiled equipment appropriately (see Chapter 3, section on 'Waste disposal'). Washbowls should be stored upside down to reduce colonisation by microorganisms, which prefer horizontal surfaces. Also, if washbowls are not dried properly and are stacked together bacteria multiply in the moisture trapped between the bowls; contaminated washbowls have been implicated in infection outbreaks, Gram-negative bacteria being most likely to be found (Ayliffe *et al.* 2001).
- Patients' own washcloths need to be washed thoroughly after use and stored so that they can dry. They should *not* be wrapped around the soap (Parker 2004).
- Document any observations made, and the care given, in the care plan or nursing notes.

Summary

- It is important to assess the suitability of a bed-bath for the individual patient, and negotiate involvement by the patient and family, as desired.
- Respect for the individual's privacy and dignity, and maintenance of comfort, should be promoted.
- Adherence to infection control procedures and safe moving and handling techniques is vital.

WASHING A PERSON'S HAIR IN BED

LEARNING OUTCOMES

By the end of this section you will be able to:
1 state the circumstances under which hairwashing in bed may be carried out;
2 describe the procedure for hairwashing, considering infection control, and patient comfort and safety needs.

Learning outcome 1: State the circumstances under which hairwashing in bed may be carried out

Many people will not be confined to bed long enough for hair washing to become a problem, and will be able to visit the bathroom where hairwashing will be more easily accomplished. In the short term, a dry shampoo can be brushed through the hair, to absorb grease and sebum and remove dead skin cells. However, if patients remain in bed for long periods their hair will need washing. This could be necessary for Bill, who, as his disease becomes more advanced, might need to have his hair washed in bed. Some hospitals have a visiting hairdresser who washes patients' hair in bed. Find out if this facility is available in your area.

You may have been introduced to the Roper–Logan–Tierney model of nursing (Roper *et al.* 2000). Which activity of living is hairwashing associated with?

Hairwashing is associated with the 'Personal cleansing and dressing' and 'Expressing sexuality' activities of living. In many cultures, hair and hairstyles play a large part in defining and advertising sexual identity. Hair can be an important part of a person's body image, and its condition may improve or lower self-esteem. These issues are considered in Chapter 2.

Learning outcome 2: Describe the procedure for hairwashing, considering infection control and patient comfort and safety needs

As with bathing in bed, think ahead about what you will need. Box 8.3 suggests suitable equipment.

Positioning

First remove the head of the bed, and assist the patient to lie flat.

Consider patient safety and comfort. Which patients might not be able to lie flat?

Examples include people who are breathless (like Bill), people with arthritis of the neck, or patients on skull traction. It is therefore very important to assess the individual before commencing hairwashing. If the patient cannot lie down, hair can be washed over a bowl on a bed table.

Procedure

- Place the empty bowl on a chair or bed table at the head of the bed, at a lower level. Consider your own comfort at this point: is the bed at a comfortable height for you to work without stooping?

Box 8.3 Preparing to wash hair in bed: equipment required

- Large jug or bowl of hand hot water
- Empty bowl
- Shampoo guard if available
- Plastic sheeting if available
- Small jug
- Shampoo and conditioner, as requested by the patient
- Towels and flannel
- Brush/comb and hairdryer
- Plastic apron

- Arrange the plastic sheet to protect the mattress and a towel to protect the patient's shoulders.
- Move the patient, using a slide sheet, so that their head is over the bowl. An assistant may be required to support the patient's head.
- Having checked the temperature of the water, wet the hair using the small jug. The patient may like to protect their eyes with a clean flannel.
- Apply shampoo, massage gently into the scalp, and rinse off. Repeat this if desired. Apply conditioner, if used, comb through, leave for a minute or two, and rinse off until the hair feels clean. You may have to empty the bowl at intervals, before it gets too full.
- Be aware of health and safety issues: mop up any spills immediately.
- Wrap the patient's hair in a clean towel and move the bowl out of the way.
- Slide the patient back on to the bed, and remove the plastic sheet. Make sure the bottom sheet is not damp; replace if necessary.
- Replace the head of the bed, and assist the patient to sit up if able, using a safe moving and handling technique.
- Empty the bowl of water once the patient is comfortable.
- Towel the hair dry, and style the hair as desired, using a hairdryer if necessary.

ACTIVITY   What health and safety issues should be considered when using hairdryers?

It is important to make sure that:
1. the hairdryer is not too hot;
2. there are no trailing flexes;
3. the equipment is checked regularly by an electrician;
4. the electric hairdryer and water are not in contact.
Finally:
- Wash and dry the bowls and jug, and dispose of all equipment in accordance with hospital policy. Leave the patient comfortable, with bed table, locker and call bell within reach. Document the care given in the care plan or nursing notes.

Summary

- If hairwashing in bed is required, carefully assess the patient's suitability first.
- Be aware of individual preferences in hair care.
- Maintain health and safety for both yourself and patients.

BATHING AND SHOWERING IN THE BATHROOM

If people are able to visit the bathroom to meet their personal hygiene needs, this is usually preferable for various reasons. For some people, actually going in the bath or shower may not be possible, but they may be able to at least sit and wash at the sink, which is usually preferable to washing in, or by, the bed.

On completion of this section you will be able to:
1 state the particular benefits and possible problems of meeting hygiene needs in the bathroom rather than at the bedside;
2 describe the procedure for assisting with bathing/showering in the bathroom, discussing health and safety issues.

Learning outcome 1: State the particular benefits and possible problems of meeting hygiene needs in the bathroom rather than at the bedside

ACTIVITY

Which of the people in this chapter's scenarios may be able to visit the bathroom to meet their hygiene needs?

> Health Action Plan
> A personal action plan developed for each individual with a learning disability, containing details of their health interventions, medication taken, screening tests etc. See *Valuing People* (DH 2001c).

All should be able to at some stage, but as previously mentioned, Bill may be too weak, tired or in pain to do so at present. Miss Smith will be able to visit the bathroom but will require mobility aids. Ellen will carry out her hygiene care in her own bathroom, but the nurse must revisit her knowledge and skills and reinforce the importance of good hygiene and a bathing routine. Underlying causes of her incontinence must be investigated using a specific tool which addresses physical, psychological and environmental dimensions. The nurse can support Ellen in accessing the necessary services (e.g. continence advisor). The aim should be for Ellen to regain continence and her ability to maintain her hygiene so her Health Action Plan should be amended to address these issues. The nurse should broach the subject sensitively; it is important to ensure that this short-term problem does not impact on her social integration and relationships in the longer term. Perhaps a carer could visit in the mornings and evenings, to help Ellen structure her day and ensure that her hygiene needs are being met.

Ellen will probably not require physical assistance in the bathroom, but she needs prompting, encouragement and praise for success in meeting her hygiene needs plan. As she re-establishes her skills, support can reduce until Ellen is self-caring once more.

The presence of a wound is not a contraindication to a shower or bath, as long as the skin edges of the wound are sealed (Briggs 1997). However, a shower is preferable to a bath for a person with a wound as there is less risk of cross-infection from a previous user (Gilchrist 1990).

ACTIVITY

Why might it be preferable for hygiene needs to be met in the bathroom if possible, rather than at the bedside?

• The bathroom is a more familiar environment for hygiene, which is important for someone who is confused, or who is preparing for discharge home. Ellen's teaching programme to meet her hygiene needs will be more effective if carried out in her own familiar bathroom. The bathroom is the most appropriate environment for Miss Smith to re-establish a routine of hygiene care.

- Privacy can be more easily maintained in a bathroom than behind curtains at the bedside.
- There is a continuous supply of water which may be desirable for cultural and/or religious reasons. For example in Hinduism, washing in running water, as a shower or by pouring water from a jug, is very important (Holland and Hogg 2001). This is easier to achieve in the bathroom.
- For older people, going into a bath is a familiar activity. Some people, for example those with muscle spasm, find a bath relaxing and therapeutic, particularly when used with bathwater additives (Tarling 1997).

ACTIVITY

While there are good reasons why people can better carry out hygiene in the bathroom, you may be able to think of some possible problems. List these.

- Patients can become chilled if a suitable temperature cannot be maintained. It can also be exhausting for people with few reserves of strength, like Bill. There are various health and safety hazards; these are discussed later.
- A bathroom may cause problems for a person whose condition is unstable – physically and mentally. Unless a nurse stays with them, observation is more difficult in a bathrooms than when they are behind curtains in the ward.
- Brawley (2002) points out that for a person with dementia, particularly if they have a visual or hearing impairment, bathrooms can be noisy and disorientating, causing fear and confusion.

The Essence of Care (DH 2001a) emphasised the importance of providing an appropriate environment for hygiene needs to be met in the benchmark of best practice: 'Patients/clients have access to an environment that is safe and acceptable to the individual' (p. 52). People with impaired mobility, like Miss Smith, have special moving and handling requirements and need suitable equipment to enable them to access baths or showers. Nurses must maintain sound moving and handling practices within bathrooms to prevent injury to patients and themselves. Occupational therapists can advise on equipment. There are shower trolleys available, which can be useful for people with spinal injuries or other neurological conditions such as cerebral palsy. There is a wide range of other equipment available to assist with bathing and showering (Collins 2001).

Learning outcome 2: Describe the procedure for assisting with bathing/ showering in the bathroom, discussing health and safety issues

As with washing a person in bed, you should introduce yourself and build a rapport prior to assisting with personal care. Miss Smith was initially resistant to going to the bathroom, but as a relationship with the staff was established she became more accepting of their help. Nurses should be patient and understanding in such situations. Assisting with hygiene in the bathroom provides opportunities to further the nurse–patient/client relationship, as it involves one-to-one interaction in a private environment.

The carers of some adults might wish to continue to be involved in bathing. A person with dementia, for example, may be more comfortable if their usual carer assists. This involvement in care should be negotiated by nurses and not taken for granted, as some informal carers may be exhausted and might appreciate a break. Involving relatives in bathing can be important preparation for discharge, particularly where a person has a new disability. Nurses can teach relatives about use of equipment and skin observation and care for example.

Equipment

As always, it is important to plan ahead, gathering all equipment likely to be needed. Having to leave the bathroom to fetch items when the person is undressed could lead to chilling and exposure; and if a person is unsafe to leave, the nurse would have to ring the call bell and wait for help to arrive. The toiletries required vary between individuals, so always ask about preferences, which some people may indicate through non-verbal rather than verbal communication. You are likely to need towels, soap/shower gel or other cleansing agent, shampoo/conditioner (if hair washing is to be carried out), clean clothing (of the person's choice), brush/comb, toothbrush and toothpaste, and flannel/disposable washcloths. Some people are prescribed specific skin care agents for use in the bath or afterwards.

Preparing the bathroom

After assembling the equipment, check that the bathroom is free, and has been cleaned after any previous user.

ACTIVITY

Why is it necessary to check the bathroom prior to taking your patients/ clients there?

Apart from any physical soiling, you should consider cross-infection risk. Always adhere to the relevant infection control policy for your practice setting regarding cleaning of baths/showers between uses. You should also check that the floor is not wet or slippery, and that any extra equipment, such as a hoist or shower stool, is available and in safe working order. Also check the temperature of the bathroom, as some people are susceptible to the cold, particularly if underweight like Bill or older people like Miss Smith. Warm the bathroom first if necessary.

Bathing or showering procedure

The following steps provide a suggested procedure that will maintain comfort and safety. As with bed-bathing, nurses must be sensitive and respectful when assisting with hygiene in the bathroom.

- If bathing, fill the bath with warm water, using your elbow or a bath thermometer to check the temperature.
- Assist the person to the bathroom, offering them the opportunity to use the toilet first if necessary.

- Give consideration to people who have sensory impairment. People with visual impairment can find bathrooms difficult as there are often white walls and white bathroom suite, making it difficult to locate the sink or bath. Therefore always take time to orientate them to the environment, showing them where everything is.
- Assist with undressing, maintaining dignity and comfort and avoiding unnecessary exposure by using towels.
- If the person has a urinary catheter *in situ,* a shower is preferable. However, if a bath is used, then the catheter should be clamped if the catheter has to be lifted above bladder level (e.g. when assisting the person in and out of the bath), to prevent reflux of urine back into the bladder (Pratt *et al.* 2007).
- If bathing, check the bathwater temperature again and allow the patient to check for themselves if they are able. Remember that some people have impaired sensation in their feet and will not be able to feel the temperature accurately.
- Using suitable equipment if necessary, help the person into the bath, or on to the shower chair. If the shower is being used, check the temperature before use.
- Promote independence by supporting/enabling people to wash themselves as far as possible. Miss Smith's independence should be encouraged to rebuild her confidence in meeting her hygiene needs. Ellen will need gentle prompting without being patronising.
- As with bathing in bed, particular attention should be given to skin creases, and areas susceptible to becoming sore – for example under breasts, palms of hands which are fixed in tonic flexion. Remember from the earlier section 'Bathing a person in bed', the importance of foot care for some people, particularly those with diabetes. Check Box 8.2, to remind yourself of the essential observations and care. Miss Smith's feet could be in a poor condition as she might not have been able to reach them for some time. She may need to be referred to a podiatrist.
- You should only leave a person alone in the bath or shower if you have assessed that it is safe to do so. For example, people who have epilepsy should not be left alone and neither should people who are confused. Always check with the registered nurse, if unsure. If it is safe to leave a person, ensure that the call bell is within reach, and working, before leaving.
- Remember, skin condition can be specifically observed, as well as psychological and physical condition – for example, any pain or breathlessness on movement, level of motivation to assist. These will all be important observations when assisting Miss Smith.
- If hairwashing is required, as for Miss Smith, use clean water in a washbasin or bowl, and a jug, or shower attachment. Wet the hair, allowing the person to protect their eyes with a flannel. Apply shampoo, and massage gently into the scalp. Rinse and repeat, if necessary, and apply conditioner, as needed. Rinse again, and dry with a clean towel.
- Before assisting the person out of the bath, it may be easier to let some water out, and dry the upper body. This minimises the time for the person to become chilled. Assist the person out of the bath or shower, using equipment as necessary, and assist with drying as needed, again thinking about maintaining comfort and

dignity by avoiding unnecessary exposure. Talcum powder and other toiletries can be applied if liked at this point. Can you recall the safety points about applying talcum powder which were discussed in the section on bathing in bed?

- Assist the person to dress in clean clothes, to clean teeth (see oral hygiene section), and to brush/style hair as desired. Once again, assess the person's ability to participate in these activities. Both Miss Smith and Ellen may need verbal encouragement and reinforcement. A structured, behavioural approach may be needed.
- Dispose of used equipment in accordance with waste disposal policy, and leave the bathroom clean and ready for the next user.
- Document the care given in the care plan or nursing notes.

Summary

- Meeting hygiene needs in the bathroom is preferable for many reasons, for example privacy and the availability of running water.
- When assisting with hygiene in the bathroom, always assemble all equipment beforehand, to avoid leaving people alone.
- The bathroom is potentially hazardous. It is important to take active steps to avoid accidents, such as falls or scalding, and only leave people alone if you have assessed that it is safe to do so.
- Maintain privacy and dignity throughout, and promote independence.

FACIAL SHAVING

LEARNING OUTCOMES

On completion of this section you will be able to:
1 discuss the rationale for shaving patients/clients who are unable to do this for themselves;
2 list the equipment needed and describe the procedure for shaving.

Learning outcome 1: Discuss the rationale for shaving patients/clients who are unable to do this for themselves

Facial hair has important social and cultural meanings. In some religions, for example Sikhism, neither facial nor hair on the head may be cut. In many Western European cultures, a wide variety of facial hair is socially acceptable, and contributes to maintaining self-esteem. While facial shaving is usually associated with men, some females (particularly older women) have unwanted facial hair which they prefer to remove. This is important to their body image. If a female patient requests assistance with shaving, always approach this sensitively and matter-of-factly.

ACTIVITY

Talk to a male relative or friend who is usually clean shaven. Ask him how he would feel if unable to shave himself.

For many men, being clean shaven is important and being unable to self-care in this way would be distressing. In addition, people visiting relatives can be upset to find them unshaven if they are usually clean shaven, and would view such a lack of care as neglectful, leading to a loss of confidence in staff. For some people shaving may be hazardous. For example, individuals receiving anti-coagulant medication can be at risk of bleeding from minor cuts, so it is safer to use an electric razor rather than carrying out a wet shave.

Learning outcome 2: List the equipment needed and describe the procedure for shaving

Equipment

You need:

- either a razor, with shaving soap/foam and shaving brush, or the person's own electric razor (communal razors pose a high risk of cross-infection);
- towel and flannel/disposable washcloth;
- bowl of hand-hot water;
- aftershave, if desired.

Procedure

Assemble the equipment and assist the person to sit up if possible. Protect the person's chest with a towel. Assess to what extent the person can assist. For some men, careful positioning, provision of a shaving mirror and having all equipment to hand may enable them to be independent with shaving. Shaving requires very fine motor control so it is important to assess the person's capability. The individual's care plan should clarify this and any particular precautions needed.

Wet shaving

- Wet the brush and apply the soap to the face, or use the foam, working up a good lather.
- Work in the direction of the hair growth, starting with the cheeks and moving on to the neck and around the mouth.
- Hold the skin taut and avoid any sores or moles. The person may be able to help by tightening his facial muscles. However, this would not be possible for all men, for example if facial weakness is present.
- For some men the facial skin can be hypersensitive and therefore great care should be taken.
- Rinse the razor after each stroke.
- When you have finished, rinse the face with clean water and dry, apply aftershave if used. Dispose of used equipment safely. Document your care in the care plan or nursing notes.

Dry shaving

- The skin should be clean and dry; a little talcum powder may help. Work with circular strokes, keeping the skin taut as for wet shaving.

- Assist the person to rinse his face when finished, apply aftershave if desired, and clean the razor ready for the next occasion. Document your care in the care plan or nursing notes.

ACTIVITY

Find a willing male friend, relative or colleague and practise both a wet shave and a dry shave. Even if you shave yourself, you may find this more difficult than you expect. Ask your 'patient' to comment on your technique.

Although this section has concentrated on facial shaving, remember that some people may wish to have other parts of the body shaved, for example legs and armpits. The nurse needs to assist with this as appropriate.

Summary

- Facial shaving is important to many people. Nurses should assist if people are unable to self-care, thus maintaining self-esteem.
- A gentle and careful technique should be used, using the person's preferred equipment.

ORAL HYGIENE

Maintaining oral hygiene is an important aspect of nursing care, as it can do much to enhance quality of life and promote health. Jones (1998) advocates that nurses should include mouth care as part of daily hygiene for people who are debilitated, but should also promote effective oral hygiene in people who can self-care. *The Essence of Care* (DH 2001a) includes benchmarks for best practice in oral hygiene, which will be referred to in this section. NHS Quality Improvement Scotland (QIS) (2005) presents best practice statements for good oral health for older people.

LEARNING OUTCOMES

By the end of this section you will be able to:
1 discuss the rationale for maintaining good oral hygiene;
2 identify factors that increase vulnerability to poor oral hygiene, and consider how those at risk can be identified;
3 understand how oral hygiene can be carried out safely and based on best evidence.

Learning outcome 1: Discuss the rationale for maintaining good oral hygiene

Oral hygiene aims to maintain a healthy oral mucosa, teeth, gums and lips, by using toothpaste, brush or other cleansing agents. A dry mouth causes people considerable distress (Kaye 1992).

ACTIVITY

What problems may arise if oral hygiene is poor, as in Miss Smith's case?

You may have considered:

- mouth and gum infections such as candidiasis ('thrush'), which is a fungal infection (Torrance 1990);
- inability to eat and malnutrition (NHS QIS 2005);
- halitosis leading to social withdrawal;
- systemic spread of infection in immunocompromised patients (Corbett 1997);
- low self-esteem (Huff *et al*. 2006).

NHS QIS (2005) also highlights a link between pneumonia and poor oral health in older people.

Learning outcome 2: Identify factors that increase vulnerability to poor oral hygiene, and consider how those at risk can be identified

ACTIVITY

You already know that Miss Smith's oral hygiene is poor. What might be the reasons for this? Now consider the other people in this chapter's scenarios. Do you think any of them are at risk of poor oral hygiene too?

Miss Smith's poor mobility has affected her ability to carry out her usual hygiene care as she cannot get to the bathroom. Although she could clean her teeth at the kitchen sink she might not have been able to adapt her routine in this way, perhaps because of her depression. She may not have been able to access a dentist or buy the necessary equipment to carry out oral hygiene. Her poor oral hygiene might have led to poor oral intake of food and fluids, thus worsening her mouth condition.

Bill is at risk of oral hygiene problems. He has an ill-fitting denture, he can drink only small amounts and he is generally debilitated. Oral *Candida* infections are common in people who are debilitated (Ayliffe *et al*. 2001).

Ellen may be maintaining good oral hygiene but the community nurse for learning disabilities could check that she is coping with her oral hygiene. Some people with learning disabilities can have oral hypersensitivity, making it uncomfortable to clean their teeth. The DH (2001c), in *Valuing People*, acknowledges that people with learning disabilities often have poor oral health leading to chronic dental problems. Davies *et al*. (2000) identify various reasons for this, including fear of dental treatment (particularly where there is difficulty understanding the need for treatment), the need to be accompanied, difficult access to healthcare facilities and negative professional attitudes. The health facilitator should provide support in overcoming these barriers and regular visits to the dentist must be included in Ellen's Health Action Plan. Tooth decay would adversely affect her quality of life, leading to pain, the need for dental treatment and poor food intake.

There are many factors that can lead to poor oral hygiene (see Table 8.1). Looking at this table might prompt you to identify further risk factors for the people in the scenarios. For example, Bill is taking morphine, which causes mouth dryness. Thurgood (1994) notes that most seriously ill people have mouth problems, which cause further discomfort and distress. The Alzheimer's Society identify how Alzheimer's disease can affect oral health and offer useful advice (see www.alzheimers.org.uk).

Health facilitator
A member of the community learning disabilities team (often a nurse) who supports a person with learning disabilities to access the healthcare they need. See *Valuing People* (DH 2001c).

Table 8.1: Factors predisposing to mouth problems (adapted from Thurgood 1994).

Drugs	• Cytotoxic drugs (reduce autoimmune response) • Corticosteroids (affect tissue healing) • Antibiotics (alters oral bacterial balance, allowing infection by *Candida albicans*) • Antihistamines, antispasmodics, anticholinergics, psychotropics, antidepressants, and tranquillisers (reduce salivary production) • Diuretics (increase fluid loss) • Morphine (causes mouth dryness)
Treatments	• Radiotherapy of head/neck (causes localised inflammation, affects ability to eat/drink normally) • Oxygen therapy, particularly if given unhumidified at high flow rates (dries oral mucosa) • Suction (can damage oral mucosa) • Restricted oral intake, such as 'nil by mouth' pre- or post-op (potential for dehydration and dry mouth)
Mental or physical health problems or disability	• Diseases: diabetes, thyroid dysfunction, oral disease/trauma, cerebrovascular disease • Mental health problems: confusion, depression • Terminal illness • Acute/chronic breathing problems • Unconsciousness • Lack of manual dexterity

People's ability to self-care for oral hygiene can change quickly, so nurses should regularly reassess this and other risk factors. *The Essence of Care* (DH 2001a) emphasises the importance of assessing individuals regarding how their oral hygiene can be maintained with its best practice benchmark:

> All patients/clients are assessed to identify the advice and/or care required to maintain and promote their individual oral hygiene.

Further benchmarks of best practice advise that the care planned and the level of assistance provided should be based on this assessment and individual needs.

ACTIVITY

What aspects would you consider when assessing oral hygiene needs?

You may have thought of the following:
- condition of the teeth – plaque, cavities;
- condition of the tongue – coated, clean;
- condition of the lips;
- ability to undertake oral care;
- ability to eat;
- whether patients have their own teeth or plates/dentures.

Assessment tools can be helpful for assessing the need for, and frequency of, mouth care. They incorporate scoring systems indicating levels of risk and several have been published (Freer 2000; Lockwood 2000; Dickinson *et al.* 2001). Factors commonly included are current mouth condition, nutritional status and special risk factors, like those in Table 8.1 (e.g. certain medication, oxygen therapy).

ACTIVITY Find out whether an oral assessment tool is used in your current clinical area and, if so, look at the aspects included and ensure you understand any scoring systems used.

Learning outcome 3: Understand how oral hygiene can be carried out safely and based on best evidence

Bowsher *et al.*'s (1999) systematic review indicates that oral care is not always evidence-based. For example, there is clear evidence *against* the use of hydrogen peroxide mouthwashes, lemon and glycerine swabs, and using foam swabs for teeth cleaning, yet they can still be found used in practice. As with any other nursing practice, best available evidence should be used for oral hygiene. A variety of equipment may be needed, depending on the care identified as appropriate for the individual. Possible items are listed in Box 8.4.

Rationale for choice of equipment

A small, soft-bristled toothbrush is the most effective agent for removing plaque and debris from the mouth, teeth and tongue (Thurgood 1994). A trial comparing the ability of foam swabs and toothbrushes in removing plaque confirmed that toothbrushes perform substantially better (Pearson and Hutton 2002). Fluoridated toothpaste should be used (NHS QIS 2005).

Jones (1998) advises that toothpaste has a generally drying effect so it should be used sparingly – about the size of a pea. Most antiseptic mouthwashes have a very transient effect so they are of limited value (Jones 1998). However, those containing chlorhexidine gluconate, for example Corsodyl, if used for 1 minute, can reduce bacterial counts by up to 80 per cent (Schiott *et al.* 1970, cited by Jones 1998). Its use is therefore worthwhile in very vulnerable people, for example immunocompromised, very sick or frail older people. Mouthwash is also useful in areas that are hard to reach (Xavier 2000).

Jones (1998) advises that, for cleansing and moistening oral mucosa, pH-balanced swabsticks are preferable; but if foam swab sticks are used, they are best when coated with Corsodyl gel, which is gentler to the delicate oral mucosa. There

Box 8.4 Equipment for oral care

- Spatula and pen torch (to inspect the oral cavity)
- Small, soft-bristled toothbrush (for teeth cleaning)
- Mouthwash, e.g. chlorhexidine (to prevent dental plaque) or water (for teeth cleaning)
- Toothpaste
- Container for dentures, if needed
- Lip lubricant, e.g. soft paraffin, to prevent dry lips
- Beaker and receiver (for mouth rinsing)
- Disposable gloves and plastic apron
- Towel, tissues

are also saliva substitutes available for people with dry mouths (Jones 1998). If foam mouth swabs are used, always check that the foam head is firmly attached to the stick before using and do not soak it before use as this can reduce the strength of the attachment; if the foam head detaches during use it could be a choking hazard (Medicine and Healthcare products Regulatory Agency 2008).

ACTIVITY

Drawing on your practice experience, how could nurses approach promoting oral hygiene for each of the people in this chapter's scenarios?

Bill may be able to carry out his own oral hygiene if equipment is placed within his reach. Perhaps he could sit at a sink to carry out his oral care, which will include cleaning his teeth and dentures. Due to his mouth's current poor condition, and if his condition worsens, he may need regular oral hygiene carried out in between teeth cleaning. This is discussed later.

Ellen can be verbally encouraged and supported in carrying out her own oral hygiene in the bathroom. For Miss Smith, equipment for oral hygiene will need to be provided and nurses should support her and encourage her to re-establish teeth cleaning, which can be done in the bathroom at the sink. She should be approached sensitively about visiting a dentist.

Teeth cleaning should be carried out twice daily (British Dental Health Foundation; see www.dentalhealth.org.uk). Cleaning of dentures should be carried out at least daily but ideally after meals too. If patients are unable to carry this out independently, nurses must provide the necessary equipment and assistance. Some people, who are more dependent and debilitated, require nurses to carry out oral hygiene on a regular basis by the bedside. The frequency of oral care should be determined on an individual basis. This care, which may be necessary for Bill, is described below.

Oral hygiene procedure: key points

- After explaining the procedure and gaining consent, the person should be assisted into a sitting position or, if unconscious, on their side to prevent inhalation of solutions or secretions.
- Protect the person's chest with a towel, or the bed with the waterproof sheet. Provide a receiver for spitting into.
- Assemble the equipment. Any mouthwash solution should be freshly prepared, and renewed after 24 hours.
- Wash your hands and put on gloves and apron, if required. Ayliffe *et al.* (2001) recommend that gloves should be worn as some infectious agents (e.g. herpes, hepatitis B) can be present in the mouth or saliva. However, oral hygiene is a hygienic procedure rather than an aseptic one; it does not breach body defences but instead enhances them (Ayliffe *et al.* 2001). Therefore gloves need not be sterile.
- Lip crusting can be removed by gently sponging with warm water (Jones 1998). Observe for any breaks in the skin or signs of *Herpes simplex* (cold sore), which would require treatment with acyclovir cream.

Box 8.5 Denture care (adapted from Jones 1998)

- Wash hands and wear gloves.
- Remove dentures into a container and rinse to remove loose debris.
- Use the person's special denture brush, scrubbing all surfaces, using denture paste or a little soap, to remove all debris.
- Rinse thoroughly.
- When dentures are not being worn, store in a marked container filled with clean water.
- Soaking plastic dentures 2–3 times per week in dilute sodium hypochlorite will help to prevent oral candidiasis. Always rinse thoroughly before replacing in the mouth.
- Dentures with a metal portion should be soaked in dilute hypochlorite for only about 20 minutes, because of the danger of corrosion.

- Remove the person's dentures, if worn. They should be brushed well to remove debris using denture paste – ordinary toothpaste is too abrasive – and rinsed well. Box 8.5 lists key points for effective denture care.

- If the person has their own teeth, they should be brushed using the toothbrush and paste. Box 8.6 explains how teeth cleaning should be carried out, and Fig. 8.1 illustrates teeth cleaning. If people can clean their own teeth it is better to facilitate this.

- Assist the person to rinse the mouth thoroughly with the chosen mouthwash solution, or use a rinsed toothbrush to do this if they are unable. Suction can be used to remove excess fluid from the mouth if they are unconscious, or have dysphagia (swallowing difficulty), as it is essential to prevent choking or aspiration of fluid (Jones 1998). A conscious person who is nursed flat, for example after a spinal injury, can use a straw to suck fluid into the mouth to rinse and to spit through afterwards.

- Replace any dentures, top set first. Some patients use denture fixative.

- Apply lip lubricant, if lips are dry. Use tissues to blot any excess water or lubricant.

- Leave the person comfortable, and dispose of equipment according to waste disposal policy. Document the care given in the care plan or nursing notes. The British Dental Health Foundation's website (www.dentalhealth.org) covers all aspects of oral hygiene and is a useful source.

ACTIVITY

With a friend or colleague, take turns to clean each other's teeth, using your own toothbrushes and the instructions in Box 8.6 and Fig. 8.1.

Summary

- Effective oral care makes an important contribution to people's physical, psychological and social well-being.
- Nurses should ensure that best evidence is used as a basis for assessing and implementing oral care.

Box 8.6 Teeth cleaning (adapted from Jones 1998)

- Explain the procedure and gain consent.
- Wash hands, wear gloves and maintain privacy.
- It may be best to work at the side of the person, cradling the head.
- Remove any partial dentures into a bowl.
- Start at the front of the mouth in the upper jaw.
- Use a soft brush with a small amount of toothpaste pressed into the surface (to avoid it dislodging into the mouth and possible aspiration).
- Place the brush sideways against the teeth overlaying the gum edges with bristles pointing towards the teeth roots.
- Use a side-to-side motion, moving the brush head just a fraction of an inch at a time, using light pressure to squeeze the gum tissue against the teeth.
- Move around the upper teeth, replacing the brush section by section against the teeth.
- Try to use the same action inside the upper jaw.
- Repeat for the outer and inner surfaces of the lower jaw.
- Finally, scrub the chewing surfaces of the upper and lower teeth with a forward and backward motion.
- Teeth should be cleaned for a minimum of 90 seconds.
- Ask the person to rinse the mouth with warm water to remove debris, paste, etc., or use foam sticks moistened with water to gently sweep away the debris and toothpaste.
- Wash toothbrush well and leave it to dry in the air. Do not store in a sponge bag or container. Toothbrushes should be replaced every 6–12 weeks.

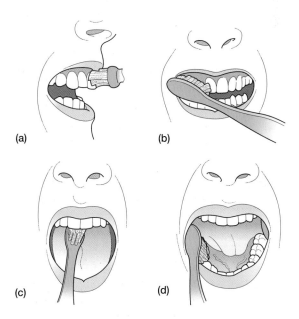

(a)   (b)

(c)   (d)

Figure 8.1: How to clean teeth.

LAST OFFICES

Last offices is the term given to meeting the final hygiene needs of a deceased patient. There are a variety of points to consider when assessing the extent of the care required. The practice of preparing the body of a deceased patient for removal to the mortuary or undertaker is the last caring act that nurses can perform for their patients and it may be regarded as an expression of holistic care and respect. The management of people who are dying and their families is beyond the scope of this section; there are many textbooks that focus on this topic. Chapter 12 addresses managing pain and comfort.

LEARNING OUTCOMES

By the end of this section you will be able to:
1 discuss the rationale for performing last offices;
2 identify religious and cultural factors affecting the performance of last offices;
3 understand the procedure for performing last offices and be prepared to carry it out safely.

Learning outcome 1: Discuss the rationale for performing last offices

Last offices are part of a long human tradition in the ritual of marking the transition between life and death (Quested and Rudge 2003). Relatives may find that viewing the body of their loved one, with a clean and cared-for appearance, helps them to accept the reality of death and aids the grieving process (Nearney 1998). It is also important that the body does not pose a risk to staff who come into contact with it. After death has apparently occurred, it must be confirmed, usually by a doctor, or senior nurse as locally agreed policy permits. The relatives, if not present, must be informed as soon as possible. In cases where death is expected, relatives may be asked if they wish to be informed immediately if the death occurs at night or would prefer to wait until morning.

Places where people die

Bill is terminally ill and can be expected to die in the fairly near future, perhaps in the acute setting where he is currently cared for. However, depending on his condition following his blood transfusion, and on how he and his wife feel about him continuing to be cared for at home, he might be discharged with appropriate support. Alternatively he may be cared for in a hospice for his final days.

ACTIVITY

What difference might the care setting and the circumstances of a death make to what happens to the body after death?

If Bill dies in an acute care setting, last offices will be carried out by nursing staff and his body will initially be moved to the hospital mortuary by porters, and at a later stage collected by an undertaker. However, if he dies at home, care of his body after his death may be minimal prior to his body being removed by an undertaker. After death in a non-acute care setting, for example a care home or hospice, local policies affect procedures, but again the body is likely to be removed by an undertaker. In some instances legal constraints dictate what care may be given. For example, following an unexpected death or one that takes place within 24 hours of an operation, in England the Coroner's office must be informed and a post-mortem may be required.

What hazards may a body present to those who handle it after death?

There may be leakage of body fluids or sharp objects such as cannulae attached to the body (see also Chapter 3 on preventing cross-infection). There will also be moving and handling issues. Therefore staff caring for a body after death should take appropriate measures to prevent problems arising.

Learning outcome 2: Identify religious and cultural factors affecting the performance of last offices

Regardless of the deceased person's cultural and religious background, privacy and dignity must be maintained for them and their relatives. Drawing the curtains around the bed in an open ward is the least requirement. Where possible, the body may be moved to a side room for greater privacy, and to minimise distress to other patients.

The patient's religious and cultural background must be considered at this point. Many of the world's major religions have specific rules and rituals concerned with death, for example about who can touch the body. However, it is important not to assume that the patient or their relatives will wish these rules to be followed to the letter. As with all human activities, there are many shades of opinion and belief. Ascertaining these beliefs in advance, if possible, is part of sensitive, holistic care. Houley (2002) writes that as a student she witnessed a senior nurse placing an open bible in the hands of an older woman who had died. The woman followed the Islamic faith and her family, understandably, reacted with great distress. Such insensitivity is clearly indefensible.

ACTIVITY

Find out the differing needs of cultures and religions in relation to the care of the body after death.

You will find that there are particular practices associated with different religions and cultures. Nurses should familiarise themselves with these so that all interventions are spiritually and culturally acceptable and do not cause offence (Sewell 2002).

ACTIVITY

Have you been involved in the death of a patient/client? Did the other patients/ residents show awareness of what had occurred? What comments did they make? How can you respond?

In most settings other than the patient's own home there will be other patients/ clients or residents around. At least some of them will be aware of the event and may ask, directly or indirectly, about the deceased person. It is important to answer questions sensitively and honestly, but without revealing confidential details.

ACTIVITY

Regarding Bill, who can be expected to die fairly soon, what would you expect his religious/cultural background to be?

From his name, you might assume that he will have a Western/Christian background, but such assumptions can be dangerous. Always ask, don't assume. And even among Christian religions there are variations, with different religious practices around the time of death.

ACTIVITY

Do you know how to contact the local chaplain, rabbi, imam or other religious leaders, so that you can gain advice about any special requirements at the time of death and when carrying out last offices?

Nurses need to be aware of how to contact local religious leaders, as referring to, and liaising with, them is an important contribution to people's spiritual support when in hospital. You may find there is a folder produced by the hospital chaplaincy with contact details and information regarding different religions. In many instances patients and their relatives, if they follow a particular religion, will have their own contacts.

Learning outcome 3: Understand the procedure for performing last offices and be prepared to carry it out safely

Immediate care after death

In whatever setting a death takes place there are a few actions that should be carried out very soon afterwards.

- Close the eyes by gently applying pressure to the eyelids for about 30 seconds (Carter 2004).
- Lay the person down flat, leaving one pillow, and straighten the body and limbs into neutral positions (Nearney 1998).
- Insert dentures, if usually worn (for example with Bill, we know he likes to wear his denture).
- Close the mouth and support the jaw with a pillow, to ensure it remains closed.

The body starts to become rigid soon after death and all these actions become more difficult to perform later.

In a hospital setting it is usual to leave the body for about an hour before full last offices are carried out. During this period relatives may visit and sit with the person, holding their hand if they wish. Therefore immediately after death the surrounding environment should be tidied up, equipment removed and the bed-linen attended to so that the person looks peaceful and comfortable. Houley (2002) writes that when she and her mother visited her grandmother after she had died they were horrified to find that her bloodstained nightdress had not been changed nor her teeth replaced. This upset them greatly as they felt that she would not have wanted to be seen like this. Relatives need to be given time and support and will, before they leave, need written information about what to do next (e.g. when and how to collect property, register the death, arrange the funeral).

Last offices procedure

Before commencing the procedure, you should gather the equipment required, including items for washing the patient (see Box 8.1), cleaning the mouth (see Box 8.4) and for shaving a male patient if required.

ACTIVITY

What other items do you think might be needed in addition to those in Boxes 8.1 and 8.4?

If the person is not to be dressed in their own nightclothes, a shroud (long white gown) might be required. Local hospital policies vary on this however; sometimes hospital nightclothes are used if patients' own are not available as some people consider shrouds, which were traditionally used, to be upsetting to relatives.

The patient's property needs to be listed and packed ready for collection by the relatives, so the appropriate documentation (Property Book) will be needed. If the patient has a wound, a waterproof dressing is required. If there are tubes to be left in, spigots will be needed to plug the tubes. Additional name bands and identity labels may be needed according to the setting and local policy. A disposable receiver may also be required.

The procedure described below includes usual practice, but always be guided by local policy, people's individual circumstances and particular religious and cultural requirements. Sometimes a close relative of the deceased may wish to be involved, perhaps helping with washing or hairbrushing. Ensure privacy as previously described. Two nurses are usually required for this procedure due to the moving and handling required.

- Protect yourself against possible infection by using plastic apron and gloves (see Chapter 3 on preventing cross-infection). For patients with a communicable disease, the existing infection control measures should continue.
- Wash the person as described in 'Bathing a person in bed', as culturally appropriate.
- Cover any wounds with waterproof dressings. Check local policy relating to removal of drains, tubes, cannulae or catheters. If a post-mortem is to take place these should be left in unless advised otherwise but can be spigotted. If no post-mortem is going to be performed these tubes can usually be removed, but always check if unsure.
- If leakage from any orifice seems likely to continue, insert packing, according to local policy, or an incontinence pad can be applied.
- Manually express the urinary bladder into a disposable receiver, if necessary and as per local policy.
- Place a clean sheet under the patient, using safe manual handling techniques.
- Remove and/or record the whereabouts of any jewellery as previously discussed with relatives (or patient). This should always be done in the presence of a witness. Jewellery left on the body should be secured with tape to prevent it being lost.
- Dress the patient in clean personal clothing or a shroud according to local policy and relatives' wishes.
- Shave a male patient as necessary, and brush hair.
- Clean the mouth and replace any dentures.
- If relatives have not yet viewed the body, this could be an appropriate point for them to do so.
- Attach identification labels to the patient according to local policy.

- Wrap the body in a clean sheet, securing it with tape.
- A body bag may be required if there are infection control issues. Consult local infection control policy or contact the infection control nurse for advice.
- Dispose of used equipment according to infection control principles and wash your hands.
- Make a list of and store property and jewellery according to local policy, in the presence of a witness.
- Arrange for the porters to collect the body, or the undertaker in a residential setting.

ACTIVITY   Find and compare the local policy on last offices with what you have read above.

As with any other clinical practices there will be a local policy, probably developed by a multidisciplinary group including the hospital chaplaincy, and which takes the local situation into account.

Summary
- Meeting the hygiene needs of a deceased patient in a safe and culturally sensitive way is an essential part of patient care.
- The extent to which last offices is carried out may vary according to the setting and will be influenced by local policy and the individual family.

CHAPTER SUMMARY

Giving personal care, with attention to the individual's dignity, privacy and personal needs, is a fundamental and essential skill for nurses, and this extends to the care of a patient's body after death. Further key principles include cultural sensitivity and prevention of cross-infection. It is important to assess carefully how hygiene needs can be met for each individual, maintaining and promoting independence where possible. People with physical and mental health problems may be able to regain self-care skills with appropriate aids, encouragement and support. Teaching people to manage personal hygiene and dressing can be an important part of rehabilitation, and should involve the multidisciplinary team and an individualised approach.

ACKNOWLEDGEMENT

This chapter has been revised and updated. The author acknowledges the contribution of Chrissie Major to this chapter in the second edition of this book.

REFERENCES

Ayliffe, G.A.J., Babb, J.R. and Taylor, L.J. 2001. *Hospital-acquired Infection: Principles and prevention*, 3rd edn. London: Arnold.
Baxter, C. 2002. Nursing with dignity. Part 5: Rastafarianism. *Nursing Times* **98**(13), 42–3.
Bowsher, J., Boyle, S. and Griffiths, J. 1999. Oral care. *Nursing Standard* **13**(37), 31.

Brawley, E.C. 2002. Bathing environments: how to improve the bathing experience. *Alzheimer's Care Quarterly* **3**, 38–41.

Briggs, M. 1997. Principles of closed wound care. *Journal of Wound Care* **6**, 288–92.

Carter, N. 2004. Last offices. In Dougherty, L. and Lister, S. (eds) *The Royal Marsden Hospital Manual of Clinical Nursing Procedures,* 6th edn. Oxford: Blackwell, 391–401.

Christmas, M. 2002. Nursing with dignity. Part 3: Christianity 1. *Nursing Times* **98**(11), 37–9.

Clegg, A. 2003. Older South Asian patient and carer perceptions of culturally sensitive care in a community hospital setting. *Journal of Clinical Nursing* **12**, 283–90.

Collins, F. 2001. Choosing bathing, showering and toileting equipment. *Nursing and Residential Care* **3,** 488–9.

Collins, F. and Hampton, S. 2003. The cost effective use of Bagbath: a new concept in patient hygiene. *British Journal of Nursing* **12**(16), 984–90.

Corbett, C.O. 1997. Mouth care and chemotherapy. *Paediatric Nursing* **9**(3), 19–21.

Davies, R., Bedi, R. and Scully, C. 2000. Oral health care for patients with special needs. *British Medical Journal* **321**, 495–8.

Department of Health (DH) 2001a. *The Essence of Care: Patient-focused benchmarking for health care practitioners.* London.

— 2001b. *National Service Framework for Older People.* London.

— 2001c. *Valuing People: A new strategy for learning disability for the 21st century.* London.

— 2006a.*From Values to Action: The Chief Nursing Officer's review of mental health nursing.* London.

— 2006b. *About the Dignity in Care campaign.* Available from www.dh.gov.uk

Dickinson, H., Watkins, C. and Leathley, M. 2001. The development of THROAT: the holistic and reliable oral assessment tool. *Clinical Effectiveness in Nursing* **5**, 104–10.

Edwards, V. 1998. A multidisciplinary approach to foot care in diabetes. *Nurse Prescriber/ Community Nurse* **4**(2), 53–5.

Foster, A. 1999. Diabetes care: getting your patients on a sure footing. *Nursing Times* **95**(37), 51–2.

Freer, S.K. 2000. Use of an oral assessment tool to improve practice. *Professional Nurse* **15,** 6357.

Geraghty, M. 2005. Nursing the unconscious patient. *Nursing Standard.* **20**(1), 54–64.

Gilchrist, B. 1990. Washing and dressing after surgery. *Nursing Times* **86**(50), Suppl, 71.

Gill, B.K. 2002. Nursing with dignity. Part 6: Sikhism. *Nursing Times.* **98**(14), 39–41.

Hancock, I., Bowman, A. and Prater, D. 2000. 'The day of the soft towel?' Comparison of the current bed-bathing method with the Soft Towel bed-bathing method. *International Journal of Nursing Practice* **6**, 207–13.

Henderson, V. 1960. *Basic Principles of Nursing Care.* Basel: S. Karger, for International Council of Nurses.

Henley, A. and Schott, J. 1999. *Culture, Religion and Patient Care in a Multiethnic Society.* London: Age Concern.

Holland, K. and Hogg, C. 2001. *Cultural Awareness in Nursing and Health Care.* London: Arnold.

Houley, C. 2002. A duty of dignity. *The Lamp* **59**(2), 22.

Huff, M., Kinion, E., Kendra, M.A. *et al.* 2006. Self-esteem: a hidden concern in oral health. *Journal of Community Health Nursing* **23**(4), 245–55.

Jones, C.V. 1998. The importance of oral hygiene in nutritional support. *British Journal of Nursing* **74**, 76–8, 80–3.

Kaye, P. 1992. *A–Z of Hospice and Palliative Medicine.* Northampton: EPL Publications.

Lentz, J. 2003. Daily baths: torment or comfort at end of life? *Journal of Hospice and Palliative Nursing* **5**, 34–9.

Lockwood, A. 2000. Implementing an oral hygiene assessment tool on an acute ward for older people. *Nursing Older People* **12**(7), 18–19.

Medicine and HealthCare Products Regulatory Agency 2008. *Medical Device Alert MDA/20008/17.* Available from www.mhra.gov.uk

National Institute for Health and Clinical Excellence (NICE) 2004. *Type 2 Diabetes: Prevention and management of foot problems.* London: NICE.

Nearney, L. 1998. Last offices, Part 1 (Practical Procedures for Nurses). *Nursing Times* **94**(26), 2p.

NHS Quality Improvement Scotland 2005. *Working with Dependent Older People to Achieve Good Oral Health.* NHS QIS: Edinburgh

Parker, L. 2004. Infection control: maintaining the personal hygiene of patients and staff. *British Journal of Nursing* **13**(8), 474–8.

Pearson, L.S. and Hutton, J.L. 2002. A controlled trial to compare the ability of foam swabs and toothbrushes to remove dental plaque. *Journal of Advanced Nursing* **39**, 480–9.

Pratt, R.J., Pellowe, C., Wilson, J.A. *et al.* 2007. National evidence-based guidelines for preventing healthcare-associated infections in NHS England. *Journal of Hospital Infection* **65**, Suppl, S1–64.

Quested, B. and Rudge, T. 2003. Nursing care of dead bodies: a discursive analysis of last offices. *Journal of Advanced Nursing* **41**, 553–60.

Rader, J. 1994. To bathe or not to bathe: that is the question. *Journal of Gerontological Nursing* **20**(9), 53–4.

Rassool, G.H. 2000. The crescent and Islam: healing, nursing and the spiritual dimension. Some considerations towards an understanding of the Islamic perspectives on caring. *Journal of Advanced Nursing* **32**, 1476–84.

Renwick, P., Vowden, K., Wilkinson, D. and Vowden, P. 1998. The pathophysiology and treatment of diabetic foot disease. *Journal of Wound Care* **7**, 107–10.

Roper, N., Logan, W.W. and Tierney, A.J. 2000. *The Roper–Logan–Tierney Model of Nursing: Based on activities of living.* Edinburgh: Churchill Livingstone.

Scott, H. 2001. Nursing care is given too narrow a definition. *British Journal of Nursing* **10**(18), 1164.

Sewell, P. 2002. Respecting a patient's care needs after death. *Nursing Times* **98**(39), 36–7.

Sloane, P., Rader, J., Barrick, A. *et al.* 1995. Bathing persons with dementia. *Gerontologist* **35**, 672–8.

Tarling, C. 1997. Washing and bathing. In *The Guide to Handling of Patients: Introducing a safer handling policy,* 4th edn. London: National Back Pain Association, 172–80.

Thompson, J. 1999. Foot problems and care of feet. Pt 2: Common disorders. *Community Practitioner* **72**, 178–9.

Thurgood, G. 1994. Nurse maintenance of oral hygiene. *British Journal of Nursing* **3**(7), 351–3.

Torrance, C. 1990. Oral hygiene. *Surgical Nursing* **13**(4), 16–20.

Valk, G.D., Kriegsman, D.M.W. and Assendelft, W.J.J. 2001. Patient education for preventing foot ulceration. *Cochrane Database of Systematic Reviews Library,* Issue 4.

Winkworth, J. 2003. Bathing is an intimate and valuable aspect of care. *Nursing Standard* **17**(21), 30.

Xavier, G. 2000. The importance of mouth care in preventing infection. *Nursing Standard* **14**(18), 47–51.

CHAPTER 9

Meeting Elimination Needs

Lesley Baillie and Rachel Busuttil Leaver

Elimination of urine and faeces is an essential bodily function which we usually become independent in within the first few years of life. Elimination is then usually a private function, but when disability or physical or mental health problems are present, independence in elimination is often affected. Patients and clients can then need help from nurses to prevent problems and maintain their comfort. Wherever possible a return to independence in meeting elimination needs is aimed for. Promoting dignity and privacy is integral to meeting people's elimination needs; it requires great skill and sensitivity to carry out this care while preserving patients' self-esteem. Many other chapters in this book are relevant to this care, particularly Chapter 2, which focuses on communication, and Chapter 3 on preventing cross-infection.

This chapter includes:
- Assisting with elimination: helping people to use the toilet, bedpans, urinals and commodes
- Urinalysis
- Collecting urine and stool specimens
- Caring for people who have urinary catheters
- Preventing and managing constipation
- Stoma care
- Promoting continence and managing incontinence

Recommended biology reading:

The following questions will help you to focus on the biology underpinning this chapter's skills. Use your recommended textbook to find out:
- What are the components of the urinary system?
- Within the kidney, blood is filtered. What forces are involved in filtration?
- Where does filtration occur? Which substances are not filtered out and why?
- What is the role of the juxtaglomerular apparatus?
- What happens to the glomerular filtrate as it passes along the nephron?
- How and why does the concentration of urine vary?
- What factors affect renal function?
- Urine is stored in the bladder. How does the bladder expand as it fills up?

- What is micturition and how does it occur?
- What is cystitis? Why is it generally more common in females than in males?
- How can urinalysis be used to assess health?
- What factors can increase the risk of urinary tract infection (UTI)?
- What are the signs of UTI?
- What are the different regions of the digestive tract and their functions?
- How does food move through the digestive tract?
- How are peristalsis and segmentation distinguished?
- What is the consequence of increased gut motility? When might this occur?
- What is the gastrocolic reflex?
- What do stools/faeces consist of?
- How do we defecate?
- What is constipation?
- What factors increase the risk of constipation?
- How does the digestive tract respond to local infection or irritation?
- How does stress affect the digestive tract?

PRACTICE SCENARIOS

The following scenarios illustrate situations where assistance with elimination is needed and they are referred to throughout this chapter.

Adult

> **Rheumatoid arthritis**
> A chronic, progressive and disabling autoimmune disease which can affect any joint causing pain, swelling and disability. It is a systemic disease and can affect the whole body, including the lungs, heart and eyes.

> **Stoma**
> An artificial permanent opening on the body such as those made in the abdominal wall during a surgical procedure to form a colostomy, ileostomy or urinary conduit.

> **Ileostomy**
> The end of the small intestine, the ileum, is surgically brought out through an opening (stoma) in the abdomen.

Jean is a 68-year-old woman who was diagnosed with cancer in the large bowel. Jean has **rheumatoid arthritis** and she has difficulty mobilising. She uses a motorised wheelchair and is cared for by her husband who is 75. He is well but has problems with his sight as he has cataracts. They live in a ground-floor council flat which has been adapted to enable her to be as independent as possible. Jean is able to transfer unaided. Jean has been admitted for surgery to have the tumour removed. She is distressed that she has cancer and is having to have drastic surgery and a **stoma** formed because of this. She is worried that she will not cope afterwards and does not want to be 'more of a burden' on her husband.

The stoma care specialist spends time with Jean to reassure her and answer her questions. The nurse also marks the site on Jean's abdomen where the stoma will be placed during surgery. Jean has a total large bowel resection with formation of an **ileostomy**. On return to the ward Jean has a stoma bag over the newly formed stoma and a urinary catheter in her bladder. The discomfort from the abdominal wound means that Jean is having trouble moving and cannot transfer herself independently. Due to her lack of mobility it is decided that the catheter should be left in the bladder until she regains the ability to transfer to the toilet. She develops a UTI which is treated with antibiotics.

Once she has recovered from surgery Jean and her husband start to learn how to care for her stoma. She will not be discharged until she is able to do this, but she is finding it difficult to get used to the change and her progress is slow.

Learning disability

Mark is 28 years old and has a syndrome that includes a learning disability, impaired renal function and deteriorating sight. He eats with some assistance and can walk short distances. He has very limited verbal communication and he also has frequent UTIs and bowel disturbances – both constipation and diarrhoea. He is cared for by his mother, who manages his physical health needs. Mark is usually continent but requires prompting and support, due to his visual impairment. When he is ill or in new surroundings he can become incontinent of both urine and faeces and wears continence pads at these times. His mother has contacted the Community Learning Disability Nurse (CLDN) as she has noticed blood in his urine, which he is infrequently passing even though she is encouraging fluids. Mark is also not eating, has a raised temperature and his mother believes he is in pain. The nurse arranges to take samples of both urine and faeces, liaises with the GP and Renal Consultant, who decide to admit Mark to hospital for further investigations. The CLDN acts as Mark's **health facilitator** and coordinates his care plan.

> **Health facilitator**
> A member of the community learning disabilities team (often a nurse) who supports a person with learning disabilities to access the healthcare they need. See *Valuing People* (DH 2001a).

Mental health

Bob is 58 years old. He has a long history of psychosis. During an acute psychotic episode, while admitted to an acute psychiatric ward, he was prescribed an atypical antipsychotic drug, clozapine, which is licensed for treatment of resistant schizophrenia only, due to its known side-effects. These include effects on white blood cell levels, thus causing vulnerability to infection. After six weeks there was a marked improvement in Bob's mental state, but he developed urinary incontinence at night (nocturnal enuresis). He found this extremely embarrassing and distressing, never having been incontinent before. Unfortunately urinary incontinence is known to be another side-effect of clozapine, the exact reasons for which are unknown. A urinalysis performed on admission had shown no abnormalities.

ASSISTING WITH ELIMINATION: HELPING PEOPLE TO USE THE TOILET, BEDPANS, URINALS AND COMMODES

LEARNING OUTCOMES

By the end of this section you will be able to:
1 identify why a person might need help with elimination and what equipment you could use to give assistance;
2 discuss important principles that you need to consider when assisting with elimination.

Learning outcome 1: Identify why a person might need help with elimination and what equipment you could use to give assistance

ACTIVITY

Reflect back on your practice experiences and write down all the reasons why a person might need help with elimination.

There are many situations where a person might need help with elimination. A patient's assessment should include identifying any elimination problems and assistance. For example, patients who are temporarily confined to bed following orthopaedic surgery, or people who are very weak, unwell or confused need help with elimination. Mark needs assistance as he is in the strange environment of a hospital and has impaired eyesight.

ACTIVITY

What equipment is available to assist with elimination? There may be examples of equipment in the skills laboratory or within your practice setting.

The toilet

Whenever possible a person should be helped to reach the toilet. NHS Quality Improvement Scotland (2005) highlights that all patients should have access to appropriate toilet facilities. The toilet is a more familiar environment for elimination (helpful if people are confused, disorientated or, like Mark, have a learning disability). It is also more private; to eliminate in a ward, behind closed curtains, may not feel very private as noise and smell may be obvious. This potential embarrassment can lead to patients ignoring the need to defecate, leading to constipation. You might need to accompany the person, who may need to use sticks, a frame or crutches (see Chapter 6, section on 'Assisting with mobilisation and preventing falls'). If a patient is unable to walk, you would use a wheelchair to take them to the toilet.

The commode

If a patient is very ill or weak it may be unwise for them to leave the bedside. When making these decisions, check their care plan and seek advice if you are unsure. If a patient is able to get out of bed, a commode is preferable to a bedpan, as it promotes a more conducive position for elimination and feels more comfortable. A commode has a pan underneath, which is removed after use and either macerated (if disposable) or cleaned in the washer–disinfector if reusable. There are many types of commode available, but those that are a good size, easy to manoeuvre, and have arms that are easy to remove are preferable (Ballinger *et al.* 1996).

Bedpans/urinals

Some people must stay in bed for medical reasons, so bedpans/urinals are required. You must choose between a standard bedpan, which the patient will sit up on, and a flat 'slipper' pan, which is rolled on to – essential when someone is unable to sit up. There are both male and female urinals for passing urine. Male patients sometimes find passing urine sitting or lying down difficult so they may need assistance to stand up instead, if their medical condition allows. Female urinals are useful for women lying flat (e.g. following back surgery) or where changing position is difficult, perhaps due to pain. There are a wide variety of female urinals available (Vickerman 2003).

Learning outcome 2: Discuss important principles that you need to consider when assisting with elimination

ACTIVITY

If you are assisting someone with elimination, what do you think would be important principles of care? Consider what you would want if in that position.

Box 9.1 lists the principles which you could have identified and they will now be discussed.

Approachability and communication

People needing help with their elimination invariably describe it as embarrassing and even distressing. The authors have known patients admit to reducing their fluid intake, thus increasing their risk of complications such as a UTI, just so that they need not call for a bedpan or commode so often. In Koch and Kelly's (1999) study, women with multiple sclerosis talked of the 'humiliation' of having to ask for help with elimination. Wareing (2005) highlighted the embarrassment of men who had frequency, which is a common symptom arising from conditions such as enlarged prostate and UTI. If a nurse does not appear approachable, then people may not feel able to ask for help, leading to emotional and physical discomfort, incontinence, retention of urine or constipation.

If people have communication difficulties, nurses must observe for non-verbal cues (e.g. restlessness or agitation). Sometimes a picture board (with a picture of a toilet) can be used to help communicate. Mark's mother is familiar with his needs and how he communicates, and nurses in his admitting ward should find out from her how Mark communicates that he needs to go to the toilet, which may be through a signing system including gestures. If the nurses ask Mark if he needs to go to the toilet, they should give him enough time to answer, as processing information may take longer for people with learning disabilities. Verbal communication when assisting with elimination should include clear and appropriate use of language.

Privacy and dignity

If these important principles (discussed in Chapter 1) are not maintained, people may feel embarrassed, degraded and experience a loss of self-esteem. Always ensure

> **Frequency**
> Passing urine more frequently than about seven times in 24 hours.

Box 9.1 Principles to follow when assisting with elimination
- Approachability and communication
- Privacy and dignity
- Promptness
- Prevention of cross-infection
- Observation
- Prevention of accidents
- Promotion of independence
- Promotion of hygiene and comfort

that bedside curtains are pulled shut properly, or the toilet door closed, and that patients are covered up while on the bedpan or commode. The British Geriatrics Society (2006) has produced *Dignity Behind Closed Doors*, which sets out standards relating to good practice in toilet provision. The aim of the campaign is 'to raise awareness that people, whatever their age and physical ability, should be able to choose to use the toilet in private in all settings'. The standards address accessibility, timeliness, equipment, safety, choice, privacy, cleanliness and hygiene.

Some people may want a nurse of the same sex to help them (Chur-Hansen 2002). Nurses should approach each person as an individual, being sensitive to non-verbal cues and being aware of possible cultural issues. For example, within some South Asian cultures modesty is very important (Holland and Hogg 2001). Nurses should also speak privately and quietly when assisting with elimination. Appropriate use of non-verbal communication may reduce the amount of verbal communication needed, minimising the risk of other patients overhearing.

Promptness

People with certain types of incontinence (urge incontinence) will not be able to wait to pass urine (see later section). In Wareing's (2005) study, men who experienced severe urgency described that 'having to hold on' was associated with panic and embarrassment. Resnick *et al.* (2006) found that care home staff contributed to residents' incontinence by not attending to them quickly enough. Clearly, such a situation is unacceptable as incontinence is distressing for people (see later section).

If patients cannot attempt to open their bowels when they feel the need, faeces are pushed back into the sigmoid colon or remain in the rectum, where water continues to be reabsorbed. Thus faeces become harder, more painful and difficult to pass, which may lead to constipation. Nurses should prioritise meeting elimination needs as patients are in a powerless position, dependent for help with this basic need. When patients have finished eliminating, nurses should respond promptly, to avoid discomfort and maintain safety. Patients should be provided with a call bell and shown how to use it.

Prevention of cross-infection

When helping people with elimination, cross-infection is a high risk. Inpatients are often particularly vulnerable to infection owing to their medical conditions (see Chapter 3 for more information).

Equipment used to assist with elimination must be cleaned effectively. Disposable bedpans and urinals are disposed of in macerators. Non-disposable urinals and bedpans should be disinfected by thermal disinfection (exposure to hot water or steam) (Ayliffe *et al.* 2001). As multi-use equipment, commodes and plastic bedpan supports must be decontaminated appropriately after each usage (Pratt *et al.* 2007). Careful handwashing is the most important measure when assisting with elimination. Ayliffe *et al.* (2001) found that after handling bedpans nurses' hands often showed *Staphylococcus aureus* and/or Gram-negative bacilli, but handwashing was effective in removing these organisms. As per personal protective equipment guidelines (Pratt *et al.* 2007), nurses should wear non-sterile gloves and aprons to prevent hands and uniform being contaminated when assisting with elimination.

Urine is normally sterile, but it is often contaminated while voiding by bacteria present around the urethral opening (Gould 1994). Urine provides an excellent medium for bacterial growth, especially Gram-negative bacteria (*Pseudomonas, Klebsiella, Escherichia coli, Proteus*), which can survive only when water and inorganic ions are present (Gould 1994). Urine passed into a bedpan or urinal should therefore be disposed of quickly, as standing at room temperature allows any bacteria present to divide rapidly, doubling approximately every 30 minutes (Gould 1994), thus becoming a reservoir of infection.

When a patient has diarrhoea, prevention of cross-infection is essential as it could be infective. As well as prompt disposal of the diarrhoea, and handwashing, nurses should employ source isolation techniques, nursing the patient in a single room and use of gloves and aprons (see Chapter 3). When caring for people with diarrhoea caused by *Clostridium difficile*, alcohol handrub is ineffective against the spores produced, so wearing non-sterile gloves, with handwashing following glove removal, is essential.

Observation

There are many useful observations you can make when assisting with elimination, such as assessing the patient's ability to move, or about the condition of their skin (see Table 9.1). If the person's urine output is measured, the jug used must be

Table 9.1: Observations to make when assisting with elimination.

Observation	Explanation
Mobility	Patient's ability to lift on to a bedpan, to transfer on to a commode or toilet, or stand to use a urinal Whether any apparent discomfort/pain, breathlessness or weakness when moving
Skin condition	Redness or broken areas on sacrum or buttocks; soreness of groins, perineum, penis or vulva
Self-care ability	Physical/mental ability to remove or adapt clothing, before and after elimination, and to carry out hygiene afterwards
Amount and frequency of urine output	A fluid input/output chart may be maintained if there are concerns about fluid balance Urine will be measured in a jug and recorded in millilitres Pads can be weighed: 1 g = 1 mL Poor urine output (oliguria) could occur in dehydration or shock No urinary output (anuria) could mean retention of urine Frequent small amounts of urine might indicate a urinary tract infection (UTI) Monitoring of frequency and amount may be part of a bladder re-education programme
Appearance of urine	See Urinalysis, next section Very dark, concentrated urine might indicate dehydration, and smoky offensive urine might indicate UTI Presence of blood may be due to kidney trauma or disease
Appearance of stools	Consistency and frequency of stools; hard and infrequent, which could indicate constipation, or frequent and loose (diarrhoea), which could be infected A stool chart to record frequency, appearance and consistency might be maintained: the Bristol stool cart is often used so that descriptions of stools are reliable (see Fig. 9.1) If infection is suspected, a stool specimen will be collected and sent (see later section)

disposed of or cleaned in the bedpan washer and a fluid chart will be used to record fluid balance. The **Bristol stool chart** can be used to record stool type (see Fig. 9.1).

ACTIVITY

When next in placement, look at any charts used for monitoring urine output and stools. What are the types of fluids listed for input and output? Does the stool chart incorporate the Bristol stool chart, as shown in Fig. 9.1?

Prevention of accidents

Thompson's (2007) falls and continence audit found that 36.8 per cent of falls were related to toileting or incontinence. Therefore a moving and handling risk assessment should be carried out (see Chapter 6 for more information).

Type 1		Separate hard lumps, like nuts (hard to pass)
Type 2		Sausage-shaped but lumpy
Type 3		Like a sausage but with cracks on its surface
Type 4		Like a sausage or snake, smooth and soft
Type 5		Soft blobs with clear-cut edges (passed easily)
Type 6		Fluffy peices with ragged edges, a mushy stool
Type 7		Watery, no solid pieces ENTIRELY LIQUID

Figure 9.1: Bristol stool chart. Reproduced by kind permission of Taylor & Francis Ltd (www.tandf. co.uk/journals). From Lewis, S.J. and Heaton, K.W. 1997. Stool form scale as a useful guide to intestinal track time. *Scandinavian Journal of Gastroenterology* **32**, 920–4.

The patient's moving and handling plan, developed following assessment, should specify the equipment needed and how many staff are required. If patients are using bedpans in bed you must ensure that they do not topple over. Balancing on a bedpan can be difficult so it may be safer for the bed or trolley rails to be up for support. The National Patient Safety Agency (2007) recommended that organisations should have a policy about bedrail use – a risk assessment form may be required as they can be hazardous. You must be sure about your reasons for using them (i.e. not using them as a form of restraint).

Using the commode by the bedside is potentially hazardous. You must ensure that brakes are on securely and that there are no fluids or slippery substances on the floor. You must consider whether the person is safe to leave: are they confused and likely to try to stand up alone, leading to a fall? Privacy is a very important principle when assisting people with elimination but has to be balanced against safety. A fall risk assessment scale can help to identify people who are at risk of falls. Find out whether such risk assessment tools are used in your local practice setting. Chapter 6 looks at causes and prevention of falls.

Promotion of independence and patient participation

The Essence of Care (DH 2001b) includes benchmarks of best practice for 'self-care' which highlight the importance of assessing people's self-care abilities and facilitating their skills and knowledge to promote self-care ability. You should therefore assess ability and promote independence while also maintaining hygiene and safety. Learning how to use the toilet unaided, after a **stroke** for example, may take some time, and both short- and long-term goals may be necessary. Clark and Rugg's (2005) study highlighted the importance of gaining independence in using the toilet for people following stroke to prevent decreased self-esteem. Nurses can liaise with occupational therapists to facilitate a return to people's normal methods and if that is not possible, how to assist patients to adjust. Teaching people how to manage transfers safely (e.g. from chair to commode), how to remove clothing, and walk to the toilet on crutches, are situations where education is needed.

For people with learning disabilities, independence will be promoted if they are well orientated to their environment and where the toilet is and are taken to the same toilet by the same route each time. Ideally, Mark's bed would be situated near the toilet. The ward nurses could show Mark where the toilet is and how the facilities work. For example, Mark may be used to a toilet with a pull handle and separate taps, while the ward might have a toilet with a button to press for flushing and a mixer tap. Mark's mother will know the best way of explaining this to him. These steps could also be helpful for people who have dementia.

Promoting hygiene and comfort

You must ensure hygiene is promoted for people whose elimination needs are met by their bedside, ensuring that you enable them to wash hands, and their perineal and genital area where necessary. When you take people to the toilet, ensure that

> **Stroke**
> Cerebral damage caused either by decreased blood flow or by haemorrhage. Effects vary, but a stroke often causes paralysis down one side of the body (hemiplegia), speech and swallowing difficulty, and elimination difficulties.

they can wash their hands at the sink afterwards. Always leave access to toilet tissue, and if people are unable to wipe themselves, then you must do this for them, or give assistance to people who are learning or relearning this skill. With female patients always wipe the vulval area from front to back to prevent transmission of bowel bacterial flora (such as *E. coli*) from the anal area to the urethra (Nazarko 1995). Females have a short urethra (4 cm), which can easily lead to contamination by such bacteria.

Within Asia, the left hand is traditionally reserved for washing underneath after using the toilet, the right hand being used for eating and other activities (Holland and Hogg 2001). These rules may be important to some Asians living in Britain so nurses should be aware of this. Muslims prefer to wash their genitals with running water after using the toilet (Akhtar 2002).

Make sure that the patient does not become cold during elimination, by covering their legs with a blanket. Ensure that anyone using a bedpan is comfortably supported with pillows. Psychological comfort will be promoted by your attitude and communication (see Chapter 2 for more information).

Summary

- Many health problems lead to people needing help with elimination.
- Various items of equipment are available to assist people who are unable to get to the toilet. Nurses must assess which is appropriate for each individual.
- There are important principles that must be followed when helping people with elimination to ensure that care is therapeutic, effective and safe.

URINALYSIS

Urinalysis is the testing of urine for the presence of a variety of substances. This simple, non-intrusive test provides useful information about an individual's renal and urinary function (Beynon and Nicholls 2004).

LEARNING OUTCOMES

By the end of this section you will:
1 understand the process of urinalysis;
2 show insight into the meaning of urinalysis results and what action to take if abnormal results are obtained;
3 identify when urinalysis should be performed.

You should be able to access urinalysis equipment either in the skills laboratory or your practice setting.

Learning outcome 1: Understand the process of urinalysis

Look at the reagent strips that are used to test urine, in the skills laboratory, or in a practice placement. Find the expiry date on the bottle and note the substances that are tested for and the timings for reading the results, on the side of the bottle.

Reagent strips must be in date, and stored and used properly (Rowell 1998), otherwise results may not be accurate. The Medicines and Healthcare Products Regulatory Agency (MHRA) (2006) advises that the strip container lid must be closed immediately after removal of a strip to prevent deterioration of the remaining strips. The full range of substances which can be tested in a urinalysis are leucocytes, nitrite, urobilinogen, protein, pH, blood, specific gravity, ketones, bilirubin and glucose. The reagent strips that you looked at may include this full range, but there are strips available that test for only a selection or even just one substance, such as blood.

Conducting a urinalysis

Bayer (1998), who produce the reagent strips, give detailed explanations about how to conduct a urinalysis accurately. Key points are summarised in Fig. 9.2, with some additional explanatory notes and rationale given below.

Urine for analysis should be collected in a clean, dry, preservative-free container and infection control aspects should be adhered to throughout the procedure (MHRA 2006). First-voided morning urine is best for a urinalysis as it is most concentrated. Ideally the urine should be tested immediately, or within 4 hours. Otherwise you can refrigerate the specimen, but you must let it return to room temperature before testing. It is particularly important to use fresh urine when testing for bilirubin and urobilinogen as these compounds are relatively unstable when exposed to room temperature and light. Bayer (1997a) advise that to test for nitrite it is best to use a first morning sample (when urine will have been in contact with bacteria, if present, for at least 3 hours).

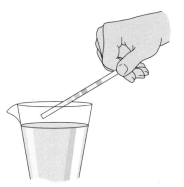

Requirements
- Reagent strip and bottle
- Freshly voided urine in a clean (preferably sterile) container

Procedure
- Observe urine for colour, consistency and smell
- Immerse all reagent areas in fresh urine and remove immediately
- Run the edge along the rim of the container to remove excess urine
- Hold the strip horizontally to prevent mixing of the chemicals from adjacent areas and prevent soiling of hands with urine
- Compare the test areas with the corresponding colour chart at the specified time or analyse in electronic reader following reader's instructions

Figure 9.2: Conducting a urinalysis: key points (Bayer 1998).

Jaundice
A condition characterised by yellowness of skin, whites of eyes, mucous membranes and body fluids due to the presence of bile pigment resulting from excess bilirubin in the blood.

When testing urine always observe the appearance of the urine sample first. Bayer (1997a,b) explain the appearance of normal urine and the cause of some abnormalities. Normal fresh urine is pale to dark yellow or amber in colour, and clear. If the urine is red or red–brown this could be from a food dye, eating beetroot, a drug, or the presence of haemoglobin. If there are many red blood cells present, the urine will be cloudy as well. A strongly yellow sample could indicate **jaundice**. The smell of the urine should also be noted. Freshly voided, non-infected urine should be virtually odourless, but if urine is infected it may smell offensive.

The strips must be read accurately as per the timings given on the bottle. Rowell (1998) reports that reading of the reagent strips may not always be done reliably. Nurses on a busy ward may not wait the correct amount of time before reading the result, and lighting and colour vision may affect readings. The MHRA (2006) advises that coloured charts used for reading results must be stored away from direct sunlight to prevent fading, and the strip must be read at the correct time in good light.

There are electronic readers available (e.g. the Clinitek 50 analyser) which can help to minimise reader error; these readers also print the results. The printout includes the time and date, and asterisks abnormal readings. These readers should lead to greater uniformity and consistency in readings. The MHRA advises that the readers should be maintained and cleaned correctly and checked regularly. Clement *et al.* (2004) found the Clinitek 50 analyser was highly reliable in identifying which patients did not have a UTI and when a specimen should be sent to the laboratory for investigation.

Learning outcome 2: Show insight into the meaning of urinalysis results and what action to take if abnormal results are obtained

If you look on the side of the urinary reagent bottle you will find the key as to what each colour is testing for. It is clearly indicated which are the normal results, and which are the abnormal. Abnormal results should be reported. Table 9.2 indicates the significance of abnormalities and suggests some possible actions. A nursing dictionary will help you with some of the technical terms included.

When to collect a urine specimen for microscopy and culture

An important reason for urinalysis is to identify whether to send a urine specimen for microscopy, culture and sensitivity (MC&S). In this laboratory test, the urine is examined under the microscope, and the urine is cultured to see whether bacteria grow and what antibiotics the bacteria are sensitive to. Studies have confirmed that urinalysis can help to screen out the unnecessary ordering of urine cultures (Panagamuwa *et al.* 2004; Manisha *et al.* 2007).

Urine should first be assessed visually and if obviously infected (cloudy and offensive) or blood-stained, then it should be sent for MC&S. However if urine is visually inspected and found to be clear this does not rule out a UTI (Bullock *et al.* 2001). A urinalysis will show whether there are leucocytes, nitrites, protein or blood present. Over 90 per cent of urinary pathogens can reduce urinary nitrate

Table 9.2: Clinical significance of test results (adapted from Bayer 1997b, 1998 with kind permission).

Significance of positive results	Commonest causes of abnormalities, and possible action to take
Glucose Not normally detectable in urine Found when its concentration exceeds the renal threshold	• In people with raised blood glucose concentration: diabetes mellitus or glucose infusion • In people without raised blood glucose concentration: pregnancy or renal glycosuria. *Action:* If positive, a blood glucose measurement should be performed, and further action may follow
Bilirubin Presence in urine indicates an excess of conjugated bilirubin in plasma Note that stale urine may give a false-negative result	• Liver cell injury: e.g. viral or drug-induced hepatitis, paracetamol overdose, late-stage cirrhosis • Biliary tract obstruction: e.g. by gall stones, carcinoma of the head of pancreas *Action:* Should always be reported as further investigations will be needed
Ketones Indicates accumulation of acetoacetate secondary to excessive breakdown of body fat Some drugs (e.g. L-dopa) may give a false-positive result	• Fasting, particularly with fever and/or vomiting • Diabetic ketoacidosis *Action:* Urgent action is needed if the person is known or suspected to have diabetes
Specific gravity A measure of total solute concentration in urine In health, varies widely according to the need to excrete water and solutes	• High values found in dehydration, or in impaired kidney function (e.g. chronic renal failure) • Low values found in people with intact renal function and high fluid intake, diabetes insipidus, chronic renal failure, hypercalcaemia, hypokalaemia *Action:* Depends on likely cause and results of other investigations
Blood May be haematuria (intact blood cells) or haemoglobinuria (free haemoglobin, excreted from plasma or liberated from red cells in the urine)	*Haematuria:* • Due to kidney disorders (e.g. glomerulonephritis, polycystic kidneys, tumour) • Due to urinary tract disorders (e.g. stones, tumour, infection, benign prostatic enlargement) *Haemoglobinuria:* • Severe haemolysis (e.g. sickle cell disease crisis) • Breakdown of red cells in urine (especially when urine is dilute and testing is delayed) *Action:* Should be reported; follow-up will depend on other tests and the clinical picture
pH In health, the pH of uncontaminated urine ranges from 4.5 to 8.0 A high pH will be found if testing stale urine, so *such specimens should not be used*	• Low values found in acidaemia as in diabetic ketoacidosis; also starvation or potassium depletion • High values found in stale urine, alkalaemia (except when due to potassium depletion) e.g. due to vomiting and consumption of large amounts of antacids, renal tubular acidosis, urinary tract infection with ammonia-forming organisms *Action:* Depends on other test results
Protein A range of proteins can be detected but the reagent is most sensitive to albumin, so a negative result does not rule out presence of other proteins	• Albuminuria may be found in acute and chronic glomerulonephritis, urinary tract infection, glomerular involvement in systemic lupus erythematosus, nephrotic syndrome, pre-eclampsia, fever, heart failure and postural (orthostatic) proteinuria *Action:* Transient results are seldom important but persistent positive results need investigating for underlying cause Other test results and clinical picture should be considered

(Continued)

Table 9.2: (Continued)

Significance of positive results	Commonest causes of abnormalities, and possible action to take
Urobilinogen Urinary excretion of urobilinogen reflects the combined effects of conversion of bilirubin to urobilinogen in the gut, and reabsorption into the bloodstream Note that false-negatives are found in stale urine	*Increased secretion:* • May be due to increased production (e.g. in red blood cell disorders such as sickle cell disease), or due to decreased uptake by the liver (e.g. in viral hepatitis and cirrhosis) *Decreased secretion:* • May be due to biliary tract obstruction (e.g. gallstones, carcinoma of pancreas), or due to sterilisation of the colon by unabsorbable antibiotics (e.g. neomycin), which prevents bacterial conversion of bilirubin to urobilinogen *Action:* Urgent investigation is needed
Nitrite Most organisms which infect the urinary tract contain an enzyme system that catalyses the conversion of dietary nitrate, which is normally present in urine, to nitrite, which is not found in urine unless there is a urinary tract infection	• Presence indicates urinary tract infection due to nitrite-producing organisms • However absence does not exclude infection, as some organisms are unable to convert dietary nitrate to nitrite • False-negatives are also found if there is insufficient dietary nitrate, or urine has not been in the bladder long enough (4 hours is ideal) for the conversion to take place *Action:* Specimen should be sent for microscopy and culture
Leucocytes Will be present when some of the leucocytes that have entered inflamed tissue from the blood are shed in the urine	• Indicates a urinary tract infection, especially when it is accompanied by acute inflammation of the urinary tract *Action:* Specimen should be sent for microscopy and culture

to nitrite if they are in contact with urine in the bladder for a minimum of 3 hours (Panagamuwa *et al.* 2004). Therefore a positive nitrite test indicates infection but some cases may be missed. Positive tests for leucocyte esterase (an enzyme within white blood cells), blood or protein may also indicate UTI. If all four tests (for nitrites, leucocytes, blood and protein) are negative it is highly likely that there is no infection, and therefore sending urine for MC&S is not indicated.

The National Institute for Health and Clinical Excellence (NICE) (2006) recommends that all women with urinary incontinence should have a urinalysis performed and if it is positive to leucocytes and nitrites, and they are symptomatic of UTI, a mid-stream specimen (see next section) should be sent for MC&S. Midthun *et al.* (2004) highlight that typical symptoms of UTI, such as pain on micturition (dysuria), frequency, fever and sometimes loin or suprapubic pain may not be present in older people. Other client groups may also not have 'typical' UTI signs and symptoms, for example people with spinal cord injury (SCI) who are susceptible to UTI and are more likely to be infected with bacteria that are not detectable or occur at lower levels than can be detected on dipstick testing (Hoffman *et al.* 2004). Hoffman *et al.* (2004) found that *Enterococcus,* which is not capable of reducing nitrate to nitrite, was often found in SCI patients' urine so urine culture is still needed for these patients.

ACTIVITY

For each of the people in the scenarios at the start of the chapter, identify why you would want to do a urinalysis.

A urinalysis gives many clues about a person's health and well-being so a nursing assessment of a newly referred or admitted person should always include a urinalysis. Urinalysis is also performed for other people at risk of developing health problems that can be indicated through a urinalysis. Examples include during pregnancy (when presence of protein or glucose may be particularly significant), and after an abdominal injury (to screen for blood which might indicate renal damage).

When Bob was first admitted, a urinalysis would have been performed as part of a general health screen. He should be reassured that this is routine and nothing to be worried about and given a clean container in which to pass the urine the morning after admission. When he developed urinary incontinence, he should have been asked for a further morning specimen to rule out UTI, which can predispose to, or compound, urinary incontinence. Remember that taking clozapine has rendered him more vulnerable to infection.

Mark is known to have a renal impairment and frequent UTIs. The community learning disability nurse has already collected a urine specimen. On admission to the ward, a urinalysis will give immediate information about his renal function and whether he currently has a UTI. Jean's urine would have been tested on admission to hospital as part of her assessment to indicate the likelihood of a UTI preoperatively. Panagamuwa *et al.* (2004) concluded that urinalysis was a safe and efficient alternative to laboratory culture for detecting UTI during pre-admission assessment of patients for arthroscopy, with specimens sent for MC&S only if urinalysis was positive. Postoperatively, Jean has a urinary catheter which is accompanied by a risk of UTI, which the scenario states did occur. A catheter specimen of urine (see Box 9.3) would be obtained to test her urine initially before sending a sample for MC&S.

Summary

- Urinalysis is a non-invasive and frequently performed practical skill which can provide very useful information about people's health status.
- To obtain an accurate result, the steps in a urinalysis must be carried out carefully with an appropriately collected specimen.
- It is important to understand the significance of abnormal results and subsequent action to take.

COLLECTING URINE AND STOOL SPECIMENS

In this section common types of urine specimen and the collection of a stool (faeces) specimen are discussed. It is often necessary to obtain specimens such as

> **Box 9.2 Collection of specimens: key points**
>
> - Adherence to infection control standard principles (hand hygiene, personal protective equipment)
> - Clear explanations
> - Maintenance of patient/client privacy, dignity and comfort
> - Avoidance of contamination of the specimen
> - Prompt transportation to the laboratory, or refrigeration for up to 24 hours
> - Clear labelling
> - Correct and comprehensive accompanying information
> - Documentation in patient/client notes of the date and time of the specimen collection

these from patients/clients as they can provide important diagnostic information, which impacts on management and care. General principles of specimen collection were considered in Chapter 3, but key points can be found in Box 9.2.

LEARNING OUTCOMES

By the end of this section you will be able to discuss the collection of:
1 a catheter specimen of urine;
2 a mid-stream specimen of urine;
3 a 24-hour specimen of urine;
4 a stoma urine specimen;
5 a stool specimen.

Learning outcome 1: Discuss the collection of a catheter specimen of urine

A catheter specimen of urine (CSU) is often taken for bacteriological examination to find out if treatment is required when symptoms of a UTI are present in a person who is catheterised. However, a person with a catheter may not display these symptoms, and in an older and/or confused person the symptoms can be still less apparent. As discussed earlier in the chapter, a CSU may have to be collected from Jean if a UTI is suspected. The risk of infection increases by 5–8 per cent each day of catheterisation (Mulhall *et al.* 1988; Saint and Lipsky 1999), so the longer the catheter is left in place, the more likely the patient will have bacteriuria. Bacteria prefer to live on surfaces rather then in a solution like urine. A catheter provides this surface and bacteria can coat it and form what is called a **biofilm.** Bacteria that live in a biofilm are more resistant to treatment, so that even if eliminated in urine by using antibiotics the ones on the catheter will persist and recontaminate the urine (Wilson 1997; Saye 2007).

It is important to distinguish between bacteriuria and a 'clinical infection'. Bacteria can colonise the urinary tract without invading the surrounding tissues (bacteriuria), often do not cause clinical symptoms, and may not be susceptible to treatment. However, clinical infection involving invasion of surrounding tissues, often producing symptoms in infected people, requires treatment.

Box 9.3 Collection of a catheter specimen of urine: equipment and key points

Equipment
- Alcohol swab, receiver, syringe (20 mL) and needle (21 g bore), specimen pot and request form
- A gate clamp may be required.

Key points
- Adhere to general points outlined in Box 9.2.
- Locate the sample port on the catheter bag tubing. Some drainage bags have a latex port which requires a needle and syringe to aspirate the urine. Others have a needleless port and a syringe can be attached directly to this to withdraw the urine.
- If there is no urine present in the catheter tubing, clamp the tubing below the sample port until sufficient urine collects. Never clamp the actual catheter, as this could damage it.
- Swab the sample port with alcohol swab and allow the port to dry. Insert the needle into the port at an angle of 45 degrees to prevent going straight through the tubing.
- For needleless sampling ports follow the same procedure, but attach the syringe directly to the sampling port.
- Withdraw the required amount of urine, remove the top from the specimen pot and fill the pot with urine. Dispose of the needle and syringe into a sharps box immediately. Replace the cap on the pot.

Whatever the classification of the infection, if a specimen is considered necessary then nurses must use aseptic technique and sterile equipment. This is to reduce the risk of further contaminating the specimen and potentially introducing different bacteria to those from the patient. This is particularly important since the treatment is based on the results of the bacteriological examination of the urine.

Urine should be obtained from the special sampling port on the drainage system; the catheter and drainage system should never be disconnected to take a specimen. You should adhere to manufacturers' instructions concerning the number of times the port may be punctured safely. Urine should never be taken from the catheter bag because the bag acts as a reservoir where microorganisms can multiply. It is thus likely to contain greater numbers of microorganisms than urine accessed via the port. The bag can also be heavily contaminated from environmental sources. Box 9.3 outlines the key principles to follow when taking a catheter specimen of urine.

Learning outcome 2: Discuss the collection of a mid-stream specimen of urine

The mid-stream specimen of urine (MSU) is collected if a UTI is suspected in a non-catheterised patient, and is obtained using a clean procedure. It is a useful aid in diagnosis and the aim is to collect the mid-stream, which is not contaminated by microorganisms outside the urinary tract.

How MSUs should be collected has been the subject of much research but the evidence base for best practice remains unclear. People have often been asked to undertake perineal cleansing with sterile swabs and saline prior to giving an MSU, to prevent contamination. However, a Canadian study concluded that contamination of urine specimens from women with acute dysuria who cleaned the perineal area prior to collection did not differ from those who did not (Lifshitz and Kramer 2000). A more recent study on toilet-trained children, on the other hand, found that those who did not clean their genital area did have a higher contamination rate then those who did (Vaillancourt *et al.* 2007).

It is debatable whether results on children are transferable to adults, however, and current advice is that perineal cleaning is not necessary (Dougherty and Lister 2004). It is theorised that the first part of the stream flushes away microorganisms from the first part of the urethra, and that the urine does not flow over the perineum as long as there is sufficient urine in the bladder to produce a good stream. If there is insufficient urine in the bladder the specimen should be collected later. The equipment required and key points of the procedure are listed in Box 9.4.

If a urine specimen is being collected because of suspected tuberculosis (TB) or cancer of the urinary tract, then an early-morning specimen is preferable because it is more concentrated and it is most likely to contain the tubercle bacillus or malignant cells (Beynon and Nicholls 2004). Usually, three consecutive early-morning specimens are required.

ACTIVITY

Read through Box 9.4. As you can see, the person's cooperation and understanding would be needed. Look at the practice scenarios: to what extent might you achieve understanding and consent from Bob and Mark?

You are more likely to gain informed consent and cooperation from anyone if you explain the procedure and its importance carefully and confidentially. You should respect the person's right to privacy and dignity throughout the whole episode of care. Remember that what may be a simple and routine procedure in your eyes

---

Box 9.4 Midstream specimens of urine: equipment and procedure

Equipment
- A toilet/commode/bedpan/urinal as appropriate, specimen pot and request form, disposable gloves

Procedure
- Adhere to key points in Box 9.2.
- Explain to the person to start passing urine as usual, then catch some urine (about 20 mL: about 2.5 cm up the pot) in the specimen pot, and then finish voiding into the toilet or commode. Wear gloves and assist the person if necessary.

may feel quite different to the person concerned. It is likely that Bob would be able to produce the specimen with little assistance. Mark may have become used to giving urine samples at his GP's surgery because of his frequent urine infections. One approach would be for his mother or a nurse to take him to the toilet about 30 minutes after a drink (assuming he is not being kept 'nil by mouth'), and try to collect the specimen in a clean receptacle in the toilet or, if possible, catch the mid-stream in a pot for him, while wearing gloves. This approach can also be used for people who are confused.

It can be difficult to produce an MSU, especially if patients are confined to bed. Adaptations will need to be made, for example, placing a waterproof pad beneath the patient to soak up any possible spillage, helping to diminish fears of wetting the bed. Allowing people plenty of time and not rushing is also important.

Learning outcome 3: Discuss the collection of a 24-hour specimen of urine

Sometimes it is necessary to collect the total volume of urine passed within a 24-hour period. This is then analysed within the laboratory so that the 24-hour excretion of a variety of key metabolites (e.g. protein, creatinine) can be assessed (Beynon and Nicholls 2004). Box 9.5 outlines the equipment needed and the procedure.

Box 9.5 24-hour urine collection: equipment and key points

Equipment
- A jug, a 24-hour urine collection container, gloves

Procedure
- Assess the person's ability to participate in the collection. When the person next passes urine, it is discarded. This marks the beginning of the 24-hour period for collection.
- Label the container with the person's details (name, ward and hospital number) and the time and date the collection started.
- Put a sign on the bed or door of the room belonging to the person indicating that a 24-hour urine collection is in place, the date and time it started and when it will finish.
- Every time the person passes urine it is collected and poured into the container. The person may be able to do this independently or may need assistance. Check their understanding and ability.
- Ask the person to empty their bladder just before the end of the 24-hour collection period.
- Advise that this ends the collection period.
- Remove the sign from the door or bed.
- Clean or discard the jug used.
- Record the completion time and ensure that the urine collection and laboratory request forms are dispatched correctly as soon as possible.

Note: If one sample of urine becomes contaminated or is accidentally discarded, the test must be discontinued and restarted.

Learning outcome 4: Discuss the collection of a stoma urine specimen

In learning outcome 1, the importance of not obtaining a catheter specimen of urine from the drainage bag was stated. The same rationale applies to patients who have had an ileal conduit (i.e. urinary stoma) formed (see section on stoma care later). If taken from the stoma bag this urine will have multiple bacteria and may be contaminated.

The correct method of collecting a stoma urine is by passing a small intermittent catheter into the stoma (see Box 9.6). This is a sterile procedure. The catheter is introduced into the opening of the stoma and gently pushed in (2.5–5 cm deep only) until urine starts to flow down the catheter into the waiting collection pot (Fillingham and Fell 2004). Occasionally this may be difficult as the stoma may be narrow or very long, or the patient may not be able to tolerate a catheter being used. In these instances a non-touch technique can be used with a sterile collecting pot held under the stoma, making sure that the rim does not touch the stoma or the surrounding skin. Urine should start to drip out of the stoma and into the pot. This may take a few minutes but should ensure the specimen is not contaminated. Alternatively a clean new bag can be put onto the abdomen over the stoma and the urine collected within a few minutes. The bag is not sterile but it will be clean and therefore there is less risk of contamination or multiple bacteria.

Box 9.6 Collection of a stoma urine specimen: equipment and key points

Equipment
- Sterile pack containing gloves and sterile gauze, sterile single-use catheter (8–14Ch), sterile specimen pot, disposable plastic apron, water or normal saline, clean stoma appliance (if required), disposal bag, incontinence pad or paper towel

Procedure
- Adhere to general points in Box 9.2.
- Prepare a new stoma bag if this needs to be replaced after procedure.
- Position an incontinence pad or paper towel under the patient.
- Remove the stoma bag and dispose of it.
- Cover stoma with sterile gauze.
- Wash and dry hands.
- Open sterile pack and prepare sterile field. Put on sterile gloves. Open sterile catheter and place on sterile field.
- Clean around stoma with sterile water or saline and gauze using strokes from the centre outwards. Dry area.
- Insert the catheter tip into the stoma opening and gently push it in to a depth of 2.5–5 cm only. Wait for urine to start to drain out into the sterile container. A minimum of 2–5 mL is sufficient, though more is preferable.
- Remove catheter and seal specimen container.
- Clean around stoma again if needed. Make sure skin is dry. Reapply stoma bag.
- Dispose of equipment as per local policy.

Learning outcome 5: Discuss the collection of a stool specimen

When do you think it might be necessary to collect a stool specimen? Thinking about a 'normal' stool will help you begin to answer this question.

You may have identified that a stool specimen is collected if a person has complained of abnormal stools, or you have observed an abnormality (e.g. diarrhoea) which may be caused by gastrointestinal infection. Infection is particularly likely if the stool is offensive and has an abnormal colour such as green. In these instances the stool is sent for MC&S, to detect the causative microorganism and identify any antibiotics to which it is sensitive.

Normal frequency of passing stools varies from person to person, but if frequency is altered this can be a reason to collect a specimen. Altered consistency might also be a reason. For example, lots of mucus can indicate disease such as ulcerative colitis, whereas fatty, offensive-smelling and floating stools sometimes indicate gall bladder disease.

Stool specimens are sent for examination for occult (hidden) blood, if rectal bleeding is suspected but not obvious. If the colour of a stool is different from that normally seen, this too can be suggestive of disease, indicating that a specimen should be taken. Bright red fresh blood must be reported and may indicate the presence of haemorrhoids or other disease. Stools that are black and tarry in consistency can indicate digested blood from the alimentary tract (termed **malaena**). Sometimes stool specimens are sent for examination for parasites. Additionally, if a person experiences pain or discomfort associated with defecation, or flatus is a problem, then a stool specimen might be taken.

See Box 9.7 for key points on collecting a stool specimen. There are stool specimen collectors available that have a spoon attached to the lid. Although these

Ulcerative colitis
Ulceration of the mucosa of the colon, causing offensive, watery stools with mucus and pus. Can cause haemorrhage and perforation.

Haemorrhoids
Dilated blood vessels in the rectal mucosa. The common term is 'piles'.

Box 9.7 Collection of a stool specimen: equipment and key points

Equipment
- Bedpan, gloves, apron, sterile stool specimen pot or sterile specimen pot and spatula, specimen bag, laboratory request form

Procedure
- Adhere to general points in Box 9.2.
- If possible the patient should be helped to a toilet rather than use a commode. A disposable bedpan can be placed under the toilet lid. Otherwise a bedpan or commode is used to catch the specimen.
- When the stool is available, take the bedpan to the sluice, open the sterile container and using a spatula, fill the container about a third full with faeces, and then secure the lid.
- Refrigerate the specimen if it cannot go to the laboratory immediately. In infections such as amoebiasis, the stool must be fresh and warm (Mead 1998), thus special arrangements for collection must be made with the laboratory.
- Remember to complete the stool chart if a record is being kept.

are easy to use when collecting the specimen, they can be difficult for laboratory staff to handle without getting contaminated. Also, pots should not be overfilled as the contents may ferment and build up sufficient pressure to force off even a tightly fitting lid (Gould and Brooker 2000).

Summary

- Explaining the procedure and its importance carefully, while maintaining dignity, privacy and respect for people, is of prime importance when collecting specimens.
- It is essential to be certain about the purpose for collecting the specimen so that it is collected appropriately.
- Great care should be taken when collecting urine and stool specimens to prevent their contamination, which would invalidate results.
- Precautions to prevent cross-infection must be adhered to when collecting urine and stool specimens.
- It is essential to label specimens accurately and to document their collection in patients' notes.

CARING FOR PEOPLE WITH URINARY CATHETERS

Urinary catheterisation involves the insertion of a hollow tube into the bladder for evacuating or instilling fluids. The catheter may be inserted intermittently, or left *in situ* (termed 'in-dwelling') and emptied intermittently via a catheter valve. In these instances, the bladder then retains its function as a reservoir. In many cases an in-dwelling catheter continuously drains the bladder within a closed system into a bag, in which case only a small volume of urine will be present at the base of the bladder. This method was used as a temporary measure for Jean immediately postoperatively.

Some people are taught to self-catheterise intermittently, termed 'intermittent self-catheterisation', often to manage incontinence or incomplete emptying in those with neurological disorders such as multiple sclerosis. Teaching a person to self-catheterise requires specific skills and knowledge (Getliffe and Fader 2007).

Urinary catheters are usually passed along the urethra, but sometimes a suprapubic catheter is passed directly through the mid suprapubic region of the anterior abdominal wall into the bladder. This is a surgical procedure, performed under anaesthesia, and may be used for people who need a long-term urinary catheter or after certain surgical procedures and in pelvic/urethral trauma or disease. The principles of catheter care for patients who have suprapubic catheters are the same as for those with urethral catheters (Colpman and Welford 2004). However, as the catheter is inserted into a tract into the skin, this can result in infection, bleeding and encrustation around the catheter site. Any secretions that form around the catheter site can be removed with soap and water. Most patients prefer not to wear a dressing around this site, though some may prefer to to do so to prevent staining of clothing.

By the end of this section you will be able to:

1 identify the main indications for urinary catheterisation;
2 show awareness of equipment commonly used for catheterisation;
3 state the main complications associated with urinary catheterisation;
4 understand the principles underpinning urethral catheterisation;
5 discuss the care required for people who have an in-dwelling urinary catheter.

You may be able to access a urinary catheter in the skills laboratory. An opened one would be particularly useful. If not, see if you can look at equipment in your practice setting.

Learning outcome 1: Identify the main indications for urinary catheterisation

It has been estimated that up to 25 per cent of people in hospital have an in-dwelling catheter (Patel and Arya 2000, cited by Wazait *et al.* 2003), with up to 28 per cent of patients residing in care homes and 4 per cent in the community having long-term in-dwelling catheters (Getliffe 1995).

ACTIVITY

Make a list of the reasons why people are catheterised. Thinking back to your practice experience will give you some clues.

Neurogenic bladder
Commonly results from lesions of the central nervous system (e.g. spinal injury, multiple sclerosis). Effects include urinary retention, overactive, underactive or uncoordinated detrusor activity.

Cytotoxic drugs
Drugs that have a destructive effect on cells and are used to treat cancer.

You may have identified the following:

- to relieve retention of urine (e.g. because of enlarged prostate or **neurogenic bladder**);
- before pelvic surgery and certain investigations, to minimise the risk of damage to the bladder;
- to measure urine output accurately postoperatively and in very ill patients (e.g. major trauma, shock) – Jean's urethral catheter was originally inserted for this reason;
- to empty the bladder during labour
- to introduce fluids into the bladder for irrigation purposes;
- to introduce drugs as direct therapy (e.g. **cytotoxic drugs**);
- to facilitate bladder healing;
- following certain pelvic, urethral or bladder neck surgery.

Incontinence is not given as a primary reason for catheterisation above because long-term catheterisation is rarely free of complications and should, therefore, only be considered when other options have failed, or are no longer appropriate. The major complications of catheterisation are considered in more detail later in this section.

Learning outcome 2: Show awareness of equipment commonly used for catheterisation

ACTIVITY

In the skills laboratory there may be a sterile or non-sterile (for demonstration purposes) urinary catheter complete with packaging material. See Fig. 9.3 for examples. Take note of the following:
* the manner in which it is packaged, batch number, expiry date;
* size;
* length;
* balloon capacity;
* the catheter material.

If you have access to a non-sterile catheter, try inflating and deflating the balloon using a syringe and water. Some catheters are manufactured pre-filled with water for inflation. Now read through the following points and relate them to your observations.

Packaging

Catheters are packaged to enable ease of insertion into the bladder. With the exception of self-catheterisation, a strict aseptic technique is employed. The way in which the catheter is packaged, including double wrapping, assists in maintaining sterility. There is a batch number and expiry date on the packaging which must be entered into patients' documentation. Many packets have removable sticky labels printed with these details which are put on the patient's notes for future reference.

Catheter size

The catheter size is measured according to its external diameter and is measured in Charrière (Ch) or French gauge units (Fg). One Ch unit equals 0.3 mm, and the catheters range in size from 6–8 (for paediatric use) to 30 Ch. A size 12 Ch catheter is 4 mm in diameter and is usually adequate for urine drainage for both men and women. The key general rule to follow is that the smallest size catheter should be

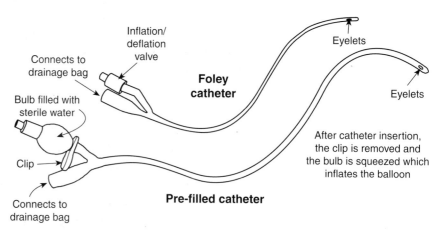

Figure 9.3: Examples of urinary catheters.

used that will allow free urinary outflow (Pratt *et al.* 2007). Large catheters are associated with complications including urethral irritation, urethral trauma, bladder spasm, urinary bypassing, pressure necrosis and increased infection risk (Getliffe 1996; Laurent 1998).

Catheter length

Catheters are usually manufactured in three lengths: standard catheters (sometimes referred to as 'male-length') are 40–44 cm, female catheters are 30–40 cm, and paediatric catheters are 30 cm (Robinson 2001). The standard catheter is often used for women, particularly if obese, because it allows easier access to the junction of the catheter and the drainage bag (Colpman and Welford 2004). Female catheters must never be used urethrally in a male as they are too short for the male urethra and would not reach the bladder. If inflated in the urethra the balloon may cause this to rupture and haemorrhage and may lead to severe trauma (Getliffe and Fader 2007).

Balloon

The Foley catheter is the design most frequently used for in-dwelling urethral catheterisation (Getliffe and Fader 2007). It has a rounded tip with two drainage eyes and an integral balloon, which, when inflated, holds the catheter *in situ*. There are two channels, one for drainage and the other for inflating the balloon. The balloon sits at the sensitive base of the bladder and can potentially cause irritation, spasm and mechanical damage to the bladder. Retention balloons come in various sizes: 10 mL is recommended for adults, but larger 30 mL balloons are sometimes used after some urological procedures (Pratt *et al.* 2007). Inflation valves are colour-coded according to the Charrière size (Robinson 2001).

Catheters for intermittent use are usually a simple tube design and do not have an inflatable balloon as there is no requirement for them to be retained in the bladder. Some suprapubic catheters do not have a balloon, but are secured by a flange and held in place by skin sutures.

Material

Catheters are available in various materials. The choice of which type to use depends on the clinical experience of the practitioner, patient assessment and the length of time it is envisaged the catheter will remain *in situ* (Pratt *et al.* 2007).

For short-term use, plastic, latex (up to 7–10 days) and Teflon-coated latex (up to 28 days) are commonly used; these materials are considerably cheaper than long-term catheter materials. Some patients are allergic to latex, and screening is advisable if latex is to be used (Woodward 1997). Plastic catheters have been found to exert low toxicity because of the inert nature of plastic. Also, the rate that this material absorbs water is low and so the catheter retains the widest internal diameter, making these catheters a common choice for drainage of postoperative blood clots and debris. However, plastic catheters can remain rigid at body temperature and have been associated with bladder spasm, pain and leakage of urine (Blannin and Hobden 1980, cited by Macauley 1997). The Department of Health (DH) (2003) recommends that in-dwelling catheters used for long-term use should have low allergenicity. Silicone, silicone elastamer-coated latex and hydrogel-coated catheters are suitable products (Laurent 1998).

Recent research has focused on developing catheters with properties specifically to reduce infection incidence. These tend to have special coatings such as silver ions or aloe vera along their length. The aim is to either stop or limit biofilms forming (Godfrey and Fraczyk 2005). These substances have been found to have anti-infection properties. However, a review found that very few trials have compared different types of catheter for long-term use and most were carried out on small numbers of patients (Jahn *et al.* 2007). The reviewers concluded that the evidence was too weak to provide reliable evidence about which type of catheter is best for which patients. The cost of the catheter should not be the primary factor in the selection process but nurses should be aware of the different costs when selecting.

Urine drainage bags and catheter valves

In-dwelling catheters are normally used in conjunction with an attached collection bag to allow periodic emptying. This is known as a **closed system.** Figure 9.4 shows a catheter attached to a leg bag, which would be secured to the patient's leg with straps. Figure 9.5 shows a urinary catheter attached to a bed bag supported on a stand, which will be suitable for when the person is in bed. A catheter valve (see Fig. 9.6) may provide an alternative for some patients but an adequate bladder capacity is required. Unless a committed carer is available, the user also requires good manual dexterity for manipulating the valve, and sufficient cognitive function to understand the need to release the valve regularly to prevent over-distension (Fader *et al.* 1997). Catheter valves are also unlikely to be suitable if the person has uncontrolled detrusor overactivity, ureteric reflux or renal impairment (Fader *et al.* 1997).

When selecting a bag, factors to consider are capacity, length of inlet tube and type of outlet tap for emptying. Bags vary in capacity from 350 to 750 mL and up to 2 L for use overnight or postoperatively. Some bags are specially designed for wheelchair users. Outlet taps are usually of a lever-type design or push-across mechanism, but other designs are available. The manual dexterity of patients and

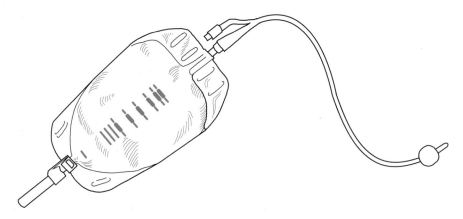

Figure 9.4: A urinary catheter attached to a leg bag.

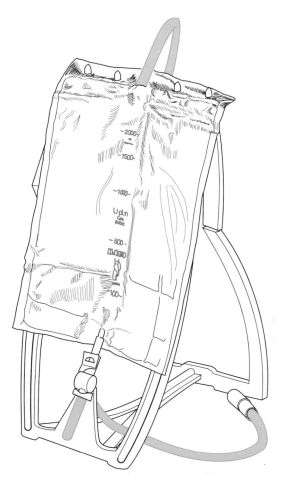

Figure 9.5: A bed bag on a stand.

carers needs to be considered. There are catheter supports available for people with restricted mobility which aim to provide firm support to prevent tugging, without restricting movement or impeding drainage.

Whatever equipment is used, you must document details of the catheter and drainage system used in the patient's records carefully. You should also provide the person with adequate information about the rationale for insertion, the insertion itself, and the maintenance and removal of catheter.

ACTIVITY

What sort of drainage bag might be suitable for Jean?

Following discussion with Jean you may decide to use a leg bag. The length of the inlet tube selected would depend on whether Jean found it most comfortable to position the bag on her thigh, knee or calf. At night the nurses will be able to attach a night bag on a stand, directly to the leg bag. For most patients, body-worn bags are preferable because their attachment to the person's leg or suspended from the waist allows maximum freedom and at the same time can be concealed beneath clothing. This reduces discomfort and promotes dignity for people like Jean who

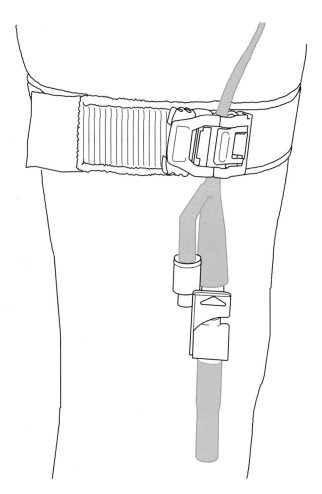

Figure 9.6: A urinary catheter strapped to the leg, with a valve in place, for emptying.

find themselves in the difficult and sometimes embarrassing situation of needing a urinary catheter *in situ*. A body-worn bag will help Jean as she begins to mobilise as she will not have to contend with carrying the bag or long trailing drainage tubes. Once she is comfortable moving and fully mobile the catheter can be removed.

Did you know?

Prior to the use of closed drainage systems almost all patients developed UTIs within 96 hours (Kass 1957, cited by Macauley 1997). As closed drainage systems have been shown to reduce this rate of infection, they are now accepted as good practice (Macauley 1997). However, many healthcare-associated infections are related to urinary catheterisation, causing significant morbidity and even mortality. Therefore, care for people with catheters must aim to prevent infection, as well as promoting comfort and understanding.

ACTIVITY

Figure 9.7 shows a diagram of a closed urinary drainage system. Where do you think bacteria could enter into the system?

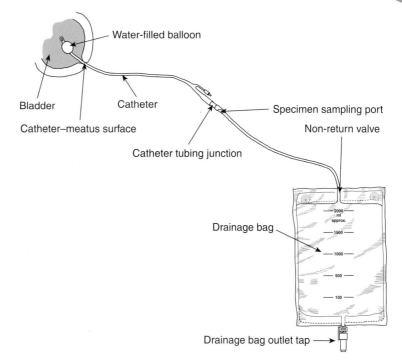

Figure 9.7: A closed urinary drainage system.

The following are potential ports of entry:

- the catheter tip during catheterisation;
- the urethral meatus around the catheter;
- the junction between the catheter and the tubing to the catheter bag;
- the specimen sampling port;
- the drainage outlet.

Bacteria are believed to enter the bladder at the time of catheterisation also via the peri-urethral space. Coagulase-negative staphylococci or micrococci can normally be found in the anterior urethra, and these are a common cause of infection immediately following catheterisation (Ayliffe *et al.* 2001).

Some systems now have a tamper-evident seal at the junction between the catheter and the connection tube aimed at preventing bacteria entering here.

Early infections are often **endogenous** (self-infection), but cross-infection (**exogenous** infection) occurs later in patients with in-dwelling catheters (Ayliffe *et al.* 2001).

Learning outcome 3: State the main complications associated with urinary catheterisation

ACTIVITY

Look back over this section and see whether you can name one major complication associated with catheterisation. Try to identify some other complications.

You probably identified that infection is a major complication of catheterisation. Encrustation and eventual blockage are also problems associated with urinary catheterisation (Burr and Nuseibeh 1997; Laurent 1998). Other complications include urethral strictures, pressure necrosis, spasm, discomfort and pain (Winn 1996).

With a catheter *in situ* the bladder's normal closing mechanism is obstructed and the natural flushing mechanism of micturition is lost. Additionally the close proximity of the catheter to the bowel presents a risk of infection, because bacteria can be mechanically transferred across skin surfaces from anus to urethral meatus (Meers *et al.* 1995). As discussed earlier, bacteria having entered the urinary system may cling to the surface of the catheter, which creates a living biofilm that is almost impossible to remove and that is highly resistant to antibiotics (Getliffe 2002). The bacteria can cause the urine to become more alkaline than usual and encrustation on the catheter surface then occurs, which can lead to blockage and then to retention of urine or to leakage and pain. These outcomes are distressing for patients, and can result in loss of comfort and dignity (Laurent 1998).

When tissue is invaded by bacteria, problems include local infection, which may result in foul-smelling urine, or systemic infection leading to pyrexia (raised body temperature). Catheterising patients places them in significant danger of acquiring a UTI, and the longer a catheter is in place, the greater the danger. Of patients with a catheter-associated UTI, 1–4 per cent develop bacteraemia and of these 13–30 per cent die (Pratt *et al.* 2007). Therefore catheterisation is best avoided if at all possible (NICE 2003; Pratt *et al.* 2007), and catheters should be removed as soon as possible if no longer needed.

Learning outcome 4: Understand the principles underpinning urethral catheterisation

Catheterisation is a skilled aseptic procedure and should be carried out only by healthcare personnel who are trained and competent to carry it out (Pratt *et al.* 2007). Catheterisation is an invasive procedure and the effects on patients may be many: physical, psychological and social.

ACTIVITY	Before reading the following section, refer to Chapter 3 for an explanation of the aseptic technique. These principles underpin the procedure of urinary catheterisation.

Appropriate and effective communication and sensitivity are essential when catheterisation takes place (see Chapter 2 for more information). Care should be taken to explain where the catheter is inserted, and why the procedure is necessary, ensuring that verbal consent is gained. This could be difficult with a person who is confused. Also, catheters should not be changed unnecessarily or as part of routine practice.

Box 9.8 outlines the equipment needed and key points when undertaking female urethral catheterisation. In many NHS Trusts additional training must be undertaken

Box 9.8 Female urethral catheterisation: equipment and procedure

Equipment

- A catheterisation pack if available, or a dressing pack and sterile receiver, sterile gloves, an appropriate catheter, sterile sodium chloride, catheter bag and stand or holder, sterile single-patient-use lubricant or anaesthetic gel, syringe and sterile water of appropriate size to inflate the balloon (often included with catheter), disposable waterproof absorbent pad, specimen pot (if required), a good light source

Note: A second nurse may be needed to help position the patient, who needs to be preferably flat with legs apart to allow good access and visibility.

Procedure

- Aseptic technique should be strictly adhered to throughout (see Chapter 3 sections on 'Hand hygiene' and 'Aseptic technique').
- Explain the procedure and ensure consent.
- Maintain privacy and reassure the patient throughout.
- Place the disposable pad under the patient's buttocks.
- Open the catheter bag and arrange at the side of the bed, ensuring the attachment tip remains sterile.
- Open the catheterisation or dressing pack, and open the catheter on to the sterile field but do not remove it from its internal wrapping.
- Draw up the sterile water to inflate the balloon (unless pre-filled syringe supplied or catheter is pre-filled).
- Pour sodium chloride into the gallipot.
- Open sterile gloves, wash hands and apply gloves.
- Place sterile towels over patient's thighs and between legs.
- Cleanse the perineal area with the sodium chloride, and then using non-dominant hand, separate labia minora and cleanse the meatus.
- Carefully locate the urethra and insert single-patient-use lubricant gel to minimise urethral trauma and infection (NICE 2003). Some gels contain anaesthetic too. Inserting the gel directly into the urethra opens up and lubricates the length of the urethra. Lubricating the tip of the catheter only is ineffective as the lubricant is quickly wiped away on insertion. Wait for the time recommended by the manufacturer, usually 5 minutes.
- Place a receiver with the catheter on the sterile towel between the patient's legs.
- Expose the tip of the catheter by pulling open the wrapper at the serrations.
- Hold the catheter so that the distal end remains in the receiver and gradually advance it out of its wrapper as you insert it into the meatus in an upward and backward direction along the line of the urethra.
- Advance the catheter 5–7 cm or until urine flows out of the catheter.
- Advance the catheter a further 5 cm. Never force the catheter. If resistance is encountered stop and seek medical advice.
- Inflate the balloon with the correct amount of sterile water, generally 10 mL for adults (NICE 2003). Incorrectly filled balloons can inflate irregularly and irritate the bladder mucosa (Wilson 1997).
- Attach the urinary drainage bag, and make the patient comfortable.
- Send a urine specimen if indicated and measure and record the urine collected.
- Document the catheterisation in the patient's notes, including date of insertion, catheter size and amount of water used to inflate the balloon. The catheter packaging may have an adhesive label with the catheter's details which can be used.

by trained nurses to perform male urethral catheterisation. However, many of the principles are synonymous with female urethral catheterisation. Suprapubic catheterisation is usually a medical procedure, and is not considered here.

Once the catheter has been inserted, dietary advice, including fluid intake and avoidance of constipation, is an important part of patient education (Getliffe 1996). Further explanations and instructions concerning why and how the catheter has been inserted, its maintenance requirements and discussion of removal will be required if the person goes home with a urinary catheter *in situ*. Patients and carers should also be educated about techniques to prevent infection (DH 2003). The district nurse will probably be involved.

Learning outcome 5: Discuss the care required for people who have an in-dwelling urinary catheter

| ACTIVITY | What specific care might be needed in relation to catheter care for Jean? |

You may have thought of:
- maintaining hygiene;
- emptying the catheter bag;
- appropriate positioning of the catheter bag;
- adequate fluid intake.

These issues will now be discussed.

Maintaining hygiene

The main aim of cleansing is to remove secretions and encrustation and prevent infection. Where possible, patients should be encouraged to attend to their own meatal and perineal hygiene needs, thus reducing the risk of cross-infection while promoting self-care and dignity. Maintaining routine daily hygiene is all that is needed, with the meatus being washed with soap and water (NICE 2003). However, for people unable to maintain their own hygiene, nurses should carry this out, wearing gloves, and with a gentle and sensitive manner. Vigorous cleansing may increase the risk of infection (Pratt *et al.* 2007).

Cleansing of the perineum and the area surrounding the catheter–meatus junction is essential after faecal incontinence and should be carried out using clean wipes. For female patients, you should clean from front to back to prevent possible movement of bacteria from the anal area and perineum to the catheter–meatus junction. The catheter should be gently wiped in one direction, away from the vulva. In male patients the foreskin should be retracted before cleansing and the same principles of cleaning the catheter away from the catheter–meatus junction should be adhered to. The foreskin must be replaced afterwards. With a suprapubic catheter, once the wound has healed around the catheter, simple cleansing with soap and water is usually sufficient to maintain hygiene.

Emptying the catheter bag

ACTIVITY

You may recall that microorganisms can be introduced into the drainage system at the junction between the catheter and bag or via the drainage tap. Bearing this in mind, work out the equipment you would need, and how you would use it, to safely empty a catheter bag. Compare your answer with Box 9.9.

Unless hands are thoroughly washed between patients and a clean container used to collect the urine, microorganisms are readily transferred to the next patient. Although disinfection of hands with 70 per cent alcohol is rapid and effective, hands that are visibly soiled or potentially grossly contaminated with dirt or organic material must be washed with soap and water (see Chapter 3, section on 'Hand hygiene').

The urinary drainage bag should be emptied frequently enough to maintain urine flow and prevent reflux, and to prevent it becoming so heavy that its weight pulls on the catheter and causes urethral trauma. There is no evidence that bags need to be changed at specific intervals, but as well as being changed when full, bags should also be changed when damaged or blocked with deposits. Bags should be changed when clinically indicated and/or in line with the manufacturers' recommendations (NICE 2003; Pratt *et al.* 2007). But the key principle – and the way to prevent bacteria or other harmful organisms entering the system – is to

---

Box 9.9 Emptying a catheter bag: equipment and procedure

Equipment
- Non-sterile gloves and apron, a heat-disinfected or disposable container, e.g. a urinal or jug, paper towel to cover, alcohol swabs

Procedure
- Explain the procedure to the patient and ensure privacy.
- Wash hands and put on apron and gloves.
- If the drainage bag is on a stand it may not need removing. If it is hanging on the bed, you may need to access it by removing the bag and placing it over the jug.
- Clean the outlet port with alcohol swab and allow it to dry.
- Open the port and drain the urine into the receptacle, ensuring that the port does not touch the side of the receptacle.
- Close the port and wipe with alcohol swab.
- Reposition bag.
- Cover the container and take to sluice for disposal. Measure the urine first if a fluid balance chart is being kept.
- The container should be disinfected, or macerated if disposable.
- Remove gloves and apron and wash hands.

leave the closed system alone as much as you can. NICE (2003) recommends that the connection between the catheter and the drainage system should not be broken except for sound clinical reasons.

Jean has a leg drainage bag attached to her catheter which can remain unchanged for up to a week as per the manufacturer's advice. A night drainage bag can be attached to the open tap of the leg bag for overnight drainage. This can be removed and discarded during the day as Jean goes back to draining into her leg bag. This process ensures the closed drainage system is not broken. Disconnection of the catheter from the drainage bag significantly increases the risk of introducing bacteria into the system and should therefore be avoided if possible (Wilson 2006). Patients with a catheter on drainage who live at home where the risks of cross-infection are low can reuse the night drainage bag for up to one week if rinsed with water and allowed to dry between use. However, in hospital and other institutional settings patients should have a new night drainage bag each time as the risk for cross-contamination and infection is too great to allow reuse. Adding antiseptic or antimicrobial solutions into drainage bags is not recommended (Pratt *et al.* 2007).

Appropriate positioning of the catheter bag

Catheter bags should be positioned to avoid reflux and facilitate the use of gravity, and positioned clear of floors or other sources of contamination (NICE 2003). Drainage bags should always be positioned below the level of the bladder and the catheter and the inlet tubing secured in a downward position (Colpman and Welford 2004). This is because reflux urine is associated with infection, so bags must be positioned to prevent backflow of urine. Where it is difficult to maintain the level of the bag below the bladder, for example when moving and handling, then clamp the urinary drainage bag tube and remove the clamp as soon as dependent drainage can be resumed (Pratt *et al.* 2007). The catheter itself should never be clamped as this can easily be damaged.

The catheter in females should be secured to prevent movement of the catheter within the urethra, which may introduce infection (Ayliffe *et al.* 2001). A variety of straps, 'net' sleeves, holsters and sporrans are available to suspend the drainage bag. Securing the catheter also ensures it does not pull on the urethra and cause ulceration or cleaving where pressure from the tube can split the urethra. In extreme cases the whole urethra may be split open and require surgical repair (Colpman and Welford 2004).

Adequate fluid intake

If the patient's condition allows, encourage oral fluids. This has traditionally been believed to result in dilute urine containing fewer nutrients, thus discouraging the growth of bacteria in the drainage bag and encrustation of components. It is believed that the larger volume of urine maintains a constant flow through the drainage system, making it more difficult for bacteria to multiply in the drainage bag (Wilson 2006). Getliffe and Fader (2007) identified that although there is no clear evidence that drinking large quantities of fluid will prevent infection, in practice it is sensible to promote good fluid intake to prevent dehydration and constipation.

Catheter removal

ACTIVITY

Think about how you would prepare Jean, or any other patient, for catheter removal.

A clear explanation should be given, emphasising that the procedure is not normally painful but that there may be a feeling of discomfort. Box 9.10 outlines equipment and key points for removing a catheter.

If a catheter is removed without insertion of a new catheter, Chillington (1992) suggests removal at midnight rather than early morning. This increases the length of time before passing urine, leading to a greater initial volume and a faster return to normal voiding, decreasing levels of anxiety. You should ensure that urine is passed satisfactorily after catheter removal and observe for problems such as incontinence, frequency and retention. A person who is confused may need prompting to pass urine (see later section on promoting continence). Some people, particularly men who have had prostate surgery, should perform pelvic floor exercises to help them to regain control (see later section). People with long-term catheters for specific medical reasons will need the catheter changing periodically depending upon clinical need, such as any problems experienced, and/or in line with manufacturers' recommendations (Pratt *et al.* 2007).

Summary

- Urinary catheterisation is experienced by many patients/clients and may be a short-term or long-term measure.
- Catheterisation is an invasive procedure and there are many complications associated with it, infection being particularly common. Therefore catheterisation should be performed only if there is a clear indication.
- Strict asepsis should be maintained, and the catheter should be removed as soon as possible, using the correct technique.
- Nurses should be aware of the different types of equipment available, and make appropriate choices regarding types of catheter and drainage bag.
- The closed system should not be broken except for good clinical reasons.
- Care should be taken to reduce physical and psychological discomfort for people with urinary catheters.

Box 9.10 Removal of a urethral catheter: equipment and procedure

Equipment

- Non-sterile gloves and apron, syringe of sufficient volume to remove the water from the balloon, disposable absorbent pad, receiver and waste bag. If a catheter specimen of urine is required: specimen pot, 20 mL syringe, needle and alcohol swab

Procedure

- Give explanation, ensure privacy and position the person comfortably. For a female the knees and hips should be slightly flexed and apart.
- Wash and dry hands and apply gloves and apron.
- Obtain a specimen of urine from the sampling port if indicated (see Box 9.3).
- Place the disposable pad under the patient's buttocks and then place the receiver between the thighs.
- Check the balloon volume, and attach an appropriately sized syringe to the balloon port of the catheter. Withdraw the water from the balloon via the syringe.
- Ask the patient to breathe in and out, and as they exhale, the catheter is gently withdrawn and placed in the receiver. If problems are encountered, stop and seek medical advice.
- Remove gloves and apron and wash hands.
- The patient should be made comfortable and because frequency may be experienced the nurse should ensure that a toilet or commode is close by. If the patient needs help with mobility, ensure a call bell is nearby.
- Document the date and time of catheter removal in the clinical notes and record the amount of urine in the catheter bag.
- The patient may be encouraged to increase fluid intake to 'flush' out the bladder.
- Monitor whether the person is passing urine satisfactorily. A chart may be kept so that frequency and amount can be monitored. Also ask the patient to inform a nurse if any unusual symptoms are experienced, e.g. dysuria (pain when passing urine).

Getliffe and Fader (2007) cover catheterisation in depth, so further reading from that source is recommended.

PREVENTING AND MANAGING CONSTIPATION

Constipation is a common condition, with multifactoral causes. People with constipation can experience various uncomfortable symptoms including headache, bloatedness, loss of appetite, nausea and vomiting (Kyle 2007a). Constipation is also a risk factor for faecal incontinence (NICE 2007). For some people constipation can be dangerous; Pellatt (2007) explains that if patients with spinal cord injury above the sixth thoracic vertebra develop bowel distension due to constipation or impaction, they can develop autonomic dysreflexia (severe hypertension) which may lead to cerebral haemorrhage, seizures or cardiac arrest. Therefore risk of constipation should be assessed so that preventative measures can be implemented, rather than waiting until constipation has developed. When constipation occurs, it should be managed effectively to relieve discomfort and prevent complications. Enemas and suppositories may be required to treat constipation, but they are also a means of medicine administration via the rectal route. Therefore, principles of medicine administration should be followed (see Chapter 5).

LEARNING OUTCOMES

By the end of this section you will be able to:
1 identify how risk of constipation can be assessed, and constipation prevented and managed;
2 understand key principles of administering suppositories and enemas.

Learning outcome 1: Identify how risk of constipation can be assessed, and constipation prevented and managed

ACTIVITY

What are likely risk factors for constipation? Think back to patients/clients you encountered in placement. Who was at risk of constipation?

There are many risk factors for constipation (see Richmond and Wright 2004; Kyle 2007b). Mark is prone to both constipation and diarrhoea. The Royal College of Nursing (RCN) (2006a) identified that constipation is more common in people with learning disabilities, particularly if they are less mobile, have inadequate nutrition and fluid intake or are taking long-term medication with constipation as a side-effect. Patients who are in hospital often experience reduced exercise alongside a changed diet, increasing their risk of constipation. Psychological and environmental factors can also contribute to constipation in hospital. Constipation is a side-effect of many medicines.

Kyle (2007a) presents the Norgine risk assessment tool for constipation (see Fig. 9.8). The tool includes all main risk factors for constipation. The assessor ticks and adds up all that apply; the higher the score, the greater the risk. The tool is designed to be used with adult patients on admission, and alerts nurses to patients' risk of constipation – leading to proactive preventative measures (Kyle 2007a).

ACTIVITY

Look back at Mark's scenario and, using the Norgine risk assessment tool in Fig. 9.8, assess his risk.

You will have found that the tool is quick and easy to use. Mark's score is 5. Under 'Medical condition' you should have ticked 'History of constipation' and 'Impaired cognition'. For 'Toileting facilities' you should have ticked 'Supervised use of lavatory/commode'; and for 'Mobility' you should have identified 'Walks with aids/assistance'. For 'Nutritional intake', Mark 'Needs assistance to eat'. If Mark is

NORGINE

Norgine® Risk Assessment Tool for Constipation

			PATIENT'S NAME	
			PATIENT'S DATE OF BIRTH	
			PATIENT'S NHS NUMBER	

Medical Condition	
Cancer	
Clinical depression	
Diabetes	
Haemorrhoids, anal fissure, rectocele, local anal or rectal pathology	
History of constipation	
Impaired cognition/dementia	
Multiple sclerosis	
Parkinson's disease	
Post operative	
Rheumatoid arthritis	
Spinal cord conditions (injury, disease or congenital)	
Stroke	✓

Current Medication	
Aluminium antacids	
Anticholinergics	
Antiparkinson drugs	
Antipsychotic drugs	
Calcium channel blockers	
Calcium supplements	
Diuretics	
Iron supplements	
Non-steroidal anti-inflammatory drugs (NSAIDs)	
Opioids	
Tricyclic antidepressants	
Polypharmacy (more than 5 drugs including ones not on this list)	

Toileting Facilities	✓
Bed pan	
Commode by bed in hospital/care home/home	
Supervised use of lavatory/commode	
Commode/raised toilet seat at home (without foot stool)	

Mobility	✓
Restricted to bed	
Restricted to wheelchair/chair	
Walks with aids/assistance	
Walks short distances but less than 1/3 mile (0.5 km)	

Nutritional Intake	✓
At nutritional risk as identified by local nutritional screening tool	
Fibre intake 6 g or less per day	
Difficulty in swallowing/chewing	
Needs assistance to eat	

Daily Fluid Intake (see below for calculation table)	✓
Minimum fluids not achieved	

Fluid Requirement Calculation
30 mls fluid per 1 kg of body weight

Patients minimum fluid intake should be:	
Weight in **kg** = x **30 ml** =	
Patients actual fluid intake is:	

INSTRUCTIONS

1. Tick all relevant categories in each table.

2. There may be more than one tick in a table.

3. ADD ALL THE TICKS TOGETHER.

4. Fill in the number of ticks in the box below.

5. Date and sign

DATE	TOTAL NO. OF TICKS	SIGNATURE

Figure 9.8: Norgine risk assessment tool for constipation. Reproduced by kind permission of Gaye Kyle, Senior Lecturer, Thames Valley University; Phil Prynn, Continence Services Manager, Berkshire West PCT; Terri Dunbar, Advanced Nurse Practitioner, Berkshire West PCT. © 2006 Norgine Pharmaceuticals Ltd.

> ### Box 9.11 Action to take when risk of constipation is identified.
>
> - Complete full bowel assessment using locally approved care pathway.
> - Monitor and record bowel movements daily using the Bristol stool chart (see Fig. 9.1) and bowel record chart.
> - For stool type 1 or type 2 on Bristol stool chart, prescribe appropriate laxative therapy.
> - Advise on toileting position.
> - Review medication, including over-the-counter medicines.
> - Advise on ways to improve mobility.
> - Encourage patients to achieve at least minimum fluid intake.
> - Improve nutrition according to nutritional intake score.
>
> Reproduced by kind permission of Gaye Kyle, Senior Lecturer, Thames Valley University; Phil Prynn, Continence Services Manager, Berkshire West PCT; and Terri Dunbar, Advanced Nurse Practitioner, Berkshire West PCT. © 2006 Norgine Pharmaceuticals Ltd

prescribed any of the medication listed, these would add to his risk. If Mark's fluid intake is inadequate, his risk increases further.

Patients who, like Mark, score more than 4 on the Norgine risk assessment tool should have further assessment and appropriate actions taken (see Box 9.11).

The main groups of laxatives are bulking agents (e.g. Isogel, regulan), stimulants (e.g. senna, bisocodyl), stool softeners and lubricants (liquid paraffin, ducoset sodium) and osmotic agents (e.g. lactulose); see the *British National Formulary* for more details (www.bnf.org). Although laxatives may be necessary to prevent and manage constipation, they are preferably a short-term measure only. The RCN (2006a) identified that, for people with learning disabilities, there has been an over-reliance on laxatives rather than promoting adequate nutrition and fluid intake. Where feasible, medicines that predispose to constipation should be avoided particularly in those who are at risk. Exercise should be increased if possible.

The first section in this chapter included many aspects relevant to preventing constipation in hospital: ensuring people feel able to ask for assistance, encouraging them to go to the toilet when the 'call to stool' occurs (often early in the morning or about 30 minutes after a meal), attending to them promptly giving assistance to go out to the toilet when possible, ensuring that they are comfortable and well-supported, and giving them unhurried time and privacy.

As regards the correct position to open the bowels, you should advise patients to:
- sit with the knees higher than the hips;
- lean forward with elbows on knees;
- bulge out the abdomen and straighten the spine.

A footstool may be needed to assist patients into this position. Any patients who can use the toilet or commode can be advised to use this position to assist them, unless there are contraindications owing to their medical condition.

Adequate fluid intake is important and dietary fibre should be increased gradually and alongside increased fluid intake to prevent bloating. High-fibre foods, fruit and vegetables should be encouraged according to people's preference. For example, if Mark likes biscuits, he could be encouraged to eat flapjacks, oatcakes, digestive biscuits or fig rolls. Depending on the risk factors, referrals to other health professionals and specialists may be helpful (e.g. doctor, continence advisor, dietician, dentist, physiotherapist, occupational therapist, speech and language therapist, pharmacist). The community nurse for learning disabilities can work with Mark and his mother to ensure that Mark has appropriate multidisciplinary support.

NICE (2007) identifies that people with faecal loading need rectally administered treatment to clear the bowel – which may need to be repeated daily for a few days. If these do not work satisfactorily, oral laxatives should be given and a plan developed to prevent recurrence. A digital rectal examination (DRE) might be carried out to check for faecal impaction, and for abnormalities such as blood, pain or obstruction. DRE involves observing the perianal area and inserting a gloved and lubricated finger into the rectum (Kyle 2007c). Manual removal of faeces (using a lubricated, gloved finger) is sometimes carried out for faecal impaction (severe constipation when there is a mass of faeces in the rectum which cannot be passed) or incomplete defecation, inability to defecate, when other bowel emptying methods have failed, in neurogenic bowel dysfunction (e.g. multiple sclerosis), and for patients with spinal cord injury (RCN 2006b). While it is usually a last resort, for some patients it will be part of their bowel management regime.

DRE and manual removal of faeces can be carried out only by registered nurses who can demonstrate competence in these skills, but they can also delegate these procedures to carers or patients if their competence has been assessed (RCN 2006b). These procedures are invasive and patients must have given consent; the RCN (2006) discusses these procedures and consent issues. Irwin (2002) explains both procedures in detail. There are contraindications to these procedures and potential risks and many organisations have developed their own policies.

In some instances, suppositories or enemas may be needed to treat constipation – these are considered in learning outcome 2.

Learning outcome 2: Understand key principles of administering suppositories and enemas

An **enema** is a liquid that is inserted into the rectum, while a **suppository** is a medicated solid formulation, usually torpedo-shaped, and is inserted into the rectum, where it dissolves at body temperature. An enema that should be retained following administration is termed a 'retention enema' and is primarily used for its local effect. For example, a steroid enema may be administered to people with ulcerative colitis for its anti-inflammatory effect. An 'evacuant enema' is given to initiate bowel emptying and is used for constipation or to empty the bowel prior to surgery or investigations of the gastrointestinal tract. Suppositories are often administered for evacuant purposes, but they are also often used to administer medication and may be administered as a local treatment, as for haemorrhoids.

Drugs commonly prescribed rectally include paracetamol (for its analgesic and/or antipyretic effect) and anticonvulsants. What are the advantages and disadvantages of this route of drug administration?

You might have thought of the following advantages:

- The rectum is an alternative route for when people cannot take oral medication because they are vomiting, unable to swallow or are 'nil by mouth' (e.g. preoperatively).
- The rectum is very vascular so rectal medication is absorbed rapidly as liver metabolism is avoided (Addison *et al.* 2000). For example, a person who is fitting cannot take oral medication and rectal administration is safer and more rapid than intramuscular injections. As faecal impaction can inhibit rectal drug absorption, constipation should be prevented in people who might require emergency rectal medication.

Disadvantages include:

- Suppository and enema administration is more invasive and embarrassing than oral administration and involves some discomfort, undressing and moving into the correct position.
- Schmelzer and Wright's (1996) review reports that there have been traumatic and even fatal side-effects of enemas, including inflammation, electrolyte imbalance and perforation of the colonic mucosa. Newer, pre-packaged enemas aim to prevent such problems. Therefore enemas should only be used if there is no alternative.

Prior to administering an enema or suppository the nurse should carefully assess the appropriateness of this route.

Can you think of any physical problems that might be contraindications?

Anal fissure
A painful crack in the mucous membrane of the anus, generally caused by hard faeces.

Contraindications might include recent colorectal or gynaecological surgery, malignancy or other pathology of the perineal area, and a low platelet count, as this predisposes to bleeding. Thus the nurse should check with both the patient and the case notes for any previous anorectal surgery or abnormalities. Further checks should also be made visually immediately prior to administration. The perianal region should be checked for abnormalities, including haemorrhoids, anal fissure and rectal prolapse.

Rectal prolapse
A protrusion of rectal mucosa through the anus.

When giving an enema or suppositories for evacuation purposes, there can be a choice of products.

ACTIVITY Find out what types of enemas and suppositories are available to evacuate the bowel. There may be examples in the skills laboratory, or you can look at them in your practice setting.

Suppositories may be of the type that will simply soften the stools, or they may have a stimulant effect. Greenstein (2004) recommends that glycerol suppositories are satisfactory and other types offer no advantage. There are **microenemas** available containing only 5 mL of solution which act as a colon stimulant. For more vigorous bowel cleansing (e.g. prior to a bowel investigation) a larger **phosphate enema** may be used.

Phosphate enemas work through osmosis – by extracting water from the bowel to draw into faeces, thus increasing the faecal mass (Bowers 2006). Bowers asserts that there is a lack of evidence to support use of phosphate enemas for constipation above other products, but that they are an effective way of clearing the colon prior to flexible sigmoidoscopy. Complications of phosphate enemas are rare but can be serious. Patients with severe constipation often have other underlying conditions that may make them more at risk of complications. It is important to check the manufacturer's instructions when administering a phosphate enema. There are a number of contraindications and Addison *et al.* (2000) advises that they are unsuitable for older or debilitated patients. Mendoza *et al.*'s (2007) systematic review of sodium phosphate enema administration identified that side-effects (mainly water and electrolyte disturbances) were rare, mainly occurring in the very young (under 5 years) or people older than 65 years. Patients suffering side-effects often had conditions such as neurological, gastrointestinal or renal disorders.

Box 9.12 provides guidance for safe administration of suppositories/enemas based on the evidence available.

> **Flexible sigmoidoscopy**
> The sigmoid colon is examined with a lighted scope, usually for bleeding, non-cancerous growths (polyps) or colorectal cancer.

Summary

- Constipation is a common condition that can cause considerable discomfort. The causes are multifactorial and a risk assessment tool can help nurses to identify people at risk.
- Prevention of constipation involves adequate fibre and fluid intake, exercise and avoiding constipation-inducing medicines if possible. Laxatives can be used but should be a short-term measure.
- Suppositories or enemas may be given to administer medication or to evacuate the bowel. Careful assessment should precede administration as there are contraindications.
- Preparation of the patient/client should include explanation and gaining consent, correct choice of enema/suppositories and other equipment, maintenance of dignity and privacy, and correct positioning of the person to prevent damage to the wall of the rectum.

Box 9.12 Administration of enemas and suppositories: equipment and procedure

Equipment

- An absorbent under pad, tissues, lubricating gel, the enema or suppository/ies, gloves and apron
- Ensure that a good light source is available and that privacy can be maintained.

Procedure

- Local medicine policy should be followed (see Chapter 5). Check expiry date of suppositories/enema.
- Explain the procedure and gain consent. If the person is known to regularly require rectal anticonvulsants, consent should be obtained in advance and documented.
- Some people can insert a suppository themselves; if so, carefully explain the procedure.
- Ensure privacy, dignity and sensitivity throughout the procedure.
- Maintain infection control procedures throughout: hand hygiene, use of gloves and aprons, correct waste disposal (see Chapter 3).
- Give explanations, encouragement and reassurance and feedback (Schmelzer and Wright 1996).
- Some enemas should be warmed before administration – check the manufacturer's instructions. Warm by placing the enema in a jug of warm water. The temperature should be slightly higher than body temperature, feeling warm to the wrist (Schmelzer and Wright 1996).
- Position the person on the left side to allow easy flow of the fluid into the rectum by following the patient's anatomy. Place the under-pad under the patient's buttocks, and ask them to lie at the edge of the bed with knees flexed, and covered by a blanket. This position aids the passage of the nozzle of the enema through the anal canal. This position may need adapting for someone with a physical disability.
- Examine the area around the anus (see discussion on contraindications).
- **Enemas**: Remove the enema cap, expel any air from the enema container (if introduced into the colon this can cause distension and discomfort). Lubricate the nozzle of the enema (some enemas have a pre-lubricated tip). Part the buttocks and gently insert into the anal canal. Squeeze the fluid gently into the rectum from the base of the container to prevent backflow. Some enemas include one-way valves which prevent backflow. Then slowly withdraw the container nozzle to avoid reflux emptying of the rectum. Clean the peri-anal area and make the patient comfortable.
- **Suppositories**: Lubricate the end of the suppository with the gel. Bradshaw and Price (2006) found conflicting evidence about which end of a suppository should be inserted first. Most manufacturers suggest the pointed end is inserted first; follow manufacturer's advice unless local policy advises otherwise. One study's results indicated that inserting the blunt end first allowed the contracting sphincter to close tightly around the anus, aiding retention (Abd-el-Maeboud *et al.* 1991). Wipe the patient's peri-anal area.
- If the enema or suppository/ies were given to empty the bowel, ask the patient to retain it inside for as long as possible (Schmelzer and Wright 1996). The patient may find it more comfortable to remain lying down. An enema, however, can be very difficult to hold on to for long as the effect is likely to be rapid. The person should be assisted to the toilet or other receptacle as necessary.
- Medication administered as a suppository should be retained by the patient. With a retention enema, the patient should remain lying down for the amount of time prescribed on the manufacturer's instructions. A call bell must be near at hand.
- Document that the enema/suppository/ies have been administered in the nursing notes or prescription chart if a medication.
- If the enema or suppositories were given to empty the bowel you will need to note the result, using the Bristol stool chart (see Fig. 9.1).

STOMA CARE

Some patients have to cope with major changes to the way they empty their bladder or bowels. In some cases the only remedy is the removal of the malfunctioning or diseased bladder or intestine. A stoma is formed and the patient wears an appliance that attaches to the abdomen to collect and dispose of the elimination products. There are three main types of stoma:

- *ileal conduit* – formed to drain urine into the stoma bag if the bladder is removed or bypassed;
- *ileostomy* – formed when the whole of the large bowel is removed (liquid stool is collected by the stoma bag);
- *colostomy* – formed when only part of the large bowel is removed (faeces are usually more formed and solid or semi-solid).

Colostomies are the most common types of stoma with more than 11 000 formed a year, compared to approximately 6500 ileostomies and just over 2000 ileal conduits (Coloplast 1999).

Having this surgery requires careful planning and major input by stoma care nurses and other members of the multidisciplinary team. Their roles are to ensure that the individual is able to recover and reintegrate into society and the family and cope with everyday life (Parascandolo *et al.* 2001). Not all surgery can be planned and sometimes a stoma is formed after emergency surgery. These patients therefore have no preparation or stoma nurse involvement prior to surgery, making it more difficult for them to come to terms with the changes and learn to look after their stoma (Erwin-Toth 2003; Richbourg *et al.* 2007). Whether planned or not, caring for this group of patients is always a challenge (Erwin-Toth 2003). This section focuses on key aspects of nursing care. Other specialist textbooks should be consulted for further detail.

LEARNING OUTCOMES

By the end of this section you will be able to:
1 identify the main indications for stoma formation;
2 show awareness of the range of equipment commonly used for the different types of stoma;
3 discuss the care required for people who have a stoma.

Learning outcome 1: Identify the main indications for stoma formation

ACTIVITY

Make a list of some diseases that may result in someone's bladder or small or large bowel having to be removed or bypassed, resulting in stoma formation.

Ileal conduit

This is formed when the patient's lower urinary tract is malfunctioning. The most common cause is bladder cancer, where the bladder is removed. However, ileal conduits are also an option for patients with intractable incontinence or post-pelvic trauma. The ureters are attached to a segment of small bowel (ileum), which is brought to the surface of the body forming a stoma, and draining into a urostomy bag. It is usually sited in the right iliac fossa or, though rarely, this can be on the left.

Ileostomy

This can be formed for cancer of the bowel but most commonly for individuals with inflammatory bowel disease such as ulcerative colitis. When the disease progresses to the point when the pain and diarrhoea and urgency becomes debilitating and interferes with quality of life, then sometimes an ileostomy is recommended. The stoma is usually in the right iliac fossa (Black 2000). The stoma is made of the small bowel. Nowadays some patients opt to have an ileoanal pouch formed instead of having a permanent ileostomy. In this case a temporary ileostomy is usually formed first. An ileoanal pouch is an internal reservoir made of bowel in which faecal matter collects and is emptied out by a catheter inserted into a continent stoma. The ileostomy is formed to allow the pouch to heal before being reversed and allowing faecal matter to move into the pouch.

Colostomy

Partial resection of the large intestine means that the stoma is formed of the patient's large bowel. Colon cancer may result in partial bowel resection and stoma formation. Unlike the ileostomy or the ileal conduit, this stoma can be positioned in different parts of the abdomen, depending on which part of the colon is being removed. The stoma can be placed in either the sigmoid, descending, ascending or transverse colon. This can be a permanent stoma (called a 'permanent end-colostomy') or a temporary one. A temporary colostomy is used when the bowel is not being resected but may need time to heal. Collecting faeces in the stoma bag rather then allowing it to move down the colon promotes this healing. The bowel is partially opened and both ends are brought through the stoma still attached on one side. A plastic 'bridge' is fixed in place under the bowel stoma to stop it slipping back into the abdomen. The stoma is reversed when the two sections of bowel are reattached to each other and pushed back into the abdomen before closing the wound.

Learning outcome 2: Show awareness of the range of equipment commonly used for the different types of stoma

ACTIVITY

In the skills laboratory there may be sterile or non-sterile (for demonstration purposes) stoma appliances complete with packaging material. See Fig. 9.9 for examples. If you can access 'real' equipment take note of the following:
* the manner in which it is packaged, batch number, expiry date;
* the difference between one- and two-piece bags and emptying devices;
* the different materials forming the base-plate and how these affect the flexibility of the appliance.

There are a huge number of appliances available for patients to choose from. Most bags are made specifically to cope with the output of a particular type of stoma. They come in one- or two-piece format:

- The **one-piece** (Fig. 9.9a,d) has the bag and flange or base-plate (i.e. the flat part that sticks to the patient's abdomen) attached to each other. To change the bag the whole appliance is peeled off the abdomen and replaced by a new one.
- The **two-piece** (Fig. 9.9b,c) has a separate bag which clicks on to the base-plate (similar to a Tupperware lid) (Fig. 9.9e). In some products a locking system can be activated to ensure greater security. If the bag needs changing it can simply be clicked off and replaced by a new one. As the base-plate remains in place rather than being peeled off the skin each time it is kinder to the skin. If a patient has to change bags more than once a day (e.g. for religious reasons), then a two-piece appliance allows them to do this without compromising the skin by having to change the base-plate each time.

The base-plate is usually made of a hydrocolloid (natural or artificial) with an integral adhesive area. This can have an extra taped area surrounding it for extra

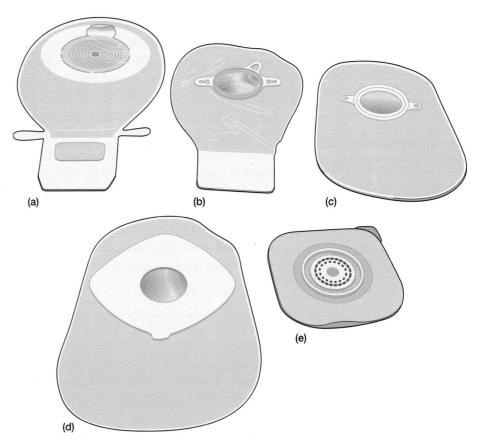

Figure 9.9: Types of stoma appliances. (a) One-piece drainage bag; (b) two-piece drainage bag; (c) two-piece non-drainable bag; (d) one-piece non-drainable bag; (e) flange/base-plate for fitting with two-piece systems, e.g. b and c.

security. This taped area is also more flexible than the hydrocolloid area and can fit to the body's contours more easily (Black 2000). The bags can be clear plastic or flesh coloured.

Bags may be drainable or non-drainable:

- **Drainable bags** (Fig. 9.9a,b). As ileal conduit and ileostomy stomas produce constant liquid output, bags are used which can be emptied via a tap (if urine) or via an opening device like a clip (if stool; see Fig. 9.9a,b). This means patients do not need to change their bags each time, especially if they choose to wear a one-piece bag. Bags have to be able to hold a reasonable capacity to avoid patients constantly having to empty the bags. Bags come in different sizes – from paediatric (holding as little as 100 mL) to adult holding anything up to 750 mL. If the colostomy is in the ascending or hepatic flexure of the transverse colon then the output is semi-solid and a drainable bag should be used.

- **Non-drainable bags** (Fig. 9.9c,d). These are used for the more formed output of colostomies sited in the descending or sigmoid colon. Patients simply change the bag once they have had their bowels open and dispose of it with its contents. Some companies now produce biodegradable colostomy bags that can be flushed down the toilet. Many patients can anticipate when they are going to have their bowels open because, if regular, most people have them open at a certain time of day (e.g. morning, before or after breakfast) and usually only once a day. Thus bags need not be large or bulky as the patient can anticipate when a larger bag is warranted.

Some patients prefer not to wear a colostomy bag. They wear a small pouch or cap to cover the stoma. To ensure they do not have their bowels open unexpectedly they opt to perform a washout or irrigation of the bowel. This is similar to a rectal washout but performed via the stoma instead. Ensuring the bowel is clean in this way means that elimination is predictable and most patients achieve complete continence in between washouts. The whole procedure can take 30–60 minutes, though experienced patients can complete it in 15 minutes (Collett 2002; Karadag *et al.* 2005).

If a patient becomes constipated then it is possible to use suppositories or an enema down the stoma to either lubricate or stimulate the bowel to pass a motion (Collett 2002).

Learning outcome 3: Discuss the care required for people who have a stoma

ACTIVITY

Try to put yourself in the place of a patient who has to have stoma surgery. What feelings or fears do you have? What skills do you think you will have to learn to be able to care for yourself once you recover?

Preoperative preparation

Effective preoperative preparation is essential and patients should therefore be referred to a stoma care nurse specialist well in advance. There may be psychological issues such as coping with a change in body image. Meeting a patient who has already had a stoma can help patients to see what living life with an appliance is really like. Bowel preparation is necessary only if the patient is impacted with faeces which cannot be cleared by restricting food intake and only allowing fluids to drink.

Siting the stoma is an extremely important consideration. The stoma care nurse specialist will address both physical and social aspects during assessment, ensuring that the bag will not hinder the patient's daily activities. It is also important to ensure the patient is not allergic to the adhesive or hydrocolloid in the base-plate, the plastic material or cover of the drainage bag, so a patch test should be carried out.

Postoperative care

The most vital part of the postoperative care is to ensure that the stoma is viable and healing well. Besides the usual postoperative care after major abdominal surgery, the stoma should be checked to ensure it is pink and warm and should adhere to the abdominal wall. The stoma should not look blue or black, or feel cold as this means that the circulation is compromised and if allowed to deteriorate the stoma may become sloughed, black and necrotic. The output should be checked; if it is an ileal conduit then the output should be urine, if a colostomy then there may be flatus though not necessarily stool, and an ileostomy should have some liquid faecal matter.

Sometimes there is a delay in the stoma becoming active. Any prolonged delay should be reported as the patient may need more surgery. Diet following stoma formation needs consideration, both postoperatively and in the longer term (see Floruta 2001).

Teaching self-care

Ideally patients are discharged from hospital only when they have learnt how to care for their stoma. Usually patients are ready to start to learn how to empty and change the bags after the first week following surgery. The patient must also learn what a normal stoma looks like, how it should function and what complications to look out for, as well as how to clean the stoma area and safe disposal of the output and the appliances. Ideally the patient should have the support of district nurses or community stoma care nurses on returning home to help adjust to living with a stoma in a non-hospital environment (Richbourg et al. 2007).

Managing the appliance

The stoma is usually swollen postoperatively but it slowly shrinks to a more normal size as the patient recovers. The base-plates which adhere to the abdomen need a central aperture cut out to fit around the stoma. These base-plates are usually all one size but are made so that the hydrocolloid area varies in size, allowing it to be cut to fit all sizes of stoma. The nurse specialist will provide a template of the correct size which the patient can use to cut out a hole in the centre of the base-plates. This must fit snugly around the stoma without being too tight or cutting off circulation to the stoma. Correct fitting ensures the skin under the base-plate is protected from the effluent produced by the stoma which otherwise may cause excoriation and leakage and result in the bag not adhering securely and falling off. As the stoma shrinks this template may have to be altered.

Stoma appliances are available on prescription and are free to stoma patients in the UK. They can be obtained from pharmacies, though many patients prefer to use supply companies who deliver the appliances in discreet packages directly to their homes. Delivery in most cases is within 24 hours of placing an order and many companies provide extras such as cleaning wipes and disposal bags at no extra cost. If patients find it difficult to cut the template openings then these companies also provide a cutting service using a personalised template which the patient can send in or which the nurse specialist can fax to the company.

| ACTIVITY | What equipment do you think you will need to change an appliance? |

The materials needed to change a stoma appliance are as follows:
- a new appliance;
- wipes for cleaning and drying skin;
- warm water;
- a waste disposal bag (at home the patient may use a nappy sac);
- scissors (if the base-plate is not pre-cut);
- measuring guide, to measure the size of stoma and cut out correct size in template for base-plate;
- gloves and apron.

Once the old base-plate and bag are removed, the skin and stoma are cleaned using warm water and a soft wipe. The skin around the stoma is dried thoroughly to ensure the new base-plate sticks to the abdominal skin securely. Applying gentle but firm pressure over the base-plate helps this process. If the base-plate cannot lie flat on the abdomen then there are products (e.g. stoma paste) and appliances that can help – the stoma care nurse specialist can advise.

Patients with ileal conduits may wish to clip a larger drainage bag to the tap at the bottom of the stoma bag at night. Once the tap is open urine will drain out of the stoma bag and into the larger drainage bag. This ensures that the stoma bag will not leak or come off if it becomes too full of urine when the patient is in bed.

Colostomy bags come with built-in flatus outlets to let gas out as it builds up in the bag. This allows the bag to lie flat under clothes and not come off or leak because of the build-up.

| ACTIVITY | What steps would you follow to teach Jean to empty her stoma bag? |

Jean should be encouraged to do this for herself as soon as possible following recovery from the effects of having surgery. She should be supervised as she goes through the following steps:
- Encourage her to find the best position, such as sitting on the toilet or kneeling or standing beside it.
- Put toilet paper in the toilet bowl to avoid splashback.

- Open the tap/clip/velcro end of bag and drain into the toilet bowl.
- Squeeze out all the contents.
- Close and clean the tap/clip/velcro on the outside to avoid staining clothing
- Flush the toilet and wash her hands (Stoma Care 2007).

ACTIVITY   How should you dispose of used stoma equipment in a hospital? How would Jean dispose of used stoma equipment at home?

In hospital, hand hygiene and use of gloves and apron are necessary (see Chapter 3) and the equipment should be disposed of in the infective waste bag unless local policy advises otherwise. The DH (2006) advised that, in the community, stoma-care waste can be disposed of in the black-bag waste stream. Accordingly, Stoma Care (2007) advises that disposal at home does not require any special arrangements and suggests that, after emptying, the appliance can be wrapped in newspaper, put in a nappy sac and disposed of in normal household refuse. However, if when at home Jean developed any type of gastrointestinal infection or the site became infected, her bag must be disposed of as infectious waste – the community nurse should advise her about this.

Most bags can stay on for up to 3 days as long as the patient is comfortable. Some patients may prefer to change the bags daily, so regimes must be tailored to individuals (Erwin-Toth 2003). If the skin becomes sensitive there are specially developed non-greasy lotions to sooth it and protect it from the adhesive. There are also lotions or wipes that dry on application to the skin forming a plastic barrier layer to protect the skin under the base-plate.

Teaching patients how to change bags and care for the stoma can be time-consuming. Patients with learning disabilities or physical problems with dexterity or eyesight may need a lot of time and input from nurses and carers. If Jean, the patient in our scenario, cannot change the bag and care for the stoma herself, her husband may have to do it instead. Even if Jean is successful she will need his help and support as someone will have to take over this part of her care should she become ill and unable to cope. This may be problematic for her husband who has problems with his sight. It is imperative, therefore, that Jean learns how to care for this herself no matter how much time it takes for her to become confident and competent. Patients should not be rushed; support and continued teaching should ideally continue after discharge.

Stomas all have similar management problems for patients. Patients should be followed up regularly by the stoma nurse to continue supporting the patient and to identify and deal with any problems. Richbourg et al. (2007) found that patients who had been counselled by nurses both before and after surgery suffered fewer complications – or at least found they coped with them more effectively. Patients who had their stoma sites marked preoperatively and were assessed by a stoma nurse also suffered fewer problems with sore skin and badly fitting appliances (Parascandolo et al. 2001; Ratliff et al. 2005). However, complications such as stenosis, prolapse, incisional or bowel hernias or disease progression could not be predicted or avoided by nursing intervention.

Nurses should be aware of other complications which often occur, including sexual dysfunction (e.g. after cystectomy for bladder cancer), problems with body image, decrease in social activities and interaction, isolation, anxiety and depression (Ratliff *et al.* 2005), and have strategies in place to help patients cope. This may include counselling or regular visits to nurse clinics to reinforce teaching and offer support. The likelihood of long-term complications (e.g. upper urinary tract changes in ileal conduit patients) increases the longer the patient has a stoma (Madersbacher *et al.* 2003).

Summary

- Having stoma surgery is life-changing and patients can find it traumatic and have serious psychological consequences such as problems with body image.
- Planned individualised preoperative preparation, and postoperative care and teaching, minimise complications and help patients cope and achieve self-care.
- Understanding these problems and having good knowledge of stoma appliances and accessory products will help offer acceptable solutions to patients and in some cases avoid further surgery.
- However, complications cannot always be anticipated and tend to increase the longer a patient has a stoma.
- Continued support of the patient and/or carer and long-term follow-up will help ensure the patient continues to have a good quality of life and ultimate survival.

PROMOTING CONTINENCE AND MANAGING INCONTINENCE

The DH defines incontinence as 'the involuntary or inappropriate passing of urine and/or faeces that has an impact on social functioning or hygiene' (DH 2000). This section focuses on developing understanding of the causes and effects of incontinence and practical issues of management, but not specialist interventions. Continence is a huge topic to which whole books are devoted; for example, Getliffe and Dolman (2007) cover all aspects in detail.

LEARNING OUTCOMES

By the end of this section, you will be able to:

1 identify the causes, prevalence and effects of urinary and faecal incontinence;
2 demonstrate understanding of how incontinence might be assessed;
3 identify interventions for promoting urinary continence;
4 identify appropriate nursing interventions for promoting faecal continence and managing faecal incontinence;
5 discuss the nursing management of incontinence.

Learning outcome 1: Identify the causes, prevalence and effects of urinary and faecal incontinence

Continence is a complex skill, requiring hormonal, muscular and neurological control (Nazarko 1997). Continence relies on being able to recognise the need to eliminate faeces and/or urine, identify an appropriate place in which to eliminate and being able to wait until arriving there. When any of these fail, incontinence occurs.

ACTIVITY

Reflect back on patients/clients you have been in contact with. From your experience, what causes urinary and faecal incontinence?

Causes are diverse and varied – see Table 9.3 for a summary of causes and types; you may see different classifications in different texts. Urinary incontinence can also be mixed, where there is involuntary urine leakage associated with both urgency and exertion, effort, sneezing or coughing (NICE 2006). Overactive bladder syndrome is

Table 9.3: Summary of causes and types of incontinence.

Type	Description	Causes
Causes of urinary incontinence (adapted from Colley 1996)		
Stress	Urine leakage associated with, for example, coughing, sneezing or exercise	Weakness of the sphincter mechanism. Most common in women (e.g. after childbirth). Can occur in men after a prostatectomy
Urge	Leakage occurring with urgency: little or no warning of the need to void. Symptoms of frequency and nocturnal enuresis may accompany	Detrusor instability (motor urgency) due to bladder neck obstruction. Hypersensitive detrusor muscle (sensory urgency) due to infection or bladder stones, for example
Overflow	Urinary leakage caused by incomplete bladder emptying	May be due to: • Outflow obstruction (e.g. faecal impaction) • Atonic or hypotonic bladder (one which does not produce adequate detrusor contraction for micturition); e.g. in diabetic neuropathy • Detrusor–sphincter dyssynergia (lack of coordination between detrusor contraction and relaxation during bladder emptying); e.g. in spinal injury
Functional	Bladder emptying when the person is unable to reach the toilet, adjust/ remove clothing, and use it appropriately	Physical impairment (e.g. lack of mobility or dexterity). Mental impairment such as confusion. An unconducive environment and unsupportive carers also contribute
Causes of faecal incontinence (Jensen 1997)		
Group 1:	People with intact anal function; e.g. stroke, diarrhoea, faecal impaction	
Group 2:	People with compromised anal sphincter function; e.g. congenital malformation, obstetric trauma	

urgency that occurs with or without urge incontinence and usually with frequency and nocturia.

Some medicines can contribute to incontinence (Bob's incontinence was probably caused by clozapine). Studies have indicated an association between urinary incontinence and diabetes (Lewis *et al.* 2005; Jackson *et al.* 2005). People with a physical disability may not be able to independently reach and use the toilet, and if carers do not assist effectively, functional incontinence results. Bar and Sowney (2007) identified that incontinence rates are often higher among people with learning disabilities due to accompanying physical disabilities and impaired mobility. People with learning as well as a physical disability may not be able to communicate that they need to be taken to the toilet, especially if staff are not familiar with their method of communicating this need, which may be through signing or symbols.

NICE (2007) identifies that faecal incontinence is a sign or symptom, not a disease. NICE lists high-risk groups for faecal incontinence as including people who are old and frail, have loose stools/diarrhoea from any cause, have a neurological or spinal disease/injury, have severe cognitive impairment, urinary incontinence, pelvic organ prolapse or rectal prolapse following colonic resection or anal surgery, people with learning disabilities and women following obstetric injury in childbirth.

To accurately assess the underlying cause and therefore possible management of incontinence, a thorough assessment is necessary (see learning outcome 2).

Box 9.13 presents statistics about the prevalence of incontinence.

ACTIVITY	Why might it be difficult to accurately identify the prevalence of incontinence?

Box 9.13 Estimated prevalence of incontinence

Urinary incontinence (DH 2000)

Women living at home
15–44 years: between 1 in 20 and 1 in 14
45–64 years: between 1 in 13 and 1 in 7
Aged 65 years plus: between 1 in 10 and 1 in 5

Men living at home
15–64 years: over 1 in 33
Aged 65 years plus: between 1 in 14 and 1 in 10

Both sexes living in institutions
One-third of those in residential homes
Nearly two-thirds of those in nursing homes
One-half to two-thirds in wards for older people, or older people with mental health problems

Faecal incontinence (NICE 2007)
- Up to 10 per cent of adults are affected by faecal incontinence.
- Between 0.5 and 1 per cent of adults have regular faecal incontinence affecting their quality of life.

You might have identified that people with incontinence may not seek help (Koch 2006), so the true prevalence of incontinence may be much higher. There are two main reasons for non-reporting of incontinence: embarrassment, and the belief that nothing can be done to help. MacDonald and Butler (2007) identified the isolation of women with incontinence who did not talk to anyone about it as they felt it was not a socially acceptable topic of conversation and that it was untreatable. NICE (2007) identified that faecal incontinence is largely a hidden problem due to its social stigma.

Wells and Wagg (2007) found that Bangladeshi women saw bladder weakness as a loss of self-control and a personal problem rather than a medical problem, so they did not seek professional help. People's definitions of incontinence vary so they may not interpret their problem as incontinence. Bush *et al.* (2001) found that almost half of the women they surveyed believed urinary incontinence was normal. Studies have found that older people with urinary incontinence consider it to be an inevitable part of ageing (Avery *et al.* 2006; Palmer and Newman 2006). However, urinary incontinence is not a disease or a normal result of ageing, but a symptom of an underlying condition.

You read in the scenario that Bob was distressed and embarrassed about his urinary incontinence.

ACTIVITY   How might incontinence affect people: physically, psychologically and socially?

The many effects include physical (e.g. increased falls, skin problems), social (e.g. impact on relationships and employment) and psychological (e.g. embarrassment, lack of self-esteem). Therefore, effective assessment and management of incontinence is essential to relieve distress.

Learning outcome 2: Demonstrate understanding of how incontinence might be assessed

As people are often too embarrassed to report incontinence to health professionals, staff should therefore ask about bladder and bowel problems during initial assessments of patients and clients; for example, 'Does your bladder or bowel ever cause you a problem?' (DH 2001b). If the answer is 'Yes' then an initial bladder or bowel continence assessment should be offered. NICE (2007) recommend that healthcare professionals should ask people in high-risk groups for faecal incontinence sensitively about symptoms.

As discussed under learning outcome 1, there are many possible underlying causes of incontinence. Temporary causes of urinary incontinence, such as UTI, confusion, medication, faecal impaction, impaired mobility and depression, should be identified. In Bob's case, staff investigated further the side-effects of clozapine and discovered that incontinence was a recognised side-effect but it was also important that their assessment included a urinalysis.

Assessment includes interviewing, observation and measurement. Keeping these in mind, think about how a nurse might assess incontinence. Have you seen any specific assessment documents used in practice for assessment of incontinence? When you have thought about this, look at Box 9.14, which identifies some key points, and these are expanded on below.

Many practice settings have a specific incontinence assessment tool that will help to identify both the cause and possible management of incontinence. The DH (2001b) advises that the assessment should be carried out by a 'suitably trained individual' and should include a review of symptoms and their effect on quality of life, physical examination (for example perineum), urinalysis, and assessment of manual dexterity and environment. NHS Quality Improvement Scotland (2005, pp. 4–5) lists items for assessment. If a UTI is suspected, following the urinalysis, a urine specimen should be sent for MC&S. NICE (2006) recommends bladder diaries should be completed for a minimum of 3 days to help with assessing urinary frequency and incontinence episodes.

When using interviewing skills to assess incontinence, approach and terminology used need careful consideration. Palmer and Newman (2006) identified that questions should be worded carefully (e.g. 'Do you lose water when you don't want to?') rather than asking if they are incontinent. Rassin *et al.* (2007) found that women often did not perceive they had incontinence but described 'leaking'. Woodward (1996) also stressed phrasing questions clearly in understandable terms. For example, the term 'frequency' may not be understood, so it is preferable to ask 'How often do you go to the toilet to pass urine during the day?'

For cognitively impaired adults who may be unable to give a clear history, Thompson and Smith (1998) emphasise the importance of observing for clues to indicate frequency and severity, and involving carers in assessment. Nurses can

---

Box 9.14 Assessment of continence: key points

- Use of an assessment tool will promote a systematic approach.
- Referral to a continence advisor may be needed.

Interviewing

- Sensitive, empathetic approach
- Careful and appropriate use of language
- Involvement of carers

Observation

- Physical factors, e.g. obstructive symptoms
- Psychological factors, e.g. confusion
- Environmental factors, e.g. access to toilet

Measurement

- Urinalysis
- Charting frequency and amount

observe for signs of pain, obstructive symptoms, such as hesitancy, intermittent stream, dribbling after voiding and straining to void, urge symptoms, and functional barriers, such as being unable to undress.

The RCN (2006a) warn that incontinence may be attributed to a person's learning disabilities rather than other causes, including ill-health. This is termed **diagnostic overshadowing**, where signs and symptoms are attributed to the learning disability rather than investigating for other causes. Bar and Sowney (2007) recommend that when assessing a person with a learning disability, the nurse should observe what the person is able to do, and ask questions such as 'How do you get on with using the toilet?', or ask a carer 'How does he manage with the toilet?' Closed negative questions asking whether the person is incontinent should be avoided. People with a physical disability and a communication difficulty may know when they want to go to the toilet, but carers will not be able to recognise this need if a method of communication has not been established. Stanley (1997) explains that incontinence in people with a learning disability should be assessed by carrying out a functional analysis, considering the person, their situation or environment, and the significant people in their life. Stanley (1997) emphasises that this individualistic approach is complex, and requires careful observation and a good knowledge about the person and their life; structured instruments are available to help the assessment.

NICE (2007) recommends that a baseline assessment for people with faecal incontinence should comprise relevant medical history, a general examination, an anorectal examination and a cognitive assessment if appropriate.

Some people with urinary and/or faecal incontinence require a more specialist assessment and should be referred to the continence service, to see a continence specialist nurse for example. Specialist investigations are sometimes necessary.

> **ACTIVITY**
>
> Find out about how referrals are made to a continence advisor in your area of practice.

Learning outcome 3: Identify interventions for promoting urinary continence

How urinary continence is promoted obviously depends on the underlying cause, which is why an understanding of causes and careful assessment is important. The DH (2000) recommends that everyone should have access to integrated continence services managed by a director of continence services (normally a specialist continence nurse or physiotherapist). Mark's community learning disability nurse, as his health facilitator, should have empowered him to access continence services and could carry out a joint assessment with a continence advisor. Mark's continence should be addressed in his Health Action Plan. Smith and Smith (2007) examine continence training for people with learning disabilities in detail.

> **ACTIVITY**
>
> What methods have you seen used to promote continence for people in practice settings?

The methods you have seen should have been chosen to address the type of incontinence, based on the person's assessment. You might have seen lifestyle advice (e.g., fluid intake, weight loss) being given, pelvic floor muscle exercises being taught (for stress or mixed incontinence), or have assisted with bladder training (for urge or overactive bladder syndrome) or voiding programmes. You might also have seen staff taking measures to prevent functional incontinence, and nurses should refer patients and liaise with the multidisciplinary team as appropriate. Physiotherapists can help with mobility and balance, enabling quicker transfers; and occupational therapists help with making the environment and dressing and undressing easier. Clothing adaptations, such as replacing trouser zips or buttons with Velcro, can be helpful. Vickerman (2003) asserts that many people are rendered incontinent by a poorly adapted environment and advises that the heights of chairs, beds and toilets should be assessed and adjusted, as well as considering lighting, signs, floor coverings, grab rails and provision of commodes and hand-held urinals. You may also have seen medical interventions which can include pharmacology (Rigby 2007) or surgery (when conservative measures have failed).

NICE (2006) recommends that, at initial assessment of women, urinary incontinence (UI) should be categorised as either 'stress UI', 'mixed UI' or 'urge/overactive bladder syndrome' so that appropriate interventions can be planned. NICE (2006) provides algorithms for each type of incontinence. The NHS Quality Improvement Scotland's (2005) best-practice statement, *Continence: Adults with urinary dysfunction,* also provides very useful guidance for managing all the different types of urinary incontinence, the aim being to restore continence.

Pelvic floor muscle training

Pelvic floor muscle (PFM) exercises aim to strengthen the pubococcygeal muscle, resulting in increased urethral closure pressure and stronger reflex contractions when there is a sudden rise in intra-abdominal pressure, such as when sneezing (Dolman 2003). Hay-Smith and Dumoulin's (2007) review recommended that PFM training should be included in first-line conservative management programmes for women with stress, urge or mixed urinary incontinence NICE (2006) suggests a trial of supervised pelvic floor muscle training for at least three months as the first-line treatment for women with stress or mixed urinary incontinence, which should involve at least eight contractions performed three times a day. Men can also benefit from PFM exercises: improving post-prostatectomy urinary incontinence (Dorey 2005; Zhang *et al.* 2007) and stress urinary incontinence and post-micturition dribble (Dorey 2007). Dorey (2007) details exercises that can be taught to men to perform at home in different situations and positions, but states that they should be taught by a specialist to ensure that they are performed correctly.

Bladder re-education

Bladder re-education involves re-educating the bladder to an improved pattern of voiding and has several variations, suitable for different client groups. All staff should be fully aware and motivated towards these programmes, so that they are implemented consistently. Roe *et al.* (2006) explained that bladder training is used for cognitively and physically able adults, while prompted voiding, habit retraining and timed voiding – collectively known as voiding programmes – are generally used for people with cognitive or physical impairments in institutional settings.

Bladder training

Bladder training aims to increase the interval between voids (Wallace *et al.* 2007). For example, the person might initially be asked to go to the toilet every hour. This is then gradually extended by half an hour at a time. NICE (2006) recommends that, for women with overactive bladders, with or without urge incontinence, bladder training for a minimum of six weeks should be offered. Education of patients and carers, use of a continence chart and continuous encouragement are all important elements. Carers need to praise to build up confidence and reinforce behaviour and they should be patient and understanding.

Timed voiding

Timed voiding is also referred to as scheduled, fixed, routine or regular toileting/ voiding. The main feature is voiding to a fixed time pattern; for example, 2-, 3- or 4-hourly. Ostaszkiewicz *et al.* (2007a) identified that timed voiding is used for managing people with urinary incontinence who cannot participate in independent toileting. It is often used for people with a neurogenic bladder, such as those with spinal cord lesions, and for people with a physical or mental disability. It can include techniques to trigger voiding, such as tapping over the suprapubic region or running water. In a Cochrane review, Ostaszkiewicz *et al.* (2007a) found insufficient evidence to draw conclusions about this intervention's effectiveness.

Habit retraining

In habit retraining, caregivers identify the person's natural voiding pattern and develop an individualised toileting schedule which pre-empts involuntary bladder emptying (Ostaszkiewicz *et al.* 2007b). A record of voiding and incontinent episodes is kept so that the schedule can be adjusted, with voiding intervals lengthened if the person is dry, and reduced if incontinence occurs. Ostaszkiewicz *et al.*'s (2007b) Cochrane review found insufficient studies of adequate quality to provide a firm base for practice and so could draw no conclusions.

Prompted voiding

Prompted voiding is a behavioural therapy aiming to improve bladder control for people with or without dementia using verbal prompts and positive reinforcement (Eustice *et al.* 2007). NICE (2006) recommended prompted voiding programmes to reduce urinary leakage for women who have urinary incontinence and cognitive impairment. Prompted voiding has been used with people with learning disabilities too. Ostaszkiewicz (2006) found that prompted voiding was more sustainable than habit retraining or timed voiding but it needed more resources to implement. Eustice *et al.*'s (2007) Cochrane review found suggestive evidence that prompted voiding increased self-initiated voiding and decreased incontinent episodes in the short term, and might be an appropriate strategy for Mark in our scenarios.

Smith (1998) provides tips for using prompted voiding with people with dementia:

- Have the word 'toilet' on the door, with a picture.
- Increase environmental safety, e.g. hand rails.
- Use simple verbal or behavioural clues.
- Use pleasant distraction such as singing.
- Keep to a routine and, where possible, a familiar nurse.
- Use clothes that are easy to remove.
- Stay pleasant and avoid hurrying or confrontation.

Learning outcome 4: Identify appropriate nursing interventions for promoting faecal continence and managing faecal incontinence

NICE (2007) includes a comprehensive flow chart for managing faecal incontinence in adults. Underlying conditions should be addressed and, if faecal incontinence continues, people should be referred for specialised management, which may include PFM training, bowel retraining, specialist dietary assessment and management, biofeedback, electrical stimulation or rectal irrigation. Interventions recommended are identified below.

Diet

There should be a balanced nutrient intake and at least 1.5 litres of fluid intake daily for people with hard stools or dehydrated (unless contraindicated). Hansen *et al.* (2006) found that diet modification was central to managing faecal incontinence: restricting foods that exacerbated faecal incontinence, avoiding gas-producing foods, and limiting portion or meal size.

Bowel habit

Predictable bowel emptying should be promoted by encouraging bowel emptying after a meal, ensuring toilet facilities are private, comfortable and safe, allowing sufficient time, encouraging people to adopt a sitting/squatting position and avoiding straining. Akpan *et al.* (2006) highlighted that many older people, especially those who were dependent, lacked privacy during bowel movements.

Toilet access

Staff can ensure that toilet location is clear, equipment/help is given to access and advise about easily removable clothing. A home/mobility assessment may be necessary.

Medication

Alternatives to those contributing to faecal incontinence should be considered. Anti-diarrhoeal drugs (e.g. loperamide) may be appropriate.

Coping strategies

These include continence products (disposable body-worn pads, bed pads, anal plugs), skin care, odour control, laundry advice and support. Learning outcome 5 addresses incontinence pads and skin care. Herbert (2008) explains the use of anal plugs, suggesting that, although not suitable for everyone, they can improve quality of life.

Palmieri *et al.* (2005) studied use of a bag to collect stools in faecal incontinence and found no adverse reactions, that it was well tolerated and it was not painful to remove or apply. The 'Flexi-Seal faecal management system' is a temporary containment device, consisting of a soft, flexible silicone catheter with a low-pressure balloon that is filled with water or saline to aid retention. The device is inserted into the patient's rectum and attached to a catheter bag. It can collect liquid or semi-liquid stools and is most suitable for bed-bound patients, for example in critical care. In Padmanabhan *et al.*'s (2007) evaluation of this system, skin condition was maintained or improved in most patients. As well as diverting faeces from the skin, the system also assists with infection control and allows more accurate fluid balance monitoring.

Targeted patient/carer education improved bowel dysfunction symptoms in Harari *et al.*'s (2004) study. Chelvanayagam and Stern (2007) found that group therapy facilitated by experienced therapists improved both physical and psychological well-being of people with faecal incontinence.

Learning outcome 5: Discuss the nursing management of incontinence

Incontinence should be managed in a manner that is unobtrusive, reliable and comfortable. Incontinence aids should preserve hygiene, psychological and social comfort.

Urethral catheterisation is rarely appropriate for managing urinary incontinence as it may lead to catheter-related problems such as UTI (see section 'Caring for people with urinary catheters'). However, NICE (2006) recommends that catheterisation should be considered for women with persistent urinary retention that causes incontinence, symptomatic infections or renal dysfunction that cannot be corrected. NICE suggests that the risks and benefits should be discussed and areas of consideration are urine contamination of skin wounds, pressure ulcers, irritation, distress and disruption caused by bed and clothing changes, and women's preference. Intermittent urethral catheterisation is another option and can be taught to the person or their carer.

ACTIVITY

If you find that a patient/client has been incontinent, what would your priorities of care be?

The person should be attended to quickly, to prevent skin damage, relieve discomfort and restore dignity. Many of the principles discussed earlier related to dealing with a person's elimination needs are relevant, in particular: approachability and communication, privacy and dignity, promptness, prevention of cross-infection, observation, hygiene and comfort. The nurse's approach when dealing with incontinence is crucial to the level of distress experienced. Nurses dealing with Bob's urinary incontinence should be discreet and matter-of-fact in changing his bed while reassuring him that the cause would be investigated. In faecal incontinence, in particular, prompt changing of soiled pads or clothing is essential to help to prevent odours and skin excoriation (Norton 1997).

How skin is cleaned is very important. If incontinence cannot be prevented, then a suitable containment method is needed, for example pads, or for a man with urinary incontinence, possibly a penile sheath. As mentioned in the previous section there are also anal pugs, faecal collection bags and systems.

Skin cleansing

Box 9.15 lists some key points about skin cleansing for people who have been incontinent.

ACTIVITY

Compare Box 9.15 to skin cleansing for incontinence that you have seen in practice. Have you seen skin cleanser rather than soap used?

Ersser *et al.* (2005) identified that urinary incontinence is an important cause of skin vulnerability and that older people are a high-risk group for skin damage as their skin is more permeable, enabling external moisture to infiltrate epidermal layers and increasing the friction coefficient at the skin's surface. Ersser *et al.* (2005) highlight the problems caused by urinary incontinence as being:

- wetness of skin encouraging maceration, disrupting the skin barrier leading to breakdown;
- decomposition of the urinary urea by microorganisms, releasing ammonia to form the alkali ammonium hydroxide, thus altering the skin's pH (the pH of normal skin ranges from 5.4 to 5.9, providing an acid mantle);
- chemical irritation of the skin arising from urine, the rise in alkalinity and bacterial proliferation;
- the presence of faecal urease, resulting in breakdown of the urinary urea, causing increase in pH, increasing activities of faecal proteases and lipases.

Box 9.15 Skin care after incontinence: key points

- Ensure prompt action, with privacy, dignity and sensitivity.
- Observe infection control: hand hygiene, gloves and apron, correct waste disposal.
- Use skin cleanser rather than soap (Bale *et al.* 2004; Nix and Ermer-Seltun 2004; Bliss *et al.* 2006; Hodgkinson *et al.* 2007). Wash gently, avoiding friction.
- Cleanse from front to back, and least soiled area to most soiled area.
- Start with the labia with females, and the tip of the penis with men.
- Cleanse the anal area last.
- Observe the skin condition.
- Dry skin carefully to avoid maceration and undue cooling, maintain comfort and permit dressing. Pat rather than rub to reduce friction (Ersser *et al.* 2005).
- Apply barrier cream, or for moderate/severe incontinence dermatitis, barrier film (Bale *et al.* 2004; Baatenburg de Jong and Admiraal 2004).

Super-absorbent pads aim to prevent mixing of urine and faeces by keeping skin dry (see section on 'Pads'). Soap, which is designed to remove dirt and grease, removes natural skin lipids and water-holding substances and weakens the epidermis. Therefore as incontinence leads to frequent washing, soap is best avoided. Skin cleansers have evaluated well in several small studies (Whittingham and May 1998; Cooper and Gray 2001; Bale *et al.* 2004; Bliss *et al.* 2006).

Pads

NICE (2006) recommends that absorbent products (pads) should not be considered a treatment for urinary incontinence and should only be used to help patients who are waiting for treatment, as an adjunct to other therapies, and for long-term management if other treatments have failed. Pads for managing incontinence can be all-in-one body-worn products or pads worn with elasticated pants. Under-pads are also available but should be used only as a procedure pad when a clean (not sterile) field is needed, for extra chair/bed protection, for example after administration of an enema, or where a body-worn pad is not practical or possible as with a very obese person, or for persistent diarrhoea in bed which cannot be contained with alternative methods (e.g. faecal collector). The DH (2000) advises that all types of pads should be available as part of the integrated continence services and individual choice should be considered in their selection.

ACTIVITY	Find out what incontinence pads are available in your practice setting.

There is a wide range of incontinence pads available but there is a lack of high-quality research into their effectiveness, making evidence-based selection difficult (Dunn *et al.* 2002). Hodgkinson *et al.*'s (2007) systematic review identified that disposable body-worn pads may prevent deterioration of skin condition better than non-disposable under-pads or body-worns. Although most pads used are disposable, washable pads are also produced but evaluations have proved disappointing in respect to leakage and social impact (Clarke-O'Neill *et al.* 2002; Macauley *et al.* 2004). Box 9.16 summarises key points in the choice and use of incontinence pads.

Pads are produced for all situations, ranging from light to severe and night-time use:
- *light* – when there is only occasional voiding of a few drops of urine;
- *moderate* – when there is frequent voiding of small to moderate amounts of urine;
- *severe* – for uncontrolled daily voiding of moderate to large amounts.

Differently shaped pads are available for men and women. It is important to read manufacturers' instructions for the optimal fitting of these pads as correct fitting of the product is essential to contain urine and faeces, and will reduce skin contact with excreta to the minimum (Gibbons 1996). As urine is broken down into its constituents – ammonia and urea – on contact with air, fitting the pads closely ensures that urine and air are not mixed. Additional features, which some pads have, are wetness indicator strips, and adhesive strips for extra security.

Box 9.16 Choice and use of incontinence pads: key points

Choice of pad
- Disposable, super-absorbent pads are preferable.
- Body-worn pads (either all-in-ones, or pad and pants) should be used rather than under-pads.
- Choose the correct pad for the individual client, considering gender, size, and extent and frequency of incontinence.

Fitting
Always follow manufacturer's instructions for fitting, but the following general principles normally apply:
- Maintain privacy, dignity and prevention of cross-infection during pad changes.
- If using pants, ensure the seams are on the outside, and pull up to mid-thigh.
- Fold the pad lengthways and create a cupped shape.
- Place the pad from front to back with largest area at the back.
- Ensure pad is smoothed out both front and back, and fitted into the groin well.
- If using pants, pull up; or if all-in-ones, seal the tapes firmly. Lower tapes should be sealed first.
- Check the pad is as close to the body as possible.

When changing a pad, it should never be referred to as a 'nappy', which is demeaning. Nurses should take care not to show annoyance or embarrass patients (see Chapter 2). It is important to ensure that people have a clean pad at mealtimes and before going out anywhere. When changing the pad, maintain privacy by shutting curtains, and change any wet or soiled clothing. To prevent cross-infection use of gloves and aprons; hand hygiene and correct waste disposal are essential (see Chapter 3).

Fader *et al.* (2004) found that incontinence pads had an adverse effect on pressure redistribution properties on mattresses, with pad folds contributing to this effect. Thus patients who are incontinent and wearing pads may be at increased risk of pressure damage, but smoothing out the folds reduced interface pressures.

Getliffe and Fader (2007) address absorbent products for containment in detail, fully illustrated; further reading from that source is recommended.

Penile sheaths

Penile sheaths (see Fig. 9.10) channel the urine into a collection bag. They avoid the complications of long-term in-dwelling urethral catheters and, by diverting urine into a bag, prevent odour and contact of urine on skin (Pemberton *et al.* 2006). In Saint *et al.*'s (2006) study, urinary sheaths reduced adverse outcomes such as infection and patients reported that they were comfortable and less painful than catheters. They are sometimes used by men who manage their continence using intermittent self-catheterisation, to avoid leakage in between (Doherty 2000). Many people are allergic to latex (Le Lievre 1996) so use of a silicone sheath avoids this risk. A clear sheath as opposed to an opaque one allows observation of the penile skin.

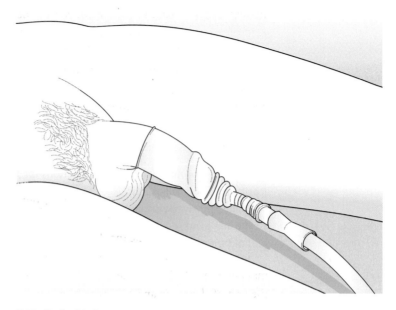

Figure 9.10: Penile sheath.

Sheaths are most suitable for men who have a moderate to severe degree of incontinence and/or have frequency and urgency and are not able to get to the toilet easily (Medical Devices Agency 1995). The Medical Devices Agency report that assessment for suitability should include assessing manual dexterity of the user (or carers), independence/availability of carers and the user's skin condition. Penile sheaths are inappropriate for people who have retention of urine (Pomfret 2000).

Sheaths may be two-piece or one-piece. The two-piece sheath requires application of an adhesive strip to the penis before rolling the sheath on, while the one-piece sheath has an integral adhesive coating. One-piece sheaths have been rated more highly than two-piece, but acceptability of different products has been found to be highly individualised (Medical Devices Agency 1995). Thus men for whom a sheath might be appropriate should be encouraged to try different products before deciding on one for long-term use.

Pemberton *et al.* (2006) identified that the most important requirements of a sheath are that it stays in place and does not leak, thus relieving embarrassment and promoting men's confidence. Security of the sheath depends on proper assessment, sizing, application and quality of the adhesive (Pemberton *et al.* 2006).

A clear explanation should be given to patients about the sheath because a positive attitude is necessary for successful use (Doherty 1998). Application of a urinary sheath is an intimate procedure, which may be embarrassing for both patient and nurse (Doherty 1998). Wearing gloves reduces the intimacy and thus embarrassment, as well as being protective for infection control purposes (Pemberton *et al.* 2006). Privacy must be provided and infection control principles adhered to.

Doherty (1998) outlines steps to ensure effective use of urinary sheaths in some detail. These include choice of the correct size, by measuring the circumference of the penis at its widest point and measuring the length. If the sheath is too tight it could cause sores and discomfort, while if it is too big it will lead to leakage as urine will seep under the sheath. Doherty (1998) notes, however, that penile size can vary and that sheath measurement should allow for expansion, although both latex and silicone are flexible materials. Williams and Moran (2006) explain that sheaths are available in a variety of widths (20–40 mm) and lengths (50–80 mm) and that each manufacturer has a defined size range and provides their own measurement guide which must be used together.

The penis and surrounding area should be washed and dried. Powder, cream or spray deodorants should not be used as they will inactivate the adhesive. If necessary, pubic hair should be trimmed but should not be shaved. A piece of paper/card, sometimes supplied by the manufacturer, can be held over the penis to keep back pubic hair while the sheath is applied.

If using a two-part sheath, apply the adhesive strip to the penile shaft in a spiral manner. When fitting the sheath, roll it over the penis, leaving a small space between the end of the penis and the cup of the sheath to allow for changes in the size of the penis while wearing. If the patient is uncircumcised, ensure that the foreskin remains over the glans and is not retracted. Pomfret (2000) suggests the sheath should be rolled back one turn prior to application to an uncircumcised penis in order to form a space of 1–2 cm between the end of the penis and the outlet of the sheath. Once the sheath is in place, gently squeeze it to ensure adhesion, and then attach it to a urine drainage bag. Never apply sticky tape as it is inflexible and could lead to restriction of the blood supply, leading to sores or gangrene.

Urinary drainage bags should be chosen carefully according to individual need. Ensure that the tubing is not kinked, thereby allowing collection of urine and pressure on the sheath, weakening the adhesive. The urine bag must be kept lower and be well supported. The sheath should be removed daily by gently rolling it off (preferably in the bath), and the skin washed and dried before reapplying.

A patient with reduced or absent sensation will not be able to feel if the sheath is too tight or a sore is developing, so the patient and his carers need to be observant for any such problems. In many cases patients can manage the system themselves.

ACTIVITY

Can you think of any patients for whom this method of dealing with urinary incontinence might be particularly unsuitable?

Patients with any soreness of the penis should not have a sheath applied. Patients with a small or retracted penis may not be suitable. Williams and Moran (2006) identify that penis retraction is affected by changes in temperature, neurological deficits following stroke, and the integrity of blood supply in patients with diabetes. For men with significant retraction, a urinary sheath is unlikely to be successful as it will roll off the shaft of the penis; alternatives for these men are more specialised devices, such as penile pouches. With mild penis retraction, short sheaths can be used. Finally, patients with cognitive impairment may pull the device off, causing trauma (Williams and Moran 2006).

Support for people with continence problems

People with continence problems can benefit from support and advice, but may often be unaware of what support is available, and where it can be accessed. Nurses should be aware of the resources available so that they can advise people with continence issues.

There are many local self-help support groups that can be very beneficial to participants. They give people the opportunity to meet informally, and share ideas and experiences; the DH (2001b) recommends that support be actively promoted. The Bladder and Bowel Foundation (www.bladderandbowelfoundation.org) provides information and support to people affected by bladder and bowel problems and the website includes a moderated chatroom and active message board. There are Independent Living Exhibitions which display materials to promote continence alongside other equipment for living with a disability. Many organisations have developed information leaflets for people who have continence problems, for example the Alzheimer's Disease Society (www.alzheimers.org.uk) and Help the Aged (www.helptheaged.org.uk).

ACTIVITY

Investigate advice and support within your area. Find out where your nearest Independent Living Exhibition is, and if possible, arrange to visit so that you can see the resources available.

Summary

- Nurses within almost any setting are likely to encounter people with continence issues, so an understanding of the underlying causes and the wide-ranging effects on people is important.
- Nurses should have knowledge about specialist services, such as the continence advisor and support organisations, so that they can advise and refer people accordingly.
- Promoting continence and managing incontinence requires careful assessment of each individual, and knowledge about appropriate strategies and products. Care for people with continence problems should be based on the best evidence available.

CHAPTER SUMMARY

This chapter has focused on assisting people with elimination, emphasising that quality care requires a sensitive and empathetic approach, effective communication skills, and a sound, evidence-based knowledge. Implementing measures to prevent cross-infection, while assisting people with elimination, are also paramount. Urinalysis and specimen collection are very common investigations but if not carried out with care they can lead to misleading results and inappropriate treatment. Constipation is a common problem and preventing and managing constipation was addressed.

Urinary catheterisation is invasive and potentially harmful, but is nevertheless often necessary as a short- or long-term measure. An understanding of this procedure, and particularly how potential complications can be reduced, is also important.

Nurses may encounter people with stomas in a range of acute and long-term settings and key aspects of stoma care were considered.

Continence is a huge topic, and may require specialist involvement. Here, the practical skills in dealing with continence have been explored; students wishing to extend their knowledge should access the referenced material. To conclude, nurses need to value the care given in relation to patients/clients' elimination needs as, if effective, it can do much for comfort, well-being and self-esteem.

ACKNOWLEDGEMENT

This chapter has been revised and updated. The author acknowledges the contribution of Vickie Arrowsmith to this chapter in the previous two editions of this book.

REFERENCES

Abd-el-Maeboud, K.H., el-Naggar, T., El-Hawi, E.M.M. *et al.* 1991. Rectal suppositories and mode of insertion. *Lancet* **338,** 798, 800.

Addison, R., Ness, W., Abulafi, M. *et al.* 2000. How to administer enemas and suppositories. *Nursing Times NT Plus: Continence* **96**(6), 3–4.

Akhtar, S.G. 2002. Nursing with dignity. Pt 8: Islam. *Nursing Times* **98**(16), 40–2.

Akpan, A., Gosney, M.A. and Barrett, J. 2006. Privacy for defecation and fecal incontinence in older adults. *Journal of Wound, Ostomy and Continence Nursing* **33**(5), 536–40.

Avery, J.C., Wilson, I. and Braunack-Mayer, A.J. 2006. Beliefs and barriers about seeking help for incontinence. *Australian and New Zealand Continence Journal* **12**(1), 6.

Ayliffe, G.A.J., Babb, J.R. and Taylor, L.J. 2001. *Hospital-acquired Infection: Principles and prevention,* 3rd edn. Oxford: Butterworth–Heinemann.

Baatenburg de Jong, H. and Admiraal, H. 2004. Comparing cost per use of 3M Cavilon No Sting Barrier Film with zinc oxide oil in incontinent patients. *Journal of Wound Care* **13**(9), 398–400.

Bale, S., Tebble, N., Jones, V. And Price, P. 2004. The benefits of implementing a new skin care protocol in nursing homes. *Journal of Tissue Viability* **14**(2), 44–50.

Ballinger, C., Pain, H., Pascoe, J. and Gore, S. 1996. Choosing a commode for the ward environment. *British Journal of Nursing* **5,** 485–6.

Bar, O. and Sowney, M. 2007. Inclusive nursing care for people with intellectual disabilities using urology services. *International Journal of Urological Nursing* **1**(3), 138–45.

Bayer 1997a. *Urinary Tract Infection,* Technical Information Bulletin 8. Newbury: Bayer.

Bayer 1997b. *Urine Analysis: The essential information.* Newbury: Bayer.

Bayer 1998. *A Practical Guide to Urine Analysis.* Newbury: Bayer.

Beynon, M. and Nicholls, C. 2004. Urological investigations. In Fillingham, S. and Douglas, J. (eds) *Urological Nursing,* 3rd edn. Edinburgh: Baillière Tindall, 25–42.

Black, P.K. 2000. *Holistic Stoma Care.* London: Baillière Tindall, in association with the Royal College of Nursing and Harcourt Brace.

Bliss, D.Z., Zehrer, C., Savik, K. *et al.* 2006. Incontinence-associated skin damage in nursing home residents: a secondary analysis of a prospective, multicenter study. *Ostomy/Wound Management* **52**(12), 46–55.

Bowers, B. 2006. Evaluating the evidence for administering phosphate enemas. *British Journal of Nursing* **15**(7), 378–81.

Bradshaw, A. and Price, L. 2006. Rectal suppository insertion: the reliability of the evidence as a basis for nursing practice. *Journal of Clinical Nursing* **16,** 98–103.

British Geriatrics Society 2006. *Dignity Behind Closed Doors.* Available from www.bgs.org.uk Accessed 10 Mar 2008.

Bullock, B., Bausher, J.C., Pomerantz, W.J. *et al.* 2001. A clear urine specimen on visual inspection cannot totally exclude a diagnosis of urinary tract infection. *Evidence-based Nursing* **4**(55), 106, e60.

Burr, R.G. and Nuseibeh, I.M. 1997. Urinary catheter blockage depends on urine pH, calcium and rate of flow. *Spinal Cord* **35,** 521–5.

Bush, T.A., Castellucci, D.T. and Phillips, C. 2001. Exploring women's beliefs regarding urinary incontinence. *Urologic Nursing* **21,** 211–18.

Chelvanayagam, S. and Stern, J. 2007. Using therapeutic groups to support women with faecal incontinence. *British Journal of Nursing* **16**(4), 214–18.

Chillington, B. 1992. Early removal advances discharge home. *Professional Nurse* **8**(2), 84–9.

Chur-Hansen, A. 2002. Preferences for female and male nurses: the role of age, gender and previous experience – year 2000 compared with 1984. *Journal of Advanced Nursing* **37,** 192–8.

Clark, J. and Rugg, S. 2005. The importance of independence in toileting: the views of stroke survivors and their occupational therapists. *British Journal of Occupational Therapy* **68**(4), 165–71.

Clarke-O'Neill, S., Pettersson, L., Fader, M. *et al.* 2002. A multicentre comparative evaluation: washable pants with an integral pad for light incontinence. *Journal of Clinical Nursing* **11,** 79–87.

Clement, S., Young, J. and Munday, E. 2004. Comparison of a urine chemistry analyzer and microscopy, culture and sensitivity results to detect the presence of urinary tract infections in an elective orthopaedic population. *Contemporary Nurse* **17**(1–2), 89–94.

Collett, K. 2002. Practical aspects of stoma management. *Nursing Standard* **17**(8), 45–52, 54.

Colley, W. 1996. Charting new waters. *Nursing Times* **92**(24), 59–60, 62, 64.

Coloplast 1999. *An Introduction to Stoma Care: A guide for health care professionals.* Peterborough: Coloplast.

Colpman, D. and Welford, K. 2004. *Urinary Drainage Systems.* In Fillingham, S. and Douglas, J. (eds) *Urological Nursing.* Edinburgh: Baillière Tindall, 67–92.

Cooper, P. and Gray, D. 2001. Comparison of two skin care regimes for incontinence. *British Journal of Nursing* **10,** Tissue Viability Supplement: S6, S8, S10.

Department of Health (DH) 2000. *Good Practice in Continence Services.* London.

— 2001a. *Valuing People: A new strategy for learning disability for the 21st century.* London.

— 2001b. *The Essence of Care: Patient-focused benchmarking for health care practitioners.* London.

— 2003. *Winning Ways: Working together to reduce healthcare associated infection in England and Wales.* London.

— 2006. *Environment and Sustainability: Safe management of healthcare waste.* Health Technical Memorandum 07-01. London.

Doherty, W. 1998. The clear advantage urinary incontinence sheath for men. *British Journal of Nursing* **7,** 730, 732–4.

Doherty, W. 2000. Urinary sheaths and drainage bags from Manfred Sauer. *British Journal of Nursing* **9,** 514–17.

Dolman, M. 2003. Mostly female. In Getliffe, K. and Dolman, M. (eds) *Promoting Continence: A clinical research resource,* 2nd edn. London: Baillière Tindall, 53–79.

Dorey, G. 2005. Restoring pelvic floor function in men: review of RCTs. *British Journal of Nursing* **14**(19), 1014–21.

Dorey, G. 2007. Why men need to perform pelvic floor exercises. *Nursing Times* **103**(26), 40–6.

Dougherty, L. and Lister, S.(eds) 2004. Elimination: urinary catheterisation. In *The Royal Marsden Hospital Manual of Clinical Nursing Procedures.* London: Blackwell, 330–347.

Dunn, S., Kowanko, I., Paterson, J. and Pretty, L. 2002. Systematic review of the effectiveness of urinary continence products. *Journal of Wound, Ostomy and Continence Nursing* **29**(3), 129–42.

Ersser, S.J., Geliffe, K., Voegeli, D. and Regan, S. 2005. A critical review of the interrelationship between skin vulnerability and urinary incontinence and related nursing intervention. *International Journal of Nursing Studies* **42,** 823–35.

Erwin-Toth, P. 2003. Ostomy pearls: a concise guide to stoma siting, pouching systems, patient education, and more. *Advances in Skin and Wound Care* **16**(3), 146–52.

Eustice, S., Roe, B. and Paterson, J. 2007. Prompted voiding for the management of urinary incontinence in adults. *Cochrane Database of Systematic Reviews,* Issue 4.

Fader, M., Pettersson, L., Brooks, R. *et al.* 1997. A multicentre comparative evaluation of catheter valves. *British Journal of Nursing* **6,** 359, 362, 364, 366–7.

Fader, M., Bain, D. and Cottenden, A. 2004. Effects of absorbent incontinence pads on pressure management mattresses. *Journal of Advanced Nursing* **48**(6), 569–74.

Fillingham, S. and Fell, S. 2004. Urological stomas. In Fillingham, S. and Douglas, J. (eds) *Urological Nursing.* Edinburgh: Baillière Tindall, 207–26.

Floruta, C.V. 2001. Dietary choices of people with ostomies. *Journal of Wound, Ostomy and Continence Nursing* **28**(1), 28–31.

Getliffe, K. 1995. Long-term catheter use in the community. *Nursing Standard* **9**(31), 25–7.

Getliffe, K. 1996. Which catheter? A guide to catheter selection. *Professional Nurse* **12**(2), insert.

Getliffe, K. 2002. Managing recurrent urinary catheter encrustation. *British Journal of Community Nursing* **7,** 574–80.

Getliffe, K. and Dolman, M. 2007(eds) *Promoting Continence: A clinical and research guide,* 3rd edn. Edinburgh: Baillière Tindall.

Getliffe, K. and Fader, M. 2007. Catheters and containment products. In Getliffe, K. and Dolman, M. (eds) *Promoting Continence: A clinical and research guide,* 3rd edn. Edinburgh: Baillière Tindall, 259–308.

Gibbons, G. 1996. Skin care and incontinence. *Community Nurse* **2,** 37.

Godfrey, H. and Fraczyk, L. 2005. Preventing and managing catheter-associated urinary tract infections. *British Journal of Community Nursing* **10**(5), 205–12.

Gould, D. 1994. Controlling infection spread from excreta. *Nursing Standard* **8**(33), 29–31.

Gould, D. and Brooker, C. 2000. *Applied Microbiology for Nurses.* London: Macmillan.

Greenstein, B. 2004. *Trounce's Clinical Pharmacology for Nurses,* 17th edn. Edinburgh: Churchill Livingstone.

Hansen, J.L., Bliss, D.Z. and Peden-McAlpine, C. 2006. Diet strategies used by women to manage fecal incontinence. *Journal of Wound, Ostomy and Continence Nursing* **33**, 52–62.

Harari, D., Norton, C., Lockwood, L. and Swift, C. 2004. Treatment of constipation and fecal incontinence in stroke patients: randomized controlled trials. *Stroke* **35**(11), 2549–55.

Hay-Smith, E.J.C and Dumoulin, C. 2007. Pelvic floor muscle training versus no treatment, or inactive control treatments, for urinary incontinence in women. *Cochrane Database of Systematic Reviews,* Issue 4.

Herbert, J. 2008. Use of anal plugs in faecal incontinence management. *Nursing Times* **104**(13), 66–8.

Hodgkinson, B., Nay, R. and Wilson, J. 2007. A systematic review of topical skin care in aged care facilities. *Journal of Clinical Nursing* **16,** 129–36.

Hoffman, J.M., Wadhwani, R., Kelly, E. *et al.* 2004. Nitrite and leucocyte dipstick testing for urinary tract infection in individuals with spinal cord injury. *Journal of Spinal Cord Medicine* **27**(2), 128–32.

Holland, K. and Hogg, C. 2001. *Cultural Awareness in Nursing and Health Care: An introductory text.* London: Arnold.

Irwin, K. 2002. Digital rectal examination/manual removal of faeces in adults. *Journal of Community Nursing* **16**(4) 16–20.

Jackson, S.L., Scholes, D., Boyko, E.J. *et al.* 2005. Urinary incontinence and diabetes in postmenopausal women. *Diabetes Care* **28**(7), 1730–8.

Jahn, P., Preuss, M., Kernig, A., Seifert-Huhmer, A. and Langer, G. 2007. Types of indwelling urinary catheters for long-term bladder drainage in adults. *Cochrane Database of Systematic Reviews,* Issue 3.

Jensen, L.L. 1997. Faecal incontinence: evaluation and treatment. *Journal of Wound, Ostomy and Continence Nursing* **24,** 277–82.

Karadag, A., Mentes B. and Ayaz, S. 2005. Colostomy irrigation: results of 25 cases with particular reference to quality of life. *Journal of Clinical Nursing* **14**(4), 479–85.

Koch, L.H. 2006. Help-seeking behaviours of women with urinary incontinence: an integrative literature review. *Journal of Midwifery and Women's Health* **51**(6), e39–44.

Koch, T. and Kelly, S. 1999. Identifying strategies for managing urinary incontinence with women who have multiple sclerosis. *Journal of Clinical Nursing* **8,** 550–9.

Kyle, G. 2007a. Bowel care. Pt 1: Assessment of constipation. *Nursing Times* **103**(42), 26–7.

Kyle, G. 2007b. Norgine risk assessment tool for constipation. *Nursing Times* **103**(47), 48–9.

Kyle, G. 2007c. Bowel care. Pt 5: A practical guide to digital rectal examination. *Nursing Times* **103**(46), 28–9.

Laurent, C. 1998. Preventing infection from indwelling catheters. *Nursing Times* **94**(25), 60–6.

Le Lievre, S. 1996. Incontinence dermatitis. *Primary Health Care* **6**(4), 17–19, 21.

Lifshitz, E. and Kramer, L. 2000. Outpatient urine culture. *Archives of Internal Medicine* **160,** 2537–40.

Lewis, C.M., Schrader, R., Many, A. *et al.* 2005. Diabetes and urinary incontinence in 50–90 year old women: a cross-sectional population-based study. *American Journal of Obstetrics and Gynaecology* **193**(6), 2154–8.

Macauley, M. 1997. Urinary drainage systems. In Fillingham, S. and Douglas, J. (eds) *Urological Nursing,* 2nd edn. London: Baillière Tindall, 90–130.

Macauley, M., Clarke-O'Neill, S., Fader, M. *et al*. 2004. A pilot study to evaluate reusable absorbent body-worn products for adults with moderate/heavy urinary incontinence. *Journal of Wound, Ostomy and Continence Nursing* **31**(6), 357–66.

MacDonald, C. and Butler, L. 2007. Silent no more: elderly women's stories of living with urinary incontinence in long-term care. *Journal of Gerontological Nursing* **33**(1), 14–20.

Madersbacher, S., Schmidt, J., Eberle, J. and Thony, H.C. 2003. Long-term outcome of ileal conduit diversion. *Journal of Urology* **169**(3), 985–90.

Manisha, J., Tinetti, M., Perrelli, E. *et al*. 2007. Role of dipstick testing in the evaluation of urinary tract infection in nursing home residents. *Infection Control and Hospital Epidemiology* **28**(7), 889–91.

Mead, M. 1998. Stool culture. *Practice Nurse* **16**(3), 170.

Medicines and Healthcare Products Regulatory Agency (MHRA) 2006. *Urine Dipsticks: Top tips*. London: MHRA.

Meers, P., Sedgwick, J. and Worsley, M. 1995. *The Microbiology and Epidemiology of Infection for Health Science Students*. London: Chapman & Hall.

Medical Devices Agency 1995. *Penile Sheaths: An evaluation*, no. A15. Norwich: HMSO.

Mendoza, J., Legido, J., Rubio, S. and Gisbert, J.P. 2007. Systematic review: the adverse effects of sodium phosphate enema. *Alimentary Pharmacology and Therapy* **26**(1), 9–20.

Midthun, S.J., Paur, R. and Lindseth, G. 2004. Urinary tract infections: does the smell really tell? *Journal of Gerontological Nursing* **30**(6), 4–9.

Mulhall, A.B., Chapman, R.G. and Crow, R.A. 1988. Bacteriuria during indwelling urethral catheterisation. *Journal of Hospital Infection* **11**(3) 253–62.

National Institute for Health and Clinical Excellence (NICE) 2003. *Infection Control: Prevention of healthcare-associated infection in primary and community care*. London.

— 2006. *The Management of Urinary Incontinence in Women*. London.

— 2007. *Faecal Incontinence: The management of faecal incontinence in adults*. Quick reference guide CG49. London.

National Patient Safety Agency 2007. *Using Bedrails Safely and Effectively*. NPSA.

Nazarko, L. 1995. The therapeutic uses of cranberry juice. *Nursing Standard* **9**(34), 33–5.

Nazarko, L. 1997. Continence: the whole story. *Nursing Times* **93**(43), 63–4, 66, 68.

NHS Quality Improvement Scotland 2005. *Best Practice Statement. Continence: Adults with urinary dysfunction*. Edinburgh: NHS Quality Improvement Scotland.

Nix, D. and Ermer-Seltun, J. 2004. A review of perineal skin care protocols and skin barrier product use. *Ostomy/Wound Management* **50**(12), 59–67.

Norton, C. 1997. Faecal incontinence in adults. Pt 2: Treatment and management. *British Journal of Nursing* **6**, 23–6.

Ostaszkiewicz, J. 2006. The clinical effectiveness of systematic voiding programmes: results of a metastudy. *Australian and New Zealand Continence Journal* **12**(1), 5–6.

Ostaszkiewicz, J., Bobston, L. and Roe, B. 2007a. Timed voiding for the management of urinary incontinence in adults. *Cochrane Database of Systematic Reviews*, Issue 4.

Ostaszkiewicz, J., Bobston, L. and Roe, B. 2007b. Habit retraining for the management of urinary incontinence in adults. *Cochrane Database of Systematic Reviews*, Issue 4.

Padmanabhan, A., Stern, M., Wishin, J. *et al*. 2007. Clinical evaluation of a flexible fecal incontinence management system. *American Journal of Critical Care* **16**(4), 384–93.

Palmer, M.H. and Newman, D.K. 2006. Bladder control: educational needs of older adults. *Journal of Gerontological Nursing* **32**(1), 28–32.

Palmieri, B., Benuzzi, G. and Bellini, N. 2005. The anal bag: a modern approach to fecal incontinence management. *Ostomy/Wound management* **51**(12), 44–52.

Panagamuwa, C., Glasby, M.J. and Peckham, T.J. 2004. Dipstick screening for urinary tract infection before arthroscopy: a safe alternative to laboratory testing? *International Journal of Clinical Practice* **58**(1), 19–21.

Parascandolo, M.E. and Doughty, D. 2001. Multiple Ostomy complications in a patient with Crohn's disease: A case study. *The Journal of Wound, Ostomy and Continence Nursing* **28**(5), 236–243.

Pellatt, G. 2007. Clinical skills: bowel elimination and management of complications. *British Journal of Nursing* **16**(6), 351–5.

Pemberton, P., Brooks, A., Erikson, C.M. *et al.* 2006. A comparative study of two types of urinary sheath. *Nursing Times* **102**(7), 36–41.

Pomfret, I.J. 2000. Urinary incontinence management: urinary sheaths. *Journal of Community Nursing* **14**(4). Available from www.jcn.co.uk.

Pratt, R.J., Pellowe, C., Wilson, J.A. *et al.* 2007. National evidence-based guidelines for preventing healthcare-associated infections in NHS England. *Journal of Hospital Infection* **65** Suppl, S1–64.

Rassin, M., Dubches, L., Libshitz *et al.* 2007. Levels of comfort and ease among patients suffering from urinary incontinence. *International Journal of Urological Nursing* **1**(2), 64–70.

Ratliff, C., Scarano, K.A., Donovan, A.M. and Colwell, J.C. 2005. Descriptive study of peristomal complications. *Journal of Wound, Ostomy and Continence Nursing* **32**(1), 33–7.

Resnick, B., Leilman, L.J., Calabrese, B. *et al.* 2006. Nursing staff beliefs and expectations about continence care in nursing homes. *Journal of Wound, Ostomy and Continence Nursing* **33**(6), 610–18.

Richbourg, L., Thorpe, J.M. and Rapp, C.G. 2007. Difficulties experienced by the ostomate after hospital discharge. *Journal of Wound, Ostomy and Continence Nursing* **34**(1), 70–9.

Richmond, J.P. and Wright, M.E. 2004. Review of the literature on constipation to enable development of a constipation risk assessment scale. *Clinical Effectiveness in Nursing* **8**(1), 11–25.

Rigby, D. 2007. Medication for continence. In Getliffe, K. and Dolman, M. (eds) *Promoting Continence: A clinical and research guide,* 3rd edn. Edinburgh: Baillière Tindall, 239–58.

Robinson, J. 2001. Urethral catheter selection. *Nursing Standard* **15**(25), 39–42.

Roe, B., Ostaszkiewicz, J., Milne, J. and Wallace, S. 2006. Systematic reviews of bladder training and voiding programmes in adults: a synopsis of findings from data analysis and outcomes using metastudy techniques. *Journal of Advanced Nursing* **57**(1), 15–31.

Rowell, D.M. 1998. Evaluation of a urine chemistry analyser. *Professional Nurse* **13**, 553–4.

Royal College of Nursing (RCN) 2006a. *Meeting the Health Needs of People with Learning Disabilities: Guidance for nursing staff.* London.

— 2006b. *Digital Rectal Examination and Manual Removal of Faeces: Guidance for nurses.* London.

Saint, S. and Lipsky, B.A. 1999. Preventing catheter-associated bacteriuria. Should we? Can we? How? *Archives of Internal Medicine* **159**, 800–8.

Saint, S., Kaufman, S.R., Rogers, M.A.M *et al.* 2006. Condom versus indwelling urinary catheters: a randomized trial. *Journal of the American Geriatrics Society* **54**(7), 1055–61.

Saye, D.E. 2007. Recurring and antimicrobial resistant infections: Considering the potential role of biofilms in clinical practice. *Ostomy/Wound Management* **53**(4), 46–52.

Schmelzer, M. and Wright, K.B. 1996. Enema administration techniques used by experienced registered nurses. *Gastroenterology Nursing* **19,** 171–5.

Smith, D.B. 1998. A continence care approach for long-term care facilities. *Geriatric Nursing* **19**(2), 81–6.

Smith, P. and Smith, L. 2007. Continence training in intellectual disability. In Getliffe, K. and Dolman, M. (eds) *Promoting Continence: A clinical and research resource,* 3rd edn. Edinburgh: Baillière Tindall, 173–202.

Stanley, R. 1997. Treatment of continence in people with learning disabilities: Part 3. *British Journal of Nursing* 6, 12, 14, 16, 18, 19, 22.

Stoma Care 2007. *An Educational Resource for Stoma Care Nursing,* DVD. Burdett Institute of Gastrointestinal Nursing and Dansac Ltd.

Thompson, J. 2007. Falls and incontinence: evaluation of a quality management project. *Australian and New Zealand Continence Journal* **13**(1), 18, 20–1.

Thompson, D.L. and Smith, D.A. 1998. Continence restoration in the cognitively impaired adult. *Geriatric Nursing* **19**(2), 87–90.

Vaillancourt, S., McGillivray, D., Zhang, X. and Kramer, M.S. 2007. To clean or not to clean: effect on contamination rates in midstream urine collections in toilet-trained children. *Pediatrics* **119**, e1288–93.

Vickerman, J. 2003. The benefits of a lending library for female urinals. *Nursing Times* **99**(44), 56–7.

Wallace, S.A., Roe, B., Williams, K. and Palmer, M. 2007. Bladder training for urinary incontinence in adults. *Cochrane Database of Systematic Reviews,* Issue 4.

Wareing, M. 2005. Lower urinary tract symptons: a hermeneutic phenomenological study into men's lived experience. *Journal of Clinical Nursing* **14**, 239–46.

Wazait, H.D., Patel, H.R.H., Veer, V. *et al.* 2003. Catheter-associated urinary tract infections: prevalence of uropathogens and pattern of antimicrobial resistance in a UK hospital (1996–2001). *British Journal of Urology International* **91**(9), 806–9.

Wells, M. and Wagg, A. 2007. Integrated continence services and the female Bangladeshi population. *British Journal of Nursing* **16**, 516–9.

Whittingham, K. and May, S. 1998. Cleansing regimens for continence care. *Professional Nurse* **14**, 167–71.

Williams, D. and Moran, S. 2006. Use of urinary sheaths in male incontinence. *Nursing Times* **102**(47), 42–5.

Wilson, J. 1997. Control and prevention of infection in catheter care. *Nurse Prescriber/ Community Nurse* **3**(5), 39–40.

Wilson, J. 2006. *Infection Control in Clinical Practice,* 3rd edn. Edinburgh: Baillière Tindall.

Winn, C. 1996. Basing catheter care on research principles. *Nursing Standard* **10**(18), 38–40.

Woodward, S. 1996. Impact of neurological problems on urinary continence. *British Journal of Nursing* **5,** 906–13.

Woodward, S. 1997. Complications of allergies to latex urinary catheters. *British Journal of Nursing* **6,** 786, 788, 790, 792–3.

Zhang, A.Y., Strauss, G.J. and Siminoff, L.A. 2007. Effects of combined pelvic floor muscle exercise and a support group on urinary incontinence and quality of life of postprostatectomy patients. *Oncology Nursing Forum* **34**(1), 47–53.

CHAPTER

10

Assessing and Meeting Nutritional Needs

Lesley Marsh

Good food in a balanced diet is important in everyone's life, and sound nutrition is an essential prerequisite for health and well-being. Nutrition is a concern to nurses working in any setting and should be regarded as central to patient/client care: 'The provision of food and fluids is a nursing role' (Florence Nightingale 1859, cited in 1980 edition).

Good nutrition for people in healthcare settings is increasingly influenced by health policy initiatives and recommendations. For example, the Department of Health's (DH) *The Essence of Care* (DH 2001a) includes a section on nutrition with benchmarking statements for good practice. Providing food and drink to patients/clients in care environments is a complex process involving a range of staff. Nurses are well placed to promote healthy eating because, within the caring team, they spend most time with the people who require this support.

According to the European Nutrition for Health Alliance (ENHA) (2005), up to 14 per cent of people aged over 65 years in the UK are malnourished, and four out of ten older people admitted to hospital are malnourished on arrival. This has implications for healthcare as patients who are malnourished stay in hospital longer, need more medications and are more likely to acquire infection (Edington *et al.* 2000). Sound nutritional care is therefore paramount in nursing practice to promote the health of patients and clients.

The Nursing and Midwifery Council's (2007a) Essential Skills Clusters comprehensively detail nutrition-related skills which students must develop.

This chapter includes:
- Nutrition in healthcare: addressing the concerns
- Recognising the contribution of nutrition to health
- Promoting healthy eating in care settings
- Nutritional screening
- Assisting people with eating and drinking
- Additional nutritional support strategies
- Enteral and parenteral feeding

Recommended biology reading:

The following questions will help you to focus on the biology underpinning the skills in this chapter. Use your recommended textbook to find out:

- What are nutrients?
- Where do nutrients come from?
- What is a balanced diet?
- What is the difference between macronutrients and micronutrients?
- Why do we need these nutrients? What are their roles?
- How are macronutrients digested?
- Once digested, where do they go?
- What factors may affect the absorption of digested nutrients?
- How does nutrition affect health?
- What are the consequences of under-nutrition and over-nutrition?
- How do nutritional requirements alter across the lifespan?
- What aspects of different age groups (e.g. teenagers, young adults and older people) may impinge upon nutritional status?
- How does a 'health need' alter our nutritional demands (or supply)?

PRACTICE SCENARIOS

Nutrition is relevant for everybody. The following practice scenarios highlight situations where nutritional issues would be particularly important, and they will be referred to throughout this chapter.

Adult

Stroke
Cerebral damage caused either by decreased blood flow or haemorrhage. Effects vary, but a stroke often causes paralysis down one side of the body (hemiplegia), and speech and swallowing difficulty.

Miss Alice West is 84 years old and has been transferred from a medical ward to a rehabilitation unit following a stroke which has caused right-sided weakness. The medical ward staff who transferred her said that, although she initially had swallowing problems, she has since been assessed as being able to swallow. However, her appetite is very poor and she often eats only a few small mouthfuls, refusing any more. The staff have been keeping a food chart and a fluid chart which confirm her poor intake. She has dentures but they appear loose. Her niece is concerned that she is 'looking thin' and seems depressed. Miss West is often uncommunicative but on occasions expresses herself clearly. She is also registered partially sighted. Her weight on admission was 58 kg and is now 53 kg. Her height is 1.64 m.

Learning disability

Phillip Picton is a 31-year-old man with a learning disability who lives in a supported living scheme with three other clients. Recently he has become increasingly overweight. His obesity is beginning to interfere with his day-to-day activities. He has expressed concern about two issues: bending over to put his socks on and getting out of breath walking to the local shops. His carers took him to see his GP who referred him to the community team for people with learning disabilities.

Health facilitator
A member of the
community learning
disabilities team (often
a nurse) who supports
a person with learning
disabilities to access the
healthcare they need. See
Valuing People (DH 2001b).

Dementia
Dementia is chronic and
progressive in nature, has
many causes and commonly
presents with memory and
language impairment, decline
in self-care ability, and
behavioural and personality
changes (Jacques and Jackson
2000).

The community nurse for learning disabilities and the occupational therapist, who is Phillip's **health facilitator**, are going to visit him to carry out an assessment. Phillip does his own food shopping with support. His weight three years ago was 58 kg and is now 92 kg.

Mental health

Charles Cooper is an 88-year-old widower (his wife died 15 years ago). He lives alone in a bungalow in a small village. The village has very poor public transport services. The local shop has recently closed. Mr Cooper has a diagnosis of dementia for which he is prescribed medication. He is prompted to take this by a home carer who calls twice a day. Recently the community psychiatric nurse (CPN) noticed that Mr Cooper had lost weight. When questioned about his dietary intake Mr Cooper stated that he has a 'good appetite' and manages to prepare all his own meals. On checking the kitchen the CPN observed little evidence of recent food preparation or cooking. The refrigerator contained some dairy products, and these had all expired and were beginning to smell.

NUTRITION IN HEALTHCARE: ADDRESSING THE CONCERNS

This chapter's introduction highlighted the continuing problem of malnutrition. Age Concern (2006) asserted that insufficient attention has been given to factors contributing to the prevalence of malnutrition in hospital.

ACTIVITY

Why do you think people are at risk of malnutrition in hospital?

Compare your ideas with the problems raised by Age Concern (2006, p. 6):
* appropriateness of the food on offer;
* help with eating the food;
* monitoring of the patient for signs of malnutrition;
* involvement of patients, relatives and carers;
* knowing how and who to raise concerns with.

Age Concern highlight that these problems closely link to relationships between staff and patients and between different groups of staff, such as nurses and catering. Age Concern's *Hungry to be Heard: The scandal of malnourished older people in hospital* includes harrowing case studies of nutritional needs being neglected.

People's likes and dislikes, and cultural and religious factors can be difficult to cater for in hospital settings. An audit of patient meals found that a third of the hospital vegetarian meals failed to provide the recommended amount of protein (Fettes and Murray 1999). However, a dietetic toolkit is available so this should not be an issue if menus are checked by a dietician. A study of South Asian older people's care experiences found dissatisfaction with their hospital food and a perceived lack of understanding from staff of the food's religious significance (Clegg 2003). The mental health charity MIND reported that 45 per cent of respondents did not have access to snacks outside of mealtimes, and almost a third of people in inpatient units said they did not have enough access to hot and cold drinks (Baker 2001).

There have been many attempts to address problems with nutrition in hospital. You may be aware of some of the following.

Better hospital foods

In 2001, leading chefs were asked to advise on varied and nutritious menus for the Better Hospital Food Programme (www.betterhospitalfood.com). However, although the menus were varied and sophisticated, they were not well received by all patients owing to their unfamiliarity. Therefore, in 2006, the DH put the Better Hospital Foods programme menus on hold.

Core standards of care

The UK governments have all released policies to direct nutritional standards in the NHS. These include the nutrition benchmarks in *The Essence of Care* and core standards in *Standards for Better Health* (DH 2004). The Welsh Assembly's (2003) *Fundamentals of Care* includes practice indicators for eating and drinking. In 2003, NHS Quality Improvement Scotland identified nutritional care standards for monitoring. In Northern Ireland, the Department of Health, Social Services and Public Safety (2007) published nursing care standards for hospital food.

Clinical guidelines

The National Institute for Health and Clinical Excellence (NICE) (2006) issued a clinical guideline regarding identification of patients who are malnourished or at risk of malnutrition.

Improving mealtimes

In 2007, the NHS Institute for Innovation and Improvement (2007) produced modules to help ward staff increase time spent on direct patient care: *Releasing Time to Care: The productive ward*. The module dedicated to meals gives guidance on how to ensure the best experience for patients while making the delivery quick and easy for staff. This enables patients to be correctly assessed nutritionally and staff to have time to assist patients with eating.

Improving Nutritional Care: A joint action plan

This document was developed jointly by the DH and the Nutrition Summit stakeholders (DH 2007a). It aims to ensure that health and social care staff and managers are well informed, equipped and supported to provide good nutrition and effective nutritional care.

As you can see, there are many guidelines and developments in the UK. In addition, the Council of Europe Alliance (2007) has identified ten key characteristics of good nutritional care in hospitals (see Box 10.1).

ACTIVITY

Consider the care environment you work in. Are all the characteristics in Box 10.1 being demonstrated?

> **Box 10.1 Ten key characteristics of good nutritional care in hospitals (Council of Europe Alliance 2007)**
>
> • All patients are screened on admission to identify the patients who are malnourished or at risk of becoming malnourished. All patients are re-screened weekly.
> • All patients have a care plan which identifies their nutritional care needs and how these are to be met.
> • The hospital includes specific guidance on food services and nutritional care in its Clinical Governance arrangements.
> • Patients are involved in the planning and monitoring arrangements for food service provision.
> • The ward implements Protected Mealtimes to provide an environment conducive to patients enjoying and being able to eat their food.
> • All staff have the appropriate skills and competencies needed to ensure that patients' nutritional needs are met. All staff receive regular training on nutritional care and management.
> • Hospital facilities are designed to be flexible and patient-centred with the aim of providing and delivering an excellent experience of food service and nutritional care 24 hours a day, every day
> • The hospital has a policy for food service and nutritional care which is patient-centred and performance managed in line with home-country governance frameworks.
> • Food service and nutritional care is delivered to the patient safely.
> • The hospital supports a multidisciplinary approach to nutritional care and values the contribution of all staff groups working in partnership with patients and users.

As this section has outlined, there is considerable concern about nutritional deficits, and increasingly initiatives and guidance have been released. At the author's NHS Trust (Whipps Cross University Hospital) there is a Nutrition Action Team: a multidisciplinary team (MDT) who meet twice a month to ensure that all aspects of nutritional care are being met within the Trust.

ACTIVITY

Find out whether your care setting has an MDT group with responsibility for nutrition. If so, what do they do? Who is in the group?

The next section highlights why sound nutrition is so important for good health.

RECOGNISING THE CONTRIBUTION OF NUTRITION TO HEALTH

An adequate supply of essential nutrients is required in the diet to maintain health. The term **diet** usually refers to the total food eaten, while **nutrients** refers to components of foodstuffs which have a role in body functioning. For example, bread is composed of the nutrients carbohydrate, protein, fat and some vitamins.

It is important to understand the key components of a nutritious diet and to be able to identify factors that might prevent good nutrition.

LEARNING OUTCOMES

By the end of this section you will be able to:
1 identify the major nutrients;
2 discuss factors that might influence healthy people's nutritional needs;
3 identify situations in which an individual's nutritional status might be impaired;
4 recognise the consequences of malnutrition.

Learning outcome 1: Identify the major nutrients

Your biology reading will have helped you understand the important groups of nutrients and their role in maintaining health.

ACTIVITY

Here is a list of Miss West's recorded food and fluid intake for the day before her transfer to the rehabilitation unit. Note one cup = 200 mL. Miss West takes milk in her tea and coffee but no sugar.
- *Morning:* **8.15** – small bowl of porridge with milk and sugar (10 dessert spoonfuls), ½ cup of tea; **9.00** – ½ glass of water; **10.30** – ½ cup of coffee (declined snack).
- *Midday:* **12.30** – small amount of mince, mashed potato and peas (8 teaspoons in total), one portion of mousse, ½ glass of water, ½ cup of tea.
- *Afternoon:* **3.15** – ½ cup of tea (declined snack); **5.30** – ½ bowl of chicken soup, ½ white bread roll with butter, one portion of yoghurt, ½ cup of water, ½ cup of tea.
- *Evening:* **6.00** – ½ cup of tea (declined snack); **8.00** – ½ cup of water.

Which nutrients does Miss West's diet include and which nutrients are missing?

Miss West's diet does contain some important nutrients (e.g. fibre and carbohydrate in her porridge, protein in her mince, fat in the butter, mousse, yoghurt and milk, and vitamin C in the peas) but her portions are so small that her calorific intake and intake of most nutrients is likely to be inadequate. Healthy people can cope with inadequate nutrition occasionally, but many people admitted to hospital are already malnourished. Because Miss West's energy and protein intake are insufficient, her body will break down fat and muscle to meet its needs, leading to weight loss. Miss West's diet contains minimal iron and she is at risk of iron deficiency anaemia if her nutritional intake does not improve. Vitamin C helps absorption of iron from non-animal sources (e.g. grains) (Wardlow 1999), but her vitamin C intake is small too. Her fluid intake is about 1100 mL, which is barely sufficient to maintain her hydration.

Recording a food chart, as the nurses have done for Miss West, is a good way of seeing what someone is actually eating and it becomes clear if their diet is inadequate. Staff should record the amount taken in spoonfuls as listed above as this enables the healthcare team to have a more accurate picture and they can therefore create a more detailed plan of care.

Miss West's fruit and vegetable intake was minimal. The current recommendations are to eat at least five portions of a variety of fruit and vegetables each day, but average fruit and vegetable consumption among people in England is less than three portions a day and consumption tends to be lower among children and people on low incomes (DH 2007b). The DH's 'Five a Day' campaign encourages people to increase their fruit and vegetable consumption (see www.5aday.nhs.uk and www.dh.gov.uk/en/Publichealth/Healthimprovement/FiveADay/index.htm). Among fruit and vegetables most people have their personal favourites, but these may not be easily available in hospital.

Learning outcome 2: Discuss factors that might influence healthy people's nutritional needs

The amounts of various nutrients required for health vary from individual to individual and throughout life.

ACTIVITY

What factors might influence a healthy person's nutritional needs?

You may have thought of the following:
- **Age**. In adulthood the energy requirement decreases with age because older people have a lower metabolic rate than younger adults (Pender 1994).
- **Gender**. Men require more energy because their relatively greater muscle mass results in a higher metabolic rate than that in women (Pender 1994).
- **Height and build**. The bigger the body the greater the amount of nutrients required to maintain cells (Piper 1996).
- **Amount of physical activity**. As energy is used as fuel, the greater the physical activity the more energy is used up (Pender 1994).
- **Pregnancy**. During the second and third trimesters of pregnancy, rapid growth of the fetus alters the woman's nutritional needs, although the exact demands made on the mother by the fetus vary from individual to individual. In particular the need for energy, protein, and vitamins A, B, C and D are likely to increase (Wardley *et al.* 1997). The increased energy required by the fetus is often compensated for in part by decreased maternal activity towards the end of pregnancy, and the average British diet generally contains sufficient protein to meet the increased demands (Wardley *et al.* 1997).
- **Lactation**. A breast-feeding woman requires increased energy (as much as 500 calories/day more), increased calcium and increased vitamins A, C and D intake (Wardley *et al.* 1997).

Being aware of factors affecting nutritional demands in healthy people is important prior to considering factors that compromise nutritional status.

Learning outcome 3: Identify situations in which an individual's nutritional status might be impaired

Bond (1997) asserts that malnourishment is an overall term that encompasses:

- under-nourishment due to inadequate food intake;
- over-nourishment due to excess food consumption, leading to obesity;
- deficiency of specific nutrients;
- dietary imbalance due to disproportionate intake.

ACTIVITY

What do you think might prevent Miss West, Phillip and Mr Cooper from meeting their nutritional needs?

Miss West may not be physically able to feed herself as her weak right arm will cause difficulty manipulating eating utensils. Her dentures do not fit properly, which will affect her eating. It seems that although she can swallow she has lost interest in food. There could be many factors causing this, for example depression or dislike of hospital food. As she is partially sighted she may not be able to see her food or utensils well. According to the Stroke Association (2006) there has been little research done into taste loss after stroke (termed **dysgeusia**). Perhaps this is because taste is a relatively simple process and taste information does not appear to be vital to human survival. A loss of taste, however, can make a big difference to the quality of life, and people find it is a distressing and unexpected after-effect of a stroke.

Phillip can eat independently and can shop with help. As he is obese it might appear that his nutritional intake is more than adequate. However, he may not be eating enough of the right foods while eating too many of foods which might lead to obesity, such as a high-fat diet or excess sugar. He might be unaware of the different nutrients he needs to stay healthy.

Mr Cooper has dementia which could affect his appetite and his ability to shop and prepare food, leading to an inadequate and inappropriate intake. His access to shops to buy food is very limited.

These examples illustrate that people may be unable to meet their nutritional needs, leading to malnutrition, as a result of inadequate intake, inappropriate intake, increased nutritional demands or any combination of these factors.

Inadequate intake

ACTIVITY

What might predispose to an inadequate nutritional intake? The scenarios will give you some clues. Remember to think about psychological and socioeconomic factors as well as physical factors.

- **Loss of appetite**. Appetite loss may be caused by pain, stress, anxiety, reduced physical activity and fatigue which often accompany illness (Pender 1994). Some medicines suppress the appetite (Holmes 2003).
- **Stress**. Some people have an inadequate intake as a result of busy, stressful lives (Edwards 1998).

- **Lack of knowledge and skills**. People may not understand the importance of eating, and could be unable to buy suitable food and prepare it.
- **Dementia**. People with dementia may not be able to eat independently. They may not cooperate with attempts to encourage them to eat and drink. In very severe cognitive impairment they may no longer recognise food (Manthorpe and Watson 2003).
- **Paranoia**. Some people may not eat because of fear of being poisoned.
- **Nausea and vomiting**. These symptoms, which are caused by various illnesses and are side-effects of some medicines, prevent people from eating even if they feel hungry (Holmes 2003).
- **Nil by mouth**. Some people may be unable to eat for prolonged periods due to their condition (e.g. if they are unconscious) or treatment (e.g. following some types of surgery).
- **Physical factors**. One example is dysphagia (difficulty in swallowing), which results from delayed or absent swallow reflex (Crawley 2003). Initially Miss West had this problem. Chewing difficulty and mouth pain caused by decayed teeth or ill-fitting dentures or mouth ulcers are other physical causes of inadequate intake. Limited dexterity causing difficulty in manipulating cutlery may make eating slow and difficult (e.g. people with cerebral palsy, stroke or rheumatoid arthritis). The physical effort of eating may be too great for some people with chronic diseases such as heart failure or emphysema (Holmes 2003).
- **Dependency**. People who are dependent on others and unable to express their needs are at risk of inadequate intake. Examples would be people unable to communicate as a result of intellectual or neurological impairment, or dementia.
- **Lack of finance**. People who are living on a low income often have many demands on their limited funds, so nutrition may not be the top priority.

> **Emphysema**
> Lung disease characterised by over-inflation and destructive changes leading to lack of elasticity in the alveolar walls.

Inappropriate intake

Some people turn to food as a *source of comfort* during periods of insecurity, depression or loneliness (Edwards 1998). With Phillip it would be important to consider whether these social and psychological factors are relevant. For example, are there sufficient activities for him to be involved in?

Fad diets and erroneous health beliefs may lead people to follow *diets that are too restricted* to meet their needs. It is important that dietetic advice is sought.

Increased demands

Holmes (2003) describes how the body's reaction to injury, infection and surgery raises the basal metabolic rate and hence increases nutritional demands. Healing of wounds and fractures requires additional nutrients. Some neurological conditions, such as some types of cerebral palsy, can cause excessive body movements, using up energy and thus increasing nutritional demands.

> **Basal metabolic rate**
> The amount of energy needed by the body for essential processes when at complete rest but awake (Brooker 1998).

Learning outcome 4: Recognise the consequences of malnutrition

Malnutrition is frequently undetected and untreated, causing a wide range of adverse consequences (Stratton *et al.* 2003).

ACTIVITY What adverse effects of malnutrition can you identify? What impact could these have on Miss West?

Stratton *et al.* (2003) identify the following effects of malnutrition:

- impaired immune responses, thus increasing infection risk;
- reduced muscle strength and fatigue;
- reduced respiratory muscle function leading to difficulties in breathing and expectoration, thus increasing the risk of chest infection and respiratory failure;
- impaired thermoregulation, predisposing to hypothermia;
- impaired wound healing and delayed recovery from illness;
- apathy, depression and self-neglect;
- increased risk of admission to hospital and length of stay;
- poor libido, fertility, pregnancy outcome and mother–child interactions.

Malnutrition could thus have a serious impact on Miss West's recovery from her stroke, increasing her risk of acquiring an infection and impairing her rehabilitation due to tiredness and lack of strength. It is possible that malnutrition is contributing to Miss West's apparent depression.

Adverse effects of malnutrition increase costs to the National Health Services throughout the UK and the community as a whole:

- In the community, older people identified as at risk of malnutrition are more likely to be admitted to hospital and to visit their GP more frequently (Stratton *et al.* 2002).
- Underweight individuals (body mass index $<20 \text{kg/m}^2$) have been shown to consume more healthcare resources than those with a BMI between 20 and 25 kg/m^2, having more prescriptions (9 per cent), more GP visits (6 per cent) and more hospital admissions (25 per cent) (Martyn *et al.* 1998)
- In hospital, patients at risk of malnutrition stay in hospital significantly longer and are more likely to be discharged to healthcare destinations other than home (Wood *et al.* 2003).

Summary

- An adequate intake of the correct balance of nutrients is essential to maintain health, and prevent malnutrition.
- Many people encountered by nurses have increased nutritional demands but their ability to meet these demands is compromised due to an inadequate, and sometimes inappropriate, dietary intake.
- Malnutrition has serious consequences, predisposing to illness and delaying recovery.

PROMOTING HEALTHY EATING IN CARE SETTINGS

An important part of promoting good nutrition is encouraging healthy eating. *The Essence of Care* states that best practice is where: 'All opportunities are used to encourage the patient/client to eat to promote their health' (DH 2001a). A balanced diet contains a particular selection of foods, in the correct proportions to meet the body cells' requirements and is essential for maintaining a healthy body that functions efficiently. We have already considered the nutrients necessary for a healthy diet and factors that affect nutritional status; but in care settings, achieving a healthy diet poses particular challenges.

LEARNING OUTCOMES

By the end of this section you will be able to:
1 identify improvement initiatives for nutrition in healthcare settings;
2 assist patients/clients to select a healthy diet from a menu in a care setting.

Learning outcome 1: Identify improvement initiatives for nutrition in healthcare settings

The NHS Plan (DH 2000) produced a programme of action for the NHS to deliver high-quality food and food services to patients.

ACTIVITY   What initiatives to improve nutrition have you seen in practice settings?

Here are initiatives identified by DH (2007c) – you may have seen these or others in practice settings:

- **Protected mealtimes**. These are periods on hospital wards when all non-urgent clinical activity stops so that patients can eat their meals uninterrupted, assisted by staff. DH (2007c) suggests that protected mealtimes lead to patients eating more, being better nourished and with improved chances of recovery.
- **24-hour catering**. Previously hot food was not always available outside mealtimes, but 24-hour catering should ensure that hot food, snacks and drinks are available to patients at any time of day.
- **Sustainability and seasonality**. This includes sourcing local food, which is likely to be fresher, using organic or fairly traded goods and reducing food waste.
- **Flexi-menu systems**. These offer a fixed menu for lunch and evening meals so patients can choose food they like more than once.

In some settings a 'red tray' system is in operation whereby patients who need help to eat have a red tray so they are more easily identified. You might have seen this or other similar systems in place. You might also have seen facilities for families to bring food in, and to heat food in a microwave. All food brought in should be labelled and dated, and staff will need to be informed in case it interacts with medication being taken or any other special diet, or the person is to be 'nil by mouth' prior to a treatment. Some mental health units have canteen facilities which usually provide more choice for service users.

Best practice statements in *The Essence of Care* (DH 2001a) include:

Food that is provided by the service meets the needs of individual patients/ clients.

'Patients/clients have set meal times, are offered a replacement meal if a meal is missed and can access snacks at any time.'

The DH guidelines also advise that there should be adapted utensils available, inappropriate activity should be curtailed during mealtimes, and food provided must be in accordance with people's cultural/religious preferences. Care settings should be working towards these benchmarks of good practice and as you read in Miss West's scenario, she is being offered snacks to encourage her to eat more, so clearly this service is available at her hospital. The Patient Environment Action Team (PEAT) programme includes assessments of food and food services which are published on the Better Hospital Food website (DH 2007c).

ACTIVITY

What is your care setting doing about nutrition benchmarking? Find out what score they obtained and what their action plan is.

Learning outcome 2: Assist patients/clients to select a healthy diet from a menu in a care setting

ACTIVITY

Think about how you might assist a patient in a hospital setting to choose from the menu.

You might first spend time with the person finding out about their likes and dislikes. You should consider their religion and culture as some people's food preferences are related to religious beliefs. It is important not to make assumptions about what people might eat according to their culture/religion, but find out from the individual or family concerned. For example, a person who follows Sikhism may refrain from eating beef, eggs or fish or may be a vegetarian (Gill 2002). A person following Judaism is required to eat kosher food (food fit to be eaten in accordance with Jewish law) but there any many diverse practices about this (Collins 2002). Religion apart, people's beliefs and values may lead them to require a vegetarian or vegan diet. Be prepared to explain foods on the menu, as some choices may be unfamiliar to people.

You may need to read out menus and complete them for people. This would be necessary for Miss West, who is partially sighted. When going through the menu you can guide your patient towards appropriate foods, ensuring there is a balance of the important food groups discussed earlier in this chapter, while taking preferences into account. Miss West requires food that is not only nourishing but also weight-inducing, so you might encourage her to eat more carbohydrates and dairy products.

As well as food intake, ensure that your patient consumes sufficient fluid on a daily basis. Two to three litres of fluid daily is considered adequate for an adult; you might remember from an earlier activity that Miss West's intake falls far short of this at present. The hydration best-practice toolkit for hospitals and healthcare, *Water for Health* (Royal College of Nursing 2007), was developed through partnership working with nurses, patient groups and key stakeholders, including Water UK.

It provides practical advice for healthcare staff on how to minimise the risk and potential harm that poor hydration can cause, and offers solutions to improve the provision of water to hospital patients.

Summary

- There have been various initiatives to improve nutrition in healthcare settings.
- Hospitals should be working towards benchmarks of good practice.
- When promoting healthy eating, nurses should try to find out food preferences.
- Nurses should guide patients/clients regarding appropriate food choices, with respect for individual preferences, culture, values and beliefs.

NUTRITIONAL SCREENING

Nurses are in a unique position to identify people at risk of malnourishment and then take appropriate action. As recognised already in this chapter, there are many factors that can affect nutritional status. If nurses do not carry out nutritional screening carefully, patients can be put at unnecessary risk from the effects of malnourishment. A range of nutritional screening tools is available, but the Malnutrition Universal Screening Tool ('MUST') tool is recommended so we will focus on this. The DH defines screening as 'the process of identifying patients who are already malnourished or who are at risk of becoming so'. The benchmark of best practice is: 'Nutritional screening progresses to further assessment for all patients/clients identified as "at risk"' (DH 2001a, p. 76).

LEARNING OUTCOMES

By the end of this section you will be able to:
1 discuss how observations can contribute to nutritional assessment;
2 understand the purpose and use of nutritional screening tools;
3 carry out nutritional screening and recognise if people are at risk of malnutrition

Learning outcome 1: Discuss how observations can contribute to nutritional assessment

Assessment should include a range of observations to gain insight into nutritional status and contribute to screening.

ACTIVITY

With reference to the scenarios, what observations could be carried out to assist nutritional assessment?

You may have identified many of the aspects listed below – most would be useful in assessing the patients/clients in the scenarios.

- Observe whether clothing, rings and dentures are fitting comfortably. If not, this could suggest an alteration in weight. These could be useful indicators as to whether Mr Cooper is losing weight. You will remember that Miss West's dentures are loose and her niece might know whether her aunt's loose dentures are a new problem. Remember that patients may be deliberately trying to lose weight and so do not make assumptions.

- Look at the skin and check for excessive dryness, scaling and temperature.
- Check the eyes for brightness and whether they are sunken into their sockets, which could indicate dehydration. These would be important observations with both Mr Cooper (who may not be drinking enough) and Miss West, whose fluid intake we know is poor.
- Note the smell of the breath. Halitosis can indicate poor dental health or dehydration. This could lead you to review the state of the mouth, and to identify a problem with the teeth or gums. A sore mouth can indicate a poor diet. Chapter 8 considers oral hygiene in detail.
- Observe the level of mobility, for example, whether the person can move their arms adequately to eat independently, or can walk or manoeuvre to get access to food. This is particularly relevant to Miss West, but the CPN should also consider Mr Cooper's mobility in relation to obtaining and preparing food.
- Observe for drooling which could be a sign of poor swallowing, as well as poor lip seal. Although Miss West has been assessed as able to swallow now, these are signs that nurses should be aware of owing to her previous history.
- While the person is eating and drinking, observe their sequence of breathing and swallowing.
- Observe for non-verbal signals, gestures or signs which the person may use to communicate their wishes, such as pushing the dish away. It is important to respect people's wishes.
- In people's own homes, community nurses can observe what food there is around and whether it is within the sell-by date. Out-of-date food could indicate that food is being bought but not actually eaten. These were important observations for Mr Cooper's CPN to make. Regarding Phillip, the community nurse for learning disability and occupational therapist could observe what food he is buying and storing.
- Observe food intake, which will indicate the amount of food that is actually being consumed. Such details recorded over several days allow for any day-to-day fluctuations. It was good practice that the staff on the medical ward from which Miss West was transferred were recording her food and fluid intake on a food chart. *The Essence of Care*'s benchmark for good practice is: 'The amount of food patients actually eat is monitored, recorded and leads to further action when cause for concern' (DH 2001a). The nurses on the rehabilitation unit should check back over charts from previous days. Three days should be sufficient to assess a patient's eating habits and then a decision can be made as to what additional support is needed. This may be by the nurse or may involve the dietician.

Learning outcome 2: Understand the purpose and use of nutritional screening tools

Nutritional screening is the process of identifying people at risk of malnourishment. The Malnutrition Advisory Group (MAG), part of BAPEN, developed 'MUST' for use with adults at risk of malnutrition (Todorovic *et al.* 2003). 'MUST' is downloadable from www.bapen.org.uk along with detailed screening guidelines and is advocated as the tool that all healthcare settings should be using. The components of the tool and its usage are presented next, but do refer to the website documents for further explanation.

Nutritional screening and care planning with 'MUST'

Todorovic *et al.* (2003. p. 4) explain that:

> [Nutritional screening is] the first step in identifying people who may be at nutritional risk or potentially at risk, and who may benefit from appropriate nutritional intervention. It is a rapid, simple and general procedure used by nursing, medical, or other staff on first contact with patients so that clear guidelines for action can be implemented and appropriate nutritional advice provided.

Todorovic *et al.* point out that repeated screening may be necessary when a person's condition and nutritional risk change, and that it is always better to prevent or detect problems early by screening than discover serious problems later. Box 10.2 presents how to screen using 'MUST'. The steps in the process, summarised from Todorovic *et al.* (2003), are explained next.

Step 1: Body mass index (BMI)

The BMI provides a 'rapid interpretation of chronic protein-energy status based on an individual's height and weight' (Todorovic *et al.* 2003, p. 5). Box 10.3 explains how to measure height and weight accurately. The formula to calculate BMI is:

$$\frac{\text{Weight in kilogrammes}}{(\text{Height in metres})^2}$$

The chart in Fig. 10.1 displays BMI scores based on weight and height and the corresponding 'MUST' score. In some care settings, entering the weight and height into an electronic patient record will automatically generate the BMI measurement. Todorovic *et al.* advise that, if weight and height measurements are not available, it may be appropriate to use self-reported height or weight.

ACTIVITY

Calculate:
- Phillip's BMI, if his weight is 92 kg and his height is 1.68 m
- Mr Cooper's BMI if his height is 1.9 m and his weight is 64 kg.

Looking at Fig. 10.1, what would their BMI scores be for the 'MUST' screening? Phillip's BMI is 33. The chart classifies this as 'obese', and his score for Step 1 of the 'MUST' is 0. Mr Cooper's BMI is 18, giving his score for Step 1 of the 'MUST' as 2.

> **Box 10.2 How to screen using the 'MUST' (Todorovic *et al.* 2003, page 4). The Malnutrition Universal Screening tool is reproduced here with kind permission of BAPEN**
>
> There are five steps to follow.
> - **Steps 1 and 2**. Gather nutritional measurements (height, weight, BMI, recent unplanned weight loss). *If it is not possible to obtain height and weight, use alternative measurements.*
> - **Step 3**. Consider the acute disease effect.
> - **Step 4**. Determine the overall risk score or category of malnutrition. *If neither BMI nor weight loss can be established, assess overall risk subjectively using other criteria* (see Box 10.4)
> - **Step 5**. Using the management guidelines and/or local policy, form an appropriate care plan.

> **Box 10.3 Measuring height and weight (Adapted from Todorovic *et al.* 2003)**
>
> Height
> - Use a height stick (stadiometer) if available. Ensure it is correctly positioned against the wall.
> - Ask the person to remove their shoes and to stand upright, feet flat, heels against the height stick or wall (if height stick not used).
> - Ask the person to look straight ahead. Lower the head plate until it gently touches the top of the head.
> - Read and document height.
> - Some people's height may need to be measured while lying in bed.
>
> Weight
> - Use clinical scales wherever possible and make sure they have been regularly checked for accuracy.
> - Ensure that the scales read zero without the person standing on them.
> - Weigh the person in light clothing and without shoes.
> - Bed scales are available to weigh patients restricted to bed. Hoist scales are also available.

Step 2

Todorovic *et al.* identify that unplanned weight loss over 3–6 months is 'a more acute risk factor for malnutrition than BMI' (p. 6). You can ask the person whether they have lost weight in the last 3–6 months and, if so, how much. You can also check their records. Then calculate how much weight has been lost and use weight-loss tables (Todorovic *et al.* 2003, p. 22) to identify the weight-loss score:

- 2 if >10 per cent of body weight ;
- 1 if 5–10 per cent of body weight ;
- 0 if <5 per cent of body weight

Note: Take care when interpreting a patient's BMI or percentage weight loss in some circumstances, for example fluid disturbances, pregnancy, lactation, critical illness

Height (feet and inches)

Weight (kg)	4'10½	4'11	5'0	5'0½	5'1½	5'2	5'3	5'4	5'4½	5'5½	5'6	5'7	5'7½	5'8½	5'9½	5'10½	5'11	5'11½	6'0½	6'1	6'2	6'3	Weight (stones and pounds)
100	46	44	43	42	41	40	39	38	37	36	35	35	34	33	32	32	31	30	30	29	28	28	15 10
99	45	44	43	42	41	40	39	38	38	36	36	35	34	33	33	32	31	30	30	29	28	27	15 8
98	45	44	42	41	40	39	38	37	36	36	35	34	33	32	32	31	31	30	30	29	28	28	15 6
97	44	43	42	41	40	39	38	37	36	35	34	34	33	32	31	31	30	29	29	28	27	27	15 4
96	44	43	42	40	39	38	38	37	36	35	34	33	32	32	31	30	30	29	28	28	27	27	15 2
95	43	42	41	40	39	38	37	36	35	34	34	33	32	31	30	30	29	29	28	27	27	26	15 0
94	43	42	41	40	39	38	37	36	35	34	33	33	32	31	30	30	29	28	28	27	27	26	14 11
93	42	41	40	39	38	37	36	35	35	34	33	32	31	31	30	29	29	28	27	27	26	26	14 9
92	42	41	40	39	38	37	36	35	34	33	33	32	31	30	30	29	29	28	27	27	26	25	14 7
91	42	40	39	39	37	36	36	35	34	33	32	31	31	30	29	29	28	27	27	26	26	25	14 5
90	41	40	39	38	37	36	35	34	33	33	32	31	30	30	29	28	28	27	27	26	25	25	14 2
89	41	40	39	38	37	36	35	34	33	32	32	31	30	29	29	28	27	27	26	26	25	25	14 0
88	40	39	38	37	36	35	34	34	33	32	31	30	30	29	29	28	28	27	27	26	26	25	13 12
87	40	39	38	37	36	35	34	33	32	32	31	30	29	29	28	27	27	26	26	25	25	24	13 10
86	39	38	37	37	35	34	34	33	32	31	30	30	29	28	28	27	27	26	25	25	24	24	13 8
85	39	38	37	36	35	34	33	32	31	31	30	29	29	28	27	27	26	25	25	24	24	23	13 6
84	38	37	36	35	35	34	33	32	31	30	30	29	28	28	27	26	25	25	24	24	23	23	13 3
83	38	37	36	35	34	33	32	32	31	30	29	29	28	27	27	26	26	25	25	24	23	23	13 1
82	37	36	35	35	34	33	32	31	30	30	29	28	28	27	26	26	25	25	24	23	23	22	12 13
81	37	36	35	34	33	32	32	31	30	29	29	28	27	27	26	26	25	24	24	23	23	22	12 11
80	37	36	35	34	33	32	31	30	30	29	28	28	27	26	26	25	24	24	23	23	22	22	12 8
79	36	35	34	33	32	32	31	30	29	29	28	27	27	26	25	25	24	24	23	23	22	22	12 6
78	36	35	34	33	32	31	30	30	29	28	28	27	26	26	25	25	24	23	23	22	22	21	12 4
77	35	34	33	32	32	31	30	29	29	28	27	27	26	25	25	24	24	23	23	22	22	21	12 1
76	35	34	33	32	31	30	30	29	28	27	27	26	26	25	24	24	23	23	22	22	22	21	11 13
75	34	33	32	32	31	30	29	29	28	27	27	26	25	25	24	24	23	23	22	22	21	21	11 11
74	34	33	32	31	30	30	29	28	28	27	26	26	25	24	24	23	23	22	22	21	21	20	11 9
73	33	32	32	31	30	29	29	28	27	26	26	25	25	24	24	23	23	22	22	21	21	20	11 7
72	33	32	31	30	30	29	28	27	27	26	26	25	24	24	23	23	22	22	21	21	20	20	11 4
71	32	32	31	30	29	28	28	27	26	26	25	25	24	23	23	22	22	21	21	20	20	19	11 3
70	32	31	30	30	29	28	27	27	26	25	25	24	24	23	23	22	22	21	20	20	20	19	11 0
69	32	31	30	29	28	28	27	26	26	25	25	24	24	23	23	22	22	21	21	20	20	19	10 11
68	31	30	29	29	28	27	27	26	25	25	24	24	23	22	22	21	21	21	20	20	19	19	10 10
67	31	30	29	28	28	27	26	26	25	24	24	23	23	22	22	21	21	20	20	19	19	18	10 7
66	30	29	29	28	27	26	26	25	25	24	23	23	22	22	21	21	20	20	19	19	19	18	10 6
65	30	29	28	27	27	26	25	25	24	24	23	22	22	21	21	20	20	19	19	18	18	18	10 3
64	29	28	28	27	26	26	25	24	24	23	23	22	22	21	21	20	20	19	19	18	18	17	10 1
63	29	28	27	27	26	25	25	24	23	23	22	22	21	21	20	20	19	19	18	18	18	17	9 13
62	28	28	27	26	25	25	24	24	23	22	22	21	21	20	20	19	19	18	18	18	17	17	9 10
61	28	27	26	26	25	24	24	23	23	22	21	21	20	20	19	19	18	18	18	17	17	17	9 8
60	27	27	26	25	25	24	23	23	22	22	21	21	20	20	19	19	18	18	17	17	17	16	9 6
59	27	26	26	25	24	24	23	22	22	21	21	20	20	19	19	18	18	17	17	17	16	16	9 4
58	26	26	25	24	24	23	23	22	22	21	20	20	19	19	18	18	18	17	17	16	16	16	9 1
57	26	25	25	24	23	23	22	22	21	21	20	20	19	19	18	18	17	17	16	16	16	16	9 0
56	26	25	24	24	23	22	22	21	21	20	20	19	19	18	18	17	17	17	16	16	16	15	8 11
55	25	24	24	23	23	22	21	21	20	20	19	19	19	18	18	17	17	16	16	16	15	15	8 8
54	25	24	23	23	22	22	21	21	20	20	19	19	18	18	17	17	16	16	16	15	15	15	8 7
53	24	24	23	22	22	21	21	20	20	19	18	18	17	17	17	16	16	16	15	15	15	14	8 4
52	24	23	23	22	21	21	20	20	19	19	18	18	17	17	16	16	16	15	15	14	14	14	8 3
51	23	23	22	22	21	20	20	19	19	18	18	17	17	16	16	16	15	15	15	14	14	14	8 0
50	23	22	22	21	20	20	19	19	18	18	17	17	16	16	16	15	15	15	14	14	14	14	7 13
49	22	22	21	21	20	20	19	19	18	18	17	17	16	16	15	15	15	14	14	14	14	13	7 10
48	22	21	21	20	20	19	19	18	18	17	17	16	16	15	15	15	14	14	14	14	13	13	7 7
47	21	21	20	20	19	19	18	18	17	17	16	16	15	15	15	14	14	14	13	13	13	13	7 6
46	21	20	20	19	19	18	18	17	17	16	16	15	15	15	14	14	14	13	13	13	13	12	7 3
45	21	20	19	19	18	18	18	17	17	16	16	15	15	15	14	14	13	13	13	13	12	12	7 1
44	20	20	19	19	18	18	17	17	16	16	15	15	14	14	14	13	13	13	13	12	12	12	6 13
43	20	19	19	18	18	17	17	16	16	15	15	14	14	14	13	13	13	12	12	12	12	12	6 11
42	19	19	18	18	17	17	16	16	16	15	15	14	14	13	13	13	12	12	12	12	12	11	6 8
41	19	18	18	17	17	16	16	16	15	15	14	14	13	13	13	12	12	12	12	11	11	11	6 6
40	18	18	17	17	16	16	16	15	15	14	14	13	13	13	12	12	12	12	11	11	11	11	6 4
39	18	17	17	16	16	15	15	15	14	14	13	13	13	12	12	12	11	11	11	11	11	11	6 1
38	17	17	16	16	16	15	15	14	14	13	13	13	12	12	12	11	11	11	11	11	11	10	6 0
37	17	16	16	16	15	15	14	14	13	13	13	12	12	12	11	11	11	11	10	10	10	10	5 11
36	16	16	16	15	15	14	14	13	13	13	12	12	12	11	11	11	11	10	10	10	10	10	5 9
35	16	16	15	15	14	14	14	13	13	12	12	12	12	11	11	11	10	10	10	10	10	10	5 7
34	16	15	15	14	14	14	13	13	13	12	12	12	11	11	11	11	10	10	10	10	10	9	5 5

Overlaid diagonal band labels: Score 0 (obese), Score 0, Score 1, Score 2

| | 1.48 | 1.50 | 1.52 | 1.54 | 1.56 | 1.58 | 1.60 | 1.62 | 1.64 | 1.66 | 1.68 | 1.70 | 1.72 | 1.74 | 1.76 | 1.78 | 1.80 | 1.82 | 1.84 | 1.86 | 1.88 | 1.90 | |

Height (m)

Note : The black lines denote the exact cut off points (30, 20 and 18.5kg/m), figures on the chart have been rounded to the nearest whole number.

Figure 10.1: Body mass index score (BAPEN 2003, page 2). Reproduced here with kind permission of BAPEN.

> **Box 10.4 Other criteria (Todorovic *et al.* 2003, page 7). Reproduced here with kind permission of BAPEN**
>
> If height, weight or BMI cannot be obtained, the following criteria which relate to them can help form a clinical impression of an individual's overall nutritional risk. The factors listed below can either contribute to or influence the risk of malnutrition.
>
> *Note:* Use of these criteria will not result in an actual score for nutritional risk but will help indicate whether or not a person is at increased risk of malnutrition.
>
> BMI
> • Clinical impression – thin, acceptable weight, overweight. Obvious wasting (very thin) and obesity (very overweight) can be noted.
>
> Weight loss
> • Clothes and/or jewellery have become loose fitting.
> • History of decreased food intake, reduced appetite or dysphagia (swallowing problems) over 3–6 months and underlying disease or psychosocial/ physical disabilities likely to cause weight loss.
>
> Acute disease
> • No nutritional intake or likelihood of no intake for more than 5 days.
> **Estimate a malnutrition risk score based on your evaluation.**

(i.e. no dietary intake for >5 days) and presence of plaster casts. Adjustments of body weight can be made for amputations (for details, see Todorovic *et al.* 2003).

Step 3

If the person has an acute illness and there has been no nutritional intake, or it is likely that there will be none for more than 5 days, they score 2.

Step 4: Overall risk of malnutrition

The scores from Steps 1, 2 and 3 are added to provide the overall risk of malnutrition:

$$0 = \text{low risk;} \qquad 1 = \text{medium risk;} \qquad 2 \text{ or more} = \text{high risk.}$$

Note: If neither BMI nor weight loss could be calculated, the score is assessed taking other criteria into account (see Box 10.4). The observations discussed earlier (in learning outcome 1) will contribute to this estimation.

Step 5: Management guidelines

Table 10.1 presents action required according to the MUST score. Todorovic *et al.* (2003, p. 9) advise that a care plan should be developed as follows:

1. Set aims and objectives of treatment.
2. Treat any underlying conditions.
3. Treat malnutrition with food and/or nutritional supplements (see next chapter section). People who cannot meet their nutritional requirements orally may need artificial nutritional support (see later chapter section on enteral and parenteral nutrition). Combinations of any or all of these may be needed. For people who are overweight or obese, follow local weight management guidelines.

Table 10.1: Management plan based on 'MUST' score (Todorovic *et al.* 2003, p. 8). Reproduced here with kind permission of BAPEN.

'MUST' score (BMI + weight loss + acute disease effect)	Overall risk of malnutrition	Action
2 or >2	High	Treat, unless detrimental or no benefit from nutritional support expected; e.g. imminent death
1	Medium	Observe, or treat if approaching high risk or if rapid clinical deterioration expected
0	Low	Routine care, unless major clinical deterioration expected

In obese people, underlying acute conditions are generally controlled before treating obesity.

4. Monitor and review nutritional interventions and care plan.
5. Reassess people identified as being at nutritional risk as they move through care settings. Therefore Miss West's score should have been recalculated on admission to the rehabilitation unit.

ACTIVITY

> Compare 'MUST' with any screening tools used in your practice setting. You should find that the key features are the same.

Learning outcome 3: Carry out nutritional screening and recognise if people are at risk of malnutrition

Nutritional screening tools have been designed to enable nurses to make an accurate and quick assessment of patients/clients.

ACTIVITY

> Using the information provided about Miss West in the scenario, and 'MUST', work out her risk of malnutrition. Remember to use Fig. 10.1 to calculate her BMI score. As discussed previously, you can use weight-loss tables to calculate her percentage weight loss in Todorovic *et al.* (2003) (accessed at www.bapen.org.uk).

Your assessment should have clearly identified Miss West as being at high risk. Compare your scoring with that below:

- Step 1 – BMI. Figure 10.1 shows that Miss West's BMI is 20, so she scores 1.
- Step 2 – weight loss. Miss West has lost 5 kg since admission. The weight-loss table calculates that she has lost 5–10 per cent of her body weight, thus scoring 1. Miss West's loose dentures also suggest some weight loss.
- Step 3 – acute disease can affect risk of malnutrition. Miss West is eating small amounts but this needs to be monitored, and she has had a stroke, so she scores 2 on this step.

- Step 4 – overall risk of malnutrition. There is a scoring system incorporated into all nutritional screening tools and this helps nurses to categorise people's risk status. Overall Miss West has scored 4, so she is at high risk and therefore a plan of care needs to be initiated .
- Step 5 – management guidelines. The next sections in the chapter detail likely interventions.

ACTIVITY

Practise using 'MUST' with some other people:
- Find a willing colleague and assess his/her nutritional status by working through the screening tool. We hope the result falls into the low-risk category.
- Think back to a person you have been caring for recently and work through the tool. Are you surprised at the score you obtained?

You have now practised using the screening tool with several individuals. If you are used to using a different screening tool, you might like to try using this too. Once you have established that a person is at risk of malnutrition you need to develop a plan of action. If the person is at high risk (like Miss West), she will need referral to a dietician for an in-depth nutritional assessment, and additional nutritional support may be needed. However, there are many ways in which nurses can help people to meet their nutritional needs, based on their individual assessment.

Summary
- Observations can usefully contribute to assessment of nutritional status.
- Nutritional screening allows rapid identification of patients at risk of malnutrition, and 'MUST' is recommended for adults in all settings.
- After screening is completed, an appropriate action plan must be developed and implemented.

ASSISTING PEOPLE WITH EATING AND DRINKING

Most people eat independently. However, physical or mental impairment, debilitating illness or generalised weakness may make people physically unable to eat and drink without assistance. Some people will be able to eat independently, as long as they have been prepared well and provided with support (e.g. positioning, equipment). These aspects are discussed in detail in this section. Other patients will need complete assistance with eating and then nurses must do everything possible to make this a pleasant experience and to ensure that their nutritional intake is adequate. When handling food in care settings, good food hygiene is essential and this is also discussed.

To gain the most from this section you need the opportunity to assist someone with eating, so you might like to work through the section with a colleague, or another willing volunteer. You will also need a variety of foods: hot, cold, chewy and soft.

Learning outcome 1: Identify how food hygiene can be promoted

Chapter 3 focused on preventing cross-infection and, when involved with food, nurses must adhere to the principles discussed. This is important for people of all age groups but particularly people who are vulnerable to cross-infection, such as people who are immunocompromised and older people, like Miss West and Mr Cooper.

ACTIVITY

> When next in the practice setting, actively observe what precautions nurses and other staff take when handling food.

Good food hygiene must be practised in all areas. Food poisoning outbreaks in healthcare settings are not uncommon. The *Guide to Food Hygiene* (Food Standards Agency 2002) provides a detailed guide to safe food handling and also outlines relevant legislation. The document identifies four main defences against the growth and spread of bacteria:

- ensuring food areas are clean and good standards of personal hygiene are maintained;
- cooking foods thoroughly;
- keeping foods at the right temperature;
- preventing cross-contamination.

You should therefore have observed staff performing hand hygiene before serving meals, wearing a clean apron (perhaps a different colour to that worn for other care activities), and keeping food covered and utensils clean, with one serving utensil per menu item.

Learning outcome 2: Assist people with eating and drinking

It is important to consider the environment in which patients are eating. In *The Essence of Care* the best practice benchmark states 'The environment is conducive to enabling the individual patients/clients to eat' (DH 2001a).

ACTIVITY

> What do you think nurses can do to make the environment in a care setting conducive for eating in?

You might have considered removing any unpleasant odours and sights and making sure that the table is cleaned. Some care settings have a separate dining area, so if possible assist people to leave the bedside and sit at a dining table to eat. The table should be set properly. Ward cleaning and bed-making must never be carried out during mealtimes, and patients should not be disturbed by other healthcare professionals carrying out ward rounds.

ACTIVITY How might nurses help patients to eat and drink? Consider how Miss West can be helped to eat independently, and the correct technique for assisting her.

Oral hygiene

Ensure that your patient's mouth is clean and that dentures have been washed. Many people leave dentures in soak overnight, so prior to serving breakfast ensure that they have been cleaned, rinsed and reinserted.

Comfort and hygiene

Offer use of the toilet before eating and offer a handwash prior to meals.

Environment

Try to create a pleasant and calm environment at mealtimes. Remove obstructions from the patient's eating area (e.g. Zimmer frames, commodes, urine bottles). If appropriate, help Miss West to move to the area she wishes to eat in – patients should have freedom to choose where, and with whom, they sit.

Positioning

Miss West should be helped into a safe and comfortable position for eating. Patients should always eat and drink in an upright position, as close to 90 degrees as possible and in the midline. This lessens the risk of food passing into the respiratory tract, causing choking. Sitting out of bed in a comfortable chair is preferable to sitting up in bed. Ideally the person should sit upright with their feet on the ground, their body well supported and their head tipped slightly forward (Crawley 2003). There may be circumstances when it is not possible for people to be positioned upright, and then a side-lying position can be substituted. It is advisable to use a pillow or similar support placed behind the back to prevent accidental rolling on to the back (Shanley and Starrs 1993).

Clothing protection

Offer the patient a serviette or protection for their clothing if they would like it. Avoid using plastic bibs or paper towels because this will reduce self-esteem and dignity.

Giving food choices

Tell the patient what the choices of food are. Ideally show the patient the food as the smell can induce appetite and appearance also influences food choice. Help your patient choose their meal – ensure you understand what is on the menu, particularly when describing casseroles. Assess whether it is lamb or beef etc. Explain clearly anything they do not understand. Encourage them to eat food that is appropriate for their needs, such as soft diet, low in sugar, low in fat.

Individual dietary needs

Ensure that patients have expressed their individual dietary requirements to the staff. Do not presume about ethnic meal requirements.

Food presentation

Try to ensure that food is well presented, at the right consistency and temperature to encourage the patient. The food should be prepared on a tray that is clean with an appropriate drink, a napkin and cutlery. Try to set the meal out so that it tempts the appetite and is enticing to eat.

Condiments

Provide a range of condiments – individual sachets of salt, pepper, mustard, vinegar, mint sauce, horseradish – and allow the patient time to choose.

Portion size

Serve food in sensible portions to suit the patient's needs. For a person with a poor appetite (like Miss West), presentation and portion size might influence whether the food will be eaten. A large meal could be overwhelming, so a small portion is better. Second helpings can then be offered if wished.

Correct consistency

Ensure specific advice from the MDT is followed regarding diet as appropriate; e.g. puree diet/thickened fluids as recommended by the speech and language therapist (SLT). Many people with eating difficulties (like Miss West) need texture-modified food and fluids, for example pureed/liquidised, or thickened. Where food needs to be liquidised, each item should be liquidised separately to preserve distinctive flavours. The SLT may recommend thickened fluids to help to prevent the choking that can occur with liquid. Nurses need to be aware that such foods may lead to lower energy density meals (Crawley 2003).

Positioning of food

Ensure that the food is within Miss West's reach and inform her that the food is in front of her. This is particularly important as she is partially sighted. The Health Advisory Service 2000 (1998) reported a relative saying 'Dad often missed breakfast (he is blind and deaf) and it would be taken away uneaten – he did not know it was there and he got very distressed about it' (p. 16).

The clock method

As Miss West has a visual impairment, make her aware of the position of the food on the plate using the clock method to explain (see Fig. 10.2). Ensure that the plate is not the same colour as the table, as this helps people who have a visual impairment to identify the plate.

Providing the correct equipment

Ensure the patient has access to specialist equipment if required for eating and drinking (e.g. adaptive cutlery, plate guard, wide-spouted beaker). You may need to liaise with the occupational therapist on this. Non-slip mats prevent the plate from moving around and are useful for people (like Miss West) who can use only one hand. Lipped plates are high-rimmed plates and bowls that prevent the food from being pushed off or over the side. This allows people with erratic hand and arm movements to manage with a degree of independence. Plate guards work in a similar way. Cups with two handles or even padded handles can improve an older person's independence (Eberhardie 2003). Insulated beakers can be useful for people who are slow to eat or drink as this keeps the liquid hot for longer.

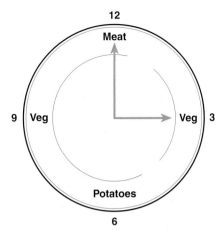

Figure 10.2: The clock method. This is a means of helping people with visual impairment to find their food. Place the food on the plate roughly at the quarter hours. Explain to the person that the meat is at the 12 o'clock position on the plate and the vegetables are at quarter past and quarter to the hour, and the potatoes are at the half-past position. Ensure that you keep the foods separate.

Assisting people to eat

You need to assess exactly how much help Miss West needs. This might range from cutting up food and giving verbal encouragement and reinforcement, to total assistance if she is unable to feed herself at all. The technique for this is discussed in detail next. With some people it is a matter of giving time and not hurrying. Do open cartons, remove lids, cut up food and spread butter on bread, because for some people this is all that is needed to eat independently. Someone who has cerebral palsy might take up to three times as long to eat. They would also need some assistance to ensure that they can safely regulate the flow of liquid. You should observe for signs of fatigue and offer to help when necessary.

Assisting people who cannot eat unaided

When assisting with eating, nurses must demonstrate a caring attitude, appreciating that people who cannot eat independently may experience feelings of helplessness and loss of self-esteem and dignity. Try to encourage social contact at mealtimes.

- Draw up a chair or stool and sit at eye level with the patient to convey a relaxed approach, indicating that you are going to spend time with the patient and value them.
- Ask the person in what order they would like the food and drink. They may communicate this through non-verbal rather than verbal communication, and it is important to observe reactions closely. Food should be cut into bite-sized proportions. If a soft diet is being given, adjust the portion according to the size of the mouth.
- Use normal cutlery/crockery appropriate to the food, as in a fork for the main course, a spoon for the pudding.
- Help your patient eat in a socially acceptable manner. If necessary, help the person to wipe away excess food from the mouth, clothes or hands after eating.

- Offer drinks that the patient may enjoy during and after mealtime. Establish when they want it (during or after) and what they would like.
- Allow patients to eat at their own pace. Allow time for the person to chew and swallow the food and drink, before offering the next mouthful. Do not hurry the person.
- Observe for any signs of choking, for example coughing or poor colour, and stop feeding if this is suspected. Be especially vigilant if you know that the person has a history of swallowing problems, which may accompany neurological impairment.
- Ensure specific safe swallowing strategies as recommended by the MDT are followed as appropriate (e.g. encourage clearing swallows, use of teaspoons etc.).
- Offer second helpings if possible.
- When the person indicates that they have finished, remove the equipment and offer further drink and the opportunity to clean their mouth and teeth. Particles of food left in the mouth may cause dental decay, or sores can develop around the gums.
- Complete documentation (discussed later), and evaluate the service provided with the patient. Are there any other care needs that are to be met?

ACTIVITY

With a willing colleague, feed each other using a variety of food and drink – cold, hot, soft and chewy. Then try some of the following positions for eating:
- sitting in a scrunched up position;
- sitting on your hands with a blindfold covering your eyes;
- lying fairly flat on your side and pretending that you cannot move. (As discussed above, this is not a recommended position for eating and should be used only for a person who, for medical reasons, has to lie flat.)

Now ask your colleague about your technique. What did they feel you did well? What do they feel you could do better? Then reflect on the experience:
- How did it feel to feed/be fed?
- What would have made the experience better?
- What have you learned from this activity?

Reporting/evaluating/documenting

After assisting a person with eating and drinking you should complete any relevant documentation, such as filling in the food chart and/or fluid balance chart. Remember to report any unusual occurrence to the nurse in charge. Review the plan of care and evaluate. Is it still appropriate? Does it need changing?

Other approaches

For people who are in non-hospital settings other approaches may be employed. For example, in some mental health units nurses eat with clients so they can encourage and prompt them to eat. For paranoid clients, it may dispel fear of poisoning if the nurse is eating the same meal from the same source. In some settings facilities to make snacks, for example sandwiches, are available and for a person with paranoia it may be less frightening to make their own food from raw materials than to eat pre-cooked food, which they may fear has been poisoned. Alternatively, they may accept food brought in by their own family.

Summary

- Good food hygiene is essential in care settings.
- When assisting with oral intake of food and drink the nurse should prepare the patient, the environment and the food carefully, and try to promote mealtimes as enjoyable and relaxed events.
- The nurse's approach should ensure that the person feels valued and does not feel rushed.
- Good hygiene should be maintained, including handwashing and oral care for the patient.
- Monitoring and recording food intake is important, especially when a patient has been assessed as at high risk of malnutrition.
- Reviewing the plan of care is vital after every meal.

ADDITIONAL NUTRITIONAL SUPPORT STRATEGIES

Nurses have a responsibility to assist and support patients in meeting nutritional needs. This section considers how the MDT can be involved to support nutrition and how the nutritional value of a person's oral intake can be improved.

LEARNING OUTCOMES

At the end of this section you will be able to:
1 identify other healthcare professionals who may be involved in the nutritional care of clients;
2 discuss how the nutritional value of a person's oral intake can be enhanced.

Learning outcome 1: Identify other healthcare professionals who may be involved in the nutritional care of clients

ACTIVITY

List healthcare professionals who might be able to help people with meeting their nutritional needs. Some have already been mentioned in this chapter. Think back to the patients/clients in the scenarios and identify healthcare professionals who might be appropriate for referrals.

Dieticians

Dieticians are experts in nutrition, able to perform comprehensive assessments of people's nutritional status and needs. They are able to offer general healthy eating advice, guidance for the use of dietary supplements and specific advice for dietary management in relation to medical disorders. Some dieticians specialise in certain age groups, for example older people.

As Miss West's screening identified she was at high risk of malnutrition she must be referred to the dietician. If Mr Cooper is found to be high-risk when nutritional screening is carried out, referral to a dietician would be appropriate for him too. A dietician can educate Phillip about eating healthily and his carers too so they can support Phillip in making healthy food choices, and also make Phillip and his carers aware of the implications of not making dietary changes.

Speech and language therapists

SLTs are able to assist people of all ages and abilities with chewing and swallowing problems (like Miss West, who had dysphagia following a stroke). It could be worthwhile asking an SLT to reassess Miss West's swallowing as she is still having problems eating. SLTs will advise on whether it is possible for people to take food orally and, if so, whether special precautions are necessary, such as using thickening agents.

Physicians

Dietary supplements may need to be prescribed by a doctor. For some people there may be an underlying medical problem affecting their nutrition, which needs to be treated. For example, in some instances weight gain, as experienced by Phillip, can be caused by an underlying medical condition, for example an underactive thyroid gland (hypothyroidism).

Pharmacists

Pharmacists may have a role in advising physicians and may also be involved in aspects of enteral and parenteral nutrition.

Dentists

Dentists may assist people with dental or denture problems. If Miss West's dentures fitted properly, this could help considerably with her eating. The CPN should check whether referral to a dentist would be appropriate for Mr Cooper too.

Community support

Some health centres have health advisors for older people, and this could be relevant to Miss West when she is discharged and for providing additional support for Mr Cooper.

Psychologists

A referral to a psychologist would be appropriate if a person has an eating disorder, for example, but could also be relevant to Miss West in relation to her possible depression.

Physiotherapists

Physiotherapists can assist people with motor problems, for example following a stroke, and help with their positioning. This is likely to be helpful for Miss West.

Occupational therapists

An occupational therapist may be able to identify suitable aids to assist with eating and drinking and positioning, thus promoting independence. Miss West would be likely to benefit from this help. The occupational therapist could assist Phillip in improving his skills in food preparation.

Social workers

A social worker would be involved in arranging home care packages, including home-carers to serve meals and shop, and meals on wheels. This may well be essential to enable Miss West to maintain her nutrition after discharge from hospital. The CPN visiting Mr Cooper will belong to a Community Mental Health Team for the over 65s, which is a MDT and includes social workers. The different members of the team will appear on his Care Programme Approach plan, with their input identified. His plan may well need reviewing and additional support planned.

Another source of help for Phillip could be to attend a 'Healthy lifestyles' course, aimed at his age group and covering a range of issues such as nutrition and exercise, which will be run by a group of professionals including the dietician, occupational therapist and community nurse for learning disabilities.

Learning outcome 2: Discuss how the nutritional value of a person's oral intake can be enhanced

Sometimes if appetite is poor or a person is very unwell, food intake may be insufficient to meet nutritional needs. Other people might have increased nutritional needs as a result of a higher metabolic rate caused by chronic illness (Moules and Ramsay 1998). Build-ups may need to be given and can be advised by qualified nursing staff; alternatively, supplements may be needed which require prescription.

ACTIVITY	What supplements have you seen in practice to increase the nutritional value of patient's or client's oral intake?

A wide range of supplements are available, some of which are designed to be added to the normal diet (e.g. powdered glucose polymers such as Maxijul and Polycal), or to be taken as a drink between normal meals (e.g. Fresubin, Fortisip and Enlive) (Holden and MacDonald 1997). The purpose of these is to increase the nutritional value of oral intake; some provide just calories while others provide proteins, vitamins and minerals in addition. A dietician can advise which is most appropriate for an individual person following a comprehensive nutritional assessment. There are a wide variety of flavours available, and for both Miss West and Mr Cooper it may be possible to find some acceptable. These supplements can be a very good way of increasing nutritional intake.

Even with the use of supplements, it may not be possible for some people to fully meet their nutritional needs with oral intake. Other people may not be able to take food and drink orally at all owing to an inability to swallow. This may be for a temporary period (e.g. if a person is unconscious for a few days) but for some people it can be permanent. In these situations, you might have seen people fed by tube (enteral feeding) or through an intravenous infusion (parenteral feeding). The next sections explore these methods.

Summary

- A multidisciplinary approach to promoting nutrition will optimise specialist skills and knowledge, giving patients and clients the best chance of having their individual nutritional needs met in full.
- If nutritional needs cannot be met through a person's usual oral diet, other alternatives must be found. These could be oral supplements, enteral feeding or parenteral feeding. The dietician's input and advice is essential in these situations.

ENTERAL AND PARENTERAL FEEDING

Enteral feeding may be achieved via a **nasogastric tube** (a tube passed via the nose down the oesophagus and into the stomach), or via a **gastrostomy tube**, which is an opening in the abdominal wall through which a tube is passed to allow feeds to enter the stomach directly. Both these procedures are invasive and consent must be gained from the patient – written consent for gastrostomy, which is a surgical procedure. A gastrostomy provides more secure nutritional provision than nasogastric tube feeding.

Enteral feeding may be used to supplement or completely replace oral intake. Examples might be to maintain adequate nutrition for a person with severe neurological impairment as a result of cerebral palsy or stroke where swallowing is extremely difficult or hazardous, or for people whose nutritional needs exceed their oral intake, owing to a health problem. Both these methods have benefits and hazards associated with them (Davies 1999). Medicines may be prescribed via the enteral tube route and this procedure is included in this section too. In some circumstances the enteral route cannot be used and this section also identifies the role of parenteral nutrition and intravenous fluid administration.

LEARNING OUTCOMES

By the end of this section you will be able to:

1 discuss nasogastric tube insertion and care;
2 explain the specific care needed following gastrostomy;
3 outline key principles for administering enteral feeds;
4 discuss the process of administering medicines by the enteral route.
5 identify the role of parenteral nutrition and intravenous fluid administration in maintaining patient nutrition.

Learning outcome 1: Discuss nasogastric tube insertion and care

Prior to nasogastric tube (NGT) insertion, key issues to consider are:

- whether the need for the tube is clinically indicated, appropriate and documented;
- whether the use of an NGT is for drainage or feeding (this section focuses mainly on NGTs for feeding although insertion of NGTs for drainage is discussed briefly);
- how to ensure the position of the tube is checked after insertion;
- what the ongoing management of the tube will entail.

Inserting an NGT for feeding

Find out what NGTs are used in your care setting. You may also be able to look at these tubes in the skills laboratory. What are their key features?

NGTs used for feeding people vary according to care setting but should be fine-bore feeding tubes. A decision must be made whether or not to insert a tube within 24 hours of identifying the need and appropriateness of enteral feeding. Consent must be gained from the patient and any potential contraindications to passing the NGT should be identified:

* previous surgery/trauma;
* oesophageal varices, stricture or other upper gastrointestinal pathology;
* complex head and neck problems (e.g. tumour, altered anatomy);
* trauma from poisoning (e.g. oral consumption of bleach);
* poor level of consciousness.

Any of the above should be discussed with the clinical team as the doctor or gastroenterology team may be required to insert the NGT under radiological guidance.

Table 10.2 and Fig. 10.3 outline the procedure for passing a nasogastric feeding tube, with the rationale explained. Checking of the NGT position is an essential element which is discussed in more detail next.

Table 10.2: Insertion of a nasogastric feeding tube (adapted from Whipps Cross University Hospital NHS Trust clinical procedure).

Wash hands and then prepare equipment:
Clinically clean tray/trolley, fine-bore nasogastric tube (NGT) with wire, sterile receiver, sterile water, 50 mL syringe, hypoallergenic tape, adhesive patch from NGT packet, glass of water, pH paper/indicator strips

Action	Rationale
Prepare the patient Arrange a signal by which the patient can communicate if he/she wants the nurse to stop (e.g. by raising his/her hand)	Reduces fear by giving the patient some control over the procedure
Assist the patient to sit in a semi-upright position in the bed or chair with head supported by pillows; or if unconscious, on their side, supported by pillows The head should not be tilted backwards or forwards	Ensures patient comfort and allows for easy passage of the tube Enables easy swallowing and ensures that the epiglottis is not obstructing the oesophagus
Ask the patient to blow his/her nose if possible	Ensures nostrils are clear, aiding insertion
Clean the mucus/encrustations around the nostrils with cotton buds, moistened with warm water	Helps with ease of insertion and ensures patient comfort
Perform hand hygiene and put on non-sterile gloves and apron	Minimises risk of cross-infection Standard principles must be observed when dealing with body fluids
Estimate the length of the tube to be passed by selecting the appropriate distance mark on the tube Measure the distance on the tube from the tip of the nose to the earlobe and then to the xiphisternum (see Fig. 10.3)	Gives the estimated length of tube required to enable the tip of the tube to rest in the stomach

(Continued)

Table 10.2: Continued

Action	Rationale
Assess if the patient has a gag/swallow reflex by consulting medical notes	Highlights the increased risk of misplacement of tube which may lead to aspiration
Lubricate the tip of the tube by dipping into the receiver of sterile water, or inject 10 mL of sterile water down the tube before inserting the NG tube	Contact with water activates coating inside tube and on the tip; this lubricates the tube assisting its passage through the nasopharynx and allows easy withdrawal of the introducer
At all times during the procedure talk to and reassure the patient	Instils confidence in the patient and allays fears
Insert the proximal end of the tube (with the guide wire introducer in position) into the clearest nostril, passing along the floor of the naso-pharynx to the oro-pharynx If any obstruction is felt, withdraw the tube and try again in a slightly different direction, or try the other nostril	Facilitates the passage of the tube into the oesophagus
As the tube passes down into the oro-pharynx, ask the patient to swallow To assist the passage of the tube ask the patient to take sips of water (if not contraindicated) If the patient is unconscious then stroking the throat can stimulate the swallow reflex	Swallowing closes the epiglottis and reduces risk of inadvertent endotracheal placement, enabling the tube to pass into the oesophagus
Advance the tube through the oro-pharynx, down the oesophagus into the stomach until the estimate mark on the tube reaches the external nares	Ensures the tube is in the correct position
If at any time the patient shows signs of distress, e.g. coughing, gasping, cyanosis, remove the tube immediately	The tube may have entered the trachea, not the oesophagus
Confirm the position of the tube by attaching the syringe to the guide wire introducer and gently aspirating a small amount of fluid (0.5–1 mL) to test with pH indicator strips The pH should be 5.5 or below; if it is 6 or above leave for 1 hour and retest (NPSA 2005b)	A pH of 5.5 or below indicates the tube is in the stomach A pH of 6 or above could indicate the aspirate is bronchial secretion See text for further discussion
If there is any doubt about the position of the tube and repeated attempts to obtain aspirate are unsuccessful, a chest X-ray may be required to verify the position of the tube	To ensure the tube is in the correct position prior to administering anything down it
Only after position has been confirmed can the guide wire be removed	While present, it makes the tube more radio-opaque, enabling repositioning of the tube if necessary
To remove the guide wire, attach a 20 mL syringe and inject 5 mL of fresh tap water down the tube	Injecting water activates the lubricant on the guide wire, enabling easy removal
Hold the tube end firmly at the tip of the nose and gently and carefully withdraw the guide wire, disposing of it appropriately	Ensures that the tube stays in position as the guide wire is removed
Secure the tube in place by taping around it and across the nose (a fixing device should be incorporated in the pack) Fix the tube to the corner of the nostril and secure the tube to the patient's cheek	Secures the tube easily and comfortably: less likely to cause nasal pressure ulcers
Using an indelible marker, mark the tube at the point where it leaves the nose	To have a visual reference point and allow easy detection of dislodgement of the tube
Document in the patient's records, including instructions regarding the commencement of feeding	To ensure there is documented evidence of insertion and confirmation of the position of the tube See text for further details

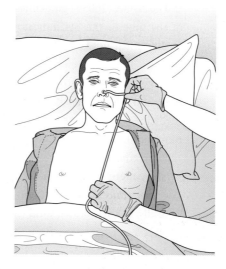

Figure 10.3: Measuring nasogastric tube length.

Checking NGT position

Potential position complications include:

- passage of the tube into the trachea;
- coiling of the tube into the posterior pharynx;
- trauma/haemorrhage or perforation of any of the surrounding tissues.

If this occurs the patient may show signs of distress or shortness of breath (cyanosis, tachypnoea, decreased oxygen saturation) and the practitioner should stop and reassess immediately.

The National Patient Safety Agency (NPSA) (2005a) reported that there have been a number of incidents where incorrect positioning of NGTs for feeding has led to patient deaths or illness. Consequently the NPSA (2005b) has provided detailed guidelines, including a flow chart, regarding how to confirm the correct position of nasogastric feeding tubes – do access these for further information. May's (2007) literature review discusses underpinning evidence for this procedure. The NPSA (2005b) advises that the tube position should be checked:

- following initial placement;
- before administering each feed;
- before giving medicines;
- at least once daily;
- following vomiting, retching or coughing;
- if the tube appears to be displaced (e.g. tape undone, tube appears to have moved).

You should also recheck if the patient complains of discomfort.

The NPSA (2005b) guidelines advise that if there is any doubt about the position of the tube or the pH indicator strip colour (particularly in the range 5–6) then feeding must not commence and further advice should be sought. The suggestion to wait 1 hour and retest if the pH is 6 or above is to allow stomach emptying after feeding and the pH to fall, but this time interval depends on the patient's clinical need and whether feeds are bolus or continuous (NPSA 2005b). Note that some medicines can increase the pH of gastric contents: antacids, H_2 antagonists, proton pump inhibitors (NPSA 2005b). If there are problems obtaining aspirate, the NPSA (2005b) advises:

• The patient should turn on their side (to enable the tip of the NGT to enter the gastric fluid pool) and then 10–20 mL of air should be injected down the tube to dispel any residual fluid (medicines, feed, water) in the tube and dislodge the NGT's exit-port away from the gastric mucosa. Then wait for 15–30 minutes and retry aspirating.

• If still no aspirate is obtained, then advance the tube 10–20 cm as this may move it into the stomach and then retry aspirating.

• If aspirate is still not obtained, seek advice and consider repassing the NGT and/ or checking the position by X-ray.

After initial insertion, subsequent tube position checks should be performed using pH strips as well as clinical judgement. You can check the external position of the tube has remained the same as documented at the time of initial insertion, and also ensure that the tube has not coiled at the back of the patient's throat.

Documentation

The type of tube, time of insertion, length to which the tube was inserted (e.g. '60 cm at right nostril') as well as who inserted the tube must be recorded in the patient records. A daily entry thereafter should be made indicating tube position, pH of aspirates and any tube-related issues until it is removed. It is the responsibility of the professional who inserted or reinserted the NGT to document:

• date and time inserted;
• type, size and batch number of tube;
• marking of the tube with an indelible pen at time of initial placement;
• expected date for review or removal;
• patency of the tube and if it has been confirmed in correct position by pH indicator strips (pH 0–5);
• any additional comments (difficulties in insertion etc.).

ACTIVITY

Take the opportunity to practise NGT insertion if available. You may have opportunity to practise on a manikin in the skills laboratory. When in practice, if a patient is to have a NGT inserted, ask if you can observe the procedure, with the patient's consent. Discuss with your mentor the reasons why the patient requires a NGT.

> ## Box 10.5 Removal of nasogastric tube
>
> - Ensure the tube is clinically no longer required or there is a clear documented reason for removal.
> - Prepare equipment – waste bag, gloves, tissues, spigot (optional).
> - Prepare the patient for the removal of the tube. Explain and discuss each step.
> - Sit the patient upright if they are able.
> - Wash hands and put gloves on.
> - Ensure feed has been stopped and detached or spigot drain if appropriate.
> - Remove tape.
> - The patient may find taking a deep breath during the removal helpful.
> - Remove the tube in one swift action and dispose of in the waste bag.
> - Wipe the patient's nose.
> - Remove gloves, wash hands and dispose of waste appropriately.
> - Document removal in the patient's medical and nursing notes.

Management of NGTs and feed administration

The tape used to secure the tube should be checked daily to highlight any inflammation, irritation, or signs of the beginnings of a nasal pressure ulcer. The tape should be changed if it is not secure or irritation has occurred. During feeding the patient should be lying at a 45-degree angle (semi-upright position) at all times. The type of feed prescribed and administered should be as recommended by the dietician. Always ensure that the feed has not expired and is in a sealed, sterile bottle. The length of time the tube is *in situ* prior to removal or reinsertion must comply with manufacturer's guidelines. Box 10.5 provides guidelines for removal of NGTs.

NGT insertion for drainage

The NGTs routinely used for drainage are larger than feeding tubes and produced in various sizes. The clinical need will determine the size of tube that is appropriate, but the smallest (i.e. narrowest) tube appropriate for the patient's management should be used.

Prior to inserting an NGT for drainage first identify whether the tube is being inserted for free drainage, aspiration, intermittent drainage or drug administration. For free drainage you will require a bile bag for attachment. Also, identify the purpose of the NGT for example, is the tube for conservative measures i.e. bowel obstruction or following surgery to prevent aspiration or relieve vomiting due to gut stasis/ileus?

As with any procedure, you should explain and obtain verbal consent from the patient. Re-check for potential contraindications: previous head, face or gut surgery or trauma including basal skull fracture, a depressed level of consciousness, oesophageal varices, cancer/tumour or complex head and neck problems, upper gastrointestinal pathology (i.e. strictures) or coagulation problems should all be taken into account. If contraindications are present the patient may need a surgeon or gastroenterology team to insert the tube under radiological guidance.

The key principles of passing an NGT for drainage are the same as for insertion of NGTs for feeding (see Table 10.2), including measuring the length of tube to be passed, checking of tube position and record keeping. However, the tube should preferably have been stored in a fridge for at least half an hour before the procedure is to begin, to ensure a rigid tube that can be passed easily. Also, have a vomit bowl available or – if there is likely to be a large gastric residual volume – ensure that appropriate suction equipment is available. Prior to passing the tube, check the patient's nostrils are patent by asking him/her to sniff with one nostril closed and repeat with the other nostril. The tube can be passed by oral route if necessary. About 15–20 cm of the tube should be lubricated with a thin coat of lubricating jelly placed on a swab, thus reducing friction between the mucous membrane and the tube.

Learning outcome 2: Explain the specific care needed following gastrostomy

Gastrostomy is indicated in patients where dysphagia has been present or is likely to be present for 28 days or more. Usually it is not required in patients who have oesophageal obstruction since other methods of treatment are available. Neurological causes of dysphagia (stroke and other chronic diseases such as motor neurone disease) are the most common reasons for referral.

> **Necrotising fasciitis**
> Rare bacterial infection of the deeper layers of skin and subcutaneous tissue.

There are two methods of placing gastrostomy; **percutaneous endoscopic gastrostomy** (PEG) is the most frequently used. **Percutaneous radiological gastrostomy** (PRG) is the other method, and is particularly indicated for patients with a high risk of pulmonary aspiration following gastro-oesophageal reflux. Both techniques can be complicated by abdominal wall sepsis (including **necrotising fasciitis**) and **peritonitis**. The type of tube placed and the date of placement are recorded in the medical notes.

> **Peritonitis**
> Inflammation of the peritoneum, which lines the inside of the abdomen and covers the internal organs, usually due to bacterial infection.

In general, gastrostomy is contraindicated where death is likely in a very short time, even if feeding were started. Survival of patients after gastrostomy is determined mainly by selection criteria. The majority of patients who receive gastrostomy feeding have had a stroke. The immediate procedure-related mortality for PEG is about 2 per cent and the 30-day mortality is about 30 per cent (Sanders *et al.* 2000, 2002). Gastrostomy placement is not a trivial decision and complications of gastrostomy can lead to death.

Box 10.6 provides guidelines for both immediate and long-term care of gastrostomy sites.

ACTIVITY

If you are caring for anyone with a gastrostomy currently, discuss the rationale for its insertion with your mentor. Also, find out about any local guidelines for immediate and long-term care following insertion.

Learning outcome 3: Identify key principles for administering enteral feeds

Most enteral feeds come prepared from the manufacturers. Feeds may be given continuously, overnight, or by bolus at regular intervals, and dieticians will decide on the most appropriate feed regimen. The feeds are administered by an enteral feed pump so the rate can be set accurately. It is increasingly common for people

Box 10.6 Gastrostomy care (adapted from Whipps Cross University Hospital NHS Trust clinical procedure)

Immediate aftercare for PEG

- One litre of sterile fluid for intravenous infusion (0.9% sodium chloride or 5% dextrose) is connected to the PEG tube in the endoscopy department to run over 12 hours.
- If there is no evidence of peritonism 12 hours after the tube is placed, then a feeding regime may be started in conjunction with the dietetic department.
- The dressing is removed from under the external retaining device at 24 hours after placement, and iodine antiseptic (e.g. Povidone iodine spray) is used twice daily for 2 days following tube placement. After removal of the initial dressing the site is kept free of any dressing.
- The patient should not immerse in water or shower for 14 days after tube placement.
- Daily cleaning should be undertaken with sterile saline and thorough drying.

Immediate aftercare for PRG

Care is the same as for PEG, except:

- No sterile fluid for intravenous infusion is started in the X-ray department.
- Standing instructions recommend commencement of feeding at 24 hours post-insertion.
- No dressing is applied to the skin, but blue nylon gastropexy sutures are present, which should be cut at skin level 14 days post-insertion. The gastropexy 'tags' will then fall into the stomach and pass through the gastrointestinal tract.

Long-term care of a gastrostomy site

- The site should be cleaned daily with non-perfumed soap and water. After washing, the site should be gently but thoroughly dried.
- From 14 days onwards, the tube should be rotated through 360 degrees once daily. This helps keep the tract in good condition. Ideally there should be a small distance (half a centimetre) between the external retaining device and the skin, and this should be checked when rotating the tube daily.
- The external rotating device should not be tight against the skin. Excessive traction on the tube by pulling or by the external retaining device being too tight against the skin leads to the internal retaining device being pulled through the gastric wall to lie within the tract ('buried bumper syndrome'). This is very painful for the patient and can lead to severe infection within and around the stoma tract.

to administer their own enteral feeds at home, with training and support from community nurses.

ACTIVITY

If a person is unable to take food or fluids orally and is being fed enterally, what special care do you think they would need?

You might have included the following:

- Observe fluid intake and output.
- Ensure the prescribed feeding regimen is adhered to. Store feeds according to manufacturer's instructions.
- Observe for and report any untoward effects (like vomiting, diarrhoea or constipation).
- Maintain mouth care (see Chapter 8).
- Ensure that the position of the tube is maintained (e.g. that a nasogastric tube is secured adequately).
- Take measures to prevent cross-infection (e.g. hand hygiene, aseptic technique when connecting the feed administration set and the feeding tube).
- Ensure that the tube remains patent. Flush with water before and after feeds and medicine are administered.
- Be aware of, and trying to minimise, the psychosocial effects of enteral feeding; for example, effects on body image (see Chapter 2) and the loss associated with inability to enjoy eating and join in with the associated social aspects.

Patients with enteral tubes may be administered medication via this route, which is discussed next.

Learning outcome 4: Discuss the process of administering medicines by the enteral tube route

Patients who are unable to take medicines orally and have a NGT or a gastrostomy tube may have some medication administered via a syringe attached to the tube's connector. Other routes (e.g. topical) should be used where possible. Community patients can learn how to self-administer their medicines via the enteral tube route.

ACTIVITY

What difficulties or risks might there be of administering medicine via the enteral tube route? Consider how these might be addressed.

You could have thought of these points:

- The NGT route can be hazardous as the tube could dislodge from its position in the stomach. Therefore the tube's position must be checked, as discussed earlier.
- Absorption and preparation of medicines for the enteral tube route may differ from oral medication. Therefore nurses must work with the pharmacist who can advise about medicines being prescribed and dispensed in a suitable format, with consideration of any drug interactions. Some liquid preparations are suspensions of small granules and are therefore not suitable and others contain sorbitol, which is a laxative (British Association for Parenteral and Enteral Nutrition (BAPEN) 2004a). The medicines will usually be prescribed as liquids or soluble tablets.
  Note: Tablets must not be crushed nor capsules opened as this could alter the medicine's therapeutic action, making it ineffective and thus invalidating the product's licence (NMC 2007b).

- Enteral tubes can become blocked. Common causes are inadequate flushing and using the wrong formulation of medicine (BAPEN 2004b). BAPEN (2004a) suggests that if blockage occurs, aspiration to remove particles can be tried followed by a warm water flush, but excessive pressure must not be applied due to risk of tube fracture.
- A syringe is used to prepare the medicine and there have been reports of enteral medicines being given intravenously by accident with serious consequences (NPSA 2007). Therefore syringes used to draw up and administer medication via enteral tubes must comply with NPSA (2007) guidance, to prevent administration errors. The syringes used must not be able to be connected to intravenous (IV) canulae, should be labelled and may be of a different colour to distinguish them from IV syringes (NPSA 2007).

ACTIVITY

Look at an enteral medication syringe – in practice or in the skills laboratory. Note how it differs from other syringes.

All safety aspects of medicine administration (see Chapter 5) must be adhered to when administering medicines by enteral tube. You must maintain infection control precautions: wash hands and put on non-sterile gloves. You should prepare the correct dose as prescribed in an enteral syringe. The pharmacist's specific instructions regarding the medicine and its preparation and administration must be followed. Liquids should be shaken well and thick liquids diluted with an equal amount of water; soluble tablets should be dissolved in 10–15 mL of water (BAPEN 2004b).

ACTIVITY

What specific aspects will be necessary when administering a medicine by the enteral tube route? Consider: the patient may have a feed in progress or the tube may be closed off with a spigot.

Remember, as discussed previously, for NGTs, if there is no feed in progress, you must first check the tube's position is in the stomach (see earlier discussion). BAPEN (2004b) advises the following method for administration:

- If the patient has a feed in progress, switch this off. Sometimes, there will need to be a break from feeding before and/or after medicine administration – the pharmacist will advise.
- Use a non-touch technique to attach the syringe to the tube's connector. Flush the tube with at least 30 mL of water (or as directed).
- Administer the medicine, flushing with 10 mL of water in between each medicine given.
- Give a final flush of at least 30 mL of water and restart the feed (unless a break is advised).

Learning outcome 5: Identify the role of parenteral nutrition and intravenous fluid administration in maintaining patient nutrition

In some instances, it may not be possible to provide nutrition enterally. Parenteral feeding (often referred to as total parenteral nutrition – TPN) may be used when a person is unable to use the gastrointestinal tract for nutrition, either temporarily or in the long term. An example would be a person who has had major surgery to the gastrointestinal tract. In parenteral nutrition, nutrients and micronutrients are administered directly into the circulation intravenously via a device in the vein and therefore only qualified nurses can administer TPN.

The aim of IV therapy is to maintain or restore normal fluid and electrolyte balance. IV therapy should always be approached with caution if fluid overload, fluid deficit, fluid shifts and unwanted alterations in electrolyte concentrations are to be avoided. It is essential that all fluid replacement regimes are tailored to the individual's requirements.

Assessment of the need for IV fluids and electrolytes should include:
- vital signs;
- fluid intake and output measurements;
- daily weight;
- skin turgor;
- jugular vein filling;
- central venous pressure (CVP) measurements (see Chapter 11, Box 11.7);
- serum electrolyte levels;
- arterial blood gas results (See Chapter 11, Box 11.3);
- urinary specific gravity.

See Metheny (2000) for further reading of fluid and electrolyte balance. IV fluid does not provide nutrition for patients, merely hydration which is crucial for life. Chapter 5 includes a section on IV fluid administration, focusing on the medicine administration aspects.

Summary
- Enteral feeding is required when nutritional needs cannot be sufficiently met through the oral route.
- NGT insertion and gastrostomy insertion are invasive procedures with potential complications. There must be good rationale for their instigation.
- NGT insertion must be carried out carefully and skilfully. It can be a difficult procedure for patients to tolerate and they need psychological support.
- Medicine administration via the enteral route must be carried out safely and in liaison with the pharmacist.
- If enteral feeding is not possible, parenteral feeding can provide nutrition. Intravenous fluid administration can maintain hydration and electrolyte balance.

CHAPTER SUMMARY

This chapter has highlighted throughout the importance of nutrition for the maintenance of health. As has been suggested, nurses are in an excellent position to screen patients/clients for nutritional risk as part of their assessment, and should work collaboratively with other healthcare professionals to identify and implement strategies to meet the differing nutritional needs of individuals.

This chapter has included general principles that apply across a range of ages and settings. Nutrition is, however, a vast subject, and you are encouraged to undertake further reading if wishing to enquire into specialist areas in more depth.

ACKNOWLEDGEMENT

Grateful thanks are due to the Whipps Cross University NHS Trust Nutrition Action Group for contributions and support to this chapter.

This chapter has been revised and updated. The author acknowledges the contributions of Kay Child and Sue Higham to this chapter in the previous two editions of the book.

REFERENCES

Age Concern 2006. *Hungry to be Heard: The scandal of malnourished older people in hospital.* England: Age Concern.

Baker, S. 2001. *Environmentally Friendly: Patients' views of conditions on psychiatric wards.* London: MIND.

Bond, S. 1997. *Eating Matters.* Newcastle: Centre for Health Services Research.

British Association for Parenteral and Enteral Nutrition 2003. *The full 'Malnutrition Universal Screening Tool'.* London: BAPEN.

British Association for Parenteral and Enteral Nutrition 2004a. *Drug administration via enteral feeding tubes: A guide for general practitioners and community pharmacists.* BAPEN. Available form www.baben.org.uk

British Association for Parenteral and Enteral Nutrition 2004b. *Administering drugs via enteral feeding tubes: A practical guide.* BAPEN. Available from www.bapen.org.uk

Brooker, C. 1998. *Human Structure and Function*, 2nd edn. London: Mosby.

Clegg, A. 2003. Older Asian patient and carer perceptions of culturally sensitive care in a community hospital setting. *Journal of Clinical Nursing* **12**, 283–90.

Collins, A. 2002. Nursing with dignity. Pt 1: Judaism. *Nursing Times* **98**(9), 34–5.

Council of Europe Alliance (UK) 2007. *Council of Europe Resolution Food and Nutritional Care in Hospitals: 10 key characteristics of good nutritional care in hospitals.* Available from www.hospitalcaterers.org.

Crawley 2003. Neurological eating disorders. In Shuttleworth, A. (ed.) *Nutrition: A practical guide.* London: EMAP Healthcare, 14–15.

Davies, S. 1999. Dysphagia in acute strokes. *Nursing Standard* **13**(30), 49–55.

Department of Health (DH) 2000. *The NHS Plan.* London.

— 2001a. *The Essence of Care: Patient focused benchmarking for health care practitioners.* London.

— 2001b. *Valuing People: A new strategy for learning disability for the 21st century*. London.

— 2004. *Standards for Better Health*. London.

— 2007a. *Improving Nutritional Care: A joint action plan from the Department of Health and Nutrition Summit stakeholders*. London.

— 2007b. *5-a-Day Introduction*. Available from www.dh.gov.uk/en/Publichealth/ Healthimprovement/FiveADay/FiveADaygeneralinformation/DH_4069924. Accessed 24 April 2008.

— 2007c. *Hospital Food*. Available from www.dh.gov.uk/en/Managingyourorganisation/ Leadershipandmanagement/Healthcareenvironment/DH_4116450. Accessed 24 April 2008.

Department of Health, Social Services and Public Safety 2007. *Get your 10 a day! The nursing care standards for patient food in hospital*. Belfast: DHSSPS. Available from www.dhsspsni. gov.uk.

Eberhardie, C. 2003. Nutrition in older people. In Shuttleworth, A. (ed.) *Nutrition: A practical guide*. London: EMAP Healthcare, 16–17.

Edwards, S. 1998. Malnutrition in hospital patients: where does it come from? *British Journal of Nursing* **7**, 954, 956–8, 971–4.

Edington, J., Boorman, J., Durrant, E.J. *et al.* 2000. *Prevalence of Malnutrition on Admission to Four Hospitals in England*. Malnutrition Prevalence Group.

European Nutrition for Health Alliance 2005. *Malnutrition within an Ageing Population: A call to action*. London: ENHA.

Fettes, S.B. and Murray, M. 1999. Audit of the nutritional content of patient meals in Ayrshire and Arran. *Health Bulletin* **57**, 374–83.

Food Standards Agency 2002. *Guide to Food Hygiene*. London: Food Standards Agency. See www.food.gov.uk.

Gill, B.K. 2002. Nursing with dignity. Pt 6: Sikhism. *Nursing Times* **98**(14), 39–41.

Health Advisory Service 2000. 1998. *'Not because they are Old': An independent inquiry into the care of older people on acute wards in general hospitals*. London: Health Advisory Service 2000.

Holden, C. and MacDonald, A. 1997. Nutritional care: the nurse's role. *Paediatric Nursing* **9**(4), 29–34.

Holmes, S. 2003. Undernutrition in hospital patients. *Nursing Standard* **17**(19), 45–52.

Jacques, A. and Jackson, G.A. 2000. *Understanding Dementia*, 3rd edn. Edinburgh: Churchill Livingstone.

Manthorpe, J. and Watson, R. 2003. Poorly served? Eating and dementia. *Journal of Advanced Nursing* **41**, 162–9.

Martyn, C.N., Winter, P.D., Coles, S.J. and Edington, J. 1998. Effect of nutritional status on use of health care resources by patients with chronic disease living in the community. *Clinical Nutrition*. **17**, 119–23.

May, S. 2007. Testing nasogastric tube positioning in the critically ill: exploring the evidence. *British Journal of Nursing* **16**(7), 414–18.

Metheny, N.M. 2000. *Fluid and electrolyte balance: Nursing considerations*, 4th edn. Philadelphia, Lippincott.

Moules, T. and Ramsay, J. 1998. *The Textbook of Children's Nursing*. Cheltenham: Stanley Thornes.

National Patient Safety Agency (NPSA) 2005a. *Patient Safety Alert: Reducing the harm caused by misplaced nasogastric feeding tubes*. Available from www.npsa.nhs.uk.

— 2005b. *How to Confirm the Correct Position of Nasogastric Feeding Tubes in Infants, Children and Adults*. Available from www.npsa.nhs.uk.

— 2007. *Promoting Safer Measurement and Administration of Liquid Medicines via Oral and Other Enteral Routes.* Available from www.npsa.nhs.uk.

National Institute for Health and Clinical Excellence (NICE) 2006. *Nutrition Support in Adults: Oral nutrition support, enteral tube feeding and parenteral nutrition.* London: NICE.

NHS Quality Improvement Scotland 2003. *Food, Fluid and Nutritional Care in Hospitals: National overview.* Edinburgh: NHS QIS.

NHS Institute for Innovation and Improvement 2007. *Releasing Time to Care: The productive ward.* London: HMSO.

Nightingale, F. 1980. *Notes on Nursing: What it is and what it is not.* Edinburgh: Churchill Livingstone.

Nursing and Midwifery Council 2007a. *Essential skills clusters.* London: NMC.

Nursing and Midwifery Council 2007b. *Standards for Medicines Management.* London: NMC.

Pender, F. 1994. *Nutrition and Dietetics.* Edinburgh: Campion Press.

Piper, B. 1996. *Diet and Nutrition: A guide for students and practitioners.* London: Chapman & Hall.

Royal College of Nursing (RCN) 2007. *Water for Health: Hydration best practice toolkit for hospitals and healthcare* London: RCN. Available from www.rcn.org.uk.

Sanders, D.S., Carter, M.J., D'Silva, J. *et al.* 2000. Survival analysis in percutaneous endoscopic gastrostomy: a worse outcome in patients with dementia. *American Journal of Gastroenterology* **95**, 1472–5.

Sanders, D.S., Carter, M.J., D'Silva, J. *et al.* 2002. Percutaneous endoscopic gastrostomy: a prospective audit of the impact of guidelines in two district general hospitals in the United Kingdom. *American Journal of Gastroenterology* **97**, 2239–45.

Shanley, E. and Starrs, T. 1993. *Learning Disabilities: A handbook of care*, 2nd edn. Edinburgh: Churchill Livingstone.

Stratton, R.J., Thompson, R.L., Margetts, B.M. *et al.* 2002. Health care utilisation according to malnutrition risk in the elderly: an analysis of data from the National Diet and Nutrition Survey. *Proceedings of the Nutrition Society* **61**: 20A.

Stratton, R.J., Green, C.J. and Elia, M. 2003. *Disease-related malnutrition: An evidence based approach to treatment.* Oxford: CABI Publishing.

Stroke Association 2006. *Taste Changes After Stroke*, Factsheet 39. Available from www.stroke.org.uk.

Todorovic, V., Russell, C., Stratton, R *et al.* 2003. *The MUST Explanatory Booklet.* Redditch: BAPEN. Available from www.bapen.org.uk.

Wardley, B., Puntis, J. and Taitz, S. 1997. *Handbook of Child Nutrition.* Oxford: Oxford University Press.

Wardlow, G.M. 1999. *Perspectives in Nutrition*, 4th edn. Boston: McGraw-Hill.

Welsh Assembly Government 2003. *Fundamentals of Care. Guidance for Health and Social Care Staff: Improving the quality of fundamental aspects of health and social care for adults.* Cardiff: WAG.

Wood, C., Stubbs, S., Warwick, H. *et al.* 2003. Malnutrition risk and health care utilisation in orthopaedic patients. *Proceedings of the Nutrition Society.*

CHAPTER 11

Assessing Physical Health and Responding to Sudden Deterioration

Sue Maddex and Tracey Valler-Jones

Recognising, monitoring, interpreting and responding to changes in a patient's health status are core nursing skills. The Audit Commission (1999) report *Critical to Success* highlighted that hospitals should review services available to acutely ill patients, recommending the availability of outreach services with ward staff being trained to deal with deterioration in a patient's condition. In 2000, the Department of Health (DH) advised that outreach teams should be an integral part of critical care services. However, the National Patient Safety Agency (2007) reported that some patients' clinical and physiological deterioration was not recognised or acted upon. The National Institute for Health and Clinical Excellence (NICE) (2007) urged hospitals to keep acutely ill patients' care at the forefront and recommended key priorities for care of acutely ill patients (see www.nice.org).

Since the publication of these reports, many hospitals have strived to address care deficits and improve acutely ill patients' care. During your practice placements you will care for many acutely ill patients in both hospital and community settings.

This chapter addresses the immediate care management of acutely ill adult patients, explaining a systematic approach to recognising and responding to sudden deterioration. The chapter then explores skills relevant to managing airway obstruction, breathlessness, circulatory problems and unconsciousness. Some relevant skills are discussed in other chapters of this book, so you are referred to them as appropriate. In particular, Chapter 4 includes monitoring vital signs (temperature, pulse, respiration, oxygen saturation and blood pressure) and neurological assessment.

This chapter includes:
- Recognising and responding to deteriorating patients/clients: an overview
- Airway obstruction problems and related skills (includes oxygen therapy and suction)
- Breathing problems and related skills (includes peak expiratory flow rate measurement, observing sputum and collecting sputum specimens)
- Circulatory problems and related skills (includes capillary refill, cardiac monitoring and electrocardiogram recording)
- Unconsciousness and related skills (includes blood glucose monitoring and managing fits)

At the beginning of Chapter 4 there were questions related to biology underpinning measurement of vital signs. Check those again to ensure that you understand the principles. The following questions will help you to focus on the biology underpinning this chapter's skills. Use your recommended textbook to find out:

- What is homeostasis?
- Why is glucose important in the body?
- What is the role of insulin in the body?

Airways and breathing

- What is the structure of the airways?
- How is oxygen transported in the body?
- What role do cilia play?
- How does the respiratory system respond to respiratory tract infection?
- What other situations could cause respiratory distress or dysfunction?
- Where is bronchial smooth muscle located?
- What is the consequence of bronchoconstriction?
- Where are the pleural membranes? What functions do they have?
- What is surfactant? How does it prevent lung collapse?
- How can lung function be assessed? What factors could affect lung function?
- What do you understand by the term acid–base balance?

Circulation

- How is blood pressure controlled within the body, and how might this be affected if a patient is in shock?
- What are baroreceptors and where are they found in the body?
- What is the basic structure of the heart? Name its layers.
- What is the electroconduction system of the heart?
- What is the function of the sino-atrial node?

Nervous system

- What is the role of the medulla oblongata in the body?
- Describe the structure of the brain.

PRACTICE SCENARIOS

The following scenarios illustrate situations where sudden deterioration in a person's condition might occur in different settings. These scenarios will be referred back to throughout the chapter.

Adult community setting: airway obstruction

Mrs Mary Wyatt, aged 89 years, is resident in a care home. She has a history of Parkinson's disease and sometimes has difficulty eating. Today during lunch she started to choke on a piece of meat. Staff initially encouraged her to cough but Mary was becoming tired and her colour was deteriorating. The staff attempted

Parkinson's disease
There is a loss of dopamine-producing neurons within the brain, causing a chronic, progressive degenerative neurological disease with symptoms such as tremor, rigidity and bradykinesia (slow movement). It affects many activities including eating, with a risk of food aspiration.

Asthma
A respiratory disorder characterised by recurrent episodes of difficulty in breathing, wheezing on expiration, coughing and viscous mucoid bronchial secretions.

Corticosteroid
Inhaled corticosteroids such as becotide are used for asthma as a preventative treatment. They reduce bronchial mucosal inflammation, thus decreasing oedema and secretion of mucus in the airway. Corticosteriods can be administered via most other routes. Prednisolone is an oral preparation.

Bronchodilator
A drug that relaxes the smooth muscle of the bronchioles to improve ventilation to the lungs. Commonly used examples are salbutamol and terbutaline.

Atrial fibrillation
A common arrhythmia where, rather than the impulse originating from the sino-atrial node, there is disorganised electrical activity in the atria, leading to irregular and often fast ventricular contraction.

Digoxin
A cardiac glycoside that increases the force of myocardial contraction and reduces conductivity within the atrioventricular node. It is commonly used to control atrial fibrillation.

first aid to clear her airway obstruction, which was not successful, and they called an emergency ambulance. The ambulance crew have used suction and given oxygen therapy. Mary has now arrived in the A&E department, where a team of staff are awaiting.

Mental health setting: breathing problem

Tina Lunn is 58 years old and has a long history of mental illness. She has been admitted to an acute mental health unit owing to her deteriorating mental state. She is known to have **asthma**, has becotide (a **corticosteroid**) and salbutamol (a **bronchodilator**) inhalers, and takes oral prednisolone (also a corticosteroid). The staff are encouraging her to manage her asthma, to monitor her peak flow and take her inhalers as prescribed. However, one morning after a restless night, her respiration is so laboured she has difficulty completing sentences and she is very distressed and wheezy. Her peak flow is about half her normal measurement. A salbutamol nebuliser (prescribed on an as-required basis) is administered via oxygen with some effect. The doctor diagnoses a chest infection and asks for a sputum specimen to be collected.

Adult hospital setting: circulatory problem

Sira Patel, a 67-year-old woman, has just returned from theatre after undergoing a left total hip replacement. She is known to have **atrial fibrillation** which is managed with 62.5 micrograms of **digoxin** daily. The anaesthetist has requested that she has cardiac monitoring for the first 24 hours postoperatively and has a 12-lead electrocardiogram (ECG) performed the following morning. She has **patient-controlled analgesia** in progress and oxygen is being delivered at 5 litres per minute via a face mask. She also has an intravenous infusion in progress. While conducting her postoperative observations, you find that her blood pressure has decreased, her heart rate is increasing and is irregular, and her respiratory rate is also rising. She has excessive drainage from her wound drain.

Learning disability setting: impaired conscious level

Enid Campbell is a 52-year-old woman with a severe learning disability and very limited verbal communication. She lives in a group home. She is overweight and **type 2 diabetes** was diagnosed six years ago. This was initially treated with oral hypoglycaemic agents; but owing to her blood glucose level being persistently high, she was started on insulin injections, which are administered by her carers. This morning the community nurse for learning disability, her health facilitator, is visiting to advise on her hydration and nutrition. When the nurse arrived, Enid's carers reported that a short while ago Enid slumped forward in her wheelchair and seemed unable to hold herself up. Some twitching of her right arm and leg was noticed. Enid has no history of epilepsy. When a staff member spoke to her she was initially unable to respond but is now responsive though 'not her usual self'. The carers checked her blood glucose and it was within Enid's usual range. Her GP has been contacted and is on her way to Enid's home.

EQUIPMENT REQUIRED FOR THIS CHAPTER

Find out what equipment is available within your skills laboratory or your practice area, for monitoring acutely ill patients. In particular, look for:

- Resuscitation Council (UK) guidelines posters (you can also look at these on the website www.resus.org.uk);
- cardiac monitoring equipment;
- 12-lead ECG;
- early-warning score (EWS) chart;
- peak-flow meter;
- blood glucose monitoring equipment.

RECOGNISING AND RESPONDING TO DETERIORATING PATIENTS/CLIENTS: AN OVERVIEW

Less than 20 per cent of patients who undergo a cardiac arrest in hospital survive to be discharged home (Peberdy *et al.* 2003). Smith and Poplett (2002) identified that medical staff and nurses do not possess adequate acute care skills to recognise deteriorating patients and monitor them effectively. Deterioration is usually preceded by changes in the physiological parameters that represent failing respiratory, cardiovascular and neurological systems. Recognition of these changes and dealing with them appropriately can help prevent further deterioration or even death.

Traditionally, the identification of critically ill and deteriorating patients relied on clinical intuition (Bright *et al.* 2004). The introduction of 'track-and-trigger' systems within healthcare has enabled staff to identify those at risk, assisting in the early detection of critical illness (Smith *et al.* 2006).

LEARNING OUTCOMES

By the end of this section you will be able to:

1 identify the components of an EWS chart, how scores are calculated and the action to be taken;

2 outline the key aspects of an ABCDE approach to assessing and managing an acutely unwell person;

3 locate and recognise emergency equipment.

Learning outcome 1: Identify the components of an early-warning score chart, how scores are calculated and the action to be taken

The **EWS**, also known as 'physiological track and trigger system', is a tool for patient evaluation based on five physiological parameters: systolic blood pressure, pulse rate, respiratory rate, temperature and **AVPU score** (Morgan *et al.* 1997; Oakey and Slade 2006). The EWS allocates points to measurements outside the 'normal' parameters, alerting staff to the patient's deteriorating condition. The use of EWS/physiological track-and-trigger systems is effective in reducing mortality

---

Sidebar:

Patient-controlled analgesia (PCA)
A pain management system in which the patient controls the dose and frequency of analgesic delivered up to a predetermined limit. PCA usually refers to an intravenous system that delivers opioids when the patient presses a demand button. See Chapter 12 for more information.

Type 2 diabetes
A form of diabetes that develops when the body makes insufficient insulin, or when the insulin that is produced does not work effectively (known as **insulin resistance**). See www.diabetes.org.uk for more information.

AVPU score
A = Alert
V = (responds to) Voice
P = (responds to) Pain
U = Unresponsive

and morbidity of acutely ill patients as well as preventing admissions to the intensive therapy unit (ITU) (Buist *et al.* 2002; Goldhill *et al.* 1999). This system is especially useful as it is not always appropriate to nurse patients in ITU or high-dependency units. If detected early enough, simple interventions such as fluid or oxygen administration can help prevent further deterioration. NICE (2007) recommended their use to monitor all adult patients in acute hospital settings. Thus, the evolvement of these EWS/physiological track-and-trigger systems continues in a move to improve acutely ill patients' care. There are many different EWS charts/systems currently in use.

ACTIVITY

Within your clinical area, find out what EWS/track-and-trigger system is used and how scores are calculated. What actions should staff take based on the score a patient receives? Who would staff need to contact?

Although protocols vary according to systems used and facilities available, in many UK hospitals if a patient has an EWS score of 3 or higher this requires an immediate review by medical personnel. If there is no improvement then referral is made to the senior doctor. This enables the ward nursing staff to refer to more senior members of staff if a patient's clinical situation is not improving. Some UK hospitals have gone further and a score of 3 results in an immediate call, by the nursing staff, directly to the ITU registrar for review (Rees 2003). Other hospitals have been more cautious and use a score of 4 or even 5 as a callout trigger (Subbe *et al.* 2003). You will need to be orientated to the chart and accompanying protocol used in your hospital.

The EWS is effective only if the information obtained is accurate and any 'triggers' (i.e. a score of 3 or more) are reported to the appropriate people. Significant variation in the reproducibility of different track-and-trigger warning systems has been found (Subbe *et al.* 2007). EWS can be used for any patient where there are concerns about their health, such as postoperatively, following severe trauma, or if the patient is diagnosed with a serious medical condition. EWSs are used in community settings as well as in hospital (Mann and Bowler 2008).

ACTIVITY

Look at Mrs Patel's scenario. When her vital signs are recorded they are:
* heart rate 112 bpm
* respiratory rate 23 pm
* blood pressure 102/63 mmHg
* temperature 37°C.

Mrs Patel is alert. Using this information and your local chart, what would her EWS score be? What would you need to do?

It is likely that her score would have indicated that you need to call for assistance and ensure that she continues to be closely monitored. You would follow local protocol on actions to take; you should be aware of who needs to be informed and when. This may be displayed on the observation chart or within the ward policy documents.

Learning outcome 2: Outline the key aspects of an ABCDE approach to assessing and managing an acutely unwell person

When a patient is acutely ill or at risk of deterioration, it is vitally important that they have an initial assessment and are frequently reassessed to evaluate interventions used and to ensure there is no further deterioration. Immediate assessment involves the ABCDE approach:
– Airway
– Breathing
– Circulation
– Disability (involves assessment of neurological status)
– Exposure (enables a full examination to be undertaken)

This order of assessment and interventions is used because airway obstructions kill faster than disordered breathing, which in turn kills faster than haemorrhage or cardiac dysfunction (Smith 2003).

The airway

A patent airway is essential to ensure that there is adequate oxygen circulating in the body. If airway compromise – or a potential for compromise – is present, you must protect and maintain it, otherwise **hypoxic brain damage** will occur. When a person becomes unconscious there is a reduction in their muscle tone, so the tongue can fall back and occlude the airway. Blood, secretions and vomit may also be present. There are various airway adjuncts available which are discussed later. If someone needs help to maintain a patent airway they must be constantly observed to ensure the airway does not become occluded.

Breathing

Once the airway is instituted and secured you must evaluate breathing. You should perform a rapid assessment of respiratory **rate** and **rhythm** and the presence of **hypo-** or **hyperventilation** and oxygen saturation. If breathing is compromised then supplementary oxygen by nasal cannulae, non-rebreathe oxygen mask or bag–valve–mask ventilation, or mechanical ventilation should be applied. Oxygen administration is considered later in this chapter.

> **Bag–valve–mask (BVM)**
> A hand-held device used to provide ventilation to a patient who is not breathing or breathing inadequately.

The circulation

Circulatory assessment must be performed rapidly in someone who is acutely ill. If perfusion is compromised then **hypoxia** and **tissue damage** occur quickly. Restoring adequate circulating blood volume is essential if oxygen deficit and inadequate tissue perfusion are present. Three of the most common indicators of inadequate circulatory function are **hypotension** (low blood pressure), **tachycardia** (increased heart rate) and **decreasing urinary output**. The pulse rate may rise for a variety of reasons and is not necessarily specific to **hypovolaemia** (low blood volume). Additionally, patients with various pre-existing medical conditions or taking medications may be tachycardic – for example, patients like Mrs Patel who has a cardiac conduction disturbance.

Note: A person with a high spinal cord injury may have **bradycardia**, not tachycardia. A simple assessment of the circulation can be obtained by the capillary refill time (see later in the chapter).

Blood pressure can be misleading or unreliable. Typical compensatory mechanisms used to maintain perfusion to the heart and brain may produce a normal systemic pressure. Loss of up to 15 per cent of the circulating volume (700–750 mL for a 70 kg patient) may produce few obvious symptoms, while loss of up to 30 per cent of the circulating volume (1.5 L) may result in mild tachycardia, **tachypnoea** and anxiety. Hypotension, marked tachycardia (pulse rate >110–120 bpm) and confusion may not be evident until more than 30 percent of the blood volume has been lost, while loss of 40 per cent of circulating volume (2 L) is immediately life-threatening (Harbrecht *et al.* 2004). If hypotension is present, it requires immediate attention and treatment.

Disability

A rapid neurological evaluation is conducted once the airway is secured, breathing is adequate and circulatory issues have been dealt with. To do this the patient's **level of consciousness** can be assessed using the Glasgow Coma Score (GCS), as described in Chapter 4. However, a more rapid assessment is the AVPU system (defined earlier in this chapter).

You should also check the **pupil reaction** to light (see Chapter 4). Pupillary responses can give important information about the causes of neurological problems. If the pupils are uniformly dilated this can denote stress, fear etc., but can also indicate that sympathetic stimulants have been taken (e.g. tricyclic antidepressants, adrenaline). If the pupils are bilaterally constricted then this can indicate opiates (e.g. morphine) or that the brain stem has been affected (Smith 2003). However, if there is a dilated pupil on one side this can suggest a unilateral **space-occupying lesion** such as haematoma, tumour or abscess which is a medical emergency and requires immediate medical attention.

A decreased level of consciousness may indicate cerebral injury. However, factors such as hypoxia, hypovolaemia, alcohol and/or drugs may alter level of consciousness. If the GCS is less than 8, the patient's level of consciousness is severely compromised and they will require help to maintain their airway. It is also important at this stage to undertake a blood glucose recording (discussed later in this chapter).

Exposure

The patient should be completely undressed to be thoroughly examined. In acute deterioration or traumatic injury, it may be necessary to cut off the clothes. Patients' dignity must be protected and they should not be exposed unnecessarily. The patient must be warmed with blankets or other warming devices to prevent the rapid onset or continued state of hypothermia. When combined with rapid infusions of cold fluids or blood products and exposure, hypothermia can have potentially fatal results if left untreated. Hypothermia is associated with arrhythmias, coagulopathies and higher mortality (Spahn *et al.* 2007). Generally, patients with a temperature of less than 32ºC should be rapidly warmed.

Remember: Always reassess ABCDE regularly and do not progress from one stage to another until you have dealt with the first.

Learning outcome 3: Locate and recognise emergency equipment.

In any new placement area, always familiarise yourself with emergency equipment and its location.

ACTIVITY	When in your next or current practice placement, locate the emergency equipment and ask your mentor to check the equipment with you.

Emergency equipment must be checked regularly to ensure it remains in working order, and rechecked after each usage. All the necessary equipment might be on a resuscitation (cardiac-arrest) trolley; or the items – including oxygen, suction, defibrillator (see Box 11.1) and pocket mask – may be available in separate locations. The Resuscitation Council (UK) (2004) advises on appropriate equipment for cardiac-arrest trolleys.

Box 11.1 The defibrillator

- A defibrillator is a device that delivers a passage of electrical current across the myocardium.
- It is used when the heart is suffering from disorganised electrical activity (e.g. ventricular fibrillation). By passing electricity through the heart in a controlled dose, the heart can be stopped briefly with the intention of restoring organised spontaneous electrical activity (Resuscitation Council UK 2006).
- The shock is administered by charging up the defibrillator to the appropriate dosage, placing the paddles or attaching pads on the patient's chest, and pressing the discharge button.
- People using defibrillators require specialist training as it is a complex and potentially dangerous skill.
- There are automatic external defibrillators (AEDs) available that can automatically recognise rhythms and give instructions for defibrillation. These are becoming increasing available both inside and outside the hospital setting.

Summary

- Patients' deterioration can be recognised through recording vital signs and calculating the EWS. Low scores must then be responded to promptly and appropriately.
- An ABCDE approach to assessing an unwell person is systematic and ensures priorities of care are addressed.
- It is essential to be familiar with emergency equipment and its location in any care setting you are working in – hospital or community.

AIRWAY MANAGEMENT PROBLEMS AND RELATED SKILLS

There are many reasons why an airway becomes compromised, including infection, smoke inhalation, allergic reaction, foreign body obstruction or trauma. Foreign bodies may cause either a mild or a severe airway obstruction and are usually inhaled bits of food such as meat, boiled sweets and fruit, or vomit or blood. Acute allergic reactions (e.g. a bee sting, peanuts, penicillin) can cause the trachea or throat to swell until it is closed.

LEARNING OUTCOMES

By the end of this section you will be able to:
1 Recognise the signs of an obstructed airway and take appropriate action
2 Identify the different types of airway adjuncts available
3 Identify reasons for oxygen administration and how it can be delivered safely
4 Explain how suction equipment is used in practice

Learning outcome 1: Recognise the signs of an obstructed airway and take appropriate action

An airway can obstruct very suddenly, so it is important to be able to recognise the signs and act on them. Your mandatory basic life-support training will address this topic.

ACTIVITY

Looking at Mary Wyatt's scenario, how do you think they knew she had an obstructed airway? What first aid should the staff have attempted?

Resuscitation Council (UK)
The Council's evidence-based guidelines are reviewed approximately every five years. For current guidance, refer to the website www.resus.org.uk.

Mary was eating at the time and she may have clutched her neck. The **Resuscitation Council (UK)** (2005) suggests that in mild airway obstruction the person is able to speak, breathe and cough, and can verbally respond to the question: 'Are you choking? However, with a severe obstruction (as in Mary's case), she would not have been able to speak but might have nodded and her attempts at coughing would have been silent.

To recognise an airway obstruction the recommended method is 'look, listen and feel' (Smith 2003).

Look

- Look to see whether there are any chest and abdominal movements. In normal respiration the chest and abdomen move outwards during inspiration and inwards during expiration, but with respiratory compromise there is a seesaw pattern of movements. Other signs include using accessory muscles: neck and shoulders and a pulling in of the trachea.
- Look at the person's colour. As hypoxia develops the peripheries gain a grey/blue tinge (cyanosis). Peripheral cyanosis is seen in areas like hands and toes. Central cyanosis (blueness in the tongue and lips) is a late sign of airway obstruction.

Listen

Listen for sounds of breathing. Normal breathing should be quiet – noise indicates a partially obstructed airway. Respiratory sounds can indicate the position of the obstruction:

- *Stridor*, a high-pitched sound usually heard during inspiration, is due to partial blockage of the trachea, larynx or pharynx.
- *Gurgling* can indicate fluids such as blood or vomit in the upper airways.
- *Snoring* indicates partial blockage of the pharynx usually by the tongue or soft palate.
- *Expiratory wheeze* can be heard when the airways collapse during expiration (e.g. asthma).

However, a silent chest is a bad sign too as it indicates a totally occluded airway.

Feel

Feel for breath by placing your cheek or your hand close to the person's mouth. You should be able to feel the air movement at the mouth.

Airway opening

You will practise airway opening in your mandatory basic life-support sessions. The steps to follow are:

- If it is possible, turn the patient onto their back.
- To perform a **head tilt and chin lift**, rest one hand on the patient's forehead and place the fingertips of your other hand on to the chin, taking care not to press on the soft tissue under the chin which can obstruct the airway. Gently push down on the forehead and lift up the chin to open the airway.
- A **jaw thrust** should be used if there is suspected neck injury. To perform this manoeuvre, kneel (or stand if they are on a bed) near the top of the patient's head. Grasp the angles of the patient's lower jaw on both sides with your fingers and lift. This displaces the mandible (jawbone) forward while tilting the head backward.

Dealing with someone who has an airway obstruction can be alarming. If the person is showing signs of a mild airway obstruction they should be encouraged to cough to help clear their airway. You should observe them closely in case they deteriorate and require intervention.

If (as in Mary Wyatt's case) the airway obstruction is severe or their cough becomes ineffective, you should help them to clear the airway. It is important to remain calm, talk to the person and explain what you are doing, as struggling to breathe can be a very frightening experience. The Resuscitation Council (UK) (2005) explains the steps to take:

- Give up to *five* sharp blows between the shoulder blades using the heel of your hand. Stand behind the person and lean them forward, so when the object is dislodged it will come out of the mouth and not back down the airway.
- If these back blows are unsuccessful, give up to *five* abdominal thrusts. Stand behind the person and put both arms around their upper abdomen. Make a fist with one hand and place it in-between the navel and the bottom end of the sternum. Clasp the other hand around it and pull sharply inwards and upwards. Ensure that you do not have your face directly behind their head as the movement can cause their head to move upwards, causing you an injury. If the person is seated or small you may need to kneel behind them.
- If after five abdominal thrusts the object has still not been expelled then give further back blows and abdominal thrusts until the object is expelled.
- If the person loses consciousness, support them to the floor and begin basic life support (see the guidelines at www.resus.org.uk).

What you are attempting to do by this is increase the intrathoracic pressure, thus forcing the object out – similar to the effect of coughing. As there is risk of internal damage, the person should always be medically assessed following abdominal thrusts.

Learning outcome 2: Identify the different types of airway adjuncts available

ACTIVITY

In the skills laboratory, look at different types of airway adjuncts. Which ones have you seen in practice? How do you think they would be used?

You may have identified any of the airway adjuncts summarised in Table 11.1. The paramedics attending Mary Wyatt may have inserted one of these. You might have seen these devices used in emergency situations or in the operating theatre. There are other methods to help secure an airway, including endotracheal tubes and tracheostomies. All airway adjuncts must be inserted by trained professionals, who will have learned how to select the correct size for each patient and how to insert them safely.

Table 11.1: Airway adjuncts

Basic oropharyngeal airway
- A rigid curved plastic tube used for unconscious patients
- The patient's mouth is checked to ensure nothing could be pushed back during insertion
- Inserted upside down until it has passed the teeth to prevent the tongue being pushed back, then rotated into the correct position
- If any signs of gagging or straining occur, it must be removed immediately

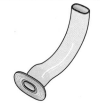

Nasopharygeal airway (NPA)
- Can be used when an oropharygeal airway cannot be tolerated, or inserted (e.g. patients with facial injuries or clenched jaws)
- Should not be used if there is a suspected basal skull fracture, owing to risk of penetrating the brain tissue (Ellis *et al.* 2006)
- The NPA, once in place, can be used for suctioning
- However, the vagus nerve can be stimulated, producing bradycardia (Pryor and Prasad 2002) – in which case, suctioning should stop and senior staff should be alerted

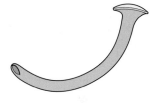

Laryngeal mask airway (LMA)
- Has an inflatable cuff that is inserted into the pharynx
- When the tube is inserted the cuff is inflated, creating an airtight seal
- Bag-valve apparatus and oxygen can be attached to ventilate the patient, which has been shown to reduce risk of gastric regurgitation (Resuscitation Council (UK) 2006)

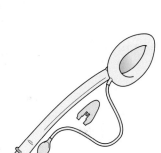

ACTIVITY

When next in your clinical area, find out what airway adjuncts are available and their location. Ensure you can recognise these pieces of equipment. Ask your mentor for guidance if necessary.

Learning outcome 3: Identify reasons for oxygen administration and how it can be delivered safely

Oxygen delivery equipment is essential in emergency situations and is available in all acute settings and many community care environments too. Oxygen delivery relies on a patent airway.

Oxygen makes up approximately one-fifth of our atmosphere at sea level. Oxygen *therapy* is the administration of extra to enable a higher inspiration of oxygen than achieved when breathing air. This may be a short-term measure in acute illness, or long-term therapy for chronic respiratory disease. For all patients, other than in an emergency situation, oxygen concentration is prescribed (see www.bnf.org) to achieve specified target oxygen saturation measurements (O'Driscoll *et al.* 2008).

Hypercapnic respiratory failure
Inadequate gas exchange by the respiratory system where there is a build-up of carbon dioxide.

For most acutely ill adults the target oxygen saturation is 94–98 per cent, but it is 88–92 per cent for people at risk of **hypercapnic respiratory failure** (O'Driscoll *et al.* 2008). Correct procedures and local guidelines must be followed for oxygen delivery.

ACTIVITY

When have you seen oxygen therapy being used within the hospital or community? When might people benefit from oxygen therapy?

Hypoxaemia
Low O_2 tension or partial pressure of O_2 (PaO_2) in the blood.

O'Driscoll *et al.* (2008) advise that oxygen is a treatment for **hypoxaemia**, not breathlessness, so oxygen saturation measurements should guide whether oxygen is administered. You may have thought of the following situations, where hypoxaemia might occur:

Chronic obstructive pulmonary disease
A chronic respiratory disease, which includes conditions such as emphysema, chronic bronchitis and chronic asthma. It causes debilitating breathlessness which affects day-to-day living.

- after a general anaesthetic;
- in emergency situations such as cardiac or respiratory arrest, shock and airway obstruction (as with Mary Wyatt);
- in chest injuries following trauma;
- in acute respiratory disease (e.g. asthma, as with Tina);
- in chronic respiratory conditions such as **chronic obstructive pulmonary disease (COPD)** and cystic fibrosis where long-term oxygen therapy may be needed, usually for a minimum of 15 hours per day.

Croxton and Bailey (2006) reported improved survival rates in people with COPD who have long-term oxygen therapy.

Oxygen supplies

In hospital, oxygen is obtained either from a cylinder (black with white shoulders) or a wall-mounted piped oxygen supply. If cylinders are used the dial showing the remaining oxygen must be checked regularly as they can run out quickly. In the home, in England and Wales, oxygen is supplied by the NHS on a regional tendering service. These companies supply the equipment and oxygen as part of an integrated service. In Scotland and Northern Ireland, supply is by local contractors. Oxygen therapy at home is usually administered from an oxygen concentrator (McLauchlan 2002), which takes in room air and removes nitrogen through filtration but without depleting the surrounding air. The concentrator runs off electricity (an emergency cylinder is supplied in case of power failure), can deliver up to 4 litres per minute, and is supplied with up to 15 metres of tubing, allowing movement around the home (Baird 2001).

Delivery devices

Different concentrations of oxygen are administered according to clinical need, which affects oxygen administration devices used. For example, for someone like Tina, who is very breathless and mouth breathing, a mask must be used.

Nurses must record details of oxygen concentration, delivery device and commencement and termination of therapy, and sign for oxygen administration on the drug chart at each drug round (O'Driscoll *et al.* 2008).

ACTIVITY	Either in your clinical setting or in the skills laboratory, look at oxygen delivery devices. How do you think different concentrations are achieved?

Oxygen therapy can be delivered at varying concentrations, often measured in percentages (e.g. 24, 28, 35, 40 per cent). Nurses should select the appropriate delivery system for each patient to achieve the target oxygen saturation level (O'Driscoll *et al.* 2008). The oxygen flow is measured in litres per minute (L/min) using a flow meter. Devices include simple oxygen masks, Venturi masks, nasal cannulae and non-rebreathing masks (see Fig. 11.1). These are disposable and packaged separately and each individual has their own equipment. Masks should be cleaned regularly (Sheppard and Davis 2000a), especially if the patient has a productive cough. Equipment should be disposed of according to local policy.

Simple oxygen masks

Mrs Patel's oxygen is currently being delivered by a simple oxygen mask. These are referred to as Hudson, MC (medium concentration) or semi-rigid. To make the mask

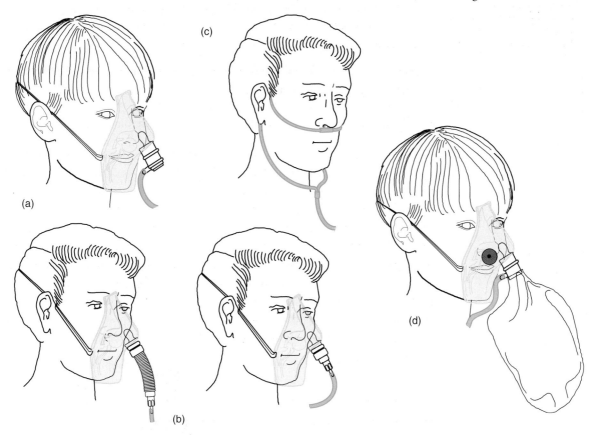

Figure 11.1: Devices for administering oxygen: (a) simple oxygen mask; (b) Venturi masks; (c) nasal cannulae; (d) non-rebreathing mask.

fit comfortably, the strap should be adjusted to fit behind the ears. The oxygen amount delivered is adjusted by using the flow meter, the exact amount delivered depending on rate and depth of breathing (Porter-Jones 2002). If a patient is breathing rapidly, large amounts of room air are drawn in and dilute the concentration (Pruitt and Jacobs 2003). Oxygen can be delivered via a simple face mask at 5–10 L/min, delivering 35–60 per cent, to achieve target oxygen saturation; rates of below 5 L/min may cause carbon dioxide rebreathing and increased resistance to inspiration (O'Driscoll *et al.* 2008).

Venturi mask system

In the Venturi system the oxygen concentration is not significantly affected by the rate and depth of breathing, so a set concentration can be achieved (Cooper 2004). The mask is supplied with different coloured fittings, each clearly marked with an oxygen percentage and the required flow rate. The device ensures that oxygen flow is accurately diluted with entrained air. You can thus administer the exact percentage prescribed by fitting the correct device and setting the correct flow rate.

Nasal cannulae

These are cheap and well tolerated (Vines *et al.* 2000), administering oxygen directly into the nostrils. Oxygen flow is adjusted by using the oxygen flow meter.

Flow rates of more than 4 L/min are not recommended owing to the drying effect on the nasal mucosa (Vines *et al.* 2000). Administration may not be very accurate, as actual oxygen intake varies according to how much the patient breathes through their mouth. To make the nasal cannulae fit closely, move the ends of the tubes through the horizontal piece of tubing across the nose and also the adaptor on the tubing below the chin.

With nasal cannulae, people can eat, drink and talk more easily than with masks. Procedures such as mouthcare can be carried out without disrupting oxygen administration. Zevola and Maiier (2001) found that nasal cannulae were considered comfortable and were better tolerated than masks. Some patients find masks claustrophobic.

Non-rebreathing masks

These have a large reservoir for oxygen (Vines *et al.* 2000), with valves to allow the patient to inhale only oxygen and prevent it mixing with expired gases. Oxygen concentration is determined by the flow meter. They provide a high concentration of oxygen (60–80 per cent), particularly for short periods of time, for example in emergencies (Mary's situation). The valve must be pressed to enable the chamber to fill with oxygen before applying the mask.

Choice of oxygen delivery system

O'Driscoll *et al.* (2008) suggest the following options for stepping dose of oxygen up or down:

- Venturi 24 per cent mask at 2–4 L/min or nasal cannulae at 1 L/min
- Venturi 28 per cent mask at 4–6 L/min or nasal cannulae at 2 L/min
- Venturi 35 per cent mask at 8–10 L/min or nasal cannulae at 4–6 L/min
- Venturi 40 per cent at 10–12 L/min or simple face mask at 5–6 L/min

- Venturi 60 per cent at 12–15 L/min or simple face mask at 7–10 L/min
- Non-rebreathe mask at 15 L/min

Fitting masks and nasal cannulae

If a mask or nasal cannulae are worn for any period of time there is a risk of pressure ulcer development, particularly on the bridge of the nose or behind the ears. Therefore masks and cannulae must be correctly fitted and skin checked regularly. Tubing can be supported by gauze or protectors to prevent sore ears.

ACTIVITY

If a hypoxic adult is confused and not tolerating oxygen therapy, what could you do?

Patients who understand how and why they need oxygen are more likely to tolerate it (Baird 2001), so clear explanations are necessary. Repositioning to improve ventilation, for example sitting upright in a chair or in bed, will be helpful. Nasal cannulae rather than a mask may be better tolerated. Support and explanations from a familiar relative may help, as well as building up a rapport with the patient and keep retrying. Remember to document your actions too. If a person with learning disabilities needs oxygen therapy, you must consider the level of understanding and learning ability. Demonstration of the mask/cannulae on a carer or nurse, and an explanation of the associated sensations and sounds, may be reassuring.

Hazards of oxygen therapy

ACTIVITY

Can you think of any hazards that might arise from oxygen therapy?

The two main hazards are fire, and the delivery of oxygen to people with chronic pulmonary disease, who are carbon dioxide retainers.

Fire hazard

You have probably attended fire lectures where a fire officer outlined the 'fire triangle'. Can you remember the three factors necessary for fire? Oxygen, fuel and heat are needed; if one of these is missing the fire cannot start or will quickly go out. Oxygen supports combustion and thus enhances the inflammable properties of other materials such as cigarettes, grease and oil (Sheppard and Davis 2000b). Administration of oxygen could therefore be a fire hazard.

ACTIVITY

What precautions will be needed to reduce fire risk during oxygen therapy?

You could have thought of:

- No Smoking signs;
- no devices that can spark;
- educating patients and relatives about the risk of smoking during oxygen administration, and alcohol-based sprays (e.g. in perfume);

- knowledge of fire procedure and equipment;
- keeping oxygen cylinders in the home away from gas fires, naked flames and hot radiators (Jones 1997).

Carbon dioxide retainers

Normally, rising levels of CO_2 stimulate respiration. However, some patients with chronic respiratory disease continuously have a high level of CO_2 in their blood, so their chemo-receptors are no longer stimulated by this. For these patients ('CO_2 retainers'), the less importzant hypoxic drive predominates, so breathing is only stimulated by lack of oxygen. These patients should carry an oxygen alert card (BTS 2008). Their target oxygen saturation will be 88–92 per cent, and they are initially administered oxygen at 28 per cent via a Venturi mask, with blood gases checked after 30–60 minutes (O'Driscoll *et al.* 2008).

Humidification

Oxygen can be drying to the mucous membranes of the upper airway (Pilkington 2004), leading to chest secretions being sticky and difficult to expectorate (Dunn and Chisholm 1998). Dryness of nostrils and mouth can be prevented through good oral hygiene, application of E45 cream and adequate fluid intake. Never use petroleum jelly near oxygen, however, because of its potentially flammable nature (Porter-Jones 2002). Oxygen administered at a high flow rate for over 24 hours should be humidified (O'Driscoll *et al.* 2008).

ACTIVITY

Either in the skills laboratory or in the clinical setting, locate humidification equipment. What sort of water would need to be used and why? What hazards might be associated with humidification equipment?

As humidification provides a moist environment there is a risk of encouraging bacterial growth. Therefore sterile water must be used to minimise bacterial contamination (Porter-Jones 2002) and the water should be changed daily. In heated-water humidifiers there is a risk of mucosal overheating or burning, and excessive condensation in the tubing can reduce oxygen flow (Porter-Jones 2002).

Learning outcome 4: Explain how suction equipment is used in practice

If the airways become obstructed (e.g. by secretions, blood, vomit), a suction device should be used. However, suctioning is a traumatic procedure and can have serious side-effects (Moore 2003). It is important to assess the patient during and after suctioning and ensure that any oxygen device is repositioned immediately. Suctioning should be done only if clinically indicated.

ACTIVITY

While in the clinical setting, locate a suction device. With your mentor, check that it is working efficiently. What attachments are there and which might you use for Mary?

> **Box 11.2 Procedure for suctioning the mouth (adapted from Day et al. 2002 and Moore 2003)**
>
> - Check that the suctioning equipment is functioning correctly and collect other equipment.
> - Maintain standard infection control precautions throughout.
> - Explain the procedure to the patient and carer.
> - Connect one end of the suction connecting tubing to the machine's suction post and the other end to a clean catheter or Yankauer sucker.
> - Set the suction machine pressure at the recommended amount, usually 80–120 mmHg.
> - Prepare the patient for the procedure and if possible ask him/her to open their mouth so that you are able to see where the secretions are.
> - Insert the catheter or sucker into the mouth but do not apply suction.
> - Gently withdraw the catheter whilst applying suction.
> - Clean the catheter by sucking through some clear water.
> - Repeat the procedure if necessary.
> - Dispose of the used equipment appropriately.
> - Rinse the suction tubing using sterile water.
> - Make sure the patient is comfortable after suctioning.
> - Assess the patient to ensure they have suffered no adverse effects from the suctioning.
> - Empty and clean the suction jar as necessary.

Suctioning devices can be wall-mounted or portable, and have a negative-pressure regulator so that the degree of suction can be altered. The recommended amount of suction is a maximum of 120 mmHg for adults (Linton 2000). It will also have a reservoir to collect the debris; this must be kept clean and clear. There should be the correct sized tubing connected, with enough length to reach the patient and a suitable suction tip. A wide-bore rigid tip, for example a Yankauer sucker, can be used to clear vomit or secretions from the mouth. A soft flexible catheter can be used in conjunction with an airway adjunct.

In Mary's case a Yankauer sucker could have been used in an attempt to remove the piece of meat initially. When she had an airway inserted it would be possible to insert a flexible suction catheter down the airway as well as using the Yankauer sucker to clear her mouth. Box 11.2 outlines the procedure for suctioning the mouth.

All suctioning equipment should be checked at least daily along with emergency equipment and before and after use to ensure it is working properly.

A suction device should only be used by staff who have had appropriate training.

Summary

- When dealing with a patient who is deteriorating it is vital to seek help immediately.

- Recognising an airway obstruction and dealing with it quickly and effectively can prevent further deterioration.
- Oxygen therapy is given to treat hypoxaemia and must be given in accordance with recommended guidelines.
- Suction should be used to clear secretions from airway but should be performed by an appropriately trained person.

BREATHING PROBLEMS AND RELATED SKILLS

Breathing problems resulting in **tachypnoea** (rapid breathing) and **dyspnoea** (difficulty in breathing) can indicate significant disease. The Royal College of Nursing (RCN) (2006) identified that respiratory disease is the main cause of death in people with learning disabilities – who are at risk of respiratory tract infections caused by aspiration or reflux if they have swallowing difficulties.

As you read, Tina Lunn has developed acute breathlessness due to her asthma, but there are many other causes of breathing problems. Some result from respiratory disease or injury. Francis (2006) offers an overview of respiratory diseases in detail. However, breathlessness also occurs in cardiac conditions, anaemia, shock (see later discussion), renal failure, drug intoxication or overdose, metabolic acidosis and allergic reactions.

All people who experience acute breathing problems should be evaluated by a healthcare professional immediately. There are a range of skills needed to assess and care for people with breathing problems. Many are included elsewhere in this book and in other sections of this chapter; you will be referred to these during this section.

LEARNING OUTCOMES

By the end of this section you will be able to:
1 consider the signs and symptoms of difficulty in breathing;
2 outline assessment skills, investigations and interventions for a person with an acute breathing problem;
3 measure and record a person's peak expiratory flow rate;
4 describe how sputum expectoration can be encouraged and sputum specimens collected.

Learning outcome 1: Identify the signs and symptoms of patients with difficulty in breathing

ACTIVITY

What are the signs and symptoms of a person who is having difficulty breathing? Consider a person, like Tina, who is acutely breathless – her scenario will give some clues.

You may have considered the following:

- tachypnoea (rapid breathing) and/or tachycardia (rapid pulse);
- noisy breathing (e.g. wheeze);
- cyanosis;
- delayed capillary refill time (explained later in this chapter);
- inability to speak in full sentences;
- use of accessory muscles;
- coughing;
- pursed lips and flared nostrils;
- leaning forward and holding of the chest
- confusion or disorientation, due to hypoxia.

In extreme situations, patients who have breathing difficulties will continue to deteriorate despite healthcare interventions. If the respiratory system suddenly ceases then **apnoea** occurs and **respiratory arrest** follows. Resuscitation Council (UK) (2005) BLS guidelines should then be followed (see www.resus.org.uk). Immediate causes of respiratory failure will be considered and treated accordingly.

Learning outcome 2: Outline assessment skills, investigations and interventions for a person with an acute breathing problem

Patients with acute breathing difficulties can use up considerable energy in trying to breathe. Prompt and careful assessment and management of their breathlessness must occur. People with acute breathing difficulties (like Tina Lunn) are often extremely anxious and frightened. You should adopt a calm and confident approach with your patient to alleviate their fears. Chapter 2 addresses communication in detail.

ACTIVITY

What assessment skills, investigations and interventions will be carried out to assess and care for a patient with an acute breathing problem? Tina Lunn's scenario will give some clues.

As discussed earlier, an ABCDE approach promotes a systematic approach. You might have included the following:

Assessment:
- airway patency (see earlier section);
- observation of effort, depth, rhythm and sound of breathing (see Chapter 4);
- pulse oximetry for measuring oxygen saturation (see Chapter 4)
- blood pressure and pulse measurement (see Chapter 4);
- capillary refill assessment (discussed later in this chapter);
- peak flow measurement (discussed later in this section);
- observation of sputum and sputum specimen collection (discussed later in this section);

- cardiac monitoring and electrocardiogram recording (discussed later in this chapter);
- temperature measurement (see Chapter 4) – as infection may be an underlying cause.

Investigations:
- chest X-ray;
- blood tests – specifically arterial blood gas analysis (see Box 11.3).

Interventions:
- oxygen therapy (see previous section);
- administration of inhalers and nebulisers (see Chapter 5);
- positioning in an upright position to aid lung expansion.

Box 11.3 Arterial blood gas analysis

- Arterial blood gas (ABG) is a blood test performed on arterial blood.
- Its purpose is to measure oxygen, carbon dioxide, bicarbonate levels and hydrogen concentration (pH) levels in the blood, thus providing an overview of the person's gaseous exchange, their respiratory status and the body's acid–base balance.
- The body's ability to regulate acid–base balance is crucial for survival; enzymes essential for biochemical reactions in cells function best within certain ranges of pH. Thus impairment of body functions results from abnormal acid–base balance.
- The results of blood gas analysis affect treatment, such as administration of medicines to adjust acidosis, and oxygen therapy.

For normal values and a discussion of ABG interpretation see Woodrow (2004).

Procedure

- Taking an arterial sample of blood is an advanced skill that is carried out by a healthcare professional who has received appropriate training – doctors or registered nurses with additional education.
- Radial and femoral arteries are commonly used.
- The test can be painful and patients undergoing the test need support.
- Local anaesthesia should be used, except in emergencies or if the patient is unconscious or anaesthetised (O'Driscoll *et al.* 2008).
- After the needle has been withdrawn, pressure needs to be applied for about 5 minutes to prevent bleeding.
- The sample is analysed and its components can offer vital evidence of the patient's well-being.
- Patients requiring regular blood gas analysis (e.g. those who are being mechanically ventilated) will have an arterial line setup, from which blood can be extracted when necessary.

See Coggan (2008a,b) for further reading.

Observation of respiration and other vital signs are relevant to all the patients in this chapter's scenarios. Mrs Patel may have a chest X-ray performed if there is concern about her developing a chest infection after having an anaesthetic, or heart failure. If Tina's condition does not improve with the nebulisers and oxygen prescribed she might need to have a chest X-ray, which could require her being transferred to the emergency department at a different hospital. Mrs Patel, Mary and Tina may have blood gas analyses performed and all will require oxygen therapy. Tina will have her peak flow rate recorded, and a sputum specimen needs to be collected.

Learning outcome 3: Measure and record a person's peak expiratory flow rate

Peak expiratory flow rate (PEFR) is a simple test of lung function. The peak flow meter measures an individual's ability to exhale. PEFR is recorded in litres per minute and is the maximum flow rate achieved on forced expiration, when starting at full inspiration. As previously identified, Tina has asthma, so the measurement of her PEFR is particularly helpful as asthma leads to a reduction of lung volume and variable obstruction of the airways. PEFR measurement is particularly useful for people who have difficulty recognising that their asthma control is worsening (McGrath *et al.* 2001).

Equipment for PEFR measurement

A peak flow meter is needed with a disposable mouthpiece for each person. Peak flow meters are often available on prescription. There are several types available, but the same peak flow meter should be used for a particular individual to ensure consistency. Figure 11.2 shows a peak flow meter that adheres to EU standard EN 13826 (see www.peakflow.com for details).

Electronic peak flow meters are now available and many patients have their own devices. The standard meter measures up to 1000 L/min, but lower reading

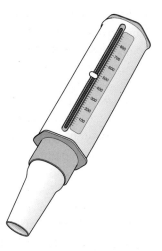

Figure 11.2: A peak flow meter which adheres to EU standard EN 13826.

or paediatric meters are also available. These should be used for children and for adults with widespread airways disease.

Access a peak flow meter and mouthpiece. Following the instructions in Box 11.4, measure your own PEFR, noting the measurements. Now work through the instructions and questions below:
- Try measuring your PEFR while in a semi-upright position. How does it compare with your original reading? What does that tell you about positioning of patients prior to PEFR measurements?
- What would you do if a measurement seemed too low?
- How could PEFR measurements be recorded?
- How often might PEFR be measured?

PEFR measurements can be misleading if the person is not positioned upright and does not use the correct technique. If a low reading is obtained you should check that the person's position and technique are correct. Then, as with any other observation, you would report the abnormal measurement to a qualified nurse. While a series of PEFR measurements is required to produce a comprehensive picture, a single low reading may need a quick response. Obviously the patient's general condition and other observations will be considered too.

In hospital, PEFR is often recorded simply as a figure at the bottom of the observation chart. There are special charts available, particularly for ongoing monitoring, and these may be used for home PEFR monitoring.

Generally, twice-daily (morning and early evening) measurements are sufficient, except during acute episodes. PEFR measurements are often used to monitor medication effects, for example with inhaled bronchodilators. The PEFR is then measured before and 30 minutes after medication (when the medication is having the maximum effect).

What are normal PEFRs?

Patients are normally advised about their baseline PEFR, according to age, height and gender. European standard EN 13826 for measuring PEFR (see www.peakflow. com) offers a chart for average PEFR readings. Generally an adult should achieve 400–600 L/min, but males achieve a higher figure than females, and greater height increases the measurement.

Box 11.4 Measuring peak expiratory flow rate

- With the mouthpiece attached, hold the peak flow meter with the scale uppermost and the pointer at zero.
- Stand upright. Take a deep breath, close your lips around the peak flow meter and blow as hard as possible as if blowing birthday candles out. Take note of the reading and return the pointer to zero. Repeat the test twice more, taking note of each reading. Record the highest result.

Asthma action plan
A personal plan given to a patient by a medical professional to advise on best treatments and management of their asthma.

Even in individuals without asthma there are variations in the measurement, with the morning figure being lower, and the highest being achieved in early evening. This tendency may be exaggerated in people with asthma (like Tina). Currie *et al.* (2005) recommend that all patients who have asthma should be aware of their own personal PEFR values and judge their deterioration or improvement on their own values rather than relying on predicted values. They also recommend that these values should form part of their asthma action plan. Tina may have her own asthma action plan; her PEFR should be compared to her 'normal' value and her immediate care should be based upon this plan.

Asthma UK, a charity that supports people with asthma, recommends that people with asthma should monitor their PEFR regularly (see www.asthma.org.uk).

ACTIVITY

Why might teaching people who have asthma to measure their PEFR be useful in managing their condition?

- They can monitor for themselves how well their asthma is being controlled by medication.
- Regular measurements may reveal a gradual – and possibly asymptomatic – deterioration that requires action (e.g. a change of medication) to prevent an acute episode. If the reading falls below 80 per cent of an individual's best level, then preventive medicine, usually an inhaled steroid, should be increased (see www.asthma.org.uk).
- Without PEFR monitoring, people can be unaware of worsening symptoms. The measurement may fall by up to 50 per cent before symptoms are noticed. Circumstances affecting measurements may be identified (e.g. contact with a cat), thus enabling asthma triggers to be recognised.
- The measurement may indicate the severity of the asthma at that particular time. The lower the measurement, the narrower the airways. A measurement of below 50 per cent of the baseline requires immediate medical attention.

BTS/SIGN (2008) emphasise that teaching people to use inhalers and volumatic spacer devices and monitor their PEFR should be only part of a comprehensive asthma management programme. This should also include instruction about avoiding asthma triggers, correct use of medication, identification of warning signs of worsening asthma, and what action to take. On-going education and monitoring can be achieved through attendance at asthma clinics where correct technique in PEFR measurement can be checked. Manual dexterity and coordination for using peak flow meters needs to be assessed. Asthma UK recommends that patients keep a peak flow diary to identify significant issues or readings. The diary also offers the patient and the healthcare team an overview of what is happening in their lungs, how effective medications are in treating breathlessness, and average PEFR readings over a given period.

Despite the potential benefits of PEFR monitoring, long-term levels of use can be low, even in motivated patients who have taken part in educational programmes.

However, the introduction of electronic devices in 2004 coupled with asthma health education programmes at asthma clinics are just some of the steps that have been taken to improve this situation.

Booker (2007) identifies how, in some instances such as non-acute settings, PEFR monitoring has been superseded by **spirometry**. The spirometer can be used for diagnosing and monitoring people with conditions such as COPD. This assessment can take place in the community setting to ensure patients are fully aware of their diagnosis and can monitor the effects of their treatment. Spirometry offers further objective feedback to people with asthma.

Learning outcome 4: Describe how sputum expectoration can be encouraged and sputum specimens collected

Adults normally produce about 100 mL of **mucus** in the respiratory tract daily, but it goes unnoticed as it is usually swallowed (Law 2000). However, in some diseases excess mucus is produced, and smoking stimulates excessive mucus production. The mucus is then expectorated from the lungs and termed **sputum**.

Sputum consists of lower respiratory tract secretions, nasopharyngeal and oropharyngeal material (including saliva), microorganisms and cells (Rubin 2002). Clearance of secretions is very important to maintain a clear airway and reduce infection risk (Rubin 2002). However, patients may deny the existence of sputum due to social stigma or lack of awareness (Law 2000). Some, particularly women, feel embarrassed to expectorate, and are more likely to swallow their sputum.

> **Spirometry**
> A test that can help diagnose lung function and identify how respiratory disease affects the lungs. It uses a spirometer, a device consisting of a mouthpiece attached to a machine which measures the amount of air exhaled.

ACTIVITY

How can you encourage Tina to expectorate her sputum?

First Tina needs to understand why it is important to clear her secretions. She will be able to cough more easily if in a well-supported, upright position, and a sputum pot and tissues should be provided. If she is well hydrated, her sputum will be less thick and therefore easier to cough up. A dry mouth makes expectoration difficult, and infected sputum can taste unpleasant. Therefore you should provide mouth care, or assist Tina to go the bathroom. Privacy should be given if there is embarrassment, and nurses should ensure that they do not show distaste even though they may feel it.

ACTIVITY

How would you describe normal sputum? What do you think might cause sputum to look abnormal?

Sputum (or mucus) is odourless, clear and thin but people who have respiratory disease may expectorate sputum that is altered in colour and consistency. When assessing, it is important to identify what the individual's sputum is like normally. Signs of respiratory infection are sputum that is green, yellow or rust-coloured and it may be odorous. Purulent green sputum in patients with an acute exacerbation of their COPD is highly associated with infection (Stockley *et al.* 2000). A *Pseudomonas* infection produces thick green sputum with a characteristic odour.

A stringy mucoid specimen often occurs with bronchial asthma (Law 2000). If blood is present the sputum will be rust-coloured or red – termed **haemoptysis**. It may be a sign of infection, but can also occur in cancer, heart failure and pulmonary embolus. Haemoptysis can be distressing to patients. It is important to check that it has actually come from the lungs and has not been vomited (**haemetemesis**) or come from the nose (**epistaxis**). Haemoptysis is worsened by vigorous coughing, chest trauma, chest physiotherapy, anticoagulant therapy and activity. When assessing the amount being produced it is best to ask in terms of teaspoons, tablespoons or cups. Patients may comment on the sputum's taste which may be unpleasant if infected or salty with cystic fibrosis.

When sputum is being produced, especially in suspected respiratory disease, a specimen is often required for laboratory examination. Tina has been asked to produce a sputum specimen as she may have a chest infection. The goal of sputum collection is to 'obtain fresh, uncontaminated secretions from the tracheobronchial tree' (Wilkins *et al.* 2005). Although the lower part of the respiratory tract is usually sterile, the upper respiratory tract, nose and mouth, are colonised by large numbers of different bacteria (Wilson 2006).

ACTIVITY	Why might a sputum specimen need to be sent to the laboratory?

A sputum specimen may be sent for microbiological examination if infection, including tuberculosis (TB), is suspected. It may also be sent for cytology – examination for abnormal (e.g. cancerous) cells. Box 11. 5 outlines the equipment needed and the procedure and additional points are discussed below.

When a sputum specimen is collected, it must come from the lower airways rather than being cleared from the throat or saliva. This needs to be explained carefully to the person, taking into account their level of understanding. You can explain that the specimen must come from the 'windpipe'. Sputum is usually more viscous and purulent than saliva; if the specimen appears to be saliva it should be discarded. A physiotherapist can assist people who have difficulty expectorating.

Box 11.5 Key points in collecting a sputum specimen

Equipment needed
- A sterile specimen container with a leakproof lid or cap, and tissues

Key points
- An early-morning specimen is best, as bacteria counts are probably highest then.
- Careful explanation is needed.
- The mouth should be rinsed with water and teeth brushed to prevent contamination with oral microbes.
- The sputum should be expectorated directly into the labelled container and the lid reapplied immediately.

When sputum is being sent for testing for tuberculosis, the specimen should be at least 10 mL. Three early-morning specimens taken on different days are required as *Mycobacterium tuberculosis*, which causes TB, may be present in small numbers only, particularly in the disease's early stages (Wilson 2006). Most bacteria grow within 24–48 hours, but *Mycobacterium tuberculosis* can take up to six weeks to grow (Wilson 2006). Nevertheless, microscopic examination of the sputum can lead to an initial tentative diagnosis.

Summary

- There are many reasons for acute breathing problems. These situations can be frightening for patients and so a calm, confident approach is necessary.
- You need to understand the assessment skills, investigations and interventions that may be needed and develop your skills to assist people with acute breathing problems.
- Peak flow measurements are important indicators of respiratory function, particularly in people who have asthma. They must be recorded accurately and consistently, as they may influence treatment.
- Nursing measures can encourage expectoration of sputum, which can then be observed for colour, consistency, amount and odour.
- Careful explanations can help to ensure that an uncontaminated sputum specimen is obtained.

CIRCULATORY PROBLEMS AND RELATED SKILLS

An effective circulation requires a functioning cardiovascular system and adequate blood volume. A range of symptoms result when abnormalities occur, so effective assessment skills and interventions are needed to support patients with circulatory problems.

LEARNING OUTCOMES

By the end of this section you will be able to:
1 identify common causes of acute circulatory problems and key aspects of assessment;
2 describe the term 'capillary refill time' and be able to perform the skill;
3 attach a patient to a cardiac monitor and recognise sinus rhythm;
4 outline how a 12-lead electrocardiograph is recorded.

Learning outcome 1: Identify common causes of acute circulatory problems and key aspects of assessment

There are many causes of circulatory problems.

ACTIVITY

Re-read Mrs Patel's scenario. Can you identify possible causes of a circulatory problem?

You read that Mrs Patel has an abnormality of her heart's conduction system (atrial fibrillation) which will affect her circulation. You also know that she would have lost

Box 11.6 Shock: key points

- Shock is a potentially recoverable but significant reduction in circulating blood volume, leading to inadequate tissue perfusion.
- The inability to deliver oxygen and nutrients to body tissues leads to metabolic and functional impairment and hypoxia.

Types of shock

- Hypovolaemia – low blood volume.
- Cardiogenic shock – due to the heart's inability to pump blood around the body efficiently (e.g. following myocardial infarction).
- Anaphylactic shock – a severe allergic reaction (see 'Preventing and managing anaphylaxis' in Chapter 5).
- Septic shock – occurs in severe infection. The systemic inflammatory response causes vasodilatation of peripheral blood vessels, increased capillary permeability and thus extravascular fluid loss.
- Neurogenic shock – rapid loss of vasomotor tone leads to vasodilation and a severe decrease in blood pressure.
- Emotional shock – emotion triggers parasympathetic stimulation leading to vasovagal syncope (unconsciousness). Spontaneous recovery usually occurs within a few minutes.

blood from her circulation during surgery and is continuing to do so. A reduction in blood volume (due to fluid loss or haemorrhage) can lead to hypovolaemia and then shock. Shock is a complex condition leading to a cascade of physiological reactions in the body. It is caused by an underlying medical condition or trauma; if left unmanaged it can be life-threatening. Your biology book will give a detailed explanation – see Box 11.6 for a few key points.

In shock, a reduction in the person's cardiac output is seen and significant changes occur in their vital signs. It is important to find the cause of shock and treat it quickly. Mrs Patel has a lot of drainage from her wound and changes in her vital signs. Thus the doctor may increase her rate of intravenous fluid administration to increase the circulating fluid volume, or order a blood transfusion (see Chapter 5).

How will you know a person is in shock?

There are four stages of shock: initial, compensatory, progressive and refractory (Hand 2001; Garretson and Malberti 2007):

- *Initial* – the body shows signs of reduced cardiac output.
- *Compensatory* – the body attempts to restore homeostasis and improve tissue perfusion.
- *Progressive* – the body loses its ability to compensate, bringing about acidosis and electrolyte imbalance.
- *Refractory* – irreversible cell damage occurs and the body organs are affected.

As the patient's condition deteriorates, their vital signs change. The body first tries to compensate by moving fluids around from within cells to the circulation, attempting to maintain blood pressure in a normal range. However, there may be a slight rise in the heart rate. As the body loses the ability to compensate, respiratory rate rises as the body tries to apply as much oxygen as possible on to the remaining red blood cells and deliver them to the cells. As this body mechanism fails, the body becomes overwhelmed. **Acidosis** and **electrolyte imbalance** follow, with the patient becoming cold, clammy, less responsive and confused.

ACTIVITY

Look back at Mrs Patel's scenario. Are there any indications that she is developing shock?

Mrs Patel has lost a lot of blood, so she will start to show signs of shock at an early stage. You read that her heart rate and respiratory rates are rising and her blood pressure falling. However, the body has an ability to compensate for a short time during shock responses and each patient responds to shock differently.

Assessment and management of a patient who is in shock should take a systematic ABCDE approach, as discussed earlier in this chapter. Driscoll *et al.* (2000) identify how measuring vital signs – including capillary refill time, conscious level, heart rate, blood pressure and urine output – are all important for patients in shock. Thus the patient in shock may have a urinary catheter inserted and hourly urine measurements would be recorded (see Chapter 9 for urinary catheterisation procedure).

A central venous catheter might be inserted so that central venous pressure (CVP) monitoring can commence. CVP monitoring assists in assessment of a patient's circulating blood volume and identification of circulatory failure. CVP measurements must be interpreted in conjunction with other vital signs, with the trend assessed rather than a single measurement. If Mrs Patel continued to deteriorate, CVP monitoring might be commenced as it would help to carefully manage fluid replacement while preventing overloading her – a particular danger with her cardiac condition. CVP monitoring is an advanced skill (see Box 11.7 for key points). Cole (2007) explains this procedure in detail.

ACTIVITY

When in the practice setting, identify whether any patients are having CVP measured. Ask your mentor to explain why the patient is having CVP monitoring and how this procedure is carried out. Discuss what the patient's CVP measurements indicate about his or her condition.

Learning outcome 2: Describe the term 'capillary refill time' and be able to perform the skill

To assess capillary refill time, cutaneous pressure is exerted on the person's fingertip for 5 seconds and released. The finger should be held at heart level or just above and the pressure should be enough to cause blanching (Resuscitation Council (UK) 2006). The test indicates capillary perfusion. Normally capillary refill time is less than 2 seconds. Situations where capillary refill time is increased include shock, dehydration, aortic aneurysm, aortic occlusion, cardiac tamponade, hypothermia and Raynaud's syndrome.

Raynaud's syndrome
A condition causing constriction of small blood vessels, usually in the hands and feet.

Box 11.7 CVP monitoring: key points

- Under aseptic conditions and local anaesthetic, a central venous catheter is inserted into a vein. The tip of the catheter will lie in the right atrium.
- Common sites for insertion are the jugular veins (external or internal) and the subclavian vein. The femoral vein and the antecubital vein can also be used.
- An X-ray is performed to check positioning of the catheter.
- CVP is the pressure in the vena cava/right atrium.
- CVP may be measured using manual equipment with a water manometer and a spirit level lined up to the person's sternal notch or mid-axilla. The position used should be consistent.
- Patients are usually positioned flat for reading CVP. If they are unable to lie flat, their position during measurement should be noted.
- Normal readings vary according to positioning: 7–12 cmH$_2$O if measured at mid-axilla, or 0–7 cmH$_2$O if measured at the sternal angle (Woodrow 2002).
- In some settings, CVP is measured using an electronic pressure transducer displaying a continual reading.
- Fluid replacement is often adjusted according to CVP readings, taking into account other indicators too (e.g. urine output, blood pressure).
- Complications include infection and air embolus. Care must be taken to ensure the catheter does not become dislodged. If this happens accidentally, immediate pressure should be applied at the insertion point.
- CVP lines must be handled aseptically. On removal the tip is often sent for microscopic culture.

ACTIVITY

Depress the tip of your finger for 5 seconds, then release the pressure and watch the blood return to your capillaries. Now repeat the test and time the return of the blood to your finger. This should be less than 2 seconds, usually the time it takes you to say 'capillary refill'.

Learning outcome 3: Attach a patient to a cardiac monitor and recognise sinus rhythm

You read that Mrs Patel had a cardiac monitor attached postoperatively. The paramedics probably attached cardiac monitoring to Mary, which will be continued on her arrival at the hospital. Cardiac monitoring is carried out for many acutely ill patients and where heart rhythm is, or may become, abnormal (e.g. cardiac conditions, electrolyte imbalance, poisoning, hypothermia). You may have seen this equipment on placement or in the skills laboratory.

The cardiac monitor detects voltage differences within the body surface and amplifies and displays these as a signal (Jones 2005). The device can offer useful information to healthcare professionals, such as indicating myocardial ischaemia and cardiac arrhythmias. The cardiac monitor consists of three standard bipolar leads, I, II and III: red, yellow and green (or black). The monitor leads are connected to adhesive electrode pads placed on the patient's chest; see Fig. 11.3 for lead placement.

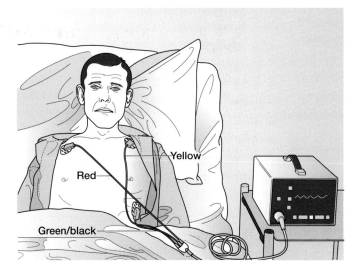

Figure 11.3: Placement of cardiac monitoring leads.

Box 11.8 Cardiac monitoring: key points

- First establish the patient's identity and rationale for cardiac monitoring.
- Inform the patient about the procedure and gain their cooperation and verbal consent.
- Check that the patient does not have a cardiac pacemaker *in situ*. If they do, seek advice before connecting any monitoring equipment, as some devices can interfere with cardiac pacemakers.
- Assemble all equipment: cardiac monitor and ECG leads, three skin-pad electrodes, alcohol wipe, razor.
- Ensure that the patient's skin is clean and free from grease as the electrodes will not adhere to the chest fully otherwise. With consent, shave or trim any chest hair to ensure that the electrodes will stick.
- Place electrodes on the chest (see Fig. 11.3 for positions).
- Turn on the monitor and adjust the setting to lead I, II or III as directed. Lead II is usually chosen as it shows a positive R wave and a clear P wave.
- Check the patient is comfortable and that the cardiac monitor is recording. Take note of the rate and rhythm of the patient's heart and report if there is an abnormality. If unsure, ask a senior colleague to review your patient with you.
- Record that you have commenced cardiac monitoring in the patient's notes.

Box 11.8 outlines key points for cardiac monitoring. The ECG produces a graphic recording of the heart's electrical impulses producing a **PQRST complex** (Jowett and Thompson 2007). Figure 11.4 shows the PQRST complex and briefly identifies what each part of the complex denotes (see Hampton 2003 for more detail).

Once connected to a monitor, you may observe that the patient has a 'normal' heart rhythm (**sinus rhythm**), portraying that electrical impulses are travelling from the sino-atrial node to the atrio-ventricular node, down the septum of the heart,

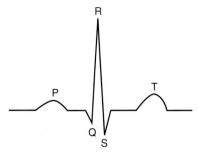

P wave: represents atrial depolarisation prior to atrial contraction
QRS: represents depolarisation of the ventricles prior to ventricular contraction:
– Q: the first downward deflection
– R: the first upward deflection
– S: the first downward deflection following the R wave
T wave: is the next positive wave which shows ventricular repolarization.

Figure 11.4: The PQRST complex.

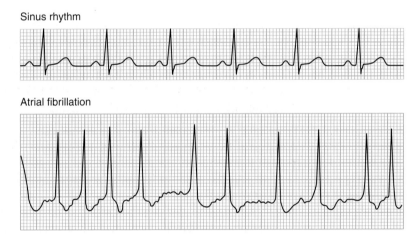

Figure 11.5: Comparison of sinus rhythm and atrial fibrillation.

into the Bundle of His and then the left and right bundle branches and the Purkinje fibres. If you need to remind yourself about this physiology, re-read the heart's conduction system in your biology book. Mrs Patel's heart rhythm, however, is known to be atrial fibrillation.

ACTIVITY

Look at the two rhythm strips in Fig. 11.5, which show sinus rhythm and atrial fibrillation. What differences can you see? Look at the following for each strip:
- the rate – frequency of the complex;
- the regularity of each complex occurring;
- whether P waves are present and precede each QRS.

Now think about what you would feel if taking Mrs Patel's pulse. How might it differ from the pulse of a person with sinus rhythm?

You will have noticed that, unlike in sinus rhythm, in atrial fibrillation 'P' waves cannot be identified. This is because the atria are 'fibrillating' rather than contracting and the impulses are conducted through the atrio-ventricular node irregularly so the QRS complexes appear irregularly. You will see that the QRS complexes occur more frequently as often uncontrolled atrial fibrillation leads to a more rapid heart rate. If you were feeling Mrs Patel's pulse, it would feel irregularly irregular. This observation is an important indicator of atrial fibrillation so should be reported.

ACTIVITY

> You may be able to practise attaching a cardiac monitor to a colleague in the skills laboratory. If so, ask them to move around and then to simulate cleaning teeth. Note how this muscle movement affects the cardiac monitor's rhythm display.

In this section you have learned how to attach a cardiac monitor, how to observe a rhythm strip and how to recognise one common arrhythmia, atrial fibrillation. There are many textbooks that look in detail at interpreting arrhythmias, so access them for further reading about arrhythmias (e.g. Hampton 2003).

Remember: Observing a cardiac monitor is no substitute for observing your patient. The observations previously discussed – vital signs and capillary refill – must also be carried out during your assessment.

Learning outcome 4: Outline how a 12-lead electrocardiograph is recorded

The 12-lead ECG is a useful diagnostic tool and can comprehensively portray the patient's heart rhythm and rate.

ACTIVITY

> Mrs Patel is to have an ECG recorded as she is known to have atrial fibrillation. In what other situations might an ECG be recorded? Think back to when you have seen an ECG recorded in practice.

ECGs are often recorded as a routine investigation before anaesthesia, particularly in older people, to identify myocardial ischaemia, in people with electrolyte imbalances and when the heart may be affected by drugs. The ECG is also recorded in emergency situations, for example patients who have collapsed, and people with a history of a fall. Therefore Enid might have one recorded, either in the community, when her GP visits, at the health centre by the practice nurse, or if she is referred to a hospital.

Electrical impulses precede cardiac muscle (myocardium) contraction so this electrical impulse is captured and recorded in an ECG. Waveforms vary in different leads placed on the person's body, and the ECG records the conduction of electrical impulses through the heart from different points. Think of taking a picture with a camera and obtaining a 360-degree view of the patient's heart from various positions around their bed. For more detail about the physiology underpinning ECGs and their interpretation, refer to your physiology textbook

---

Box 11.9 Recording ECGs: key points

- Assemble the equipment: ECG machine, alcohol wipes, tissues, razor (to trim chest hair if necessary), 10 disposable pre-gelled electrodes.
- Identify the patient, explain the procedure and gain their verbal consent.
- Ensure the patient's privacy and dignity is maintained during the procedure.
- Position the patient in a semi-recumbent position if their clinical condition allows. Otherwise record the ECG in the position they are comfortable in.
- Plug in the ECG machine to the DC power supply, or ensure that the machine's battery is fully charged
- Perform hand hygiene.
- Clean the patient's skin, where the electrodes are to be applied, with an alcohol wipe and remove excess chest hair if the electrodes will not adhere to the skin.
- Apply the electrodes to the limbs and chest (see Fig. 11.6). Connect the ECG leads to these electrodes, placing the lead box on the patient's abdomen.
- Switch on the ECG machine, check calibration of the machine and ECG size.
- Set the paper speed at 25 mm/s unless otherwise instructed
- Enter the patient's name, date of birth, date and time of procedure if the ECG machine has these facilities.
- Inform the patient you are going to now record the ECG and advise them not to move, speak or cough but to breathe normally. Print the ECG. Remember that movement will affect the reading and be seen as an artefact on the ECG, and then the test will have to be repeated.
- Advise the patient that you have completed the test. Attempt to reassure the patient as this may be an anxious time.
- Advise that the ECG will now be reviewed by a nurse or doctor trained in this procedure. Do not make any attempt to offer a diagnosis to the patient at this stage, and avoid suggesting the test was 'all right' as a patient may misinterpret this that their ECG shows no signs of disease or problem.
- Labelling – If this has not been entered before the procedure, note the patient's details now on the ECG printout. Do not allow anyone to remove the ECG from the machine before you label it. Record if the patient has chest pain or not at this stage. If this is a serial ECG, write the number on it too.
- Disconnect the ECG leads from the patient, make the patient comfortable and assist them to redress if necessary.
- Document that you have recorded an ECG.
- Clean the ECG machine before returning it to its storage place and reconnecting it to the DC power supply.
- Show the ECG to a competent practitioner and assist in any treatment that the patient now requires.

and specialist cardiology books (e.g. Jowett and Thompson 2007). The practice of recording an ECG is focused on here. Box 11.9 provides key practice points for recording ECGs.

Placement of the ECG leads

The 12-lead ECG uses ten electrodes (sometimes referred to as 'leads') to obtain the reading: six are placed on the person's chest and one on each of the four limbs. The placement of these electrodes offers 12 views of electrical activity in different areas of the heart – hence the name 12-lead ECG.

The four limb leads (which are labelled) are placed as follows:

- RA on right arm;
- LA on left arm;
- LL on left leg;
- RL on right leg – this plays no part in the actual reading other than providing an earth.

If the patient is an amputee place the electrode on the stump.

The placement of these leads forms six standard leads: three bipolar leads (I, II, III) and three augmented vector leads (aVR, aVL, aVF). These limb leads record electrical activity in the following areas (see Hampton 2003):

- I, II and aVL – the lateral aspect of the heart;
- III and aVF – the inferior aspect of the heart;
- aVR – the right atrium.

The six chest leads provide the other six views and are colour-coded and labelled: red (V1), yellow (V2), green (V3), brown (V4), black (V5) and purple (V6). These leads are placed on the torso (see Fig. 11.6):

- V1 – at the 4th intercostal space, approximately 1–2 cm right of the sternum;
- V2 – at the 4th intercostal space, approximately 1–2 cm left of the sternum.
- V4 – at the left side of the chest at the 5th intercostal space on the mid-clavicular line;
- V3 – midway between V2 and V4;
- V5 – at the 5th intercostal space at level of V4 (anterior axilla, halfway between V4 and V6);
- V6 – at the same level as V4 and V5, at the mid-axilla line.

| ACTIVITY | Try feeling for the 4th and 5th intercostal spaces on your own chest in front of the mirror. |

These chest leads record electrical activity in the following areas (see Hampton 2003):

- V1 and V2 – right ventricle;
- V3 and V4 – septum and anterior wall of the left ventricle;
- V5 and V6 – anterior and lateral walls of left ventricle.

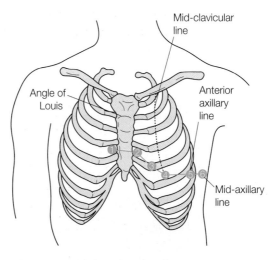

Figure 11.6: Placement of chest leads for 12-lead ECG.

ACTIVITY

If possible, while in your healthcare setting, observe an ECG being recorded and then record one under supervision. An ECG technician might be able to assist you with this activity, or a nurse. Look at the ECG recorded and observe the differences in how the PQRST complex appears in the 12 different views.

Summary

- Assessment of a patient's circulatory volume and vital signs measurement is an important part of the ABCDE assessment.
- Recognising and responding to signs of shock in patients is essential in nursing practice.
- Clinical skills such as measuring capillary refill are simple to learn and greatly assist in your patient's assessment. Practise these skills and take time in refining them.
- Cardiac monitoring and the recording of a 12-lead ECG are more complex skills that will require direct supervision at first, and then you gaining knowledge and experience in a variety of settings to become competent in these skills and understand their significance.

UNCONSCIOUSNESS AND RELATED SKILLS

Our awake state is known as consciousness, whilst unconsciousness is defined as when an individual's awareness no longer exists. Normal reflexes protecting conscious patients are lost and so healthcare professionals must maintain their safety and provide all care needed. Regarding the assessment of an unconscious person, look back to Chapter 4 for an overview of how to carry out a neurological assessment – AVPU and the GCS – and ensure that you can conduct these assessments before continuing with this section as they are necessary for anyone with altered conscious level.

By the end of this section you will be able to:-
1 identify possible causes of unconsciousness and general care required for people who are unconscious;
2 understand the principles of blood glucose monitoring;
3 describe how to deal with fits.

Learning outcome 1: Identify possible causes of unconsciousness and general care required for people who are unconscious

There are many possible causes of unconsciousness.

ACTIVITY

List all the causes of unconsciousness you can think of. Looking back at Enid's scenario might give some clues.

You may have considered the following:
- drug intoxification;
- fits;
- focal head injury (trauma);
- hypoxia (lack of oxygen to the tissues);
- hypercarbia (high levels of carbon dioxide in the circulating blood);
- hypothermia (below normal temperature) or hyperthermia (high body temperature due to loss of thermoregulatory control);
- hyperglycaemia (blood glucose above normal) or hypoglycaemia (blood glucose below normal);
- infection (e.g. encephalitis, meningitis);
- brain tumour;
- vascular events: shock, stroke.

ACTIVITY

What general care might an unconscious person require?

You should have identified that an unconscious person's airway must be maintained, and oxygen and suction could be necessary (see earlier sections). They will also need care to prevent complications of immobility (Chapter 6), hygiene care, including mouth and eye care (Chapter 8), care of their elimination (Chapter 9), and maintenance of their fluid and nutrition (Chapter 10). It is also important to consider whether they are experiencing pain, and ensure their comfort (see Chapter 12 for more information).

Communication is vital when dealing with unconscious patients. When a person loses consciousness, they may be still aware of their surroundings and sensitive to touch and speech. Thus Enid's carers should have talked to her calmly while she appeared unresponsive. It is very important to talk to unconscious patients and explain what you are going to do. Social conversation is also helpful so that the person is aware of your presence. Family members and significant others should be encouraged to talk to the unconscious person. They may need your help and support in doing this initially.

Learning outcome 2: Understand the principles of blood glucose monitoring

Hypoglycaemia or hyperglycaemia can cause unconsciousness. Glucose is generated in the body from the foods we eat and is circulated in the blood. Insulin is necessary to enable glucose to enter the cells to provide energy for cellular metabolism. Check your biology textbook for a detailed explanation about this process. If glucose levels rise or fall outside the normal range (4–7 mmol/L; 3.6–5.8 mmol/L fasting) then the person's conscious level is affected and they can become extremely unwell. Blood glucose monitoring is therefore often carried out by or for people known to have diabetes. However, other underlying medical conditions and traumatic incidents can affect a person's blood glucose levels without them having diabetes. So most unconscious patients or medically unwell people will have their blood glucose levels assessed to identify if these are within normal range.

Organisations have varying policies about who can carry out blood glucose monitoring, so you must go by local policy as to whether you can carry it out in practice. You must be trained how to use your organisation's particular blood glucose monitoring equipment.

ACTIVITY

Find out about blood glucose monitoring in your own practice setting. Investigate:
* what equipment is used;
* what training is given to use this equipment;
* whether there are training updates;
* who can carry out blood glucose monitoring.

The Diabetes UK website (www.diabetes.org.uk) is regularly updated and very informative about managing diabetes; ensure that you review this regularly as management interventions change rapidly. In particular, do look up recognition and management of hypoglycaemia on this website. Also, there are NICE guidelines about managing diabetes and National Service Frameworks and guidelines for all four UK countries, which you can access via their websites.

Blood glucose monitoring is part of the daily routine of many people with diabetes, who know their normal blood glucose levels and are aware of how to control their blood glucose. In Enid's instance, her carers know her usual blood glucose level. When a person becomes unwell due to infection, disease, trauma or a mental health problem, they may be unable to control their diabetes. Blood glucose levels are measured by carrying out a finger prick and gaining a blood sample which is then analysed using a glucose meter. There are many different types of these available. Alternatively, a blood sample can be taken to the biochemistry laboratory for glucose levels to be analysed. This test usually takes a little time to perform and is therefore not useful in an emergency situation. Treatment will need to be administered according to the blood glucose level. Box 11.10 lists key points in blood glucose measurement.

ACTIVITY

Read Box 11.10 carefully and identify possible reasons for blood glucose tests being inaccurate. Now categorise these causes under the following headings: 'Problems with technique' and 'Problems with equipment'. What could be the consequences of obtaining an inaccurate blood glucose result – either too high or too low?

You must pay attention to both technique and the equipment used to gain accurate results. Examples of technique error include failing to wash the finger (consider how the result might be affected if the person has just been eating grapes or chocolate), squeezing the finger leading to interstitial blood entering the blood sample, and insufficient blood being obtained. Equipment problems can include reagent strips that have been exposed to air or are out of date, and a machine that has not been quality checked as per manufacturer's instructions.

Gaining inaccurate results of any test is potentially very dangerous. Blood glucose monitoring directly affects treatment. For example, a sliding-scale insulin pump is adjusted according to the blood glucose result. If the result obtained was higher than it really is the person might be administered more insulin than they really need,

---

Box 11.10 Blood glucose monitoring: key points

Equipment
- Finger-pricking device, gauze/cotton wool for cleaning finger with water and drying, glucose meter, reagent strips

Technique
- Remember infection control. Always consider hand hygiene, wash your hands prior to the procedure, use non-sterile gloves to protect yourself and the patient.
- The glucometer must be maintained and checked as per manufacturer's instructions and the strips should be correctly stored (airtight container) and in-date. The user must be trained to use the specific meter and strips.
- Fingers used should be 3rd, 4th or 5th on either side of the end of the finger – but not the top, as this is more painful. This gives 12 possible sites and the site should be rotated to avoid causing neurological damage over time with repeated finger pricks. The thumb and 2nd finger are not used as these are most important for touch.
- If the hand is very cold, ensure that the patient is warm first.
- The finger site must be washed and dried with water as contamination by food etc. can affect the accuracy of the test.
- The finger should not be squeezed/milked from the base.
- After the finger has been pricked, blood is applied to the reagent strip as per the manufacturer's instructions and then inserted in the meter for reading.
- Ensure safe sharps disposal.
- Record the result in the patient's notes.
- Show the results to a competent practitioner and assist in any treatments that are necessary.

with the risk they could develop hypoglycaemia. If the result is lower than it really is they might not be administered enough insulin and could become increasingly hyperglycaemic. Recording and reporting results from the test is important because, like other information obtained in assessment, it directly impacts on care. If a blood glucose result was very high or very low, immediate action might be necessary.

<table>
<tr><td>**ACTIVITY**</td><td>Arrange to observe blood glucose being measured and, if allowed within your organisation's policy, and you have been trained on the meter used, carry out blood glucose monitoring under supervision. Ensure that you document the result and discuss its implications with your mentor.</td></tr>
</table>

Learning outcome 3: Describe how to deal with fits

> **Epilepsy**
> A tendency to have recurrent seizures (sometimes called fits). A seizure is caused by a sudden burst of excess electrical activity in the brain, causing a temporary disruption in the normal message passing between brain cells. This disruption results in the brain's messages becoming halted or mixed up. See www. epilepsy.org.uk.

Fits (sometimes caused seizures or convulsions) can be caused by medical conditions, but some people experience fits on a regular basis and are then said to have **epilepsy**. They may wear jewellery alerting that they have epilepsy, or carry a card.

All healthcare practitioners should be able to recognise and respond appropriately to a person experiencing a fit. There are thought to be around 40 different types of seizures which vary in severity. Epilepsy Action (2008) estimate that as many as 600 000 people in the UK have epilepsy and many require some form of healthcare intervention each year. Mencap (2004) identified that 22 per cent of people with learning disabilities have epilepsy compared to 1 per cent of the rest of the population.

People who experience an epileptic fit can progress through several stages of fitting. Dreifuss (1989) offers the following international classification for fits:

- *partial seizures*, either local or focal in origin;
- *generalised seizures* (convulsive or non-convulsive), involving the whole brain;
- *unclassified epileptic seizures*, including all seizures that have incomplete data to aid classification.

> **Status epilepticus**
> A seizure that lasts 30 minutes or longer, or a series of seizures without consciousness being regained in between (Epilepsy Action 2008).

When a person with epilepsy convulses or fits, it should always be treated as an emergency situation and prompt action taken. Stokes *et al.*'s (2004) guidelines recommend a systematic approach to their care. Some people who experience epileptic fits have prolonged episodes of fitting. This is known as **status epilepticus**.

Convulsive stages and interventions

Stage 1

This is referred to as from the commencement of the fit to the first 10 minutes. This may well occur in a community setting. The person should be assessed using an ABCDE approach (see earlier section) and interventions as per Resuscitation Council (UK) (2005) guidelines should be followed as required. Drug therapy may be considered; for example, midazolam may be administered rectally by an appropriately trained person (see Chapter 9).

During the convulsion, **do**:

* protect the person from further harm and provide privacy;
* maintain their airway (see earlier section);
* stay with the person and reassure them by speaking calmly.

During the convulsion, **do not**:

* restrain the person in any way;
* put any object in the person's mouth;
* attempt to rouse them.

Stage 2

This is up to 30 minutes from the commencement of the fit. This may occur in the hospital setting or in the community. At this stage, the person requires careful monitoring of their vital signs and consideration of the possible causes of the fit. After convulsions have ceased, move them into the recovery position to protect the airway. Sometimes incontinence occurs during a fit so be sensitive and promote dignity. Hospitalisation usually follows if the person does not recover spontaneously.

Stage 3

This is from the commencement of the fit to 60 minutes and involves considering the aetiology of the fit and alerting healthcare professionals to the patient's condition.

Stage 4

This stage (30–90 minutes) encompasses maintenance of vital signs (as discussed in Chapter 4). Assessment of arterial blood gases, monitoring of blood glucose levels, cardiac monitoring and recording of a 12-lead ECG, as discussed earlier in this chapter, also occur at this stage as required.

Stokes *et al.* (2004) (see www.nice.co.uk) provide full details about the management of people with epilepsy.

Summary

* Recognising the causes of unconsciousness and carrying out an accurate assessment of an unconscious patient forms an important aspect of a patient's initial assessment in the acute setting.
* Patients who are unconscious need support and monitoring for their airway, breathing and circulation as well as pressure area care, hygiene, elimination, nutrition and comfort.
* Blood glucose monitoring can assist in identifying a cause for a patient's deterioration. This skill should be observed in your practice setting and appropriate training on using specific equipment obtained before practising this skill. Local policies must be adhered to.
* Dealing with fits and recognising the stages of convulsion and responding appropriately are important skills for all nurses.

CHAPTER SUMMARY

This chapter has aimed to review how to identify, assess and manage an acutely ill adult patient. The systematic ABCDE assessment approach was discussed. Appropriate emergency skills and care interventions have been highlighted. Since ABCDE assessments are frequently performed in acute settings, you may not have an opportunity to talk to your colleagues about what is happening at the time. Try to find an opportunity to review this emergency assessment with your colleagues after the event when you will be able to learn more about the situation and the patient's assessment and management. ABCDE assessment forms part of many EWSs and you should familiarise yourself with your local organisation's charts, methods of record keeping and protocols. It can take considerable time to become confident in these acute skills. It is important that you work with your mentor to develop these skills in a practice setting.

REFERENCES

Audit Commission 1999. *Critical to Success: The place of efficient and effective critical care services within the acute hospital.* London: Audit Commision.

Baird, A. 2001. Concordance with long-term oxygen therapy. *Practice Nursing* **12**, 457–9.

Bright, D., Walker, W. and Bion, J. 2004. Outreach: a strategy for improving the care of the acutely ill hospitalized patient. *Critical Care* **8**, 33–40.

Booker, R. 2007. Understanding why we use spirometry: Part 1. *Nursing Times* **103**(45), 46–8.

British Thoracic Society/Scottish Intercollegiate Guidelines Network 2008. British Guidelines on the Management of Asthma. Available from www.brit-thoracic.org.uk

Buist, D., Moore, G., Bernard, S. *et al.* 2002. Effects of a medical emergency team on the reduction of incidence of and mortality from unexpected cardiac arrests in hospital: preliminary review. *British Medical Journal* **324**, 387–90.

Coggan, J.M. 2008a. Arterial blood gas analysis 1. Understanding ABG reports. *Nursing Times* **104**(18), 28–9.

Coggan, J.M. 2008b. Arterial blood gas analysis 2: Compensatory mechanisms. *Nursing Times* **104**(19), 24–5.

Cole, E. 2007. Measuring central venous pressure. Nursing Standard **22**(7), 40–2.

Cooper, N. 2004. Acute care: treatment with oxygen. *Student BMJ* **12**, 56–8.

Croxton, T.L. and Bailey, W.C. 2006. Long-term oxygen treatment in chronic obstructive pulmonary disease: recommendations for future research. *American Journal of Respiratory and Critical Care Medicine* **174**, 373–8.

Currie, G., Deveraux, G. Lee, D. and Ayres, J. 2005. Recent developments in asthma management. *British Medical Journal* **330**, 585–9.

Day, T., Farnell, S. and Wilson-Barnett, J. 2002. Suctioning: a review of current research recommendations. *Intensive and Critical Care Nursing* **18**, 79–89.

Department of Health (DH) 2000. *Comprehensive Critical Care: A review of adult critical care services.* London: DH.

Dreifuss, F.E. 1989. Classification of epileptic seizures and the epilepsies. *Pediatric Clinics of North America* **36**, 265–79.

Driscoll, P., Skinner, D. and Earlam, R. 2000. *ABC of Major Trauma*, 3rd edn. London: BMJ Publishing.

Dunn, L. and Chisholm, H. 1998. Oxygen therapy. *Nursing Standard* **13**(7), 57–60.

Ellis, D.Y., Lambert, C. and Shirley, P. 2006. Intracranial placement of nasopharyngeal airways: is it all that rare? *Emergency Medicine Journal* **23**, 661.

Epilepsy Action 2008. *Homepage*: www.epilepsy.org.uk. Accessed 20 May 2008.

Francis, C. 2006. *Respiratory Care: Essential clinical skills for nurses*. Oxford: Blackwell.

Garretson, S. and Malberti, S. 2007. Understanding hypovolaemic, cardiogenic and septic shock. *Nursing Standard* **50**(21), 46–55.

Goldhill, D., White, S. and Sumner, A. 1999. Physiological values and procedures in the 24 hours before ICU admission from the ward. *Anaesthesia* **54**, 853–60.

Hampton, J. 2003. *ECG Made Easy*, 6th edn. London: Churchill Livingstone.

Hand, H. 2001. Shock. *Nursing Standard* **15**(48), 45–52.

Harbrecht, B.G., Alarcon, L.H. and Peitzman, A.B. 2004. Management of shock. In Moore, E.E. *et al.* (eds), *Trauma*, 5th edn. New York: McGraw-Hill, 201–25.

Jones, I. 2005. *Cardiac Care: An introductory text*. London: Whurr.

Jones, S. 1997. Oxygen therapy. *Community Nurse* **3**, 23–4.

Jowett, N. and Thompson, D. 2007. *Comprehensive Cardiac Care*, 4th edn. London: Baillière Tindall.

Law, C. 2000. A guide to assessing sputum. *NT Plus* **96**(24), 7–10.

Linton, M. 2000. Endotracheal suctioning. In Sinha, S.K. and Donn, S.M. (eds) *Manual of Neonatal Respiratory Care*. New York: Futura.

Mann, S. and Bowler, M. 2008. Using an early warning score tool in community nursing. *Nursing Times* **104**(20), 30–1.

McGrath, A.M., Gardner, D.M. and McCormack, J. 2001. Is home peak expiratory flow monitoring effective in controlling asthma symptoms? *Journal of Clinical Pharmacy and Therapeutics* **26**(5), 311–17.

McLauchlan, L. 2002. Supplementary oxygen therapy in the community. *Nursing Times Plus* **98**(40), 50–2.

Mencap 2004. *Treat Me Right! Better healthcare for people with a learning disability*. London: Mencap.

Moore, T. 2003. Suctioning techniques for the removal of respiratory secretions. *Nursing Standard* **18**(9), 47–54.

Morgan, R.J.M., Williams, F. and Wright, M.M. 1997. An early warning scoring system for detecting developing critical illness. *Clinical Intensive Care* **8**, 100.

National Patient Safety Agency 2007. *Safer Care for the Acutely Ill Patient: Learning from serious incidents*, 5th report. London: NPSA.

National Institute for Health and Clinical Excellence (NICE) 2007. *Acutely Ill Patients in Hospital: Quick reference guide*, clinical guideline 50. London: NICE. Available from www.nice.co.uk. Accessed 20 May 2008.

Oakey, R. and Slade, V. 2006. Physiological observation track and trigger system. *Nursing Standard* **20**(27), 48–54.

O'Driscoll, B.R., Howard, L.S. and Davison, A.G. 2008. BTS guideline for emergency oxygen use in adult patients. *Thorax* **43**(Suppl VI), vi1–vi68.

Peberdy, M.A., Kaye, W., Ornato, J.P. *et al.* 2003. Cardiopulmonary resuscitation of adults in the hospital: a report of 14,720 cardiac arrests from the National Registry of Cardiopulmonary Resuscitation. *Resuscitation* **58**, 297–308.

Pilkington, F. 2004. Humidification for oxygen therapy in non-ventilated patients. *British Journal of Nursing* **13**(2), 111–15.

Porter-Jones, G. 2002. Short-term oxygen therapy. *Nursing Times Plus* **98**(40), 53–6.

Pruitt, W.C. and Jacobs, M. 2003. *Basics of Oxygen Therapy*. Available from http://findarticles. com/p/articles/mi_qa3689/is_200310/ai_n9330708. Accessed 16 May 2008.

Pryor, J.A. and Prasad, A. 2002. *Physiotherapy for Respiratory and Cardiac Problems in Adults and Paediatrics*, 3rd edn. Edinburgh: Churchill Livingstone.

Rees, J.E. 2003. Early warning scores. *World Anaesthesia* **17**, 10.

Resuscitation Council (UK) 2004. *Recommended Minimum Equipment for In-hospital Adult Resuscitation*. Available from www.resus.org.uk/pages/eqipIHAR.htm. Accessed 1 May 2008.

— 2005. *Resuscitation Guidelines*. Available from www.resus.org.uk/pages/guide.htm. Accessed 1 May 2008.

— 2006. *Immediate Life Support Course Manual*, 2nd edn. London: Resuscitation Council (UK).

Royal College of Nursing (RCN) 2006. *Meeting the Health Needs of People with Learning Disabilities: Guidance for nursing staff*. London: RCN.

Rubin, B.K. 2002. Physiology of airway mucus clearance. *Respiratory Care* **47**, 761–8.

Sheppard, M. and Davis, S. 2000a. Oxygen therapy – 2. *Nursing Times* **96**(30), 43–4.

Sheppard, M. and Davis, S. 2000b. Oxygen therapy – 1. *Nursing Times* **96**(29), 43–4.

Smith, G. 2003 *ALERT: A multiprofessional course in care of the acutely ill patient*, 2nd edn. Portsmouth: University of Portsmouth.

Smith, G.B. and Poplett, N. 2002. Knowledge of aspects of acute care in trainee doctors. *Postgraduate Medical Journal* **78**, 335–8.

Smith, G.B., Prytherch, D.R., Schmidt, P. *et al.* 2006. Hospital-wide physiological surveillance: a new approach to the early identification and management of the sick patient. *Resuscitation* **71**(1), 19–28.

Spahn, D.R., Cerny, V., Caoats, T.J. *et al.* 2007. Management of bleeding following major trauma: a European guideline. *Critical Care,* **11**, R17.

Stockley, R.A., O'Brien, C., Pye, A. and Hill, S.L. 2000. Relationship of sputum colour to nature and outpatient management of acute exacerbations of COPD. *Chest* **117**, 1638–45.

Stokes, T., Shaw, E.J, Juarez-Garcia, A. *et al.* 2004. *Clinical Guidelines and Evidence Review for the Epilepsies: Diagnosis and management in adults and children in primary and secondary care*. London: Royal College of General Practitioners.

Subbe, C.P., Davies, R.G., Williams, E. *et al.* 2003. Effects of introducing the modified Early Warning Score on clinical outcomes, cardio-pulmonary arrests and intensive care utilisation on acute medical admissions. *Anaesthesia* **58**, 775–803.

Subbe, C.P., Gao, H. and Harrison, D.A. 2007. Reproducibility of physiological track-and-trigger warning systems for identifying at-risk patients on the ward. *Intensive Care Medicine* **33**(4), 619–24.

Vines, D.L., Shelledy, D.C. and Peters, J. 2000. Current respiratory care. Pt 1: Oxygen therapy, oximetry, bronchial hygiene. *Journal of Critical Illness* **15**, 507–10, 513–15.

Wilkins, R.L., Sheldon, R.L. and Krider, S. J. 2005.*Clinical Assessment in Respiratory Care*, 5th edn. St Louis: Elsevier Mosby.

Wilson, J. 2006. *Infection Control in Clinical Practice*, 3rd edn. London: Baillière Tindall.

Woodrow, P. 2002. Central venous catheters and central venous pressure. *Nursing Standard* **16**(26), 45–51.

Woodrow, P. 2004. Arterial blood gas analysis. *Nursing Standard* **18**(21), 45–52.

Zevola, D.R. and Maier, C.B. 2001. Use of nasal cannula versus face mask after extubation in patients after cardiothoracic surgery *Critical Care Nurse* **21**(3), 47–53.

USEFUL WEBSITES

- Asthma UK: www.asthma.org.uk
- British Lung Foundation: www.lunguk.org
- *British National Formulary*: www.bnf.org/bnf
- British Thoracic Society: www.brit-thoracic.org.uk
- Diabetes UK: www.diabetes.org.uk
- Epilepsy Action www.epilepsy.org.uk
- Resuscitation Council (UK): www.resus.org.uk
- www.peakflow.com

Managing Pain and Promoting Comfort

Dee Burrows and Lesley Baillie

Clients and patients in all healthcare settings experience pain and discomfort, whether it be physical, emotional or spiritual. Studies suggest that some 72 per cent of hospital inpatients are in pain at any one time (Brook *et al.* 2002). Furthermore, 7.8 million people – or one in seven of the UK population – have chronic pain (Chronic Pain Policy Coalition 2007). Managing pain and promoting comfort are therefore essential skills in nursing practice.

Many relevant skills have already been explored in this book. This chapter aims to bring them together to help you understand how they may be used consciously to reduce pain and promote comfort. The first section of the chapter focuses on pain. Pain and its management are large topics, so the section offers an introduction to provide a foundation for future practice and learning. To develop your understanding and skills further, you should refer to literature and other sources. The second part of the chapter looks at how nurses promote comfort in a range of settings.

This chapter includes:
- Managing pain in a variety of settings – the nature of pain, pain assessment, pain management using medication, and non-pharmacological approaches to managing pain
- Promoting comfort – using presence, monitoring, touch, talking and physical actions

Recommended biology reading:

The following questions will help you to focus on the biology underpinning the skills used in pain management. Use your recommended textbook to find out:
- What is pain?
- What terminology is used to describe pain?
- Why do we feel pain? Can pain be useful diagnostically?
- What anatomical components are required to 'feel' pain?
- Identify three pain-producing substances. Where are they produced?
- What is a nociceptor?

- What effect does myelination have on the transmission of pain messages?
- Where are the substantia gelatinosa and laminae? What are their relevance to pain perception?
- What affects pain perception? How does this relate to the gate control theory?
- How does the release of endogenous opiates reduce pain?
- What is serotonin and what part does it play in pain perception?
- What physical signs may indicate when a person is in acute pain?

PRACTICE SCENARIOS

The following scenarios illustrate when managing pain and promoting comfort may be needed. They will be referred to throughout this chapter.

Adult

Radical retropubic prostatectomy
Removal of the prostate gland and surrounding tissues.

Tom Briggs is 64 years old, married, with three grown-up children, and previously fit and well though he takes medication to control hypertension. He was recently diagnosed with prostate cancer during a routine blood test. Yesterday he had a radical retropubic prostatectomy and lymphadenectomy and this is his first postoperative day. He initially had an epidural infusion to control his pain, but this was discontinued during the night as his pain was not being controlled well (pain score 7–8) and he was quite distressed. Patient-controlled analgesia (PCA) was commenced instead with effect and his pain score is now 1–2. He has an intravenous infusion of normal saline in progress and his abdominal wound is covered with a dressing. He has a urinary catheter and his urine is being measured hourly. He has flowtron boots attached to his feet and calves to prevent deep vein thrombosis. His vital signs and PCA observations are being recorded hourly. His temperature is raised but his vital signs are otherwise in a normal range. He is having oxygen administered at 2 L/min via nasal cannulae. He is now having sips of water. He is quite alert and cheerful this morning, pleased to have the operation over. He hopes to get out into a chair this morning following a wash.

Lymphadenectomy
A surgical procedure in which the lymph nodes are removed and examined to see whether they contain cancer.

Learning disability

Bony metastases
Metastases describes the spread of cancer from one part of the body to another, in this case to the bones.

Maria is a 58-year-old woman with a moderate learning disability living in a group home. She was diagnosed with breast cancer eight years ago and underwent surgery and chemotherapy. However, the cancer has returned and she now has bony metastases in her left hip, making it painful to mobilise. She also has metastases in her ovaries, lungs and liver. The community learning disability nurse is her health facilitator and is coordinating her care plan. He is working with Maria and other professionals to understand her illness and treatment plan and gain Maria's consent. He and the occupational therapist are supporting Maria, with input from her family, friends and carers, to develop Maria's 'life book', which celebrates her life's experiences and includes many photos and Maria's wishes and aspirations. The nurse is also working with the staff team, Maria's family (she has three siblings, two of whom live locally with their families), the district nurse, physiotherapist and the palliative care team to establish an individual pain assessment scale and effective pain management. Maria mobilises with difficulty and is currently taking non-opiate analgesics.

Mental health

Violet Davies, aged 76 years, has advanced Alzheimer's disease. She has been admitted to a care home, as her husband is physically and emotionally exhausted and unable to cope. He has refused help in the past as he has been determined to look after his wife, but he has now agreed to her admission. Violet is physically well but she is also known to have osteoarthritis in her right hip. She looks permanently worried and agitated and keeps repeating the same phrase over and over again. Mr Davies looks shaky and tearful.

MANAGING PAIN IN A VARIETY OF SETTINGS

LEARNING OUTCOMES

By the end of this section you will be able to:

1 discuss the nature of pain;
2 explain the differences between pain threshold, pain tolerance and pain behaviour;
3 consider the different dimensions of pain that may need to be assessed;
4 identify appropriate pain assessment tools for different client groups;
5 demonstrate understanding of the pain ladder and how it can be applied in practice;
6 explore non-pharmacological approaches to managing pain.

Learning outcome 1: Discuss the nature of pain

ACTIVITY

Reflect back on your practice experiences. Write down a few examples of people you have met with pain and the setting that you met them in.

Sadly, pain is all around us. Despite advances in medication management, up to three-quarters of postoperative patients continue to experience moderate to severe pain (MacIntyre and Ready 2007). Figures for pain in the community vary tremendously. It is probable that some 27–40 per cent of people living at home (Census 2001) and 70–80 per cent of those in residential care (Closs *et al.* 2003) are experiencing pain at any one time. It is, therefore, a key element of day-to-day nursing practice in all healthcare settings.

Pain is frequently referred to as either 'acute' or 'chronic'. However, the reality is more complex. For instance, you may have come across people in acute pain who

---

Alzheimer's disease

Also referred to as dementia of Alzheimer's type (DAT), this is the most common form of dementia. It is commoner in older people and is thought to result from neurological changes in the brain (Cheston and Bender 1999). Dementia is chronic and progressive in nature, has many causes and commonly presents with memory and language impairment, decline in self-care ability, and behavioural and personality changes (Jacques and Jackson 2000).

Osteoarthritis

A degenerative joint disorder where there is progressive loss of articular cartilage, new bone formation and capsular fibrosis. Main symptoms are pain, stiffness and restricted movement.

also have unrelated chronic pain. In addition, in your biology reading you will have learned about A-delta and C fibre transmission. If you think about what happens when you twist an ankle, you experience immediate sharp pain as a consequence of A-delta fibre stimulation, followed several hours later by deep throbbing pain arising from C fibre stimulation. This is often referred to as 'fast' (A-delta fibre) and 'slow' (C fibre) pain. As people's pain is often not clearly defined, viewing pain in this light helps to explain some anomalies that can be seen in acute and chronic care settings.

ACTIVITY

With reference to your biology reading and the scenarios, what factors may affect pain perception? How might these relate to the 'gate control' theory?

You may want to read the following paragraphs more than once to ensure that you understand the knowledge underpinning some of the practical skills that will be discussed later in this chapter. More information can be found in some of the texts included in the reference list at the end of the chapter (e.g. Mann and Carr 2006).

Pain fibres transmit pain impulses as a consequence of stimulation of the **nociceptors**. Stimuli may be mechanical, chemical, thermal, electrical, mental, social or spiritual.

Nociceptors
Receptors in the skin, mucous membranes or organs that pick up harmful stimuli.

- Tom will have pain as a consequence of the surgical incision (mechanical stimuli) and the resulting tissue damage (chemical stimuli). Although he seems cheerful he may actually be anxious, which as a mental stimulus will act through the **limbic system** and descending pathways to open the gate to pain.

Limbic system
A group of brain structures that control the emotional aspects of pain.

- Maria's metastatic pain also arises from mechanical and chemical stimuli. In addition she may be frightened of dying (spiritual stimuli).
- Violet's situation is complex, with pain caused by the mechanical stimulation of osteoarthritis and mental, social and possibly spiritual stimulation arising from her Alzheimer's disease. Violet's pain perception may be further enhanced through the **reticular activating system** as a consequence of her agitation. Both ascending and descending influences on the gate thus reduce the likelihood of the gate closing.

Reticular activating system
A network of brain cells concerned with arousal and awareness.

- Violet's husband may be suffering from social isolation in addition to his mental and physical exhaustion. He may need comforting and active support if he is going to be able to look after his wife at home again in the future.

Some of the examples given above refer to mechanical and chemical stimulation of the nociceptors – this is known as **nociceptive pain.** Pain can also occur as a consequence of peripheral or central nerve damage – when it is termed **neuropathic pain.** For example, people with multiple sclerosis may experience neuropathic pain because of demyelination of the axon and subsequent scar formation of the nerves; and nociceptive pain due to mechanical stimulation arising from altered muscle balance and muscle spasms (Multiple Sclerosis Trust 2007).

Note: Knowledge of these two different types of pain is important if you are to understand the different pharmacological and non-pharmacological approaches to pain management discussed later in this chapter.

Defining pain

ACTIVITY

Think back to a time when you have experienced pain, and write the experience down. Looking at your notes, how would you define pain?

Pain is a complex, personal experience that has been defined in various ways. For example, the International Association for the Study of Pain (IASP) defined pain as:

> An unpleasant sensory and emotional experience associated with actual or potential tissue damage, or described in terms of such damage. (IASP Subcommittee on Taxonomy 1979, p. 250)

This definition, which post-dated the publication of the 'gate control' theory, clearly recognises that pain comprises both physical and psychological components. A classical definition of pain used in nursing is that by Margo McCaffery, first published in 1968:

> Pain is whatever the experiencing person says it is, existing when the experiencing person says it does. (McCaffery 1968, cited in Sofaer 1998, p. 95)

McCaffery's definition is an *operational* definition as it aims to guide real practice. Nurses who follow this stance believe what the person says about their pain and manage it accordingly. This may appear an obvious statement, as compassion – according to Roach (2002) – includes sensitivity to pain. However, patients' descriptions are not always believed. Not believing what someone says is, of course, tantamount to calling them a liar. It would be surprising if the population were divided into two groups: honest healthcare professionals and dishonest clients and patients! As Moskow (1987) points out:

> Pain occurring in unicorns, griffins, and jabberwockies is always imaginary pain, since these are imaginary animals: patients on the other hand, are real, and so they always have real pain. (Moskow 1987, p. 68)

If pain is to be managed effectively so that patients are comfortable, nurses need to be:
* **compassionate** to patients' needs;
* willing to listen to their own **conscience**;
* **confident** in their assessment skills;
* **competent** in, and **committed** to, their chosen pain management strategies;
* aware of **comporting** themselves well – thus appearing and behaving professionally.

Chapter 1 explains Roach's *six Cs of caring* in more detail.

ACTIVITY

Return to the notes you made about your experience of pain and the people that you met in practice settings. Was your pain and their's believed? Were you and they treated with compassion? Did the nurses appear to understand the complexity of pain?

You can read in detail about the misconceptions surrounding pain in the first half of Chapter 3 in McCaffery and Pasero (1999). Before you do so, try examining your own attitudes by completing the scale at the end of this chapter (Appendix 12.1). You can then compare your answers to the views of McCaffery and Pasero. If you cannot access their text you could try looking up misconceptions, myths, attitudes and barriers in any pain management book that you can access.

Learning outcome 2: Explain the difference between pain threshold, pain tolerance and pain behaviour

ACTIVITY

- How often have you or friends commented that someone has 'a high (or low) pain threshold'? Think for a minute what you meant by this. Jot down your feelings about people with a low threshold and those with a high threshold.
- Now consider what you understand by the word 'tolerance'.

In pain management, 'threshold' refers to the level at which the population at large perceives a stimulus as painful. In other words, if everything were equal we would all feel pain at much the same level. Pain threshold, therefore, is essentially a physiological measurement.

Pain 'tolerance' refers to the amount of pain an individual can tolerate at any given time. It is linked to that person's psychological state and is, in essence, an outcome of 'gate control'. To illustrate this, imagine you are sitting in a lecture and are experiencing a really bad headache. What would you do? Perhaps you would take painkillers or go home. You still have your headache but need to get ready for a party or meal out. What would you do? It is possible that you would go to the social event and within a short space of time forget your headache!

ACTIVITY

Refer back to the gate control theory to understand more about why and how this happens.

Pain tolerance varies from one individual to the next and within an individual from one minute to the next. Some factors that open the gate to pain – and thereby increase pain perception – are listed in Box 12.1 as **gate openers**. Those that have the potential to fully or partially close the gate – and thereby modulate pain perception – are listed as **gate closers**.

ACTIVITY

Look at the scenario of Violet and list the factors that may be influencing her pain perception. Note down an explanation for each factor.

Box 12.1 Examples of factors that open and close the gate to pain

Gate openers
- Anxiety, fear, worry, tension
- Lack of control
- Tiredness
- Prolonged or recurrent pain
- Previous poor experiences with pain

Gate closers
- Information
- Relaxation, distraction
- Control
- Touch, social interaction, reassurance
- Known positive outcome
- Previous positive experience with pain

- Mr Davies's emotional and physical exhaustion, his desire to support Violet at home, and his tearfulness may be transmitted to Violet and increase her worry.
- The strange and potentially frightening environment may reduce Violet's sense of personal control and enhance her feelings of social isolation.
- The prolonged nature of Violet's osteoarthritis may have reduced her pain coping strategies.
- Violet's agitation will prevent her from relaxing and increase her tension.
- The lack of information about the immediate future may reduce Mr and Mrs Davies's abilities to maintain any sense of cognitive control.
- The pathophysiology of Alzheimer's disease may alter Violet's pain experience (covered further in learning outcome 3).

Knowing and understanding the factors that reduce pain perception can help guide your approach to pain management. The third concept you need to consider is pain behaviour.

ACTIVITY

Again, thinking about headaches:
- How do you behave when you have a headache?
- How does your best friend behave?
- How do other people you know behave?

Perhaps one of the people you thought of wants attention, while another prefers to be on their own. Maybe one frowns, grimaces and becomes irritable, while someone else tries to relax their facial expression and carry on as normal. As well as non-verbal and social responses, verbal and vocal (e.g. shouting, moaning) responses also vary. These are all different pain behaviours or pain expressions.

Pain expression and pain behaviour are learned through our families and culture. In their book *Challenge of Pain,* Melzack and Wall (1996) discuss the influence of culture in relation to the gate control theory. A study by Madjar (1985) highlighted the importance of nurses understanding cultural expression in pain management. She compared postoperative pain behaviours in 20 Anglo-Australian and 13 Yugoslav-Australian patients and found that, although there were no significant differences between vocal and motor behaviours, social and verbal differences were identified. Anglo-Australians were more likely to seek help, including analgesics, but tended to withdraw socially to cope with their pain. Yugoslavs preferred company, openly discussed their pain and yet asked for fewer analgesics.

Although published some years ago now, those findings have been supported by more recent research. Lovering (2006), for example, found that Afrikaans are stoic, often denying pain and rarely acknowledging the emotional impact. Conversely, Irish people tend to verbalise both physical and emotional pain, whereas Saudis verbalise physical pain, but prefer religious healing to narcotics. Cultural beliefs are thus a strong determinant of pain expression and behaviour.

ACTIVITY

- Think of the different pain behaviours you have seen. List the ones you think Tom, Maria and Violet might be adopting.
- Scenarios often push you into stereotyping (as do handovers). Consider the behaviours you have listed for each scenario and ask yourself why you identified those particular ones.
- Try to access Lovering's (2006) article and make some notes about the different cultural perspectives of those involved in her study.

In summary, an appreciation of the differences between pain threshold, pain tolerance and pain behaviour will help you to understand how people's pain and their reactions to it vary. The next section considers pain responses in greater depth.

Learning outcome 3: Consider the different dimensions of pain that may need to be assessed

Because there are many different factors that influence pain perception and pain behaviour, pain is regarded as a multidimensional phenomenon. A number of different multidimensional frameworks exist to help practitioners assess pain. One of the authors' clinical practice in chronic pain management is based on a psychological model that acknowledges the individual's personal situation or context and the interactions of thoughts, feelings, physical sensation of pain and behaviour. McGuire (1992), who is an American nurse, developed a framework based around six dimensions:

- physiological;
- sensory;
- affective;
- cognitive;
- behavioural;
- sociocultural.

This framework is outlined below.

Physiological dimension

The physiological dimension of pain deals with the anatomical structures (nociceptors, peripheral nerves, dorsal horn, ascending pathways, brain, descending pathways) and physiological perception of pain via the release of pain-producing chemicals in the tissues and viscera, nerve conduction, gate control mechanisms and the effects of, for example, nerve damage and neurotransmitters such as serotonin.

Surgery leads to acute postoperative pain as a result of tissue damage arising from the surgical procedure. As well as pain, noxious stimuli will increase sympathetic activity, resulting in raised blood pressure, heart rate, oxygen consumption, muscle tension and sphincter tone in the bladder and bowels (MacIntyre and Ready 2007). These are frequently cited signs and symptoms of acute pain. However, because of the way the body adapts to stress they normalise long before the pain disappears. Physiological signs and symptoms are therefore usually regarded as the least reliable way of measuring pain. However, they may be helpful in situations where verbal assessment is constrained, such as with unconscious or cognitively impaired patients, although there are an increasing number of assessment tools being developed and validated for assessing pain in these groups (see learning outcome 4).

As you read in the scenarios, Tom's vital signs were checked by the nurse and these would have helped in her general assessment of him, particularly when compared to preoperative baselines. Similarly Tom's pain was assessed as a fifth vital sign (Chronic Pain Policy Coalition 2007).

The absence of raised sympathetic signs does not mean that the person is not in pain. People with chronic pain, such as Violet with her osteoarthritis, will not have a raised pulse and blood pressure as a consequence of pain. Violet may, however, exhibit these signs due to her agitation.

Sensory dimension

The sensory dimension considers the location, intensity and quality of pain. Acute pain is usually well defined. For example, a patient with appendicitis will describe their pain as being in the lower abdomen, either in the centre or on the right. Tom is likely to tell you that his pain is localised to the incision site. Maria's pain is more widespread because of the different foci of her metastases, but is still likely to be focused. Conversely, Violet's chronic osteoarthritis pain may be diffuse, radiating into both her back and her knee.

Practitioners and the general public tend to think of acute pain as far more intense than chronic pain. However, this is not always the case. Practitioners also have a tendency to rank acute pain so that more credence is given to the pain of a mycodardial infarction (heart attack), for example, than to the pain of a kidney infection. Although there is some evidence to suggest that certain pain sensations may be more intense than others, the most important guide is to listen to what the person says about the **intensity** and **quality** of their pain.

Quality of pain refers to the way pain is described. It is influenced by whether the pain arises from A-delta fibre stimulation (e.g. sharp pain), or from C fibre stimulation (e.g. deep throbbing or aching pain), or from nerve damage (e.g. hot burning, tingling pain). Some pain assessment tools help to differentiate the quality of pain in order to inform, for example, diagnosis of pain type and medication management (see learning outcome 4).

Maria and Violet may be unable to describe their pain because of communication difficulties, confusion or deficits in cognitive processing. In Alzheimer's, the disease affects the limbic system, which impacts on the person's ability to explain the quality of their pain. However, the sensory cortex is not involved so patients are still able to perceive pain (Frampton 2003).

ACTIVITY

Look at the scenarios again and consider whether you have made any assumptions about the intensity of pain each of the people will be experiencing. On what basis did you make these assumptions?

You might have listed age, gender, emotional state, cognitive ability, level of understanding, family support, ability to verbalise pain, the acuteness of the pain and so on. Some of these factors, such as emotional state, are known to influence pain perception, while the evidence base for others is less clear. For example, there is considerable debate about whether, as a consequence of A-delta fibre demyelination, older people's ability to perceive pain is reduced. If this is the case, it may be one explanation for why older people tend to use C fibre (e.g. throbbing) rather than A-delta fibre (e.g. sharp) descriptive words to describe their pain (Chakour *et al.* 1996; Yezierski 2007).

Affective dimension

The affective dimension addresses people's emotional responses to pain. In the activity above you may have considered some of the affective factors listed earlier as gate openers or closers. For instance, we know that Violet is 'worried and agitated'. We can infer that Maria may be frightened, but the information given on Tom is that he is 'cheerful', which may or may not reflect his underlying emotional response. One of the affective factors that may be relevant to Maria's experience is helplessness. Studies indicate that the more informed a person, the less helpless they feel, the better able they are to cope with their pain and, in some cases, the less pain they experience (SIGN 44 2000; NHS QIS 2004). The input from the community nurse for learning disabilities, in explaining to Maria and her family what is happening, should help to decrease feelings of uncertainty and helplessness.

Cognitive dimension

The cognitive dimension explores the way in which pain is influenced by, and influences, people's thoughts, attitudes, beliefs and preferred cognitive strategies for coping with pain. Tom's concerns about his future may well have heightened his postoperative distress and pain perception. Violet's Alzheimer's disease will affect her cognitive processing of pain, and thus her understanding (Kovach *et al.* 1999; Forsyth 2007). Strategies for coping with pain are discussed later in the chapter.

Behavioural dimension

The behavioural dimension includes behaviours associated with pain perception and behaviours associated with attempts to control pain. Facial grimacing, moaning, supporting the painful area, rigid posture or restlessness are all recognised signs of acute pain (MacIntyre and Ready 2007). Signs associated with chronic pain include muscle tension, depression, loss of appetite, altered posture, sleeplessness and focus on self.

However, just because someone has pain does not mean they will exhibit pain behaviours. As with physiological signs, acute behavioural signs will normalise as part of general adaptation. Thus if, for example, a patient recovering from surgery appears to be sleeping, or laughing with their visitors, it cannot be assumed that they are pain-free. Tom's pain score is a more accurate assessment of pain than his cheerfulness. Similarly, people with chronic pain do not always display the pain behaviours cited above. The employment of behavioural coping strategies, such as distraction and relaxation, may further emphasise any lack of pain behaviour.

It is precisely because the physiological and behavioural signs are unreliable that pain experts emphasise the importance of verbal pain assessment. However, these signs can be helpful if verbal assessment is limited or impossible (see learning outcome 4).

Sociocultural dimension

The sixth and final of McGuire's (1992) dimensions is the sociocultural one. This deals with family, cultural, societal and environmental influences on pain. Children learn about pain, pain behaviours and coping strategies from their families and peer groups. In addition, the meaning of pain and the expression of pain differ between ethnic groups and cultures (Smith-Stoner 2003; Lovering 2006). Many years ago, one of the writers was about to give an opiate injection to a non-English speaking man who was screaming. His son arrived and informed the staff that this behaviour was a way of letting out the devils that were causing the problems – a practice that was apparently common in the man's cultural group. Within 10 minutes he was quite relaxed and peaceful. This anecdote demonstrates the importance of capturing the patient or client's perspective.

In summary, McGuire's (1992) framework offers a guide and knowledge base for the different aspects of pain that can be helpful when assessing and managing pain.

Learning outcome 4: Identify appropriate pain assessment tools for different client groups

Pain is assessed in a variety of ways in different clinical settings. It is a key aspect of pain management and research has consistently demonstrated that accurate pain assessment leads to effective pain management. All patients and clients should have their pain assessed and recorded at the beginning of each episode of care and at suitable intervals thereafter.

Pain intensity

In busy acute settings there are times when it may be appropriate to simply ask a patient:

- 'Do you have any pain?'
- 'Where is the pain?'
- 'How bad is the pain?'

To help patients respond to this last question, some nurses and doctors ask: 'On a scale of zero to ten, with zero being no pain and ten being the worse pain you can imagine, what is your pain?' Imagining a 0–10 scale when you are anxious, experiencing intense pain and possibly feeling very ill can be difficult. It is more effective to show the patient a scale and to ask them to point to the level that their pain is at. Figure 12.1 is an example of this type of numerical analogue scale.

Other types of scales are the visual analogue scale (see Fig. 12.2), the verbal analogue scale (Fig. 12.3) and combined verbal and numerical scale (Fig. 12.4). The last one tends to be the easiest to use, with some 96 per cent of cognitively sound adults able to visualise pain intensity in this way. Pain intensity in chronic pain can also be measured using these scales. However, other dimensions of pain must also be assessed.

| 0 | 1 | 2 | 3 | 4 | 5 | 6 | 7 | 8 | 9 | 10 |

Figure 12.1: A numerical analogue scale.

No   Unbearable
pain   pain

Figure 12.2: Visual analogue scale.

No   Mild   Moderate   Severe   Unbearable
pain   pain   pain   pain   pain

Figure 12.3: Verbal analogue scale.

No   Mild   Moderate   Severe   Unbearable
pain   pain   pain   pain   pain
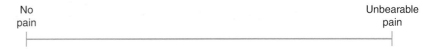

Figure 12.4: Combined verbal and numerical scale.

Categorical scales are also popular measurement tools. An example is shown in Fig. 12.5. These scales can be used either as verbal rating scales by recording the words or as numerical rating scales by assigning a number to each level as shown in Fig. 12.5. Categorical scales are simple to explain and complete. However, they lack the degree of sensitivity that can be obtained with the analogue scales.

Nevertheless they are useful for people with cognitive impairments such as Violet (Closs 2003; Closs *et al.*, 2007). Kovach *et al.* (1999) developed a categorical index of the behaviours associated with discomfort and pain in people with Alzheimer's disease. The most frequently occurring signs were tense body language, sad facial expression, fidgeting, repetitive verbalisations and verbal outbursts. Agitation, which is one of Violet's symptoms, was also listed. More recently the **Abbey Pain Scale** has gained popularity as the tool of choice for assessing pain in older people with severe cognitive impairment. A copy of this scale is available in the Royal College of Physicians, British Geriatrics Society and British Pain Society 2007 guidelines on assessing pain in older people (also at www.racgp.org.au/silverbookonline/4-6.asp). Using this scale together with discussion with Mr Davies would facilitate accurate assessment of Violet's pain.

Pain assessment has also been identified as a major issue with people with learning disabilities. Learning disability nurses should be aware of, and able to detect, subtle behavioural changes which might indicate distress (Read 1998; Davies and Evans 2001). In Maria's case the focus on family involvement and liaison across the multidisciplinary team will help practitioners determine the underlying causes of behavioural change. Davies and Evans (2001) also advocate that nurses build sufficient rapport with clients to enable intuitive nursing practice to contribute to the assessment of pain in those with profound learning disabilities.

ACTIVITY

Make some notes on how you would approach Violet to assess her pain, taking into account ways of communicating with people who have Alzheimer's disease and how you could explain the scale you choose to use to her and her husband.

Pain intensity

None	0
Mild	1
Moderate	2
Severe	3

Figure 12.5: Categorical pain assessment scale.

The tools mentioned above tend to focus on measuring and assessing the impact of pain intensity. Similar scales can also be used to measure pain distress, pain relief and anxiety.

Body charts can help to identify the location of pain and, when used with a categorical or numerical scale, can provide insight into the areas that are the most painful. It is important to be aware that just because someone is complaining of pain in one area of their body does not mean that they do not have pain elsewhere. In postoperative settings, it is not unusual for nurses to give opioids in response to a patient's complaint of pain, when the problem is a post-intubation sore throat or long-standing back pain, rather than incisional pain. Tom may also have discomfort or pain resulting from his cannula and/or catheter. Many people with chronic pain also have multiple pain foci.

Multidimensional pain assessment

Tools for multidimensional pain assessment are useful for people with complex care needs and those experiencing chronic pain. One of the best known tools is the **McGill Pain Questionnaire** (MPQ) (Melzack and Katz 1999), which is available in both long and short forms. Through the use of descriptor words, the MPQ enables practitioners to identify the nature and quality of pain (see learning outcome 3, 'Sensory dimension') and thereby best approaches to pain management (see learning outcomes 5 and 6). Pain diaries can also be a useful way of gaining insight into the activities and factors that enhance and reduce people's pain.

Another example of a multidimensional tool is the **Disability Distress Assessment Tool** or DisDAT (©2005 Northgate & Prudhoe NHS Trust and St Oswald's Hospice). The tool, which ends with the poignant words 'Distress may be hidden, but it is never silent', is available at www.mencap.org.uk/document.asp?id=1476. The community learning disability nurse might consider completing the tool with Maria and the two siblings who live nearby to gain an in-depth understanding of the way in which Maria is currently, or might in the future, express her pain. The findings can then be used to inform analgesic and non-pharmacological management as Maria moves towards the end of her life.

Psychological and coping strategies assessment

There are many tools available to assess the psychological components of pain and the ways in which people cope with their pain. These measurements are generally administered by pain experts and tend to be used in outpatient and chronic care settings. They include anxiety and depression scales, coping strategies, impact of pain on function, physical activity profiles and so on.

Figure 12.6 shows the **Pain Strategies Questionnaire** (PSQ). The tool was developed from the strategies recorded by 200 adults attending surgical outpatient clinics for the first time. The tool was then used in a randomised controlled trial to test whether identifying and supporting patients' own strategies in the hospital setting would reduce patients' postoperative anxiety, pain and distress, as well as other outcomes (Burrows 2000). The study findings are discussed later under learning outcome 6.

Pain Strategies Questionnaire

Many people use strategies at home to help relieve pain. We have found that if you continue to use them in hospital it can help to reduce the amount of pain you experience. Please help us to find out what you use by filling in the table below and handing this sheet to your nurse:

Please place a ✓ in column A, against all of the strategies that you use when in pain.

In column B, please place a ✓ against any of the strategies you would like to use in hospital.

Strategy	Column A	Column B
None/not sure		
Painkillers (state which if known)		
Distraction e.g. TV, reading etc.		
Relaxation		
Breathing exercises		
Imagery (using your senses to imagine a place or experience)		
Music		
Massage		
Warmth		
Cold		
Resting alone: e.g. lying down, trying to sleep, peace & quiet PLEASE STATE WHICH		
Grin & bear, mind over matter, positive thinking		
Mobilising: e.g. walking, moving about, exercise PLEASE STATE WHICH		
Positioning: e.g. changing position, support painful area PLEASE STATE WHICH		
Treatment: e.g. seeking medical attention to treat the cause or pain, advice or information PLEASE STATE WHICH		
Reassurance: e.g. talking about the pain, physical contact with someone else, confidence in someone else PLEASE STATE WHICH		
General help with activities		
Other: PLEASE STATE WHAT		

Thank you for completing this questionnaire

Figure 12.6: Pain Strategies Questionnaire (Burrows 2000). Reproduced with kind permission of Dee Burrows.

ACTIVITY   Complete column A of the Pain Strategies Questionnaire in Fig. 12.6.

Depending on your past experience of pain, you may or may not have been aware of some of the strategies you use when in pain. We will consider how you might support patients' own strategies later in the chapter.

In summary, there are a variety of approaches to pain assessment. Each has its place with different client groups and different dimensions of pain. Whatever the approach, the response should be recorded so that it can be compared with the pain experience following an intervention. In acute pain settings, recordings should be made at rest and upon movement: postoperatively, a patient may well stay quite rigid if experiencing pain following surgery. As deep breathing, leg movements and mobilisation are important to postoperative recovery and the prevention of complications, it is imperative that pain does not prevent movement and rehabilitation. In chronic and palliative pain, post-intervention comparisons are likely to be more wide-ranging.

ACTIVITY   Investigate what pain assessment tools are used in your locality for different client groups.

Learning outcome 5: Demonstrate understanding of the pain ladder and how it can be applied in practice

Analgesic
A drug for relieving pain ('painkiller').

Analgesia
Another word for pain relief.

Knowledge of pharmacology and analgesic management may help to enhance analgesia, decrease anxiety, improve functional activity and mood and promote comfort.

The World Health Organization (WHO) (1996) suggests that analgesic administration should be based on the pain ladder, where simple analgesics are used for mild pain, weak opioids for moderate pain, and strong opioids for severe pain. First developed for use in cancer and palliative care, the principles have been extrapolated to acute and chronic pain management. The ladder also allows for drugs from different levels of the ladder to be co-prescribed and administered as patients move from one level to another. Other key principles in promoting analgesia include:

- assessing pain at the beginning of each episode of care and at appropriate intervals thereafter;
- giving analgesics before or as soon as acute pain begins;
- giving sufficient and regular analgesics to ensure patient comfort;
- considering drugs other than the true analgesics for chronic and neuropathic pain;
- assessing pain relief and side-effects;
- balancing medication approaches with non-pharmacological strategies;
- never letting pain get out of control;
- remembering that pain is the fifth vital sign (Chronic Pain Policy Coalition 2007; see www.paincoalition.org.uk/pain5.html).

ACTIVITY   Why should you never let pain get out of control?

You may have come up with a number of ideas, such as that it is inhumane, places patients at risk of physical and emotional complications, increases the likelihood of hospital admissions for those living in the community or residential homes, and so on.

Pharmacological management of pain is a team effort, involving the person with pain, their family, the doctor, pharmacist, nurse, physiotherapist and others. Nurses should:

- Listen to patients and their relatives.
- Record patients' pain assessments.
- Manage and evaluate pain.
- Work with relevant members of the multidisciplinary team towards effective pain control.
- Ensure that their knowledge is sufficient to achieve patient comfort.
- Work to educate patients/clients and their families.

Patients should be encouraged to request analgesics, take sufficient analgesics to enable them to carry out appropriate activities, and ask for more analgesics if their pain continues. If – as in Maria and Violet's cases – it is possible that they will not do so, the family must be listened to and assessment and evaluation must be undertaken regularly.

Table 12.1 gives an example of analgesics from each level of the ladder.

Table 12.1: Examples of commonly used analgesics and their position on the ladder.

Drug	Location on ladder	Administration	Side-effects
Paracetamol	Simple analgesic. Helpful for mild pain, but effect often underestimated Potentiates (enhances) the effect of weak and strong opioids	*Adult:* One/two 500 mg tablets every 4 hours Maximum 8 per day, unless otherwise directed	Rare Potentially fatal liver damage following overdose
Codeine	Weak opioid Helpful for moderate pain	*Adult:* 30–60 mg every 4 hours Maximum 240 mg per day	Constipation Initial drowsiness or dizziness not unusual At least 8% of the population are unable to metabolise codeine
Tramadol	Weak opioid Helpful for moderate pain	*Adult:* 50–100 mg every 4–6 hours Maximum 400 mg per day	Constipation Initial drowsiness or dizziness not unusual
Morphine Oxycodone Fentanyl	Strong opioid	*Adult:* varies Note 10 mg IM/IV is equivalent to 30 mg orally	Most commonly nausea and vomiting; may also experience light-headedness, confusion, pruritus, constipation Respiratory depression

ACTIVITY Make a list of the analgesics used in your locality. Think about their location on the ladder, dosages, and possible side-effects.

You may come across drugs such as co-codamol, co-dydramol and Tramacet. These drugs combine paracetamol with a weak opioid. Although they are popular in the community, research by McQuay and Moore (1998) suggests that there is little, if any, advantage to combination drugs. You might like to talk to a pharmacist about their views on these drugs.

Studies suggest that around 20 per cent of doctors and nurses fear that patients will become addicted to painkillers (Carr and Mann 2000). In fact, hospital-prompted addiction occurs in less than 0.5 per cent of admissions (Ferrell *et al.* 1992). Addiction is caused by cravings, and this is another reason why we should ensure that patients receive sufficient analgesics to be comfortable. Not only is fear of prompting addiction a problem in healthcare generally, but it appears particularly prevalent in relation to older people.

Routes of analgesic administration

ACTIVITY List the different routes for administering analgesics that you have come across.

You may have included PCA systems on your list. PCA is an approach to pain management in which the patient controls the dose and frequency of analgesic up to a predetermined limit. When practitioners refer to PCA, they generally mean the intravenous system that delivers opioids when the patient presses a demand button. These systems are most commonly used in surgical settings and their management is covered by local protocols. Tom's protocol includes recording hourly PCA observations, such as the prescription, level of analgesia and side-effects and administering oxygen at 2 L/min via nasal cannulae.

ACTIVITY Look up your local protocol for PCA. List the recordings that must be made by nurses, and why.

The concept of PCA is an important one. It acknowledges the patient as the expert on their pain and as a partner in pain management. People living at home manage their pain on a day-to-day basis, purchasing over-the-counter painkillers or visiting their GP for prescriptions. On admission to hospital, the power and control for medication management is frequently transferred to doctors and nurses.

Entonox is a 50:50 mixture of nitrous oxide and oxygen delivered through a hand-held mask or mouthpiece. If the patient becomes drowsy (as a consequence of the drug), their hand and therefore the delivery set will fall away. As such, entonox is another form of PCA. It is effective for mild to moderate short-lasting pain and is used by paramedics, in emergency care and for procedural pain (BOC Medical 2001; MacIntyre and Ready 2007).

Epidural space
The space between the spinal canal and dura mater.

Epidurals are another route for administration, involving the infusion of a local anaesthetic, with or without an opioid, through a fine catheter into the epidural space (Middleton 2006).

Tom's epidural 'failed'. This sometimes happens if the catheter shifts or blocks and this underpins the need to monitor analgesia regularly. However, reviews indicate that epidural analgesia tends to provide better pain relief than PCA, intramuscular or oral opioids in the immediate postoperative period (Nishimori *et al.* 2007; Werawatganon and Charuluxanun 2007).

ACTIVITY

Look up your local protocols for entonox, epidurals and syringe drivers. List the recordings that must be made by nurses, and why.

Although Maria is not currently taking opioids, it is likely that as she moves towards the end of her life she will do so. Good practice principles advocate that oral medication should always be the route of choice. In recent years, fentanyl and buprenorphine **patches** have become available for pain relief. These are a method of continuous drug delivery across the skin (transdermal). Patches are available at the weak and strong opioid levels and are useful in chronic as well as palliative pain contexts.

If oral or transdermal routes are no longer feasible for those approaching end of life, appropriate conversions are made initially to subcutaneous injection – for example, 2.5–5 mg of diamorphine p.r.n. The Liverpool Care Pathway for the Dying Patient advocates that if three or more doses are required in 24 hours then a **syringe driver** should be considered. Syringe drivers involve a fine needle being inserted just under the skin of the abdomen or arm, attached to tubing, which in turn is attached to the pump. Analgesics, such as diamorphine, are made up to a 24-hour dose and delivered via the syringe driver. This enables the individual to receive a continuous dose. Other medications such as antiemetics can be added.

ACTIVITY

Access the NHS Improving End of Life Care for Adults website at www. endoflifecareforadults.nhs.uk/eolc/index.htm. Have a look at the resource packs for people with learning disabilities and those living in care homes. Write some notes on ideas you gain for managing Maria and Violet's pain and how you might involve their families.

There are a number of other drugs that are used for pain relief. A few of them are mentioned below.

Non-steroidal anti-inflammatory drugs (NSAIDs)

NSAIDs reduce inflammation and are effective for mild to moderate pain. They are commonly used postoperatively in combination with analgesics and are also the drug of choice in conditions such as arthritis and some other chronic pain conditions. Ibuprofen 400 mg and diclofenac 50 mg have been shown to be as effective as 10 mg intramuscular morphine in the treatment of acute pain (McQuay and Moore 1998). Side-effects include gastric irritation, bleeding and renal failure. Nurses need to be aware

Box 12.2 Examples of drugs used in neuropathic pain management

- Antidepressants – amitriptyline, nortriptyline
- Anticonvulsants – gabapentin, pregabalin, carbamazepine
- Local anaesthetic – lidocaine patches

of these, be conscious that a past history of asthma, gastritis, ulcers and kidney problems may exclude an individual from using NSAIDs, and be observant for side-effects.

Analgesics and NSAIDs are useful drugs in the management of nociceptive pain. However, other drugs are needed for the treatment of neuropathic pain.

Drugs for neuropathic pain

The analgesic properties of antidepressants and antiepileptic drugs have been found to be useful for neuropathic pain. Unfortunately, because many healthcare practitioners are unaware that these drugs may be used to treat pain, it is not uncommon for patients with neuropathic pain to hear themselves labelled as 'depressed epileptics' because of the medication they are taking. It is worth finding out, therefore, why someone is taking their medication, rather than assuming the 'obvious'. Chapter 2 discusses how such labelling of patients affects interactions between nurses and patients.

Recently, lidocaine patches have been made available for people with post-shingles and other similarly localised nerve pain. Another recent development is that guidelines are being produced for the diagnosis and management of neuropathic pain in primary care.

Box 12.2 shows some of the common antidepressants and anticonvulsants used in pain management.

Other medications used for pain management

You may be familiar with the use of biphosphonate drugs for osteoporosis. However, these drugs can also help with pain caused by bony metastases and may well be a drug of choice for Maria if she can tolerate taking them.

Resources

There are many resources to help nurses develop their pharmacological knowledge. These include standard pharmacological and pain management texts, specialist texts such as that by MacIntyre and Ready (2007), websites such as the *British National Formulary* (BNF) site (www.bnf.com), pharmaceutical literature, journal articles and nursing, medical and pharmacist colleagues. Understanding the way a drug works can be a rewarding addition to a nurse's knowledge base and practice.

Learning outcome 6: Explore non-pharmacological approaches to managing pain

Non-pharmacological approaches to pain management include a variety of technical, taught, self-generated, comfort care and complementary strategies. The latter include acupuncture (which is available through the NHS), reflexology, massage and aromatherapy, but it is beyond the remit of this chapter to discuss these approaches. However, two activities are listed below to help you explore these approaches further. They will also lead you to two very useful resources. The first is an excellent publication on managing pain in care home residents; the second is a social enterprise site based on patients' narratives.

ACTIVITY

Access the 'Pain in Residential Aged Care Facilities' at www.apsoc.org.au/news. php?scode=9e2c2n. Read Chapter 6 and then consider what additional strategies might benefit Violet and her husband.

ACTIVITY

Access www.patientvoices.org.uk. Listen to 'Taking my life back', which is narrated by a woman with fibromyalgia, a chronic musculoskeletal pain and fatigue condition. You will need to click on <find a story>, type Ctrl+f to bring up the search box, type in *pain,* and click on <next> until you get to the correct story.

There are three other stories on the www.patientvoices.org.uk website related to pain. One is about postoperative pain; one is about the pain experienced by a carer and his wife relating to the wife's suprapubic catheter; and one is about the pain of someone diagnosed with a chronic painful condition called 'reflex sympathetic dystrophy', or 'complex regional pain syndrome' as it is more commonly termed now.

ACTIVITY

Moving back to the hospital setting, and in particular thinking of Tom's experiences, look at the strategies that you ticked in Figure 12.6. As a nurse, how might you support someone who wanted to use these strategies in a hospital setting?

Burrows's (2000) study found that identifying and supporting patients' self-generated strategies reduced postoperative anxiety, opiate consumption, pain and distress. Many texts and articles suggest that nurses teach imagery, relaxation, distraction and exercise and administer massage, heat and cold. In fact, the evidence for the efficacy of taught strategies remains relatively weak, although further studies are currently under way. In chronic pain management there is a fairly long history of working with patients to develop their own strategies. Studies suggest that this may be more effective than using taught strategies (Rokke and al'Absi 1992).

In the activity above, you might have come up with some of the ideas offered in Table 12.2.

The nurse's caring role in the context of people using self-generated strategies is to support the person to use their strategies effectively when the experience of illness and a strange environment may disrupt their expertise. This may mean being compassionate to the person's needs by simply giving them permission to use the technique, being confident in offering ideas on how to adapt the strategy to a

Table 12.2: Examples of supporting patients in using their own pain relieving strategies.

Identify the strategies the person uses	Understand how the strategy works	Work with the person to enable them to use their strategy in the clinical setting
Distraction	Focusing on something other than pain Useful for brief periods Can increase perception of self-control and reduce pain intensity	May include watching TV, reading, listening to music, visits from family and friends Example: if a patient says they watch television help them to the day room
Relaxation	Directs attention away from pain Useful for mild to moderate pain Can reduce muscle tension, distress, anxiety and fatigue	Find out the person's technique and support them with it if asked Ensure periods of relative peace and quiet to enable them to use the strategy Teach short and long techniques
Imagery	Using imagination to create mental pictures: directs attention away from pain by imaging sights, sounds, odours, taste and touch (e.g. a garden on a warm summer's day) Can alter pain experience (e.g. when visualising cool water trickling over a hot painful area)	Find out the person's preferred image and talk them through it if asked Ensure periods of relative peace and quiet to enable them to use the strategy
Warmth	Promotes relaxation and comfort, reduces muscle tension	Hot water bottles cannot be used in hospital settings for safety reasons Wheat packs, heat pads and wraps, warm water, baths and showers are alternatives
Cold	May help reduce inflammatory pain Should not be used over wounds, as cold will decrease healing rate	Provide cold flannels, water, ice or cold packs and gels Even better, in the clinical area, show the patient/family where to access them
Positioning	Eases stiffness and enhances comfort	Help person to adopt most comfortable position, using own special pillows or cushions Encourage changes of position

clinical setting, being committed to reminding the person to use their strategy, and/or being competent to work with them to rehearse and use their techniques.

ACTIVITY

List the constraints that you are aware of in your locality in terms of allowing patients and clients to use their own strategies in clinical settings. Give some thought as to whether the rationale for any barriers is sound.

TENS (transcutaneous electrical nerve stimulation)
A battery-powered machine that delivers small electric shocks via adhesively attached electrodes, with the aim of blocking the pain messages to the brain and producing the body's natural painkillers – endorphins.

Hospital policies can sometimes present barriers, but – in a break with ward protocol – one of the authors was allowed access to a ward microwave to heat up a wheat pack for relieving back pain following unrelated surgery. The above focus upon self-generated strategies is not to deny the utility of nurses taking the lead in introducing techniques to patients. However, not all strategies are appropriate for all people, in all situations. For example, touch and massage can be painful for some people with neuropathic pain because of altered sensation, while others find TENS to be helpful.

ACTIVITY

Consider which non-pharmacological strategies you might use with each of the people in the scenarios, and why. How do these link to the different dimensions of pain and promotion of comfort care?

There are many other non-pharmacological approaches to pain management, some of which you are likely to come across during your nursing studies. For most patients, the most effective approach is to listen to what the person says about their pain and its effect on their home, leisure and work activities, to work with the multidisciplinary team to combine pharmacological and non-pharmacological strategies, and to monitor the effectiveness of pain relief.

Summary

- Pain is a subjective, multidimensional experience, unique to each individual.
- Nurses need to differentiate between the terms 'pain threshold', 'pain tolerance' and 'pain behaviour'.
- Effective pain assessment is the key to successful pain management, and pain assessment tools can facilitate communication about pain.
- Pain management comprises both pharmacological and non-pharmacological approaches. As people generally have their own pain-coping strategies, these should be incorporated into pain management.

PROMOTING COMFORT

Malinowski and Stamler (2002) assert that comfort is a basic human need. People can usually promote their own comfort, but when they are unwell, physically or mentally, their usual ways of seeking comfort may not be possible. Promoting comfort is a fundamental skill all nurses need to develop. Bottorff *et al.* (1995) observed that comforting strategies are embedded in practice and are often devalued. Yet they are a significant part of nurses' work.

LEARNING OUTCOMES

By the end of this section you will be able to:
1 discuss the nature of comfort and promoting comfort;
2 demonstrate the use of presence to provide comfort;
3 identify how monitoring can promote comfort;
4 consider how touch can be used in comfort care;
5 explore how talking can be used to promote comfort;
6 select physical actions that can be used to promote comfort;
7 integrate strategies to promote comfort in different circumstances.

Learning outcome 1: Discuss the nature of comfort and promoting comfort

To consider the nature of comfort, we will first explore *discomfort*.

Think back to the scenarios at the start of this chapter. In what ways might these people experience discomfort?

Palliative care

The World Health Organization (WHO) (2008) defines palliative care as 'an approach that improves the quality of life of patients and their families facing the problem associated with life-threatening illness, through the prevention and relief of suffering by means of early identification and impeccable assessment and treatment of pain and other problems, physical, psychosocial and spiritual.'

Violet certainly appears to be suffering discomfort and it might be assumed that this is mainly psychological due to her change of environment and her mental condition. However, it could also be physical – she could be in pain due to her osteoarthritis or need to pass urine but be unable to express this verbally. She could be too hot or too cold, or hungry or thirsty. It is important not to make assumptions about the reasons for people's apparent discomfort.

Tom has had major surgery for a serious health condition which he was unaware of until recently. During the night, due to his unrelieved pain, he experienced considerable discomfort. Tom also has the emotional discomfort of having been diagnosed with cancer and the knowledge that his treatment will continue for some time and affect his life in many ways. Wilby (2005) asserts that, for patients with cancer, relieving distress of physical symptoms and the accompanying emotional distress is a central role for nurses.

Maria has a terminal illness and could have a range of physical symptoms which cause her discomfort, including pain, breathlessness, tiredness and nausea. She needs **palliative care** to control her symptoms. Her choices for end-of-life care must be elicited and respected, and the community learning disability nurse has an important role in ensuring this happens (Foster 2006).

The NHS end-of-life care programme, mentioned in the previous section in relation to pain (see www.endoflifecare.nhs.uk/eolc), emphasises quality of care for people who are dying and that their choices of where to live and die should be enabled. Cardy (2005) emphasises that communication is central in palliative care for people with learning disabilities to aid assessment of symptoms such as pain and emotional distress. Thus, involving Maria's carers and family, who understand her specific needs and communication methods, is essential. Read (2005) outlines resources available to support carers of people with learning disabilities who need palliative care. The National Institute for Health and Clinical Excellence (NICE) (2004) presents guidelines for palliative care for adults with cancer which emphasise recognising patients' individual needs and supporting families and carers. They also highlight the importance of partnership, service user involvement, multidisciplinary working, primary and community care, and ethnically and culturally sensitive care.

Comfort care is the action taken to promote comfort, but for an acutely ill person total comfort may not be possible. Morse *et al.* (1994) argue that 'Total comfort is an elusive gold standard for the sick, for the very nature of illness disrupts the body – to be sick is to be without comfort.' They therefore suggest that nurses should aim to maintain patients within their own comfort range. In Tom's scenario, his pain is now controlled thus relieving one aspect of physical discomfort.

Kolkaba (1995) states that when comfort care is successful patients feel well cared for and comforted because the care was efficient, individualised, targeted to the whole person and creative. Several studies have indicated the importance of an individualised approach to comfort. Bland (2007) found that what constituted comfort and how it could be attained was different for each individual care home resident. In Tutton and Seers's (2004) study of older people's comfort on a rehabilitation ward, comfort was also an individual process. Rasin and Kautz (2007) emphasised the importance of staff getting to know residents with dementia, as person-centred knowledge led to staff being able to anticipate needs and know when something was 'not right' – important requirements for providing comfort care. Thus the care home staff will need to get to know Violet as a person to be able to promote her comfort. Malinowski and Stamler (2002) highlighted that comfort must be provided in a culturally relevant way, according to the patient's cultural values.

Wilby (2005) found that when patients felt comforted they were more relaxed and better able to accept their situation. She also identified actions that were *dis*comforting, which included treating patients as though they were unimportant, ordering patients to do things, forgetting to do things for patients, and giving inaccurate information. Kindness from family and staff promoted comfort, and some patients derived comfort from visits from a chaplain or priest.

Williams and Irurita (2006) studied hospitalised adults and focused specifically on emotional comfort, which patients defined as positive feelings including optimism, happiness and being high in spirit. Emotional discomfort exacerbated physical discomfort and involved feelings such as fear, frustration, sadness, worry, anger, stress, anxiety and embarrassment. A central feature of emotional comfort was personal control – the ability to influence situations or the environment. When patents had some personal control it enhanced feelings of worth and self-esteem. Williams and Irurita (2004) also found that competent staff, who portrayed ability and confidence, promoted emotional comfort by helping patients to feel secure.

ACTIVITY

Tom's scenario mentions that he was distressed in the night when he was in pain and that his method of pain relief was therefore changed. This is a physical action to promote comfort but could have taken some time to organise. Can you think of anything else that nurses might have done to promote comfort at this time?

The nurses might have used touch – perhaps holding his hand. They could have tried to be with him as much as possible – 'being there' or 'presence' is well recognised as a comfort strategy. The nurses would also have been checking and monitoring his condition – which would have been comforting as it would have helped Tom to feel safe. The nurses would have talked to Tom, perhaps giving him explanations about what was happening to him and that his method of pain relief would be changed. They could have reassured him about his condition as otherwise Tom might have been anxious that his severe pain was an abnormal sign, indicating that something was wrong. The nurses could also have attended to Tom's physical comfort, for example providing mouthcare and ensuring he was in a comfortable position as it would be difficult for him to change position unaided. Thus in promoting comfort for Tom, nurses would have used:

- presence;
- monitoring;
- touch;
- talking;
- physical actions.

The qualities of staff which promote comfort have been found to include kindness, gentleness and friendliness (Tutton and Seers 2004), and Wilby (2005) identified concern and compassion. These qualities can be displayed through the comfort care strategies listed, which are looked at in more detail in the next sections.

Learning outcome 2: Demonstrate the use of presence to provide comfort

Presence is about 'being there' with someone who is in distress and needs comfort. Zerwekh's (1997) description of presence suggests planned, professional nursing action – 'presencing' is referred to as a fundamental nursing intervention involving 'deliberate focused attention, receptivity to the other person, and persistent awareness of the other's shared humanity'. Davidson (1992) argues that it is a 'mark of one's humanity to be able to just be with someone, no matter what state they are in, without needing to act on them in some way'.

Studies have confirmed that the presence of nurses is a source of comfort (Clukey 1997; Gilje 1993; Wilby 2005). Williams and Irurita (2004) found that staff who spent time with patients, getting to know them as people and making frequent contact, promoted emotional comfort.

ACTIVITY

Think about when you sat with someone who was distressed, either in the healthcare setting or in everyday life. Were you comfortable doing this, or was it difficult in any way?

It is not always easy to be with someone who is in distress, particularly if you are unable to relieve their discomfort and, in some circumstances, this is not possible. If someone has received bad news, perhaps about a serious diagnosis or death of a loved one, nothing you can say or do can take that away. Nurses often feel more comfortable when they can 'put things right': relieve mental distress, pain, vomiting or breathlessness. If they are unable to do this, simply being with a person who, despite medication and other measures, continues to be suicidal, in pain, vomiting or acutely breathless can engender feelings of helplessness.

The presence of a relative or friend (rather than a nurse) can be the best source of comfort. Morse *et al.* (1994) gave an example of how a man with depression gained comfort from support given by family and friends. When relatives/friends are providing comfort by being present, nurses should then support them to be with their loved one, remembering that they may find it difficult to be there.

Learning outcome 3: Identify how monitoring can promote comfort

Monitoring, referred to as 'vigilance' by Hawley (2000) and as 'surveillance' by Walker (1996), is about observing and checking a distressed person's mental and/or physical condition. Monitoring is often combined with 'being there': presence. A number of research studies have identified that monitoring is comforting to patients/clients, in surgical wards (Kralik *et al.* 1997), mental health settings (Weissman and Appleton 1995), and in cancer care (Wilby 2005). Monitoring as a comfort measure might involve taking physiological measurements but also observing the person's appearance, asking about symptoms, and assessing pain, as described earlier in this chapter.

Nurses who are monitoring people need specific knowledge and skills – to be able to select, carry out and interpret physiological measurements and observations, and act appropriately. In relation to Roach's six Cs of caring (Roach 2002), explained in Chapter 1, this comfort measure particularly relates to competence, commitment and confidence. Competent and confident nurses, who show commitment to monitoring their patients, comfort the frightened and distressed people they are caring for.

ACTIVITY

Drawing on other chapters of this book and your experience in nursing to date, think about how you might monitor someone after an operation. Re-reading Tom Briggs's scenario will give you clues.

Monitoring would include checking physiological measurements (respiration, oxygen saturation, pulse, blood pressure, temperature) and fluid balance. Checking pain level would also be very important (as explained in the section on pain assessment earlier in this chapter). In Tom's case, close monitoring of his pain during the night led to his pain management being changed. You would also ask the patient about how they feel generally, for example, they might experience nausea or have a dry mouth. Did you remember that the patient might have a wound? You would therefore check the wound dressing for any bleeding. Some patients with surgical wounds have drains and so you would check these for drainage too. Some patients (like Tom) have epidural analgesia or PCA, and these devices will be checked regularly. Remember that if family are present, monitoring also involves checking on how they are managing with the situation.

Learning outcome 4: Consider how touch can be used in comfort care

The use of touch to comfort is well supported by research (Bush 2001; Chang 2001; Hawley 2000; Williams and Irurita 2004). In a vividly described example, Smith-Regojo (1995) recalls stroking the forehead of a man dying from a severe burn; she later found out that the man did not speak any English, thus highlighting the importance of touch to communicate comfort, rather than words.

There are two main types of touch used in nursing care: instrumental touch and comforting touch. **Instrumental touch** is used while carrying out nursing actions such as repositioning someone or taking their pulse. As care increasingly uses technology this type of touch is diminishing. For example, there is minimal touch involved in using electronic equipment to measure blood pressure, and using hoists to move patients. **Comforting touch** is used intentionally to comfort. In Chapter 1, Box 1.2 gives an example of how both instrumental touch (used to assist with washing and dressing) and comforting touch (touching the shoulder) were used to bring comfort to one of the authors of this chapter postoperatively.

Moore and Gilbert (1995) suggest that nurses should be encouraged to use comforting touch consciously and intentionally. Using comforting touch can be combined with other comfort measures: presence, and also monitoring. For example, the nurses looking after Tom when he was in distress during the night could have been observing his breathing while holding his hand, to comfort him. Read (1998) identified that touch may be helpful for people with learning disabilities who are terminally ill; thus touch might be an important source of comfort to Maria.

ACTIVITY	Think back to a recent experience when you were comforting someone. Did you use touch? If so, how did you use it? How comfortable do you feel about using touch to comfort? Now ask three close family members or friends about how they would feel about nurses using touch to comfort them.

People vary in how comfortable they feel about using and receiving touch; some people are much more 'touchy' than others. Some nurses use touch a great deal and feel comfortable to use touch in a variety of ways, while others shy away from using touch. In an article in *The Observer,* Colin Ludlow (2008) recalled how, when feeling 'fretful, feverish and frightened' in the intensive care unit, he asked for his wife to sit with him for comfort but that as the message never reached her, he remained alone:

> So I asked the nurses if they will hold my hand. Just for a few minutes to calm and settle me. They are tremendously caring. They tenderly manoeuvre me to change my sweaty sheets, or patiently prepare cold compresses for my burning forehead. But this request seems to embarrass them. "When I've finished this" or "When I've done that" they reply. I have no recollection of whether they ever do.

It seemed that Ludlow yearned for a comforting touch but he perceived that the nurses felt uncomfortable about using touch, while being attentive to physical comfort care actions. In contrast, in Arman and Rehnsfeldt's (2007, p. 378) study, a patient described how a particular nurse was a relief to her:

> I was so happy when she was at work . . . she gave that little bit extra, she was really sweet. She would sit and hold my hand when I was sad and in tears. It makes such a difference.

While many people respond well to touch as a means to comfort them, nurses should be sensitive to any non-verbal cues that indicate patients do not want to be touched. Maria's carers will know how she responds to touch as a means of comfort. Touch has cultural significance and also has different meanings and rules according to the gender of those involved. Giger and Davidhizar (1999) suggest that the 'message conveyed through touch depends on the attitude of the person involved and on the meaning of touch both to the person touching and to the person being touched'.

As with any care, you should evaluate the effect, so observe for responses to touch. For example, if staff attempt to use comforting touch with Violet, does she become calmer or more agitated? Does she grasp their hand tightly or snatch her hand away? In some situations it is appropriate to ask: 'Would you like to hold my hand during this [procedure]?' Also be aware that in some care situations use of touch could be misconstrued, and some people might view touch as an invasion of privacy and personal space.

Bottorff *et al.* (1995) suggest that touch can be used purely for comforting by holding a hand or stroking to reassure, soothe or calm people in acute distress. But they also identify 'connecting touch', which might be a light touch prior to a nurse leaving the bedside to reinforce interest in the patient or reassure them.

Learning outcome 5: Explore how talking can be used to promote comfort

Tutton and Seers (2004) found that nurses' interpersonal approach to patients was central in promoting comfort and, as discussed in Chapter 2, interpersonal skills comprise verbal and non-verbal communication. Studies in a range of settings have supported the role of talk in comforting. For example:

- Walters (1994) identified talking and listening to critically ill patients as important in comfort care, even with unconscious patients.
- Weissman and Appleton (1995) found that, for mental health patients, being kept informed helped to enhance comfort.
- Williams and Irurita (2004) found that explaining openly and honestly about what to expect and being encouraging provided emotional comfort.

Hawley (2000) identified four types of comforting talk which emergency unit patients described nurses using:

- *reassuring talk* – phrases like 'Don't worry, we'll take care of you';
- *coaching talk* – for example, helping patients to stay in control and cope with pain and anxiety;
- *explanatory talk* – such as giving information and answering questions;
- *empathetic talk* – which conveyed understanding and caring.

A pattern of talk – 'comfort talk' – has been identified (Morse and Proctor 1998), which nurses use to help patients get through difficult situations or painful procedures. This appears to be what Hawley (2000) refers to as 'coaching'. Penrod *et al.* (1999) describe comfort talk being used during nasogastric tube insertion to gain patient cooperation. Comfort talk is slow and rhythmic, with short simple sentences and uses phrases such as 'We're almost there', 'You're doing well' along with other emotionally supportive statements (Proctor *et al.* 1996).

Morse and Proctor (1998) suggest that comfort talk helps patients to endure the situation, allows an information exchange and communicates a sense of caring. They emphasise that nurses' comfort talk is accompanied by being face-to-face with the patient, holding the patient's hand and focusing on their eyes. Thus appropriate non-verbal communication is also important. Read (1998) suggests that, for a person with learning disabilities who is terminally ill, carers should use simple and concrete language accompanied by a range of communication methods, including pictures, photos, creative mediums such as drawing, painting, modelling, music, clay and poetry.

ACTIVITY

Think about phrases that you might use if you were supporting a patient during an uncomfortable procedure. Use one from each of Hawley's four categories: reassuring, coaching, explanatory and empathetic.

Examples in each category include:

- *reassuring* – 'Don't worry, it'll soon be over' or 'You'll be fine';
- *coaching* – 'Well done, you're getting there';
- *explanatory* – 'You'll now feel . . . Because . . .';
- *empathetic* – 'I'm sorry, I know this is uncomfortable for you'.

Wilby (2005) highlighted that the way explanations are given can be as important as the content, so you should be aware of the tone used during your verbal communication.

Williams and Irurita (2004) found that patients gained emotional comfort from 'chit-chat' and social conversation with nurses. Such chat can provide distraction and lighten the atmosphere (Bottorff *et al.* 1995), and for the patient or relative who is feeling wretched, being 'chatted to' – as one human being to another – can be comforting. For example, staff could ask Maria's sister about how her journey was. Taylor (1992) refers to the comforting nature of 'ordinariness' and how this represents a shared humanity between nurses and patients. Bottorff *et al.* (1995) identified the gentle use of humour as an often used strategy for comforting.

Talking can also be used in techniques to promote relaxation, such as guided imagery and distraction. You considered these strategies in relation to pain relief earlier in this chapter. The literature identifies these comfort measures mainly in relation to children (Pederson 1994) and pain management, but they can successfully be used with adults, and in other circumstances where comfort is needed.

Learning outcome 6: Select physical actions that can be used to promote comfort

Wilby (2005) found that, to achieve physical comfort, the relief of physical symptoms (especially pain) is necessary.

ACTIVITY

What physical actions have you used in practice, or seen used, to promote comfort?

There are a wide range of physical actions which nurses can use to promote people's comfort.

- *Administering medicines.* Obvious examples include analgesics (which you looked at earlier in this chapter), antiemetics (to prevent nausea and vomiting), antipyretics (to reduce high temperature), bronchodilators (via nebulisers or inhalers) to reduce dyspnoea, and sedatives. However, many prescribed medicines also reduce discomfort from unpleasant symptoms. Examples include drugs to regulate the heart rate and rhythm, thus stopping palpitations, and antibiotics which relieve fever-related symptoms like headache, aching and malaise by treating infection.

- *Repositioning.* Assisting a breathless person into a sitting position well supported by pillows or in a chair, turning people to provide relief from pressure, and positioning limbs to prevent contractures, are all examples of using repositioning to promote comfort.

- *Providing a comfortable bed.* For a person who is in bed for all or part of the day a comfortable bed and appropriate bedding are fundamental. A comfortable, pressure-relieving mattress should be provided (see Chapter 6). Clean, unwrinkled bed-linen, covers that are not too hot, too heavy or too cold, and sufficient supportive pillows are all essential.

- *Assisting with hygiene.* Wilby (2005) found that people were comforted by being helped with hygiene care. Chapter 8 covers all aspects of this in detail, and attention should be paid to mouth care, hair care and shaving, as well as the skin. In Bland's (2007) study, care home residents identified that being offered a refreshing shower on a hot day promoted comfort. Cairncross *et al.* (2007) found that 36 per cent of care home residents derived comfort from taking a shower or having a bath. Hygiene is an important comfort measure for people who are vomiting. Teeth cleaning, mouthwashes, hand and face washes, and changing of clothes can help patients feel more comfortable.

- *Assisting with elimination.* Incontinence causes both physical and psychological discomfort. Chapter 9 looks in detail at assisting people with elimination, and promoting continence and managing incontinence in ways that promote comfort.

- *Providing food and drink.* Hunger and thirst cause discomfort, as you will almost certainly have experienced yourself at some point. Chapter 10 looks in detail at how people can be assisted with eating and drinking. Wilby (2005) found that people were comforted by being helped with eating. For people who are 'nil by mouth' (like Tom was when he first returned from theatre), it is important to explain why they cannot eat and drink and to offer mouthwashes to reduce the discomfort of a dry mouth.

- *Modifying the environment.* You need to be observant about whether the environment is too hot or too cold for the people you are caring for. Patients who are just sitting can quickly become cold. Windows can be opened or closed and fans used to modify environmental temperature. Also pay attention to reducing excessive or unpleasant noise. Music, if to people's choice, can be comforting, as can a pleasant décor, plants and pictures. A study of mechanically ventilated patients indicated that music promoted comfort (Lee *et al.* 2005). The psychological environment is also important: a calm, confident and relaxed atmosphere where there is good teamwork can all engender comfort.

In many instances people may not request the physical actions listed above owing to communication difficulties or because they feel unable to ask, so nurses must be proactive in assessing people's needs for these comfort measures.

The way in which physical actions are carried out is also significant. In Kralik *et al.*'s (1997) study patients described being given physical care which, although it left them free of pain, physically comfortable and clean, did not leave them feeling cared for because of the depersonalised manner in which it was carried out. It is easy to see how physical actions could be combined with other aspects of comfort care: talking, monitoring, presence and touch.

Learning outcome 7: Integrate strategies to promote comfort in different circumstances

The previous sections discussed different strategies to promote comfort but, as already highlighted, combining strategies is necessary for effective comfort care. Competent physical actions and monitoring of patients' conditions are expected as fundamental aspects of the nurse's role, but to provide comfort these need to be integrated with presence, touch and talking. These latter measures are ones that nurses often feel they do not have time for, but the art of comfort care is about smoothly integrating a number of measures. As Kolkaba (2003) explains, patients remember nurses who took time to comfort them.

ACTIVITY

Identify how the use of presence, monitoring, talking, touch and physical actions could be integrated to promote comfort if Maria appears agitated and uncomfortable.

A familiar member of staff, a friend or relative could sit with her and hold her hand (presence and touch), and gently talk to her about familiar things (talking) or look at her 'life book' with her. Depending on Maria's wishes, they could read her poetry or look at photos with her. Maria's general condition should be observed – for example, does she feel too hot or too cold (monitoring)? Physical actions include assessing whether she is in pain or has other symptoms such as nausea and administering appropriate medication to control these symptoms. It will be important to communicate with Maria effectively to do this, and the staff who know Maria will be able to use their knowledge of how she communicates to find out her needs and any cause of discomfort. Repositioning may help – for example, sitting up so that breathing is easier. Perhaps Maria needs to be helped to go to the toilet or has been incontinent.

Summary

● Promoting comfort is a key role of nurses in many different settings, and is fundamental to caring.

● Promoting comfort requires a holistic approach and the integration of presence, monitoring, touch, talking and physical actions, encompassing a range of skills and knowledge, as applicable for each individual.

CHAPTER SUMMARY

Throughout this book, practical nursing skills are contextualised within a philosophy of caring. Chapter 1 introduced Roach's six Cs of caring, and these were returned to in this final chapter which has looked at some fundamental aspects of nursing: managing pain and promoting comfort.

Nurses have an important role in promoting comfort, a role recognised by Florence Nightingale who wrote in 1854:

> The benefits which this Institution [hospital] ought to afford to the sick are perhaps best seen when we are enabled to give comfort in the time of danger and to lessen the agony of death. (quoted in Verney 1970)

Pain management is a huge topic with a developing theoretical base, and this chapter's material aimed to provide a firm basis from which to build your nursing practice. Both pain management and promoting comfort require nurses to integrate a range of skills, with an appropriate attitude and a sound underpinning knowledge base.

REFERENCES

Arman, M. and Rehnsfeldt, A. 2007. The 'Little Extra' that alleviates suffering. *Nursing Ethics* **14,** 372–86.

Bland, M. 2007. Betwixt and between: a critical ethnography of comfort in New Zealand residential aged care. *Journal of Clinical Nursing.* **16,** 937–44.

Bottorff, J.L., Gogag, M. and Engelberg-Lotzkar, M. 1995. Comforting: exploring the work of cancer nurses. *Journal of Advanced Nursing* **22,** 1077–84.

BOC Medical 2001. *Entonox: Controlled pain relief reference guide.* Manchester: BOC Group.

Brook, P., Collins, P.D., Briggs, J. and Nichols, B.J. 2002. Point prevalence study of pain in a district general hospital. *Annual Scientific Meeting 2002 Poster Abstracts.* London: Pain Society.

Burrows, D. 1997. Action on pain. In Thomson, S. (ed.) *Nurse Teachers as Researchers: A reflective approach.* London: Arnold, 86–117.

Burrows, D. 2000. *Engaging Patients in their Own Pain Management: An action research study.* Unpublished PhD thesis, Brunel University.

Bush, E. 2001. The use of human touch to improve the well-being of older adults: a holistic nursing intervention. *Journal of Holistic Nursing* **19,** 256–70.

Cairncross, L., Magee, H. and Askham, J. 2007. *A Hidden Problem: Pain in older people.* Oxford: Picker Institute.

Cardy, P. 2005. Learning disability and palliative care. *International Journal of Palliative Nursing* **11**(1), 14.

Carr, E. and Mann, E. 2000. *Pain: Creative approaches to effective management.* Basingstoke: Macmillan.

Census 2001. *Health, Disability and Provision of Care.* National Statistics Online: www.statistics. gov.uk/census2001/profiles/commentaries/health.asp. Accessed 1 November 2003.

Chakour, M.C., Gibson, S.J., Bradbeer, M. and Helme, R.D. 1996. The effect of age on A-delta- and C-fibre thermal pain stimuli. *Pain* **64,** 143–52.

Chang, S.O. 2001. The conceptual structure of physical touch in caring. *Journal of Advanced Nursing* **33,** 820–7.

Cheston, R. and Bender, M. 1999. *Understanding Dementia: The man with the worried eyes.* London: Jessica Kingsley.

Chronic Pain Policy Coalition. 2007. *A New Pain Manifesto.* Available from www. paincoalition.org.uk.

Closs, S.J. 2007. Assessment of pain, mood and quality of life. In Crome, P., Main C.J. and Lally, F. (eds) *Pain in Older People.* Oxford: Oxford University Press, 11–19.

Closs, S.J., Barr, B., Briggs, M. *et al.* 2003. Evaluating pain in care home residents with dementia. *Nursing and Residential Care* **5**(1), 32–3.

Clukey, L. 1997. *'Just Be There': The experience of anticipatory grief.* Rush University, College of Nursing DNSC.

Davidson, B. 1992. What can be the relevance of the psychiatric nurse to the life of a person who is mentally ill? *Journal of Clinical Nursing* **1,** 199–205.

Davies, D. and Evans, L. 2001. Assessing pain in people with profound learning disabilities. *Learning Disability Nursing* **10**(8), 513–16.

Ferrell, B.R., McCaffery, M. and Rhiner, M. 1992. Pain and addiction: an urgent need for change in nursing education. *Journal of Pain and Symptom Management* **7,** 117–24.

Forsyth, D. 2007. Pain in patients with cognitive impairment. In Crome, P., Main C.J. and Lally, F. (eds) *Pain in Older People.* Oxford: Oxford University Press, 21–39

Foster, J. 2006. End-of-life care: making choices. *Learning Disability Practice* **9**(7), 18–22.

Frampton, M. 2003. Experience assessment and management of pain in people with dementia. *Age and Ageing* **32**(3), 248–51.

Giger, J.N. and Davdhizar, R.E. 1999. *Transcultural Nursing: Assessment and intervention,* 3rd edn. St Louis: Mosby.

Gilje, F.L. 1993. *A Phenomenological Study of Patients' Experiences of the Nurse's Presence.* PhD thesis, University of Colorado Health Sciences Center.

Hawley, M.P. 2000. Nurse comforting strategies: perceptions of emergency department patients. *Clinical Nursing Research* **9,** 441–59.

International Association for the Study of Pain Subcommittee on Taxonomy 1979. Pain terms: a list with definitions and notes on usage. *Pain* **6,** 249–52.

Jacques, A. and Jackson, G.A. 2000. *Understanding Dementia,* 3rd edn. Edinburgh: Churchill Livingstone.

Kolkaba, K.Y. 1995. Comfort as process and product, merged in holistic art. *Journal of Holistic Nursing* **13,** 117–31.

Kolkaba, K.Y. 2003. *Comfort Theory and Practice: A vision for holistic health care and research.* New York: Springer.

Kovach, C.R., Griffie, J. and Muchka, S. 1999. Assessment and treatment of discomfort for people with late-stage dementia. *Journal of Pain and Symptom Management* **18,** 412–19.

Kralik, D., Koch, T. and Wotton, K. 1997. Engagement and detachment: understanding patients' experiences with nursing. *Journal of Advanced Nursing* **26,** 399–407.

Lee, O.K., Chung, Y.F., Chan, M.F. and Chan, W.M. 2005. Music and its effect on the physiological responses and anxiety levels of patients receiving mechanical ventilation: a pilot study. *Journal of Clinical Nursing* **14,** 609–20.

Liverpool Care Pathway for the Dying Patient. See www.mcpcil.org.uk/liverpool_care_pathway. Accessed 19 April 2008.

Lovering, S. 2006. Cultural attitudes and beliefs about pain. *Journal of Transcultural Nursing* **17,** 389–95.

Ludlow, C. 2008. One couple's extraordinary story of how they both survived the same cancer. *The Observer,* 27 January, 26–32.

MacIntyre, P.E. and Ready, L.B. 2007. *Acute Pain Management: A practical guide,* 3rd edn. Edinburgh: W.B. Saunders.

Madjar, I. 1985. Pain and the surgical patient: a cross-cultural perspective. *Australian Journal of Advanced Nursing* **2**(2), 29–33.

Malinowski, A. and Stamler, L.L. (2002) Comfort: exploration of the concept in nursing. *Journal of Advanced Nursing* **39,** 599–606.

Mann, E. and Carr, E. 2006. *Pain Management: Essential clinical skills for nurses.* Oxford: Blackwell Publishing Ltd.

McCaffery, M. and Pesaro, C. 1999. *Pain Clinical Manual,* 2nd edn. St Louis: Mosby.

McGuire, D. 1992. Comprehensive and multidimensional assessment and measurement of pain. *Journal of Pain and Symptom Management* **7,** 312–19.

McQuay, H. and Moore, A. 1998. *An Evidence-based Resource for Pain Relief.* Oxford: Oxford University Press.

Melzack, R. and Katz, J. 1999. Pain measurements in persons in pain. In Wall, P.D. and Melzack, R. (eds) *Textbook of Pain,* 4th edn. Edinburgh: Churchill Livingstone, 409–26.

Melzack, R. and Wall, P. 1996. *Challenge of Pain.* Harmondsworth: Penguin.

Middleton, C. 2006. *Epidural Analgesia in Acute Pain Management.* Chichester: John Wiley.

Moore, J.R. and Gilbert, D.A. 1995. Elderly residents: perceptions of nurses' comforting touch. *Journal of Gerontological Nursing* **21,** 6–13.

Morse, J.M. and Proctor, A. 1998. Maintaining patient endurance: the comfort work of trauma nurses. *Clinical Nursing Research* **7,** 250–74.

Morse, J.M., Bottorff, J.L. and Hutchinson, S. 1994. The phenomenology of comfort *Journal of Advanced Nursing* **20,** 189–95.

Moskow, S.B. 1987. *Human Hand and other Ailments.* Boston: Little, Brown.

Multiple Sclerosis Trust 2007. *Multiple Sclerosis: Information for health and social care professionals.* Letchworth: Multiple Sclerosis Trust.

National Institute for Health and Clinical Excellence (NICE). 2004. *Improving Supportive and Palliative Care for Adults with Cancer.* Available from www.nice.org.uk.

NHS End of Life Care Programme. See www.endoflifecare.nhs.uk/eolc. Accessed 19 April 2008.

NHS QIS National Health Service Quality Improvement Scotland 2004. *The Management of Pain in Patients with Cancer: Best practice statement.* See www.nhshealthquality.org.

Nishimori, M., Ballantyne, J.C. and Low, J.H.S. 2007. Epidural pain relief versus systematic opioid-based pain relief for abdominal aortic surgery. *Cochrane Database of Systematic Reviews,* Issue 4.

Pederson, C. 1994. Ways to feel comfortable: teaching aids to promote children's comfort. *Issues in Comprehensive Pediatric Nursing* **17,** 37–46.

Penrod, J., Morse, J.M. and Wilson, S. 1999. A blend of comforting strategies and a form of team comforting were used during nasogastric tube insertion. *Journal of Clinical Nursing* **8**, 31–8.

Proctor, A., Morse, J.M. and Khonsari, S. 1996. Sounds of comfort in the trauma center: how nurses talk to patients in pain. *Social Science Medicine* **42**, 1669–80.

Rasin, J. and Kautz, D.D. 2007. Knowing the resident with dementia: perspectives of assisted facility caregivers. *Journal of Gerontological Nursing* **33**(9), 30–6.

Read, S. 1998. The palliative care needs of people with learning disabilities. *British Journal of Community Nursing* **3**, 356–61.

Read, S. 2005. Learning disabilities and palliative care: recognizing pitfalls and exploring potential. *International Journal of Palliative Nursing* **11**(1), 15–20.

Roach, S.M. 2002. *Caring, the Human Mode of Being: A blueprint for the health professions*, 2nd revised edn. Ottawa: Canadian Hospital Association Press.

Rokke, P.D. and al'Absi, M. 1992. Matching pain coping strategies to the individual: a prospective validation of the cognitive coping strategy inventory. *Journal of Behavioral Medicine* **15**, 611–25.

Royal College of Physicians, British Geriatrics Society and British Pain Society 2007. *The Assessment of Pain in Older People: National guidelines*. Concise Guidance to Good Practice Series 8. London: RCP.

Scottish Intercollegiate Guidelines Network (SIGN) 2000. *Control of Pain in Patients with Cancer*. Edinburgh. Available from www.sign.ac.uk/guidelines/fulltext/44/index.html. Accessed 19 April 2008.

Smith-Regojo, P. 1995. 'Being with' a patient who is dying. *Holistic Nursing Practice* **9**, 1–3.

Smith-Stoner, M. 2003. How Buddhism influences pain control choices. *Nursing* **33**(4), 17.

Sofaer, B. 1998. *Pain Principles, Practice and Patients*, 3rd edn. Cheltenham: Stanley Thornes.

Taylor, B.J. 1992. Relieving pain through ordinariness in nursing: a phenomenologic account of a comforting nurse-patient encounter. *Advances in Nursing Science* **15**(1), 33–43.

Tutton, E. and Seers, K. 2004. Comfort on a ward for older people. *Journal of Advanced Nursing* **46**(4), 380–9.

Verney, H. 1970. *Florence Nightingale at Harley Street: Her reports to the governors of her nursing home 1853–4*. London: J.M. Dent.

Walker, A.C. 1996. The 'expert' nurse comforter: perceptions of medical/surgical patients. *International Journal of Nursing Practice* **2**, 40–4.

Walters, A.J. 1994. The comforting role in critical care nursing practice: a phenomenological interpretation. *International Journal of Nursing Studies* **31**, 607–16.

Weissman, J. and Appleton, C. 1995. The therapeutic aspects of acceptance. *Perspectives in Psychiatric Care* **31**, 19–23.

Werawatganon, T. and Charuluxanun, S. 2007. Patient controlled intravenous opioid analgesia versus continuous epidural analgesia for pain after intra-abdominal surgery. *Cochrane Database of Systematic Reviews*, Issue 4.

Wilby, M.L. 2005. Cancer patients' descriptions of comforting and discomforting nursing actions. *International Journal for Human Caring* **9**(4), 59–63.

Williams, A.M. and Irurita, V. 2004. Therapeutic and non-therapeutic interpersonal interactions: the patient's perspective. *Journal of Clinical Nursing* **13**, 806–15.

Williams, A.M. and Irurita, V.F. 2006. Emotional comfort: the patient's perspective of a therapeutic context. *International Journal of Nursing Studies* **43**, 405–15.

World Health Organization (WHO) 1996. *Cancer Pain Relief*, 2nd edn. Geneva: WHO.

— 2008. Definition of palliative care; available from www.who.int/cancer/palliative/definition/en. Accessed 31 January 2008.

Yezierski, R.P. 2007. Effects of age on pain sensitivity: need for translational studies. *Pain in Older Persons* (newsletter of the IASP Special Interest Group on Pain in Older Persons), June.

Zerwekh, J.V. 1997. The practice of presencing. *Seminars in Oncology Nursing* **13**(4), 260–2.

USEFUL WEBSITES

- Action on Pain: www.action-on-pain.co.uk
- Alzheimer's Society: www.alzheimers.org.uk
- American Academy of Pain Management: www.aapainmanage.org
- American Pain Society: www.ampainsoc.org
- Australian Pain Society: www.apsoc.org.au
- BackCare: www.backcare.org.uk
- Bandolier, Pain Research at Oxford: www.jr2.ox.ac.uk/bandolier/painres/PRintro.html
- Centre for Pain Relief: www.painreliefforpain.com/pain_relief.htm
- Chronic Pain Policy Coalition: www.paincoalition.org.uk
- DIPEx: www.healthtalkonline.org
- End of life care: www.endoflifecare.nhs.uk
- European Federation of IASP Chapters: www.efic.org
- British Pain Society: www.britishpainsociety.org
- International Association for the Study of Pain: www.iasp-pain.org
- Medscape: www.medscape.com
- Mencap: www.mencap.org.uk
- Marie Curie Cancer Trust: www.mariecurie.org.uk
- NIH Pain Consortium: painconsortium.nih.gov/pain_index.html
- Pain Concern: www.painconcern.org.uk
- PainConsultants Ltd: www.painconsultants.co.uk
- Pain.com: www.pain.com
- Pain Support: www.painsupport.co.uk
- Pain-Talk: www.gb42.com/ynot.html
- Physiotherapy Pain Association: www.ppaonline.co.uk
- Tame the Pain: www.tamethepain.co.uk
- Pain Relief Foundation: www.painrelieffoundation.org.uk
- Welcome Trust, Pain: www.wellcome.ac.uk/en/pain/microsite/index.html

APPENDIX 12.1 – Attitude to pain – questionnaire (Burrows 1997)

	Strongly agree	Agree	Unsure	Disagree	Strongly disagree
1 Nurses can determine accurately the amount of pain a person will suffer from knowledge of the surgery					
2 Talking to patients preoperatively about pain helps reduce pain post-operatively					
3 Analgesics are always the best way of reducing pain					
4 Using pain assessment charts provides a more accurate picture of the patient's pain					
5 All real pain has an identifiable physical cause					
6 Education on pain management helps nurses recognise when patients are in pain					
7 It is best that patients should not know what is happening to them as this may cause anxiety					
8 Patients who have had surgery (of any type) in the past, know what to expect with regard to post-operative pain					
9 Patients should expect to suffer some pain					
10 A person's age affects their tolerance to pain					
11 Anxiety increases the perception of pain					
12 Patients complaining of pain 2–3 hours after an injection should be encouraged to wait a little longer for their next injection					
13 Nurses most often underestimate the severity and existence of a person's pain					
14 Patients who refuse analgesics when they are in pain are not acting in their own best interests					
15 Some ethnic groups can tolerate more pain than others					

	Strongly agree	Agree	Unsure	Disagree	Strongly disagree
16 It is possible to control pain post-operatively					
17 Talking and listening to patients can reduce their pain					
18 Patients should receive post-operative analgesics on a PRN basis only					
19 Nurses always make accurate inferences about the severity and existence of a person's pain					
20 Relaxation and distraction techniques are effective measures in relieving pain					
21 The person who uses his/her pain to obtain benefits or preferential treatment does not hurt as much as he/she says he/she does and may not hurt at all					
22 Patients should receive post-operative analgesics on both a regular and PRN basis					
23 What the person says about his/her pain is always true					
24 Patients who refuse analgesics show a great sense of character					
25 Nurses are better qualified and more experienced to determine the existence and nature of a person's pain than the person him/herself					
26 Patients should receive analgesics on a regular basis only					
27 All persons can and should be encouraged to have a high tolerance to pain					
28 Nurses learn enough about pain during their training to manage patient's post-operative pain effectively					
29 Care should be taken when giving controlled drugs post-operatively as patients easily become addicted					
30 A person's pain can always be detected by their behaviour and physiological signs					

Odd numbered questions and question 30 taken from Davis, P. 1988. Changing nursing practice for more effective control of post-operative pain through a staff initiated educational programme. *Nurse Education Today* **8**(6), 325–31.

INDEX

Note: page numbers in **bold** refer to figures, those in *italics* to tables, and those in ***bold italics*** to boxes or margin notes